Essentials of Infectious Diseases

Essentials of Infectious Diseases

Editor: Jasmine Frost

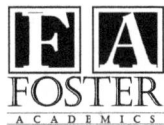

FOSTER
ACADEMICS

www.fosteracademics.com

www.fosteracademics.com

FA FOSTER ACADEMICS

Cataloging-in-Publication Data

Essentials of infectious diseases / edited by Jasmine Frost.
    p. cm.
Includes bibliographical references and index.
ISBN 978-1-63242-693-2
1. Communicable diseases. 2. Infection. 3. Diseases--Causes and theories of causation.
4. Epidemics. I. Frost, Jasmine.
RC111 .E87 2019
616.9--dc23

Foster Academics,
118-35 Queens Blvd., Suite 400,
Forest Hills, NY 11375, USA

ISBN 978-1-63242-693-2 (Hardback)

Contents

Preface

Diseases caused due to infection are known as infectious diseases. Infection is the invasion of the tissues of an organism's body by disease-causing agents, the toxins they produce, and their multiplication. Infectious agents like bacteria, viruses, nematodes, arthropods, fungi and other macroparasites can cause infections. Some common signs of infection include fever, weight loss, fatigue, night sweats, aches, pains and lack of appetite. Antibiotics, antivirals, antifungals, antiprotozoals and antihelminthics are some of the common medicines used to treat infections. This book aims to shed light on some of the unexplored aspects of infectious diseases and the recent researches in this field. It provides significant information of this discipline to help develop a good understanding of infectious diseases and related aspects. It will provide comprehensive knowledge to the readers.

This book is the end result of constructive efforts and intensive research done by experts in this field. The aim of this book is to enlighten the readers with recent information in this area of research. The information provided in this profound book would serve as a valuable reference to students and researchers in this field.

At the end, I would like to thank all the authors for devoting their precious time and providing their valuable contribution to this book. I would also like to express my gratitude to my fellow colleagues who encouraged me throughout the process.

Editor

Virologic suppression in response to antiretroviral therapy despite extensive resistance within HIV-1 reverse transcriptase after the first virologic failure

Marta Iglis Oliveira[1] (iD), Valter Romão de Souza Junior[3*] (iD), Claudia Fernanda de Lacerda Vidal[2] and Paulo Sérgio Ramos de Araújo[1,2]

Abstract

Background: Incomplete virologic suppression results in mutations associated with resistance and is a major obstacle to disease control. We analyzed the genotypic profiles of HIV-1 patients at the time of the first virologic failure and the response to a salvage regimen after 48 weeks.

Methods: This work was a cross-sectional, retrospective, analytical study based on data collected from medical records and genotyping tests between 2006 and 2016. The sample consisted of data on individuals living with HIV (PLWH) from three major reference centers.

Results: A total of 184 patients were included in the data analysis. Viral subtype B was the most common (81.3%) as well as M184 V/I (85.3%) and K103 codon mutations (65.8%). Forty-eight weeks after switching to a salvage regimen, 67.3% of patients achieved an undetectable viral load.

Discussion: The number of mutations associated with nucleos(t)ide reverse transcriptase inhibitors (NRTI(t)s) did not affect virologic suppression (9.3% for zero NRTI(t)-associated mutations vs 48.6% for 1–2 NRTI(t)-associated mutations vs 42.1% for ≥3 NRTI(t)-associated mutations, $p = 0.179$). An ARV time (the beginning of the first ARV regimen up to genotyping) of > 36 months was a protective factor for detectable viral load (PR = 0.60, 95% CI = 0.39–0.92, $p = 0.020$) and a risk factor for developing ≥3 NRTI(t)-associated mutations (PR = 2.43, 95% CI 1.38–4.28, $p = 0.002$).

Conclusions: We found that extensive resistance to NRTI(t)s at the time of the first virologic failure did not impact virologic suppression at 48 weeks after switching to a second-line therapy based on NRTI(t)s plus protease inhibitors.

Keywords: HIV-1 drug resistance, Genetic diversity, Subtypes, Antiretroviral therapy

Background

Approximately 21 million people are living with HIV (PLHIV) and receiving antiretroviral therapy [1], which is responsible for a significant decrease in their morbidity and mortality as well as in the risk of transmission [2, 3]. However, the importance of this therapy to global health has been threatened by an increased prevalence of resistance to antiretrovirals (ARVs), which has increased from 11 to 29% since 2001 [4]. Of the individuals under ARV treatment, 20% will have to switch ARVs due to virologic failure [5, 6]. Thus, drug resistance is a real obstacle to viral suppression and disease control [1].

In Brazil, approximately 60% of PLHIV receive ARVs [7] through a program by the Brazilian Ministry of Health. From 2004 to 2017, the first-line therapy in the country was based on regimens involving efavirenz (EFV), a non-nucleoside reverse transcriptase inhibitor (NNRTI). In 2013, tenofovir (TDF) became the preferred nucleos(t)ide reverse transcriptase

* Correspondence: jr_walter@hotmail.co.uk
[3]Faculdade de Medicina do Recife, Universidade Federal de Pernambuco, Av. Prof. Moraes Rego, 1235, Recife, Pernambuco, Brazil
Full list of author information is available at the end of the article

inhibitor (NRTI(t)), and it was given in a single dose combined with lamivudine (3TC) and EFV [8]. In 2017, dolutegravir (DTG), an integrase inhibitor that was administered with TDF/3TC, became the first-line therapy [9].

Genotypic and immunovirologic data from patients following the first virologic failure are scarce in Brazil, and they are limited to certain regions of the country. A recent study from the city of São Paulo[10] on patients who failed first-line therapy between 2013 and 2015 found a higher prevalence of the M184 V/I mutation (74.3%) and K103 codon (56.7%), similar to that found in other Brazilian states [11]. Among the 205 subjects who started the second-line therapy with NRTI(t)s combined with protease inhibitor/ritonavir (PI/r), 76.6% experienced virologic suppression (< 200 copies/ml), despite the extensive resistance of the virus to NRTI(t)s [10].

Low- and middle-income countries in sub-Saharan Africa, where 70% of PLHIV live [1], access 2 NRTI(t) + NNRTI as a first-line therapy [12]. This regimen has a low genetic barrier and easily results in cross-resistance. Thus, the sensitivity of NRTI(t)s may be compromised by multiple mutations that arise during the first virologic failure. In addition, NRTI(t)s have recognized risks of toxic effects. These factors are concerning and have led to the decision to retain this drug class as a second-line therapy, and they have motivated the development of randomized clinical trials to evaluate the efficacy of the salvage regimen with NRTI(t)s plus PI/r.

Mutations are associated with high reduced susceptibility or virologic response to relevant NRTIs. Mutations reduce NRTI susceptibility or virologic response, which contributes to reducing susceptibility in combination with other NRTI-resistant mutations. The impact of mutations associated with NRTI(t)s during the second-line regimen was evaluated through the SECOND-LINE, EARNEST and SELECT studies [13–15] and they were recently reevaluated in a meta-analysis [20], which showed the success of salvage regimens based on NRTI(t)s combined with PI/r. In this study, we analyzed the genotypic profile of HIV-1 in patients during the first virologic failure and the predictors of virologic success 48 weeks after switching to a salvage regimen.

Methods

This work was a cross-sectional, retrospective, multicenter study evaluating genotypic resistance tests of PLHIV during the first virologic failure in the city of Recife, the capital of the state of Pernambuco, an important medical center in Northeast Brazil. The patients were enrolled in three large centers specializing in the care of PLHIV. We reviewed tests that were performed from January 2006 to December 2016 and included patients over 18 years of age who had used ARVs for more than six

months and presented two consecutive viral load measurements, with an interval of at least 30 days, and values greater than 1000 copies/ml. Individuals who underwent ARV switching due to virologic failure without genotyping tests, those who used ARVs before receiving the first-line therapy, those showing an absence of mutations associated with resistance in genotyping, and those with insufficient data were excluded.

The immunovirologic and genotypic data and the history of ARV use were collected from genotyping tests, medical charts and through the Laboratory Test Control System (Sistema de Controle de Exames Laboratoriais - SISCEL- online platform). To identify the mutations associated with resistance, the ViroSeqTM HIV-1 Genotyping System kit (Celera Diagnostics, Alameda, CA, USA) was used from 2006 to 2008 and the TRUGENE System (Siemens, Munich, Germany) was used from 2009 to 2016 by the laboratories that served the National Genotyping Network (Rede Nacional de Genotipagem - Renageno). The viral load (VL) was measured until July 2013 using the Versant HIV-1 RNA 3.0 assay (bDNA, Siemens, USA); real-time qPCR was used after this date (Abbott Laboratories, USA). The CD4 T-cell counts (CD4) were performed by flow cytometry (BD, USA).

The Stanford HIVdb program version 8.4 (https://hivdb.stanford.edu/hivdb/by-mutations) was used to interpret the genotype resistance. The mutations were analyzed individually using a list provided by the International AIDS Society (IAS) in 2017, [16] and the Stanford HIVdb program and categorized as mutations associated with NRTI(t), NNRTI and major and accessory mutations for protease inhibitors (PI). Forty-eight weeks after switching to second-line therapy, virologic suppression was considered successful when an undetectable viral load was found by the given method. Viral load values made available 60 days before or after the date of completion (for the 48 weeks) were considered. The time on ARVs was the period between the beginning of the first ARV regimen and the performance of the genotyping test. The time in virologic failure was the period between virologic failure detection (two consecutive viral loads above 1000 copies/ml) and the switch to the salvage regimen.

The genotypic sensitivity score (GSS) was calculated individually only for the drugs used by each patient in the salvage regimen. A value of 1 was attributed to drugs with full activity, 0.75 for a low potential resistance level, 0.5 for a resistance level, 0.25 for an intermediate resistance level and zero if the drug showed a lack of activity.

SPSS 13.0 (Statistical Package for the Social Sciences) for Windows and Excel 2010 were used for the statistical analysis. The results are presented in the tables with their respective absolute and relative frequencies. The mean or median values for the quantitative variables were calculated according to the normality of their distribution. The normality of the quantitative variables was tested using the Kolmogorov-Smirnov test.

We tested for the presence of an association using the chi-square test and Fisher's exact test for categorical variables. To identify the predictive factors that independently influenced virologic suppression and the number of mutations associated with NRTI(t)s, we used the STATA/SE 12.0 programs. For the multivariate analysis, the Poisson regression model was used, taking into account the variables that obtained significance ≤0.20 in the bivariate analysis. The prevalence ratio was calculated with a 95% confidence interval. A $p < 0.05$ was considered statistically significant. Poison-regression was chosen as excellent alternative to estimate the adjusted prevalence ratio for confounding variables in cross-sectional studies compared to Cox and log-binominal logistic regression. The study was approved by the institutional ethics committee (CEP-CCS-UFPE/1.985.922).

Results

A total of 534 medical records were evaluated, of which 270 were excluded due to a lack of genotyping tests when patients switched ARVs after the first virologic failure. In 59 medical records, there was no selective pressure during genotyping. Therefore, the absence of mutation does not represent reality. Thus, 59 patients were excluded. Non-adherence to ARV use at the time of genotyping was recorded in the medical charts of the 59 excluded patients with absence of resistance-associated mutations. Furthermore, 21 patients were not either illegible or had insufficient data.

A total of 184 patients were included in the first virologic failure for analysis. The majority of the participants were male (73.4%) and the mean age at virologic failure was 41 (±9.4) years. The median CD4 ($n = 155$) and VL ($n = 141$) pre-ARV were 176 cells/m3 and 130,000 copies/ml, respectively.

This sample is representative considering the limited resources scenario. It represents a decade of genotyping in the first virologic failure in Pernambuco, Northeast Brazil. In 2016, we were able to access genotyping easily. Between 2006 and 2016, there was therapeutic rescue without genotyping due to the logistic difficulty in this region of Brazil. Therefore, more than 50% of the sample was excluded by changing the scheme without genotyping.

Factors associated with mutations, immunovirologic and ARV characteristics at the time of genotyping

The genotypic, immunovirologic and ARV characteristics at the time of genotyping are described in Table 1.

Table 1 Demographic and clinical characteristics of study participants

Variables	N	%
Age (years) (mean ± SD)	41,1 ± 9,4	
Gender		
Male	135	73,4
Female	49	26,6
Baseline CD4 count, median (Q1; Q3)	234, 0 (118, 0; 361, 0)	
CD4		
< 200	78	42,4
200 a 350	50	27,2
> 350	47	25,5
Data unavailable	9	4,9
VL (copies/ml), median (Q1; Q3)	19.812,5 (7.036,0; 78.674,2)	
VL (copies/ml)		
≤ 10.000	59	32,1
> 10.000 a 100.000	75	40,7
> 100.000	37	20,1
Data unavailable	13	7,1
Δt on ART (months), median (Q1;Q3)	54, 5 (29, 0; 90, 0)	
Δt in virologic failure (months), median (Q1;Q3)	17, 0 (10, 0; 34, 0)	
NRTI in failing regimen	184	100,0
AZT/3TC	126	68,5
TDF/3TC	48	26,1
Others	10	5,4
NNRTI in failing regimen	155	84,2
EFV	135	87,1
NVP	20	12,9
PI in failing regimen	29	15,8
LPV/r	16	55,2
ATV/r ou ATV 400 mg	12	41,4
Outros	1	3,4
Viral Subtype	171	92,9
B	139	81,3
F	31	18,1
BF	1	0,4

VL = viral load, ART antiretroviral therapy, NNRTIs nonnucleoside reverse transcriptase inhibitors, NRTIs nucleoside/nucleotide reverse transcriptase inhibitors, AZT zidovudine, 3TC lamivudine, TDF tenofovir, EFV: efavirenz, NVP nevirapine, PI protease inhibitor; LPV/r lopinavir/ritonavir, ATV/r atazanavir/ritonavir

The NRTI(t)-associated mutation M184 V/I emerged in 78.4% of the subtype B sequences and in 21.6% of the non-B subtype sequences ($p = 0.009$). Most individuals (89.7%) exhibited at least one mutation for NRTI(t). The association of the presence of ≥3 NRTI(t)-associated mutations with CD4 pre-ARVs < 200 cell/mm3 (66.7% vs 33.3% for CD4 pre-ARVs ≥200, prevalence ratio [PR] =

1.52, CI = 1.00–2.31, p = 0.041), with CD4 at the time of genotyping < 200 cells/mm3 (59.4% vs 23.4% for CD4 200–350 vs 17.2% for CD4 > 350, PR = 2.04, CI = 1.18–3.55, p < 0.011), and with a time on ARV of greater than 36 months (81.2% vs 18.8% for Δt < 36 months, p = 0.003) were significant, according to Table 2. In addition, a VL of 10,000–100,000 copies/ml was associated with the highest number of NRTI(t)-associated mutations (Table 2).

After analysis using the Poisson regression model (Table 3), only patients who were on ARVs for more than 36 months until genotyping (PR = 2.43, 95% CI = 1.38–4.28, p = 0.002) and who developed VL at the time

Table 2 Risk factors associated with HIV-1 drug resistance

Number of resistance mutations					
Factors	≥ 3 n (%)	< 3 n (%)	PR	PR 95% IC	P-value
Age (years)					0, 806[a]
18–30	7 (10, 1)	11 (11, 5)	0, 90	0, 49 – 1, 66	
31–50	52 (75, 4)	68 (70, 8)	1, 00	–	
> 50	10 (14, 5)	17 (17, 7)	0, 85	0, 50 – 1, 46	
Gender					0, 476[a]
Male	53 (76, 8)	69 (71, 9)	1, 17	0, 75 – 1, 81	
Female	16 (23, 2)	27 (28, 1)	1, 00	–	
Viral subtype					0, 771[a]
B	50 (80, 6)	74 (78, 7)	1, 00	–	
No-B	12 (19, 4)	20 (21, 3)	0, 93	0, 57 – 1, 53	
VL before ART (copies/ml)					0, 570[b]
≤ 10.000	4 (7, 5)	3 (4, 3)	1, 00	–	
> 10.000 a 100.000	17 (32, 1)	27 (38, 6)	0, 68	0, 32 – 1, 42	
> 100.000	32 (60, 4)	40 (57, 1)	0, 78	0, 39 – 1, 55	
CD4 before ART					0, 041[a]
< 200	40 (66, 7)	39 (49, 4)	1, 52	1, 00 – 2, 31	
≥ 200	20 (33, 3)	40 (50, 6)	1,00	–	
VL in virologic failure (copies/ml)					0, 042[a]
≤ 10.000	15 (24, 6)	38 (71, 7)	1, 00	–	
> 10.000 a 100.000	34 (55, 7)	33 (36, 3)	1, 79	1,10 – 2, 92	
> 100.000	12 (19, 7)	20 (22, 0)	1,33	0,71 – 2, 46	
CD4 in virologic failure					0, 011[a]
< 200	38 (59, 4)	33 (35, 9)	2, 04	1,18 – 3, 55	
200–350	15 (23, 4)	28 (30, 4)	1, 33	0, 69 – 2, 56	
> 350	11 (17, 2)	31 (33, 7)	1, 00	–	
ART regímen at NRTI baseline					0, 189[a]
TDF	12 (17, 4)	25 (26, 0)	1, 00	–	
No-TDF	57 (82, 6)	71 (74, 0)	1, 37	0, 83 – 2, 27	
Time to virologic failure (months)					0, 221[a]
< 12	13 (19, 4)	28 (30, 4)	1, 00	–	
12–24	25 (37, 3)	34 (37, 0)	1,3 4	0, 78 – 2, 29	
> 24	29 (43, 3)	30 (32, 6)	1, 55	0, 92 – 2, 60	
Time on ART (months)					0, 003[a]
≤ 36	13 (18, 8)	39 (40, 6)	1, 00	–	
> 36	56 (81, 2)	57 (59, 4)	1, 98	1, 19 – 3, 29	

ART antiretroviral therapy, *PR* prevalence ratio, *CI* confidence interval, *VL* viral load, *cell T CD4* CD4 T cell count, *TDF* tenofovir, *NRTIs* nucleoside/nucleotide reverse transcriptase inhibitors
[a]Chi-square test
[b]Fisher's exact test

Table 3 Analysis using the poisson regression model

Variables	PR	PR 95% CI	P-value
CD4 before ARTs (cells/mm³)			
< 200	1, 46	0, 95 – 2, 24	0, 084
≥ 200	1, 00	–	
HIV AIDS (Auckl)			
≥ 10.000	1, 00	–	
> 10.000 a 100.000	2, 09	1, 25 – 3, 50	0, 005
> 100.000	2, 20	1, 14 – 4, 27	0, 018
Time to failure (months)			
≤ 36	1, 00	–	0, 002
> 36	2, 43	1, 38 – 4, 28	

PR prevalence ratio, *CI* confidence interval, *CD4* CD4 + T cell count, *VL* viral load

of genotyping of 10,000–100,000 copies/ml (PR = 2.09 95% CI = 1.25–3.50, $p = 0.005$) and > 100,000 copies/ml (PR = 2.20, 95% CI = 1.14–4.27, p = 0.005) had a higher risk of having ≥3 NRTI (t)-associated mutations.

There was a trend towards the emergence of three or more thymidine-associated mutations (TAMs) when the time on ARVs was greater than 36 months (92% vs 8% for Δt on ARVs ≤36 months, $p = 0.051$). K65R emerged in 7.6% of 184 genotyping tests (Fig. 1) and was observed in 27.1% of patients who were exposed to TDF/3TC. Mutations in the K103 codon were observed in 65.8% ($n = 121/184$) of the genotyping tests. Among those who used NNRTI, this mutation occurred in 78.0% ($n = 121/155$). The NNRTI-associated mutation 90IV was more frequent in the non-B subtype (57.1% vs 42.9% for subtype B, $p = 0.024$) and the 190AS was most prevalent for etravirine.

Considering the 29 patients who used PI, 55.2% ($n = 16$) were on lopinavir/ritonavir (LPV/r) and 41.4% ($n = 12$) were on atazanavir (ATV) (Table 1). The PI-associated

major and accessory mutations were 82AF (51.7%) and 10IFV (62%), respectively.

The PI-associated major mutation 54VL emerged frequently in subtype B sequences (58.3% vs 41.7% for non-B subtype, $p = 0.05$), as did the PI-associated accessory mutations 10IFV (69% vs 31% for non-B subtype, $p = 0.019$) and 20RT (60% vs 40% for non-B subtype, $p = 0.010$).

The total number of mutations was significantly equal to or greater than seven among the users who had a CD4 count below 200 cells/m3 at the time of genotyping (52.9% vs 27.6% for CD4 200–350 cells/m3 vs 19.5% for CD4 > 350 cells/m3, $p = 0.045$).

Salvage therapy characteristics

There was a loss of follow-up in eight (4.3%) patients after the genotyping test was performed. Thus, 176 (95.7%) patients switched to the salvage regimen. Of these individuals, 109 (61.9%) patients used TDF/3TC as the NRTI(t), followed by 28 (15.9%) who used TDF/AZT(zidovudine)/3TC and 27 (15.3%) AZT/3TC. Only nine (5.1%) individuals did not have NRTI(t)s included in their salvage regimen.

PIs were present in the salvage regimen of 99.4% of the individuals; only one patient did not use PI. LPV/r was the most frequently prescribed (48.5%) followed by ATV/r (33.1%). Integrase inhibitors made up the salvage regimen of 35 (19.9%) individuals. Raltegravir (RAL) was the most frequently used one ($n = 32$). When the salvage regimen consisted of two active drugs (GSS = 2), 79.5% of this population showed genotyping with less than three NRTI(t)-associated mutations (79.5% vs 20.5% for ≥3 NRTI(t)-associated mutations, $p < 0.000$).

The susceptibility of etravirine was not associated with the use of EFV or nevirapine (NVP) or with the number of NNRTI-associated mutations. This treatment remained fully active in 63.2% of the sequences among

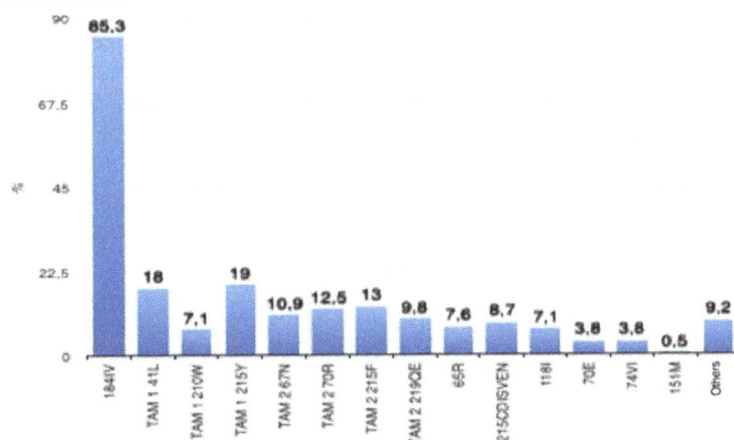

Fig. 1 The prevalence of drug resistance to NRTI among 184 HIV-1 infected patients with virologic failure

the patients who experienced a failed NNRTI therapy. We found a similar susceptibility of AZT and TDF (64.2% vs 65.9%). Among the PI/r users, darunavir/ritonavir (DRV/r) showed the highest percentage of sensitivity (69%), and ATV/r experienced the highest percentage of resistance (79.3%).

Most of the salvage regimens showed GSS equal to two (42.6%) or greater than two (44.3%). We found that in most of the regimens with a GSS greater than 2, the patient was in virologic failure for more than 24 months (46% vs 30.8% for Δt in virologic failure 12–24 months vs 23.2% for Δt in virological failure < 12 months, $p = 0.013$) and on ARV for more than 36 months (76.9% vs 23.1% for Δt in ARV 36 months, $p = 0.004$).

When virologic failure occurred during LPV/r use, the GSS of the salvage therapy regimen was significantly higher than two (85.7% vs 14.3% for GSS = 2 vs 0% for GSS < 2, $p = 0.001$). The significant majority of TDF users in virologic failure were salvaged with an ARV regimen with a GSS equal to two (62.2% vs 27.0% for GSS > 2 vs 10.8% for GSS < 2, $p = 0.023$).

Predictors of undetectable viral loads and CD4 T-cell count variation at 48 weeks after the onset of the salvage regimen

Of the 176 patients who received documented salvage therapy prescriptions, we were able to obtain the VL value 48 weeks after switching ARVs for 159 (90.3%). Of these, 67.3% ($n = 107$) experienced virologic suppression and 11.3% did not reach an undetectable VL but had below 400 copies/ml. The majority of the population with undetectable VL had more than 36 months of ARV use until genotyping (73.8% vs 26.2% for 36 months, $p = 0.022$), and 42.0% were in virologic failure for 12 to 24 months (42.0% vs 34.6% for > 24 months vs 23.4% for < 12 months, $p = 0.029$) (Table 4).

The number of NRTI(t)-associated mutations did not affect virologic suppression (9.3% for zero NRTI(t)-associated mutations vs 48.6% for 1–2 NRTI(t)-associated mutations vs 42.1% for ≥3 NRTI(t)-associated mutations, $p = 0.179$) (Table 5).

After an analysis with the Poisson regression model, only being on ARVs for more than 36 months until genotyping was a protective factor for a detectable viral load (PR 0.6, 95% CI = 0.39–0.92, p = 0.02) 48 weeks after switching to the salvage regimen (Table 6).

For the 153 patients with documented CD4 after 48 weeks, the median was 376 cells/mm3 (Q1 246; Q3 553) and the median CD4 gain was 125 cells/mm3 (Q1 47; Q3 243). In the population with virologic success, the variation in the CD4 gain above 100 cells/mm3 was significant when the VL at the time of genotyping was 10,000–100,000 copies/ml (69.8% vs 30.2% for

variation < 100 cells/mm3, $p = 0.047$) and when the CD4 at the time of genotyping was below 200 cells/mm3 (81.4% vs 18.6% for CD4 < 100 cells/mm3 $p = 0.010$).

Discussion

After evaluating 184 genotyping tests from patients during the first virologic failure, we found a higher prevalence of subtype B, of the M184 V/I and K103 N mutations, as well as a high frequency of NRTI(t) and NNRTI-associated mutations, with no impact on virologic suppression. We observed that the salvage therapy regimen was predominantly composed of PI/r and NRTI(t)s, with virologic success in most cases. Subtype B remains the most common in Pernambuco [17–19] and in Brazil [11], except in the south, where subtype C [21] is predominant. There has been an increase in the proportion of recombinant forms in Rio de Janeiro [22] and subtype F in Minas Gerais [40].

The elevated presence of M184 codon mutations is expected and arises as a consequence of the use of lamivudine as part of all the first-line regimens in our study. This drug confers a high level of resistance to cytosine analogs (lamivudine and emtricitabine), a low level of resistance to abacavir, and the increased susceptibility of zidovudine and TDF. In addition, it decreases the replication capacity of HIV-1 [23, 24]. Its presence has been associated with virologic success [10], but we did not observe this success in the present study.

Similar to our results, the high prevalence of M184 V/I mutations was reported in several regions of Brazil [11, 25, 40], in Sub-Saharan Africa [26] and in Asia [27], but to a lesser extent in western Europe [28]. This difference can be explained by the use of emtricitabine in European countries and by the use of lamivudine in low- and middle-income settings. However, in a recent meta-analysis [29], lamivudine and emtricitabine were clinically equivalent. All the genotype sequences of the non-B subtype (F and BF) had the M184 V/I mutation, probably due to the high prevalence of this mutation and the very low frequency of non-B subtypes in our study.

We found no association between the number of NRTI(t)-associated mutations and the ARVs used at the time of genotyping, including ARV regimens with or without TDF. There are studies showing a greater number of resistance-associated mutations among AZT [30] and TDF users [10, 31]. However, those studies had populations with different characteristics, especially with regard to subtype prevalence. A higher number of mutations with a TDF-based regimen was reported for both the B subtype[10] as well as with the C subtype [33]. The association between a high number of NRTI(t)-associated mutations with CD4 pre-ARV and at the time of genotyping of > 200 cells/mm3 suggests a late

Table 4 Characteristics related to the irrigation regimen, ART time and virological failure time associated with virological suppression after 48 weeks from the start of the rescue scheme

Viral load (VL)					
Characteristics	Detectable n (%)	Undetectable n (%)	PR	PR 95% IC	P-value
Time to virologic failure (months)					0, 029[a]
< 12	22 (42, 3)	25 (23, 4)	1, 00	–	
12–24	13 (25, 0)	45 (42, 0)	0, 48	0, 27 – 0, 84	
> 24	17 (32, 7)	37 (34, 6)	0, 67	0, 41 – 1, 11	
Δt on ART (months)					0, 022[a]
≤ 36	23 (44, 2)	28 (26, 2)	1, 00	–	
> 36	29 (55, 8)	79 (73, 8)	0, 60	0, 39 – 0, 92	
ART rescue NRTI					0, 711[b]
TDF/3TC	36 (69, 2)	62 (57, 9)	1, 00	–	
AZT/3TC	7 (13, 5)	18 (16, 8)	0, 76	0, 39 – 1, 50	
TDF/AZT/3TC	7 (13, 5)	19 (17, 8)	0, 73	0, 37 – 1, 45	
DDI/3TC	0 (0, 0)	1 (0, 9)	–	–	
ABC/3TC	1 (1, 9)	1 (0, 9)	1, 36	0, 33 – 5, 58	
NNRTI	1 (1, 9)	6 (5, 6)	0, 39	0, 00 – 2, 43	
ART rescue PI					0, 013[b]
LPV/r	24 (46, 1)	55 (51, 5)	2, 13	0, 71 – 6, 39	
ATV/r	20 (38, 5)	33 (30, 8)	2, 64	0, 88–7, 96	
DRV/r	3 (5, 8)	18 (16, 8)	1, 00	–	
FPV/r	5 (9, 6)	1, (0, 9)	5, 83	1, 93 – 17, 65	
ART rescue with RAL					0, 050[a]
YES	5 (9, 6)	24 (22, 4)	1, 00	–	
NO	47 (90, 4)	83 (77, 6)	2, 10	0, 91 – 4, 81	
GSS					0, 947[a]
< 2	8 (15, 4)	15 (14, 0)	1, 11	0, 57 – 2, 14	
2	22 (42, 3)	44 (41, 1)	1, 06	0, 65 – 1, 72	
> 2	22 (42, 3)	48 (44, 9)	1, 00	–	

[a]Chi-square test [b]Fisher's exact test; *PR* prevalence ratio, *CI* Confidence interval, *NNRTI* nonnucleoside reverse transcriptase inhibitors, *NRTI* nucleoside/nucleotide reverse transcriptase inhibitors, *AZT* zidovudine, *TAM* analogous thymidine mutation, *3TC* lamivudine, *TDF* tenofovir, *PI* protease inhibitor, *LPV/r* lopinavir/ritonavir, *ATV/r-* atazanavir/ritonavir, *DRv/r* Darunavir/ritonavir, *FPV/r* fosamprenavir/ritonavir, *GSS* genotypic sensitivity score

diagnosis of PLHIV in our population, with an impact on the genotypic profile. These factors did not remain significant after the analysis with the Poisson regression model.

The K103 N/S mutation was documented in most genotypic sequences, due to the frequent use of EFV as the primary NNRTI in the first-line therapy for more than a decade in Brazil. These findings are similar to the national data [10–12] and data from low- and middle-income countries [14, 15, 26, 27]. The susceptibility of etravirine, a second-generation NNRTI, was not influenced by experiencing a long period of time in virologic failure while using EFV or NVP, or by the number of NNRTI-associated mutations.

This analysis was hampered by the small number of NVP users at the time of virologic failure. However, some studies [32–34] have shown that NVP-containing ARVs have repercussions on the response to etravirine for selecting the Y181C and G190A mutations, whereas the K103 mutation associated with EFV does not interfere with etravirine susceptibility.

The median time from ARV therapy to genotyping was similar to that of recent studies in Brazil [10], 10 Africa and Europe [36]. After the Poisson regression model analysis, remaining on ARV for more than 36 months until genotyping was the only factor that impacted the virologic response 48 weeks after the onset of salvage therapy, appearing as a protective

Table 5 Genotypic and immuno-trophic characteristics at the time of genotyping associated with virological suppression after 48 weeks of initiation of the rescue scheme

Viral Load (VL)

Characteristics	Detectable n (%)	Undetectable n (%)	PR	PR 95% IC	P-value
Age (years)					0, 662[a]
18–30	6 (11, 5)	13 (12, 2)	0, 92	0, 45 – 1, 86	
31–50	40 (76, 9)	76 (71, 0)	1, 00	–	
> 50	6 (11, 5)	18 (16, 8)	0, 73	0, 35 – 1, 52	
Gender					0, 385[a]
Male	36 (69, 2)	81 (75, 7)	0, 81	0, 50 – 1, 29	
Female	16 (30, 8)	26 (24, 3)	1, 00	–	
VL on genotypic result (copies/ml)					0, 752[a]
≤ 10.000	18 (35, 3)	36 (34, 3)	1, 00	–	
> 10.000 a 100.000	20 (39, 2)	47 (44, 7)	0, 90	0, 53 – 1, 52	
> 100.000	13 (25, 5)	22 (21, 0)	1, 11	0, 63 – 1, 98	
CD4 on genotypic result (cells/mm3)					0, 796[a]
< 200	20 (38, 5)	45 (42, 9)	0, 95	0, 54 – 1, 66	
200–350	18 (34, 6)	31 (29, 5)	1, 13	0, 64 – 1, 99	
> 350	14 (26, 9)	29 (27, 6)	1, 00	–	
Number of NRTI resistance mutations					0, 179[a]
zero	6 (11, 6)	10 (9, 3)	1, 00	–	
< 3	32 (61, 5)	52 (48, 6)	1, 02	0, 51 – 2, 02	
≥ 3	14 (26, 9)	45 (42, 1)	0, 63	0, 29 – 1, 38	
N° of thymidine analogue mutation					0, 058[a]
zero	35 (67, 3)	54 (50, 4)	1, 00	–	
< 3	14 (26, 9)	34 (31, 8)	0, 74	0, 45 – 1, 24	
≥ 3	3 (5, 8)	19 (17, 8)	0, 35	0, 12 – 1, 02	
Number of NNRTI resistance mutations					0, 113[a]
≤ 2	32 (61, 5)	79 (73, 8)	1, 00	–	
> 2	20 (38, 5)	28 (26, 2)	1, 45	0,93 – 2,25	
Number of PI resistance mutations					1, 000[b]
≤ 2	4 (80, 0)	14 (77, 8)	1, 00	–	
> 2	1 (20, 0)	4 (22, 2)	0, 90	0, 13 – 6, 35	
M184 V/I mutation					0, 693[a]
Yes	44 (84, 6)	93 (86, 9)	1, 00	–	
no	8 (15, 4)	14 (13, 1)	1, 13	0, 62 – 2, 07	

[a]Chi-square test [b]Fisher's exact test, *PR* prevalence ratio, *CI* Confidence interval, *CD4: CD4 T* cells, *CV* viral load, *NNRTI* non-nucleoside reverse transcriptase inhibitor, *PI* protease inhibitor, *NRTI* nucleoside reverse transcriptase inhibitor

factor for a detectable viral load. To understand the impact of time on ARV on virologic success, factors that could influence treatment adherence would have to be identified and controlled, because the major cause of acquired virologic failure is poor adherence to ARVs [42].

A shorter time on ARV is used as the best scenario for adherence in the calculation of odds ratio in studies that seek to understand the risk factors for treatment adherence. However, after association testing, its impact on adherence is not always confirmed [43]. This finding is probably observed because adherence is a dynamic behavior and varies over time for the same individual, and it is affected by diverse factors such as psychosocial-, ARV- and clinical scenario-related factors. This finding explains why the time on ARV may be a risk or protective factor for poor adherence, with an impact on virologic success [42].

Virologic suppression in response to antiretroviral therapy despite extensive resistance...

9

Table 6 Poisson model for viral load detectable after 48 weeks of onset of rescue scheme

Variables	PR[a]	PR IC95%[b]	p-value
[c]Δt on ARV (months)			
≤ 36	1,00	–	0,020
> 36	0,60	0,39 – 0,92	

[a]PR: prevalence ratio [b]IC: Confidence interval [c]time variation on antiretroviral therapy

By contrast, more than 36 months on ARV increased the risk for the selection of three or more NRTI(t)-associated mutations, although a longer time in virologic failure did not generate the same outcome. According to the virologic failure criterion of this study, individuals with low VL (> <1000 copies/ml) were not considered to be in virologic failure, because the genotyping tests available in Brazil during the data collection period were not able to expand the genetic material when the VL was < 1000 copies/ml. However, there is evidence that having a VL of > 200 copies/ml increases the risk for virologic failure and may lead to mutation accumulation [44]. Therefore, it is possible that many individuals who are on ARV for a long period of time (> 36 months) had low VL but were not diagnosed with virologic failure, accumulating mutations.

We observed that the presence of NRTI(t)-associated mutations or TAMs at the first virologic failure did not interfere with virologic suppression 48 weeks after the switch to a second-line therapy with NRTI(t)s combined with PI/r. This finding is not only due to the high potency of PI/r or to the direct activity of NRTI(t)s, and it may reflect an effect of the NRTI(t)s on viral fitness [35]. This finding is consistent with the results of three large randomized controlled trials in which patients with extensive resistance to reverse transcriptase evolved with virologic success after salvage therapy based on NRTI(t) with PI/r [13–15].

We found no difference in the virologic response between regimens with an individual GSS of less than two and those greater than or equal to two, confirming the hypothesis that there is no difference between active, partially active or inactive NRTI(t)s in terms of virologic success [35]. In the EARNEST study [14], the group receiving inactive or partially active NRTI(t)s exhibited viral load suppression that was similar to if not better than that exhibited by the group receiving the regimen containing a fully active drug from a new class, and it was superior to that exhibited by the group using only a protease inhibitor.

It is possible that pharmacokinetic characteristics optimize the benefits of NRTI(t)s even if inactive. Thus, ARVs with a long intracellular half-life, such as TDF and lamivudine, may help the PI/r to maintain viral suppression. This effect is independent of the drug activity [41].

We were able to define the time in virologic failure until the switch to second-line therapy. Surprisingly, most of the patients with undetected viral loads were in virologic failure for more than 12 months. Because the time under virologic failure did not interfere with the number of NRTI(t)-associated mutations or TAMs in our study, we can suggest that the resistance-associated mutations arose during the first months of virologic failure. In the EUROSIDA study [37], a high number of TAM-1 mutations was observed within one year of failure, with a lower accumulation rate than what was predicted among those who stayed on the failing regimen.

The total absence of ARV selective pressure during part of the virologic failure period is another way to explain why the longer virologic failure time did not influence the number of NRTI(t)-associated mutations or TAMs. The complete withdrawal of ARVs generates fewer resistance-associated mutations than does the maintenance of sub-therapeutic doses [9]. It was not possible to determine whether the study participants were kept on sub-therapeutic doses or if they completely abandoned the treatment when they were in virologic failure.

When we analyzed the virologic response and ARVs used in salvage therapy, we observed that there was no difference between the patients who used AZT or TDF or both. The use of LPV/r was significant among those who experienced virologic success, probably because it was the most frequently prescribed PI during the study period, as directed by the Brazilian Ministry of Health. Among users of DRV/r or RAL, the majority achieved virologic success, although they were smaller in absolute numbers.

DRV/r is the newest PI and has a high genetic barrier, in addition to fewer adverse effects than LPV/r, possessing activity even with a protease mutation [38]. When the protease is not intact, adding a new ARV class is critical. This class has often been the integrase inhibitor [39]. It should be noted that this study was not designed to assess the individual power of each regimen. Among those who reached an undetectable VL, a CD4 gain above 100 cells/mm3 was significant in subjects with CD4 at the time of genotyping > 200 cells/mm3, demonstrating that when there is adherence, a significant immunologic gain is possible even in patients with a low immunologic reserve and extensive resistance in reverse transcriptase.

Our primary limitation was the difficulty in establishing cause-and-effect relationships, because this was a cross-sectional study. Our results may have been partially affected by data we were unable to collect, particularly those related to adherence to ARV therapy, and by the loss of information in some variables. However, this study has relevant points because it updates the genotypic data of an important region of Brazil with limited resources. In addition, we were able to establish the time in virologic failure and the ARV regimen before and after genotyping in the first virologic failure as well as the factors associated with the number of NRTI(t)-associated mutations and virologic success.

Conclusions

Patients in their first virologic failure who were seen at referral centers in the city of Recife, Pernambuco, Northeastern Brazil presented a high frequency of mutations pertaining to secondary resistance to the use of NRTI(t)s and NNRTIs. However, extensive resistance in reverse transcriptase did not impact the second-line virologic suppression after 48 weeks of the salvage therapy with PI/r combined with active, partially active or inactive NRTI(t)s. The time on ARVs to genotyping was an independent protective factor for a detectable viral load. Long-term follow-up is needed to support the use of partially active NRTI(t)s in salvage therapy regimens while controlling for adherence-related factors. Studies assessing the actual need for genotyping after the first virologic failure with NNRTIs are also needed.

Abbreviations
3TC: Lamivudine; ARVs: Antiretrovirals; ATV: Atazanavir; AZT: Zidovudine; CD4: CD4 T-cell counts; DRV/r: Darunavir/ritonavir; EFV: Efavirenz; GSS: Genotypic sensitivity score; IAS: International AIDS Society; LPV/r: Lopinavir/ritonavir; NNRTI: Non-nucleoside reverse transcriptase inhibitor; NRTI(t): Nucleos(t)ide reverse transcriptase inhibitor; NVP: Nevirapine; PI: Protease inhibitors; PLHIV: People are living with HIV; SPSS: Statistical package for the social sciences; TAMs: Thymidine-associated mutations; TDF: Tenofovir; VL: Viral load

Authors' contributions
All authors contributed equally. All authors read and approved the final manuscript.

Competing interests
The authors declared no potential competing interest with respect to the research, authorship, and/or publication of this article.

Author details
[1]Programa de Pós-graduação em Ciências da Saúde, Universidade Federal de Pernambuco, Av. Prof. Moraes Rego 1235, Recife 50670-901, Brazil. [2]Instituto Aggeu Magalhaes, FIOCRUZ, Av. Prof. Moraes Rego 1235, Recife 50670-901, Brazil. [3]Faculdade de Medicina do Recife, Universidade Federal de Pernambuco, Av. Prof. Moraes Rego, 1235, Recife, Pernambuco, Brazil.

References
1. 1 Joint United Nations Programme on HIV/AIDS. Global AIDS Update. 2016. http://www.unaids.org/en/topic/treatment. (Accessed Dec 20, 2017).
2. Strategies for Management of Antiretroviral Therapy (SMART) Study Group, El- Sadr WM, Lundgren J, Neaton JD, et al. CD4+ count-guided interruption of antiretroviral treatment. N Engl J Med. 2006;355:2283–96.
3. Rodger AJ, Cambiano V, Bruun T, et al. PARTNER study group. Sexual activity without condoms and risk of hiv transmission in serodifferent couples when the HIV- positive partner is using suppressive antiretroviral therapy. JAMA. 2016;316(2):171–81.
4. World Health Organization. HIV drug resistance report 2017. (https://www. who.int/hiv/pub/drugresistance/hivdr-report-2017/en/).
5. Campbell TB, Smeaton LM, Kumarasamy N, et al. Efficacy and safety of three antiretroviral regimens for initial treatment of HIV-1: a randomized clinical trial in diverse multinational settings. PLoS Med 2012; 9:e1001290. [sPubMed: 22936892].
6. Tilghman M, Tsai D, Buene TP, et al. Pooled nucleic acid testing to detect antiretroviral treatment failure in HIV-infected patients in Mozambique. J Acquir Immune Defic Syndr. 2015;70:256–261. [PubMed: 26135327].
7. Joint United Nations Programme on HIV/AIDS. Global AIDS Update. 2016. In:. Accessed 20 Dec 2017.
8. Brasil. Protocolo Clínico e Diretrizes Terapêuticas para Manejo da Infecção pelo HIV em Adultos. Data de publicação: 03/10/2013. Data última atualização: 31/07/2015. Available at https://www.aids.gov.br/tags/publicacoes/protocolo-clinico-e-diretrizes-terapeuticas. (Accessed 20 Aug 2017).
9. Brasil. Protocolo Clínico e Diretrizes Terapêuticas para Manejo da Infecção pelo HIVem Adultos. Data de publicação: 2017. Available at www.aids.gov. br/tags/publicacoes/protocolo-clinico-e-diretrizes-terapeuticas. (Accessed 01 Dec 2017).
10. Matsuda EM, Coelho LP, Romero G, et al. High prevalence of drug resistance mutations among patients failing first-line antiretroviral therapy and predictors of virological response 24 weeks after switch to second-line therapy in São Paulo state, Brazil. AIDS Res Hum Retroviruses. 2017;34(2):1–27. http://doi.org/10.1089/aid.2017.0052.
11. Brites C, Pinto-Neto L, Medeiros M, et al. Extensive variation in drug-resistance mutational profile of Brazilian patients failing antiretroviral therapy in five large Brazilian cities. Braz J Infect Dis. 2016;20(4):323–9.
12. World Health Organization. Consolidated Guidelines on the use of antiretroviral drugs for treating and preventing HIV infection. https://www.who.int/hiv/pub/arv/treatment-monitoring-info-2017/en/ (Accessed 20 Dec 2017).
13. Boyd MA, Kumarasamy N, Moore CL, et al. for the second-line study group. Ritonavir-boosted lopinavir plus nucleoside or nucleotide reverse transcriptase inhibitors versus ritonavir-boosted lopinavir plus raltegravir for treatment of HIV-1 infection in adults with virological failure of a standard first-line ART regimen (SECOND-LINE): a randomised, open-label, non-inferiority study. Lancet. 2013;381:2091–9.
14. Paton NI, Kityo C, Hoppe A, et al. EARNEST trial team. Assessment of second- line antiretroviral regimens for HIV therapy in Africa. N Engl J Med. 2014;371(3):234–47.
15. La Rosa AM, Harrison LJ, Taiwo B, et al. Raltegravir in second-line antiretroviral therapy in resource-limited settings (SELECT): a randomised, phase 3, non- inferiority study. Lancet HIV. 2016;3:e247–58.
16. 2017 Resistance Mutations Update. Volume 24, Issue 4, Dec. 2016/January 2017. Available at https://www.iasusa.org/sites/default/files/uploads/2017hiv-muta-article.pdf. Accessed in 01/20/2017.
17. Cavalcanti AM, Lacerda HR, Brito AM, et al. Antiretroviral resistance in individuals presenting therapeutic failure and subtypes of the human immunodeficiency virus type 1 in the northeast region of Brazil. Mem Inst Oswaldo Cruz. 2007;102:785–92.
18. Lacerda HR, Medeiros LB, Cavalcanti AM, et al. Comparison of the epidemiology, profile of mutations, and clinical response to antiretrovirals among subtypes B and F of the human immunodeficiency virus type 1. Mem Inst Oswaldo Cruz. 2007;102:693–9.
19. Lima K, de Souza Leal É, AMS C, Salustiano DM, de Medeiros LB, da Silva SP, et al. Epidemiological, Clinical and Antiretroviral Susceptibility Characterization of Human Immunodeficiency Virus Subtypes B and Non-B in Pernambuco, Northeast Brazil. PLoS One. 2016;11(5):e0155854.
20. Kanters S, Socias ME, Paton NI, et al. Comparative efficacy and safety of second- line antiretroviral therapy for treatment of HIV/AIDS: a systematic review and network meta-analysis. The Lancet HIV. 2017;3018(17):1–9.
21. Gräf T, Vrancken B, Maletich Junqueira D, et al. Contribution of epidemiological predictors in unraveling the phylogeographic history of HIV-1 subtype C in Brazil. J Virol. 2015;89:12341–8.
22. Velasco-de-Castro CA, Grinsztejn B, Veloso VG, et al. HIV-1 diversity and drug resistance mutations among people seeking HIV diagnosis in voluntary counseling and testing sites in Rio de Janeiro, Brazil. PLoS One. 2014;9(1):e87622.
23. Miller MD, Margot N, Lu B, Zhong L, et al. Genotypic and phenotypic predictors of the magnitude of response to tenofovir disoproxil fumarate treatment in antiretroviral- experienced patients. J Infect Dis. 2004;189(5):837–46.
24. Melikian GL, Rhee SY, Taylor J, et al. Standardized comparison of the relative impacts of HIV-1 reverse transcriptase (RT) mutations on nucleoside RT inhibitor susceptibility. Antimicrob Agents Chemother. 2012;56(5):2305–13.

Virologic suppression in response to antiretroviral therapy despite extensive resistance...

11

25. Lopes CA, Soares MA, Falci DR, Sprinz E. The evolving genotypic profile of HIV- 1 mutations related to antiretroviral treatment in the north region of Brazil. Biomed Res Int. 2015;2015:738528e.

26. Hamers RL, Sigaloff KC, Wensing AM, et al. PharmAccess African studies to evaluate resistance (PASER). Patterns of HIV-1 drug resistance after first-line antiretroviral therapy (ART) failure in 6 sub-Saharan African countries: implications for second-line ART strategies. Clin Infect Dis. 2012;54(11):1660–9.

27. Sivamalar S, Dinesha TR, Gomathi S, et al. Accumulation of HIV-1 drug resistance mutations after first-line immunological failure to evaluate the options of recycling NRTI drugs in second-line treatment: a study from South India. AIDS Res Hum Retrovir. 2017;33(3):271–4.

28. The TenoRes Study Group. Global epidemiology of drug resistance after failure of WHO recommended fi rst-line regimens for adult HIV-1 infection: a multicentre retrospective cohort study. Lancet Infect Dis. 2016;16:565–75.

29. Ford N, Shubber Z, Hill A, et al. Comparative efficacy of lamivudine and Emtricitabine: a systematic review and meta-analysis of randomized trials. PLoS One. 2013;8(11):e79981.

30. Von Wyl V, Yerly S, Böni J, et al. Swiss HIV cohort study. Incidence of HIV-1 drug resistance among antiretroviral treatment-naive individuals starting modern therapy combinations. Clin Infect Dis. 2012;54(1):131–40.

31. Van Zyl GU, Liu TF, Claassen M, Engelbrecht S, et al. Trends in genotypic HIV-1 antiretroviral resistance between 2006 and 2012 in south African patients receiving first and second-line antiretroviral treatment regimens. PLoS One. 2013;8(6):e67188.

32. Stevens WS, Wallis CL, Sanne I, Venter F. Will etravirine work in patients failing nonnucleoside reverse transcriptase inhibitor-based treatment in southern Africa? J Acquir Immune Defic Syndr. 2009;52(5):655–6.

33. Kiertiburanakul S, Wiboonchutikul S, Sukasem C, Chantratita W, Sungkanu- parph S. Using of nevirapine is associated with intermediate and reduced response to etravirine among HIV-infected patients who experienced virologic failure in a resource- limited setting. J Clin Virol. 2010;47(4):330–4.

34. Taiwo B, Chaplin B, Penugonda S, et al. Suboptimal Etravirine activity is common during failure of Nevirapine-based combination antiretroviral therapy in a cohort infected with non-B subtype HIV-1. Curr HIV Res. 2010;8(3):194–8.

35. Paton, N, Kityo, C, Thompson, J, et al. Impact of NRTI cross-resistance on second-line PI + NRTI therapy outcomes in Africa; Conference on Retrovirus and Opportunistic Infections; Seattle, WA, USA. Feb 23–26, 2015;119 (abstr).

36. Lam EP, Moore CL, Gotuzzo E, et al. Antiretroviral resistance ater first-line anti- retroviral therapy failure in diverse HIV-1 subtypes in the SECOND-LINE study. AIDS Res Hum Retrovir. 2016;32:841–50.

37. Cozzi-Lepri A, Phillips AN, Martinez-Picado J, et al. EuroSIDA study group. Rate of accumulation of thymidine analogue mutations in patients continuing to receive virologically failing regimens containing zidovudine or stavudine: implications for antiretroviral therapy programs in resource-limited settings. J Infect Dis. 2009;200(5):687–97.

38. Molina JM, Cohen C, Katlama C, Grinsztejn B, Timerman A, Pedro RD. et al. Safety and efficacy of darunavir (TMC114) with low-dose ritonavir in treatment- experienced patients: 24-week results of POWER 3. J Acquir Immune Defic Syndr. 2007;46:24–31.

39. Grinsztejn B, Nguyen B-Y, Katlama C, et al. For the Protocol 005Team. Safety and efficacy of the HIV-1 integrase inhibitor raltegravir (MK-0518) in treatment- experienced patients with multidrug-resistant virus: a phase II randomised controlled trial. Lancet. 2007;369:1261–9.

40. Duani H, Aleixo AW, Tupinambás U. Trends and predictors of HIV-1 acquired drug resistance in Minas Gerais, Brazil: 2002-2012. Braz J Infect Dis. 2017;21(2):148–54.

41. Nucleoside reverse-transcriptase inhibitor cross-resistance and outcomes from second-line antiretroviral therapy in the public health approach: an observational analysis within the randomised, open-label, EARNEST trial.

42. Horizons/Population Council, International Centre for Reproductive Health and Coast Province General Hospital, Mombasa-Kenya. Adherence to Antiretroviral Therapy in Adults: A Guide for Trainers. Nairobi: Population Council. 2004. Available from: http://www.popcouncil.org/uploads/pdfs/ horizons/mombasaarvtrainingguide.pdf. Accessed 6 Feb 2018.

43. Shigdel R, Klouman E, Bhandari A, et al. Factors associated with adherence to antiretroviral therapy in HIV-infected patients in Kathmandu District, Nepal. HIV AIDS (Auckl). 2014;6:109–16.

44. Vandenhende MA, Ingle S, May M, et al. Impact of low-level viremia on clinical and virological outcomes in treated HIV-1-infected patients: the antiretroviral therapy cohort collaboration (ART-CC). AIDS. 2015;29(3):373–83.

2

Quality control implementation for universal characterization of DNA and RNA viruses in clinical respiratory samples using single metagenomic next-generation sequencing workflow

A. Bal[1,2,3,4], M. Pichon[1,2,3], C. Picard[5,6], J. S. Casalegno[1,2,3], M. Valette[1,2,3], I. Schuffenecker[1], L. Billard[7], S. Vallet[7,8], G. Vilchez[4], V. Cheynet[4], G. Oriol[4], S. Trouillet-Assant[4], Y. Gillet[9], B. Lina[1,2,3], K. Brengel-Pesce[4], F. Morfin[1,2,3] and L. Josset[1,2,3]*

Abstract

Background: In recent years, metagenomic Next-Generation Sequencing (mNGS) has increasingly been used for an accurate assumption-free virological diagnosis. However, the systematic workflow evaluation on clinical respiratory samples and implementation of quality controls (QCs) is still lacking.

Methods: A total of 3 QCs were implemented and processed through the whole mNGS workflow: a no-template-control to evaluate contamination issues during the process; an internal and an external QC to check the integrity of the reagents, equipment, the presence of inhibitors, and to allow the validation of results for each sample. The workflow was then evaluated on 37 clinical respiratory samples from patients with acute respiratory infections previously tested for a broad panel of viruses using semi-quantitative real-time PCR assays (28 positive samples including 6 multiple viral infections; 9 negative samples). Selected specimens included nasopharyngeal swabs ($n = 20$), aspirates ($n = 10$), or sputums ($n = 7$).

Results: The optimal spiking level of the internal QC was first determined in order to be sufficiently detected without overconsumption of sequencing reads. According to QC validation criteria, mNGS results were validated for 34/37 selected samples. For valid samples, viral genotypes were accurately determined for 36/36 viruses detected with PCR (viral genome coverage ranged from 0.6 to 100%, median = 67.7%). This mNGS workflow allowed the detection of DNA and RNA viruses up to a semi-quantitative PCR Ct value of 36. The six multiple viral infections involving 2 to 4 viruses were also fully characterized. A strong correlation between results of mNGS and real-time PCR was obtained for each type of viral genome (R^2 ranged from 0.72 for linear single-stranded (ss) RNA viruses to 0.98 for linear ssDNA viruses).

(Continued on next page)

* Correspondence: laurence.josset@chu-lyon.fr
[1]Laboratoire de Virologie, Institut des Agents Infectieux, Groupement Hospitalier Nord, Hospices Civils de Lyon, Lyon, France
[2]Univ Lyon, Université Lyon 1, Faculté de Médecine Lyon Est, CIRI, Inserm U1111 CNRS UMR5308, Virpath, Lyon, France
Full list of author information is available at the end of the article

(Continued from previous page)

Conclusions: Although the potential of mNGS technology is very promising, further evaluation studies are urgently needed for its routine clinical use within a reasonable timeframe. The approach described herein is crucial to bring standardization and to ensure the quality of the generated sequences in clinical setting. We provide an easy-to-use single protocol successfully evaluated for the characterization of a broad and representative panel of DNA and RNA respiratory viruses in various types of clinical samples.

Keywords: Clinical virology, Quality control, Next-generation sequencing, Viral metagenomics, Respiratory viruses

Background

Since the development of Next Generation-Sequencing (NGS) technologies in 2005, the use of metagenomic approaches has grown considerably. It is now considered as an efficient unbiased tool in clinical virology [1, 2], in particular for the characterization of viral acute respiratory infections (ARIs). Several advantages of metagenomic NGS (mNGS) compared to conventional real-time Polymerase Chain Reaction (PCR) assays have been highlighted. Firstly, the full viral genetic information is immediately available allowing the investigation of respiratory outbreaks, viral epidemiological surveillance, or identification of specific mutations leading to antiviral resistance or higher virulence [3–5]. Secondly, a significant improvement in viral ARIs diagnosis has been reported [4, 6–9]; as the process is sequence independent, mNGS is able to identify highly divergent viral genomes, rare respiratory pathogens, and to discover respiratory viruses missed by targeted PCR [1, 4, 7].

However, the diversity in viral nucleic acid types has impaired the development of a unique viral metagenomic workflow allowing the comprehensive characterization of viruses present in a clinical sample. Most of the published viral metagenomic protocols have been optimized for the detection either of DNA viruses or RNA viruses [4, 5, 10–13]. In addition, despite the growing number of studies using a metagenomic process in clinical virology, evaluation of workflows has not systematically included both clinical samples and quality control (QC) implementation. A metagenomic protocol involves a large number of steps and all of these have to be controlled to ensure the quality of the generated sequences [6, 14–16]. Furthermore, specimen to specimen, environmental, and reagent contaminations are also a major concern in metagenomic setting and must be accurately evaluated [6, 17–19].

The objective of this study was to implement QCs in a single metagenomic protocol and to evaluate it for the detection of a broad panel of DNA and RNA viruses in clinical respiratory samples.

Methods
Clinical samples

A total of 37 respiratory samples collected from patients hospitalized in the university hospital of Lyon (Hospices Civils de Lyon, HCL) were retrospectively selected to evaluate our metagenomic approach. Selected specimens included various types of clinical samples; nasopharyngeal swabs ($n = 20$), aspirates ($n = 10$), or sputums ($n = 7$). These samples were initially sent to our laboratory for routine viral diagnosis of ARI using semi-quantitative real-time PCR assays targeting a comprehensive panel of DNA and RNA viruses (r-gene, bioMérieux, Marcy l'étoile, France). This panel included: influenza virus type A and B, adenovirus, cytomegalovirus, Epstein-Barr virus, human herpes virus 6, human bocavirus (HBoV), human rhinovirus, respiratory syncytial virus, human parainfluenza virus, human coronavirus (HCoV), human metapneumovirus, and measles virus. Twenty-two samples were positive for only one targeted virus, 6 were characterized by a multiple viral infection and 9 were negative for all the targeted viruses. These 9 samples were also found to be negative using the FilmArray Respiratory Panel (FA RP, bioMérieux). After PCR testing, the rest of samples were stored at $-20\ °C$ until mNGS analysis.

Metagenomic workflow

For sample viral enrichment, a 3-step method was applied to 200 µl of thawed and vortexed sample [20]: low-speed centrifugation (6000 g, 10 min, 4 °C), followed by filtration of the supernatant using 0.80 µm filter (Sartorius, Göttingen, Germany) to remove eukaryotic and bacterial cells, without loss of large viruses [21] and then Turbo DNase treatment (0.1 U/µL, 37 °C, 90 min; Life Technologies, Carlsbad, CA, USA). Total nucleic acid was extracted using the NucliSENS EasyMAG platform (bioMérieux, Marcy l'Etoile, France) followed by an ethanol precipitation (2 h at $-80\ °C$). As previously described, modified whole transcriptome amplification was performed to amplify both DNA and RNA viral nucleic acids (WTA2, Sigma-Aldrich, Darmstadt, Germany) [21]. Amplified DNA and cDNA were then purified using a QiaQuick column (Qiagen, Hilden, Germany) and quantified using the Qubit fluorometer HS dsDNA Kit (Life Technologies, Carlsbad, CA, USA). Nextera XT DNA Library preparation and Nextera XT Index Kit were used to prepare paired-end libraries, according to the manufacturer's recommendations (Illumina, San Diego, CA, USA). After normalization, a pool of libraries (V/V) was made and quantified using universal KAPA library quantification kit (Kapa Biosystems, Wilmington, MA, USA); 1% PhiX genome was added to the quantified library before sequencing with Illumina NextSeq 500 ™ platform (Fig. 1). In addition, it should be noticed that our wet-lab process was designed to prevent contaminations as much as possible: reagents were stored and prepared in a DNA-free room; patient samples were opened in a laminar flow hood in a pre-PCR room; after the amplification step, tubes were handled and stored in a post-PCR room.

Bioinformatic analysis

A stepwise bioinformatic filtering pipeline was used to quality filter reads using cutadapt and sickle; and to remove human, archaeal, bacterial, and fungal sequences by aligning reads with bwa mem. The databases used were GRCh38.p2, RefSeq archaea, RefSeq bacteria, and RefSeq fungi. Remaining reads were aligned on ezVIR viral database v0.1 [22] and bacteriophage genomes from the RefSeq database (downloaded on 17 February 2017) using bwa mem. Normalization for comparing viral genome coverage values was performed using reads per kilobase of virus reference sequence per million mapped reads (RPKM) ratio [4, 23]. RPKM ratio corrects differences in both sample sequencing depth and viral gene length. Viral reads (expressed in RPKM) from the No-Template Control (NTC) were subtracted from viral reads (in RPKM) of each sample within the batch prior to further analysis. A sample was considered to be positive for a particular virus when the RPKM of this virus was positive. No threshold regarding genome coverage pattern was applied nor requirement to cover a particular region of the genome. This latter requirement could be important to correctly identify RNA virus subtypes with high recombination frequencies within a species, but has to be implemented specifically for each viral family.

Quality control implementation

All respiratory specimens were spiked with internal quality control (IQC) before sample preparation. MS2 bacteriophage from a commercial kit (MS2, IC1 RNA internal control; r-gene, bioMérieux) was selected as the IQC. As positive external quality control (EQC), we used

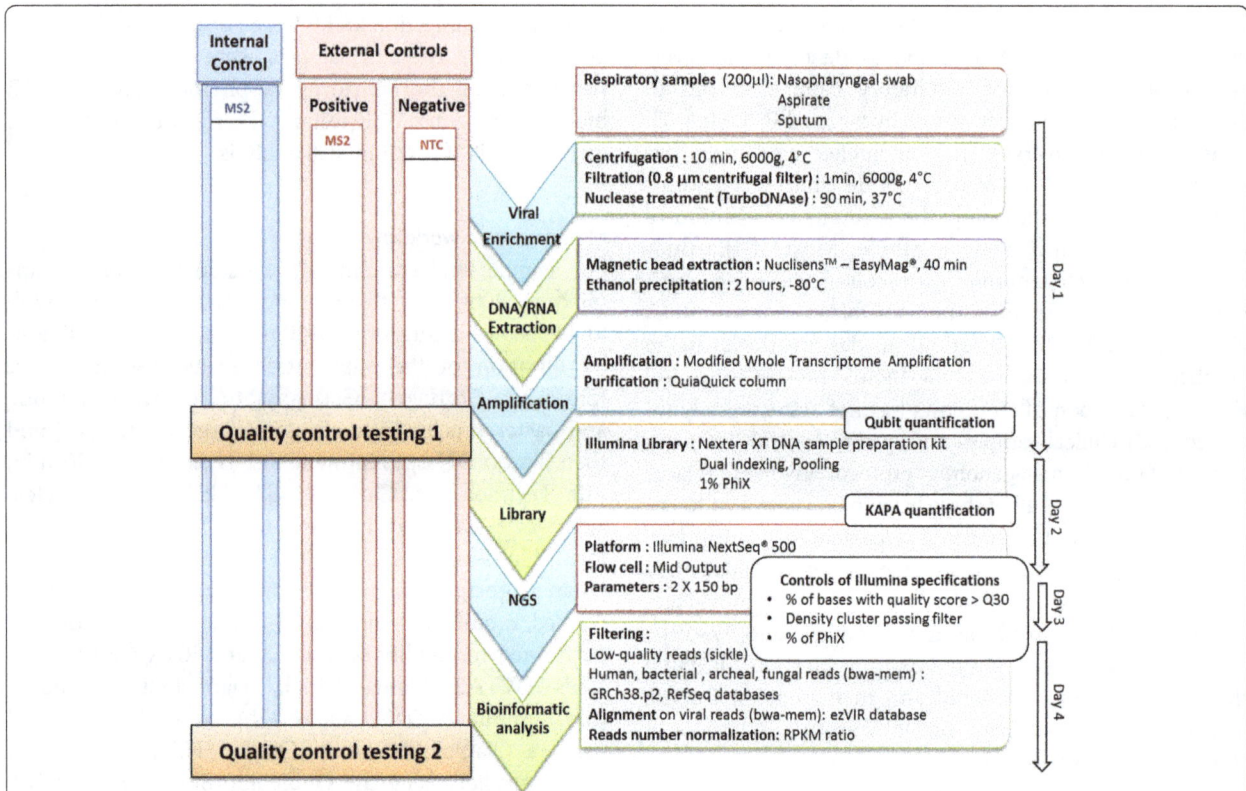

Fig. 1 Schematic representation of the metagenomic workflow and quality control steps. The whole process is summarized in the middle. On the left side, internal control (MS2 bacteriophage) is represented in blue, and external controls are represented in red, including positive control (MS2 bacteriophage spiked in viral transport medium) and No-Template Control (NTC: viral transport medium). Quality control testing 1 corresponds to MS2 bacteriophage molecular detection with commercial PCR assay. Quality control testing 2 corresponds to control by sequencing metrics (number of MS2 reads normalized with RPKM ratio and MS2 genome coverage). On the right, each technique used by phases is indicated black. In addition, on the far right the duration of each step is indicated

viral transport medium spiked with MS2 at the same concentration used for the IQC. A No-Template Control (NTC) was implemented to evaluate contamination during the process. NTC was constituted of viral transport medium (Sigma-virocult, MWE, Corsham, UK) that was processed through all mNGS steps. Two QC testing (QCT) were performed: QCT1 which was the semi-quantitative detection of MS2 using a commercial real-time PCR assay (IC1 RNA internal control, r-gene, bioMérieux,) after amplification step (Fig. 1). QCT1 validation criteria were: MS2 semi-quantitative PCR Cycle threshold (Ct) below 37 Ct for IQC and EQC, and no MS2 detection for NTC. QCT2 evaluated the sequencing performance by quantifying the number of reads aligned on the MS2 genome (in RPKM) and MS2 genome coverage (MS2 genome accession number: NC_001417.2; Fig. 1). QCT2 validation criteria were MS2 genome coverage > 95% for positive EQC, and an MS2 RPKM > 0 for IQC.

Statistical analysis

Statistical analyses were performed using GraphPrism version 5.02 applying the appropriate statistical test (associations between mNGS and viral real-time PCR assay were determined by applying the Pearson's correlation coefficient and differences between median and distributions were evaluated by the Mann–Whitney U test). A p-value less than 0.05 was considered to be statistically significant.

Results

Determination of optimal internal quality control spiking

MS2 bacteriophage (MS2), a single-stranded RNA virus (ssRNA), was used as the IQC to validate the whole metagenomic process for each sample. In order to optimize IQC spiking level, the sensitivity of the metagenomic analysis workflow for MS2 detection was first evaluated with a ten-fold serial dilutions of MS2 (from 10^{-2} to 10^{-5}) in a nasopharyngeal swab tested negative using FA RP (bioMérieux). MS2 was detected in internal QCT1 (IQCT1) for all levels of MS2 spiking (Ct ranged from 17.5 at the 10^{-2} dilution to 26.4 Ct at the 10^{-5} dilution). Full to partial MS2 genome coverage was obtained for all MS2 spiking levels in internal QCT2 (IQCT2; coverage ranged from 98% at the 10^{-2} dilution to 69% at the 10^{-5} dilution). For the highest spiking level, 66.0% of the total number of viral reads was mapped to MS2; for the lowest spiking level, 0.9% were so (Fig. 2). To limit the number of NGS reads consumed for IQC detection, the optimal spiking condition was determined to be the 10^{-5} dilution and was used for the rest of the study.

Validation of mNGS results

A total of 37 clinical respiratory samples from patients with ARIs caused by a broad panel of DNA and RNA viruses or of unknown etiology were analyzed in a single mNGS workflow. Libraries were sequenced to a mean of 5,139,248 million reads passing quality filters (range: 270,975 to 13,586,456 reads). Human sequences represented the main part of NGS reads for both positive samples (mean = 61.3%) and negative samples (mean = 67.1%), but not of NTC which was mainly composed of bacterial reads (67.8%). The proportion of viral reads ranged from 0.006 to 85.2% (mean = 9.6% for positive samples and 0.6% for negative samples, Additional file 1). Viral metagenomic results were then validated according to the criteria described in the Methods section. QCT1 (MS2 molecular detection performed before library preparation) was negative for NTC. After sequencing, viral contamination represented 0.13% (4245/3,215,616) of the total reads generated from NTC including 2 MS2 reads (MS2 RPKM = 173). For targeted viruses, 21 reads (RPKM = 480) and 185 reads (RPKM = 1.1E + 04) mapping to influenza A(H3N2) and HBoV were detected, respectively. The positive EQC was successfully detected at QCT1 (MS2 PCR positive at 25 Ct) and after the sequencing step (QCT2; MS2 genome coverage = 99.7%, MS2 RPKM = 5.5E + 05). Regarding IQC results, 37/37 samples passed QCT1 (MS2 PCR Ct values < 37) and were therefore further processed. A total of 33/37 samples passed QCT2 (MS2 RPKM > 0; Fig. 3). For these 33 samples, MS2 genome coverage ranged from 15 to 100% (Additional file 2).

The 4 samples that did not pass IQCT2 included one sputum that was previously tested negative using real-time PCR (sample # 37), one HCoV positive sputum (sample # 11, Ct = 32), one HBoV positive nasopharyngeal swab (sample # 19, Ct = 30), and one nasopharyngeal aspirate tested positive for HBoV and CMV (sample # 23, Ct = 15 and 31, respectively). For sample # 37 and sample # 19, none of the real-time PCR targeted viruses were detected after bioinformatic analysis. For sample # 19, we sequenced a replicate which similarly failed both IQC and HBoV detection. We could not test any replicate for sample # 37 owing to insufficient quantity. Viral metagenomics results for sample # 23 were validated as viral reads represented 85.2% (9,489,578/ 11,144,324) of the total reads generated (Fig. 3). For sample # 11, the number of reads mapping to HCoV was 9/ 5,125,947 with a HCoV genome coverage of 0.2%. Results were therefore not validated for this sample. Overall, mNGS results were validated for 34/37 samples including 26/28 positive samples and 8/9 negative samples.

Metagenomic workflow evaluation according to viral genome type

The evaluation of the metagenomic workflow was performed using the 26 previously validated respiratory

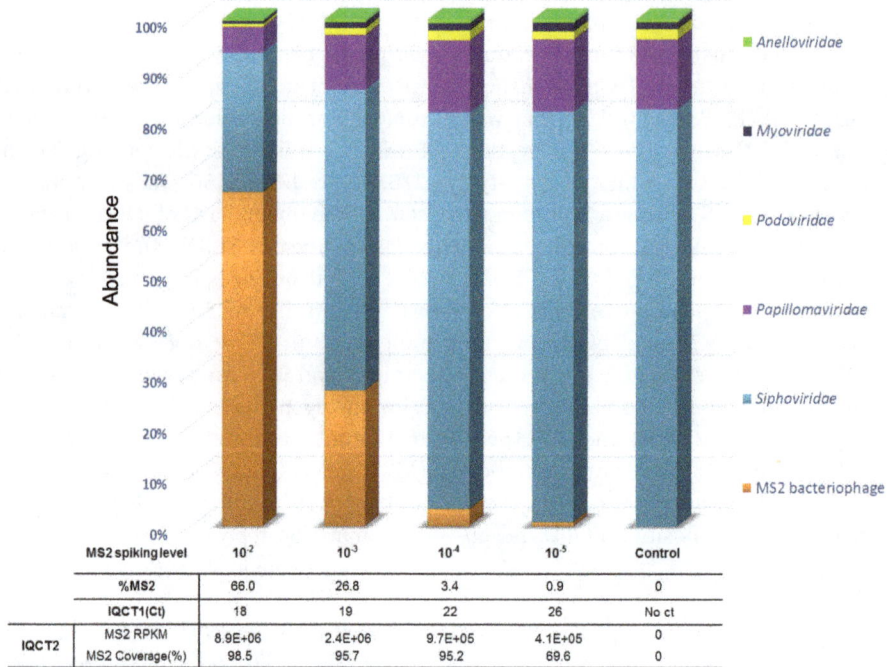

MS2 spiking level		10^{-2}	10^{-3}	10^{-4}	10^{-5}	Control
%MS2		66.0	26.8	3.4	0.9	0
IQCT1(Ct)		18	19	22	26	No ct
IQCT2	MS2 RPKM	8.9E+06	2.4E+06	9.7E+05	4.1E+05	0
	MS2 Coverage(%)	98.5	95.7	95.2	69.6	0

Fig. 2 Determination of optimal spiking level for internal quality control. The sensitivity of the metagenomic analysis workflow for MS2 bacteriophage (Internal Quality Control, IQC) detection was evaluated with a MS2 ten-fold serial dilutions in a nasopharyngeal swab tested negative with multiplex viral PCR. Relative abundance of MS2 bacteriophage and viral families are represented depending on the MS2 spiked-in concentration. IQCT1 corresponds to MS2 molecular detection with commercial real-time PCR assay after amplification step. IQCT2 corresponds to control by sequencing metrics (number of MS2 reads normalized with RPKM ratio and MS2 genome coverage)

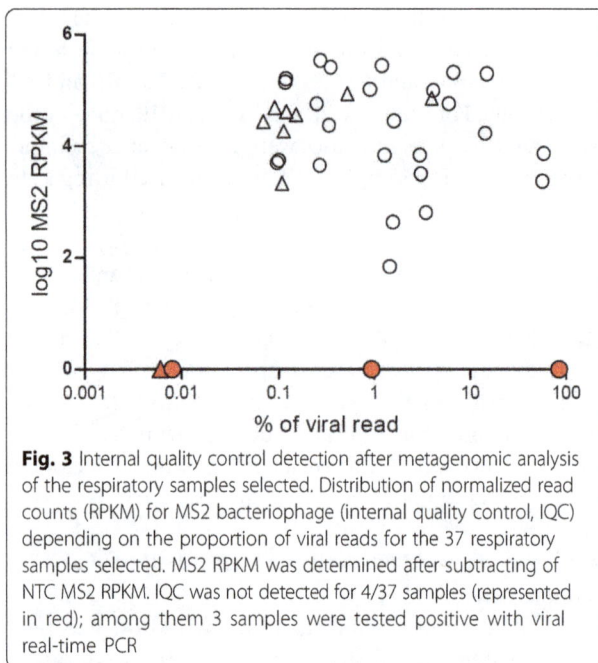

Fig. 3 Internal quality control detection after metagenomic analysis of the respiratory samples selected. Distribution of normalized read counts (RPKM) for MS2 bacteriophage (internal quality control, IQC) depending on the proportion of viral reads for the 37 respiratory samples selected. MS2 RPKM was determined after subtracting of NTC MS2 RPKM. IQC was not detected for 4/37 samples (represented in red); among them 3 samples were tested positive with viral real-time PCR

samples tested positive with viral real-time PCR targeting a representative panel of DNA and RNA viruses. For all 26 samples tested, viral metagenomic sequencing allowed the identification of the 36/36 viral genotypes matching targeted PCR results and on-target viral genome coverage ranged from 0.6 to 100% (median = 67.7%). For these 36 targeted viruses, the real-time PCR Ct values ranged from 15 to 37 Ct (median = 28 Ct). The six multiple viral infections involving from 2 to 4 different viruses were also fully characterized (Table 1). For sample # 25 (sample tested positive for 2 DNA viruses and 2 RNA viruses using real-time PCR), mNGS results were cross-checked on a duplicate which reported RPKM deviations lower than 0.5 log for each targeted virus (mNGS results for the 2 replicates are summarized in Additional file 3). Regarding mNGS results obtained from the 8 negative samples validated with IQC, no clinically relevant virus was detected. A strong correlation between mNGS and real-time PCR results was obtained for each viral genome type (R^2 ranged from 0.72 for linear ssRNA viruses to 0.98 for linear ssDNA viruses, Fig. 4a). Normalized read counts were significantly lower for linear dsDNA viruses than for other viral genome types (Fig. 4b).

Table 1 Metagenomic NGS results for the validated respiratory samples tested positive with viral real-time PCR.

Sample No.	Real-time PCR Ct values		Viral genome type	mNGS results for targeted viruses[a]			
				Identification	No. of reads	RPKM	Coverage(%)
1	HRV/EV	25	linear ssRNA	HRV-A19	13,061	5.5E + 06	97.6
2		24		HRV-A19	29,743	8.2E + 06	98.2
3		29		HRV-A63	2672	1.4E + 06	58.1
4		34		HRV-A56	453	1.4E + 04	75.2
5	RSV	27		RSV-B	14,218	1.9E + 06	91.2
6		36		RSV-A	187	1.5E + 03	22.0
7	MPV	33		HMPV-A	44,556	9.1E + 05	100.0
8	HCoV	20		HCoV NL63	73,878	2.4E + 06	94.2
9		24		HCoV 229E	19,615	1.1E + 06	99.8
10		28		HCoV 229E	20,666	2.4E + 05	100.0
12		36		HCoV NL63	1815	1.3E + 04	9.6
13	MV	23		Measles Virus	289,019	9.1E + 06	98.1
14	IBV	23	fragmented ssRNA	Influenza B	42,212	1.1E + 06	97.2
15	IAV	27		Influenza A(H3N2)	24,234	1.9E + 05	78.6
16		34		Influenza A(H3N2)	1559	1.9E + 04	21.2
17		35		Influenza A(H3N2)	258	1.8E + 03	26.5
18	HBoV	24	linear ssDNA	HBoV-1	79,504	2.7E + 06	100.0
20	AdV	17	linear dsDNA	HAdVC-1	245,2476	1.6E + 07	99.8
21		36		HAdVD-51	18	8.0E + 01	0.6
22[b]		30		HAdVC-6	284	1.0E + 03	6.2
	HHV-6	28		HHV-6B	18,411	1.4E + 04	54.8
23[b]	HBoV	15	linear ssDNA	HBoV-1	9,470,426	1.6E + 08	100.0
	CMV	31	linear dsDNA	CMV	653	2.5E + 02	5.3
24[b]	HBoV	17	linear ssDNA	HBoV-1	7,966,089	1.1E + 08	100
	MPV	29	linear ssRNA	HMPV-A	10,629	5.9E + 04	95.7
25[b, c]	AdV	26	linear dsDNA	HAdVC-2	2165	6.8E + 03	12.4
	HPIV	26	linear ssRNA	HPIV-3	17,576	1.3E + 05	66.7
	HRV/EV	34		HRV-C	446	7.0E + 03	9.2
	CMV	27	linear dsDNA	CMV	34,577	1.7E + 04	24.8
26[b]	HRV/EV	26	linear ssRNA	HRV-A78	114,684	1.4E + 07	99.9
	AdV	30	linear dsDNA	HAdVC-2	65	1.6E + 03	9.6
	RSV	30	linear ssRNA	RSV-A	586	3.5E + 04	68.7
27[b]	AdV	32	linear dsDNA	HAdVC-2	24	1.3E + 02	3.2
	HPIV	37	linear ssRNA	HPIV-2	50	6.3E + 02	2.3
28[b]	HRV/EV	31		HRV-A71	1309	3.5E + 04	61.3
	EBV	23	linear dsDNA	EBV	2556	3.0E + 03	39.3

HRV: human rhinovirus, *EV*: enterovirus, *RSV*: respiratory syncytial virus, *HCoV*: human coronavirus, *HMPV*: human metapneumovirus, *HPIV*: human parainfluenza virus, *MV*: measles virus, *HBoV*: human bocavirus, *AdV*: adenovirus, *HHV*: human herpes virus, *CMV*: cytomegalovirus, *EBV*: Epstein-Baar virus, *Ct*: Cycle threshold, *RPKM*: reads per kilobase of virus reference sequence per million mapped reads (normalization of the number of reads mapping to a targeted viral genome)
[a]Targeted viruses: viruses detected with real-time PCR
[b]Multiple viral infections
[c]Cross-checked on duplicate sample (deviation < 0.5 log)

Discussion

Over the last few years, a growing number of viral meta-genomic protocols have been published but systematic evaluation on clinical respiratory samples and validation by QC is still lacking. In the present study, we describe a process allowing the sensitive detection of both DNA

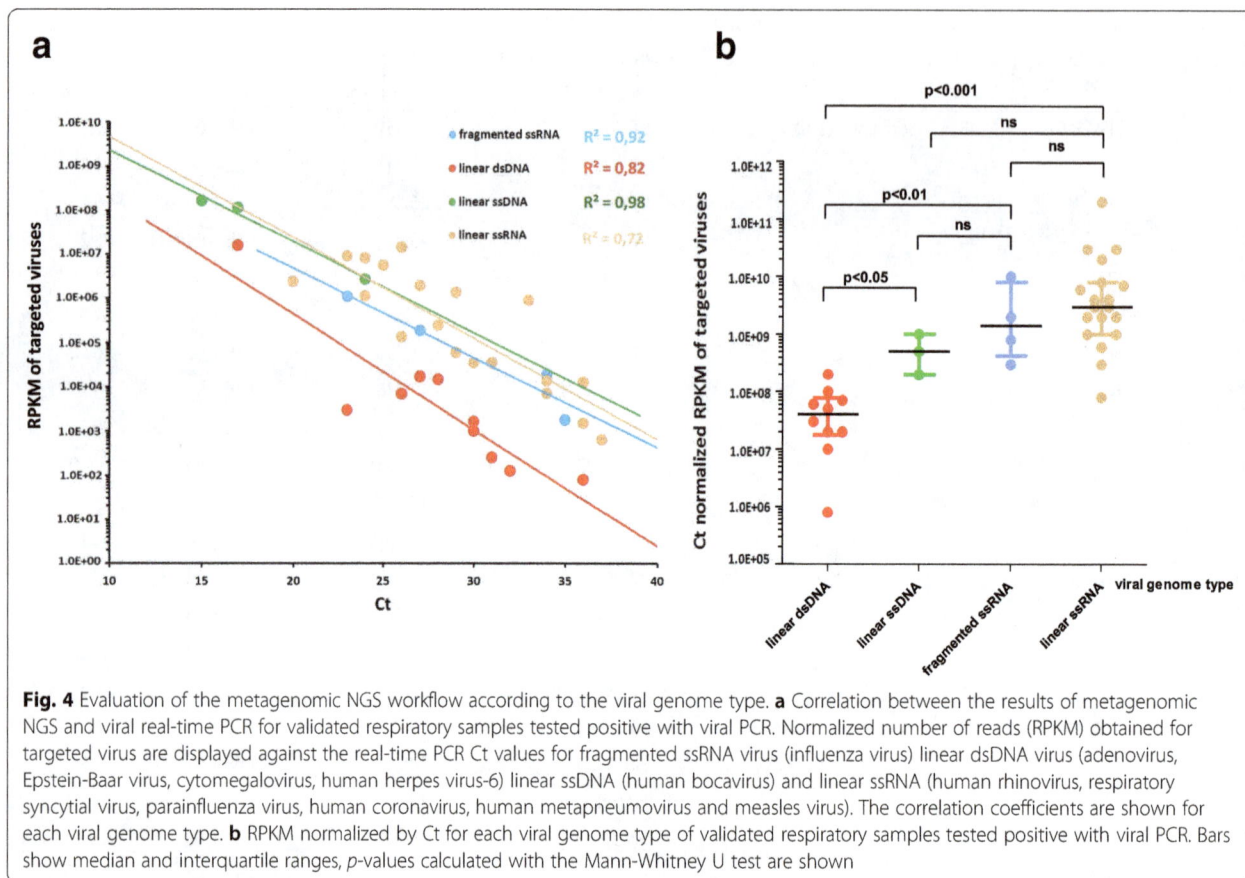

Fig. 4 Evaluation of the metagenomic NGS workflow according to the viral genome type. **a** Correlation between the results of metagenomic NGS and viral real-time PCR for validated respiratory samples tested positive with viral PCR. Normalized number of reads (RPKM) obtained for targeted virus are displayed against the real-time PCR Ct values for fragmented ssRNA virus (influenza virus) linear dsDNA virus (adenovirus, Epstein-Baar virus, cytomegalovirus, human herpes virus-6) linear ssDNA (human bocavirus) and linear ssRNA (human rhinovirus, respiratory syncytial virus, parainfluenza virus, human coronavirus, human metapneumovirus and measles virus). The correlation coefficients are shown for each viral genome type. **b** RPKM normalized by Ct for each viral genome type of validated respiratory samples tested positive with viral PCR. Bars show median and interquartile ranges, p-values calculated with the Mann-Whitney U test are shown

and RNA viruses in a single assay and implemented several QCs to validate the whole metagenomic workflow.

First, IQC was implemented to control the integrity of the reagents, equipment, the presence of inhibitors, and to allow the validation of mNGS results for each sample. The MS2 bacteriophage was selected as IQC for three main reasons; firstly MS2 is widely used as IQC during viral real-time PCR assays to control both extraction and inhibition [24], secondly, an RNA virus was required to control the random reverse transcription and second strand synthesis steps, and thirdly MS2 is a ssRNA virus with a small genome (3569-bp) that is perfectly characterized and therefore can be easily detected after bioinformatic analysis without the need for extensive NGS reads. The use of MS2 as an IQC has been previously reported for metagenomic analysis of cerebrospinal fluid specimens [25]. In another metagenomic study, RNA of MS2 was included after extraction as an IQC but the use of purified RNA does not validate the viral enrichment step [26]. In the protocol described herein, whole MS2 virions were added to each clinical sample from the beginning of the workflow. QCT1 was implemented to control the first steps of the process and to avoid unnecessary library preparation when these steps fail. At the end of the workflow, QCT2 was able to invalidate 2

samples as neither MS2 nor viruses causing ARIs were significantly detected after metagenomic analysis while routine PCR screenings detected a HBoV and a HCoV. The re-testing of these 2 samples found the same findings suggesting an inhibition or a competition issue during the process. Without the use of IQC, these samples would have been mistakenly classified as false negatives by mNGS. However, the expected competition between viruses and MS2 during the process could lead to a non-detection of IQC reads in case of high viral load. Thus, the interpretation of IQC results should consider the proportion of viral reads of each sample. Although not observed, IQC reads may also be reduced in samples with a greater numbers of patient cells which may affect the sensitivity of the assay [25].

In addition to IQC, we implemented negative external control because contamination issues are frequently reported in metagenomic studies and may lead to misinterpretation in clinical practice [17]. mNGS reads in this negative control were mainly composed of bacterial reads. However, viral reads (mainly derived from prokaryote viruses) were also detected which could be present in reagents ("kitome") or may represent laboratory contaminants or bleed-over contaminations from highly positive samples within the batch. Such contamination was observed in the present study from the highly positive HBoV sample (sample # 23, Ct = 15) which contaminated the NTC (HBoV: 185 reads, RPKM = 1.1E + 04 RPKM). In the clinical setting, subtracting NTC viral reads prior to interpretation of each sample result is therefore required.

To evaluate the workflow, clinical respiratory samples tested for a representative panel of DNA and RNA viruses using real-time PCR were selected. This workflow is based on a previous publication where a single protocol had been specifically developed for stool specimens and evaluated on mock communities containing high concentrations of spiked viruses [21]. Interestingly, 6 multiple viral infections involving both DNA and RNA viruses were fully characterized highlighting the power of our mNGS approach as a universal method for virus characterization despite the lack of common viral sequence. In addition to viruses targeted by PCR, viral reads deriving from the commensal virome, including viruses from the *Anelloviridae* family, were generated both in PCR negative and positive samples but not in the NTC.

Regarding the sensitivity of the mNGS approach, a wide range of semi-quantitative real-time PCR Ct values was covered. Thorburn et al., compared mNGS to conventional real-time PCR for the detection of RNA viruses on nasopharyngeal swabs and reported a detection cut-off of 32 Ct for the mNGS approach [27]. Our workflow allowed the characterization of both DNA and RNA viruses up to a semi-quantitative real-time PCR Ct value of 36 which is considered to be a low viral load. A major critical point in viral metagenomics is to reduce host and bacterial components. In comparison with similar studies, viral reads herein were highly represented (mean = 7.4%); for example, a study on 16 nasopharyngeal aspirates tested positive with viral PCR assays found a mean of 0.05% of viral reads [12]. In addition, a strong correlation between results of mNGS and conventional real-time PCR was obtained by regrouping viruses according to their genome types. Similar findings were reported elsewhere, suggesting that mNGS results could be used for semi-quantitative measurement of the viral load in clinical samples [3–5, 12]. A lower RPKM values for dsDNA viruses compared to the other viral genome types were noticed. As previously described for EBV and CMV, the necessary use of DNase to reduce host contamination may affect these fragile large dsDNA viruses [9, 10]. As the detection limit of mNGS analysis is mainly dependent on viral load and total number of reads per sample, this effect could be overcome by increasing sequencing depth; however, we chose to limit the costs of the workflow.

The reagent cost of this mNGS approach is relatively low and was estimated to ~€150 thanks to our viral enrichment process and the amplification method using a commercial kit which is diluted 5-fold [21]. The use of a universal workflow for both DNA and RNA viruses also reduces the reagent cost compared with metagenomic protocols targeting DNA and RNA viruses separately. In contrast, targeted NGS of specific viruses following their specific amplification by PCR can be up to 2 times cheaper based on our experience (e.g. influenza virus sequencing [28]. Due to several limitations, including its cost and a long turnaround time, viral metagenomics is currently considered to be a second-line approach and is not used as a primary routine diagnostic tool. However, with the improvement of sequencing technologies allowing real-time sequencing such as MinION sequencers (Oxford nanopore, Oxford, United Kingdom), it could be envisioned that mNGS will gradually be used for primary diagnosis in the mid-term. In case of high viral load and sufficient DNA input after amplification our workflow might be used with a MinION sequencer.

The approach described in this preliminary work is crucial to bring standardization for the routine clinical use of mNGS process within a reasonable timeframe. Further evaluation studies with a greater number of samples are urgently needed to establish IQC cut-off according to the number of viral, human and bacterial reads, and to define the performance of the workflow, including repeatability, reproducibility, as well as the detection limit for each virus. In addition, improvement of the bioinformatics pipeline are being explored, including implementation of threshold regarding genome coverage pattern [25], but their impact on performance of the workflow has to be established.

Conclusion

The potential of mNGS is very promising but several factors such as inhibition, competition, and contamination can lead to a dramatic misinterpretation in the clinical setting. Herein, we provide an efficient and easy to use mNGS workflow including quality controls successfully evaluated for the comprehensive characterization of a broad and representative panel of DNA and RNA viruses in various types of clinical respiratory samples.

Additional files

Additional file 1: Summary of clinical samples and metagenomic NGS information. (XLS 45 kb)

Additional file 2: Quality control testing results. QCT1 corresponds to MS2 bacteriophage molecular detection with commercial real-time PCR assay. QCT2 corresponds to control by sequencing metrics (number of MS2 reads normalized with RPKM ratio and MS2 genome coverage). MS2 RPKM for the 37 selected clinical samples was determined after subtracting of NTC MS2 RPKM. (XLS 37 kb)

Additional file 3: Metagenomic NGS results for duplicates of sample # 25. Sample # 25 corresponds to a clinical respiratory sample tested positive for 2 DNA viruses (adenovirus, cytomegalovirus) and 2 RNA viruses (human parainfluenza virus, human rhinovirus) using real-time PCR. This sample was analyzed twice using our single metagenomic workflow (replicate 1 and replicate 2). a) Pie charts show classification of reads into human, bacteria, viruses, fungi, archea and unknown categories (unassigned reads). b) Normalized read counts (RPKM) for each targeted virus (viruses detected with real-time PCR) and for internal quality control (MS2 bacteriophage). c) Coverage plot of targeted viral genomes and internal quality control (MS2 bacteriophage). Sequencing reads were mapped on ezVIR viral database that identified human adenovirus C-2 (accession number: KF268130.1), cytomegalovirus (accession number: GQ396662.1), human parainfluenza virus 3 (accession number: KF687321.1), human rhinovirus C (accession number: JF317014.1) and MS2 bacteriophage (accession number: NC_001417.2). (PPT 283 kb)

Abbreviations
ARIs: Acute Respiratory Infections; Ct: Cycle threshold; EQC: External Quality Control; HCL: Hospices Civils de Lyon; IQC: Internal Quality Control; mNGS: metagenomic Next-Generation Sequencing; MS2: MS2 bacteriophage; NGS: Next-Generation Sequencing; NTC: No-Template Control; PCR: Polymerase Chain Reaction; QC: Quality controls; QCT: Quality Control Testing; RPKM: Reads per kilobase of virus reference sequence per million mapped reads

Acknowledgments
We thank Audrey Guichard, Gwendolyne Burfin, Delphine Falcon and Cecile Darley for their technical assistance as well as Philip Robinson (DRCI, Hospices Civils de Lyon) for his excellent help in manuscript preparation. Part of these data has been presented at the International Conference of Clinical Metagenomic held in Geneva in October 2017.

Funding
This study was funded by a metagenomic grant received in 2014 from the French foundation of innovation in infectious diseases (FINOVI, *fondation innovation en infectiologie*).

Authors' contributions
AB, LJ, FM, KB, SA conceived the study. AB, MP, LB, CP, VC performed the sample preparations and sequencing. LJ, GO, GV performed bioinformatic analysis. LJ is the guarantor for the NGS data. YG, MV, IS, BL, SV, JSC, FM are the guarantor for clinical data and sample collection. AB was the main writer of the manuscript. All authors reviewed and approved the final version of the manuscript.

Competing interests
The authors declare that they have no competing interest.

Author details
[1]Laboratoire de Virologie, Institut des Agents Infectieux, Groupement Hospitalier Nord, Hospices Civils de Lyon, Lyon, France. [2]Univ Lyon, Université Lyon 1, Faculté de Médecine Lyon Est, CIRI, Inserm U1111 CNRS UMR5308, Virpath, Lyon, France. [3]Centre National de Reference des virus respiratoires France Sud, Hospices Civils de Lyon, 103 Grande-Rue de la Croix Rousse, 69317 Lyon, France. [4]Laboratoire Commun de Recherche HCL-bioMerieux, Centre Hospitalier Lyon Sud, Pierre-Bénite, France. [5]Unité de Biologie des Infections Virales Emergentes, Institut Pasteur, Lyon, France. [6]CIRI Inserm U1111, CNRS 5308, ENS, UCBL, Faculté de Médecine Lyon Est, Université de Lyon, Lyon, France. [7]INSERM UMR1078 "Génétique, Génomique Fonctionnelle et Biotechnologies", Axe Microbiota, Univ Brest, Brest, France. [8]Département de Bactériologie-Virologie, Hygiène et Parasitologie-Mycologie, Pôle de Biologie-Pathologie, Centre Hospitalier Régional et Universitaire de Brest, Hôpital de la Cavale Blanche, Brest, France. [9]Hospices Civils de Lyon, Urgences pédiatriques, Hôpital Femme Mère Enfant, Bron, France.

References
1. Mokili JL, Rohwer F, Dutilh BE. Metagenomics and future perspectives in virus discovery. Curr Opin Virol. 2012;2:63–77.
2. Capobianchi MR, Giombini E, Rozera G. Next-generation sequencing technology in clinical virology. Clin Microbiol Infect. 2013;19:15–22.
3. Prachayangprecha S, Schapendonk CME, Koopmans MP, Osterhaus ADME, Schürch AC, Pas SD, et al. Exploring the potential of next-generation sequencing in detection of respiratory viruses. J Clin Microbiol. 2014;52:3722–30.
4. Graf EH, Simmon KE, Tardif KD, Hymas W, Flygare S, Eilbeck K, et al. Unbiased detection of respiratory viruses by use of RNA sequencing-based metagenomics: a systematic comparison to a commercial PCR panel. J Clin Microbiol. 2016;54:1000–7.
5. Fischer N, Indenbirken D, Meyer T, Lütgehetmann M, Lellek H, Spohn M, et al. Evaluation of unbiased next-generation sequencing of RNA (RNA-seq) as a diagnostic method in influenza virus-positive respiratory samples. J Clin Microbiol. 2015;53:2238–50.
6. Schlaberg R, Queen K, Simmon K, Tardif K, Stockmann C, Flygare S, et al. Viral pathogen detection by metagenomics and Pan-viral group polymerase chain reaction in children with pneumonia lacking identifiable etiology. J Infect Dis. 2017;215:1407–15.
7. Xu L, Zhu Y, Ren L, Xu B, Liu C, Xie Z, et al. Characterization of the nasopharyngeal viral microbiome from children with community-acquired pneumonia but negative for Luminex xTAG respiratory viral panel assay detection. J Med Virol. 2017 Dec;89(12):2098–107.
8. Lewandowska DW, Schreiber PW, Schuurmans MM, Ruehe B, Zagordi O, Bayard C, et al. Metagenomic sequencing complements routine diagnostics in identifying viral pathogens in lung transplant recipients with unknown etiology of respiratory infection. PLoS One. 2017;12:e0177340.
9. Parize P, Muth E, Richaud C, Gratigny M, Pilmis B, Lamamy A, et al. Untargeted next-generation sequencing-based first-line diagnosis of infection in immunocompromised adults: a multicentre, blinded, prospective study. Clin Microbiol Infect. 2017;23:574.e1–6.
10. Lewandowska DW, Zagordi O, Geissberger F-D, Kufner V, Schmutz S, Böni J, et al. Optimization and validation of sample preparation for metagenomic sequencing of viruses in clinical samples. Microbiome. 2017;5:94.
11. Reyes A, Haynes M, Hanson N, Angly FE, Heath AC, Rohwer F, et al. Viruses in the faecal microbiota of monozygotic twins and their mothers. Nature. 2010;466:334–8.
12. Yang J, Yang F, Ren L, Xiong Z, Wu Z, Dong J, et al. Unbiased parallel detection of viral pathogens in clinical samples by use of a metagenomic approach. J Clin Microbiol. 2011;49:3463–9.
13. Kim K-H, Bae J-W. Amplification methods bias metagenomic libraries of uncultured single-stranded and double-stranded DNA viruses. Appl Environ Microbiol. 2011;77:7663–8.
14. Kozyreva VK, Truong C-L, Greninger AL, Crandall J, Mukhopadhyay R, Chaturvedi V. Validation and implementation of clinical laboratory improvements act-compliant whole-genome sequencing in the public health microbiology laboratory. J Clin Microbiol. 2017;55:2502–20.
15. Simner PJ, Miller S, Carroll KC. Understanding the promises and hurdles of metagenomic next-generation sequencing as a diagnostic tool for infectious diseases. Clin Infect Dis. 2018;66(5):778–88.
16. Ruppé E, Schrenzel J. Messages from the second international conference on clinical metagenomics (ICCMg2). Microbes Infect. 2018;20(4):222–7.
17. Miller RR, Uyaguari-Diaz M, McCabe MN, Montoya V, Gardy JL, Parker S, et al. Metagenomic investigation of plasma in individuals with ME/CFS highlights the importance of technical controls to elucidate contamination and batch effects. PLoS One. 2016;11:e0165691.
18. Thoendel M, Jeraldo P, Greenwood-Quaintance KE, Yao J, Chia N, Hanssen AD, et al. Impact of contaminating DNA in whole-genome amplification kits used for metagenomic shotgun sequencing for infection diagnosis. J Clin Microbiol. 2017;55:1789–801.
19. Gargis AS, Kalman L, Lubin IM. Assuring the quality of next-generation sequencing in clinical microbiology and public health laboratories. J Clin Microbiol. 2016;54:2857–65.
20. Hall RJ, Wang J, Todd AK, Bissielo AB, Yen S, Strydom H, et al. Evaluation of rapid and simple techniques for the enrichment of viruses prior to metagenomic virus discovery. J Virol Methods. 2014;195:194–204.
21. Conceição-Neto N, Zeller M, Lefrère H, De Bruyn P, Beller L, Deboutte W, et al. Modular approach to customise sample preparation procedures for viral metagenomics: a reproducible protocol for virome analysis. Sci Rep. 2015;5: 16532.
22. Petty TJ, Cordey S, Padioleau I, Docquier M, Turin L, Preynat-Seauve O, et al. Comprehensive human virus screening using high-throughput sequencing with a user-friendly representation of bioinformatics analysis: a pilot study. J Clin Microbiol. 2014;52:3351–61.
23. Mortazavi A, Williams BA, McCue K, Schaeffer L, Wold B. Mapping and quantifying mammalian transcriptomes by RNA-Seq. Nat Methods. 2008;5: 621–8.

24. Dreier J, Störmer M, Kleesiek K. Use of bacteriophage MS2 as an internal control in viral reverse transcription-PCR assays. J Clin Microbiol. 2005;43: 4551–7.
25. Schlaberg R, Chiu CY, Miller S, Procop GW, Weinstock G. Professional practice committee and committee on laboratory practices of the American Society for Microbiology, et al. validation of metagenomic next-generation sequencing tests for universal pathogen detection. Arch Pathol Lab Med. 2017;141:776–86.
26. Zhou Y, Fernandez S, Yoon I-K, Simasathien S, Watanaveeradej V, Yang Y, et al. Metagenomics study of viral pathogens in undiagnosed respiratory specimens and identification of human enteroviruses at a Thailand hospital. Am J Trop Med Hyg. 2016;95:663–9.
27. Thorburn F, Bennett S, Modha S, Murdoch D, Gunson R, Murcia PR. The use of next generation sequencing in the diagnosis and typing of respiratory infections. J Clin Virol Off Publ Pan Am Soc Clin Virol. 2015;69:96–100.
28. Pichon M, Gaymard A, Josset L, Valette M, Millat G, Lina B, et al. Characterization of oseltamivir-resistant influenza virus populations in immunosuppressed patients using digital-droplet PCR: comparison with qPCR and next generation sequencing analysis. Antivir Res. 2017;145:160–7.

3

Evaluation of cardiac function by global longitudinal strain before and after treatment with sofosbuvir-based regimens in HCV infected patients

Maria Mazzitelli[1†], Carlo Torti[1*†], Jolanda Sabatino[2], Greta Luana D'Ascoli[2], Chiara Costa[1], Vincenzo Pisani[1], Elena Raffetti[3], Salvatore De Rosa[2], Alessio Strazzulla[1], Alfredo Focà[4], Maria Carla Liberto[4], Ciro Indolfi[2] and the CARDIAC study group

Abstract

Background: Possible cardiotoxicity of sofosbuvir in humans has not been demonstrated yet. Also, since HCV can exert deleterious effects on hearth function, it is of interest to know whether HCV eradication provides any benefits using global longitudinal strain (GLS), a measure of left ventricular function more reliable than ejection fraction (EF).

Methods: Patients eligible for treatment with the combination therapy for HCV were invited to perform a transthoracic cardiac ultrasound at four different time points: before starting treatment, after one month, at the end of treatment and, after six month. Left ventricular function was measured with both EF and GLS.

Results: From March 2015 to December 2016, 82 patients were enrolled. Fifty-six percent patients were males. Mean age was 66.12 (SD: 9.25) years. About 20% patients did not present any cardiovascular risk factors or comorbidities. A worsening trend of GLS was observed. Variations were not found to be statistically significant when EF was studied along the follow-up. However, when GLS was studied, its variations were found to be statistically significant indicating a worsening effect, albeit with different trends in patients who underwent treatment for three months compared to six months. Worsening of GLS was found to be statistically significant even after adjusting for body mass index and liver fibrosis, independently from treatment duration.

Conclusions: Our results showed unexpected worsening of left ventricular function when measured through GLS after HCV treatment response induced by DAAs including sofosbuvir. Although this result is not proven to be clinically significant, the safety profile of sofosbuvir-based regimens needs to be studied further.

Keywords: Cardiac function, HCV eradication, DAA treatment, Longitudinal study

Background

Extra-hepatic manifestations (such as neoplastic, auto-immune and vascular diseases) occur in about 70% of patients infected by hepatitis C virus (HCV) [1–3]. Among these manifestations, cardiovascular diseases (CVD) are more prevalent in HCV infected patients, but mechanisms are currently unknown. HCV related inflammation, oxidative stress [4, 5] and direct damage due to HCV infecting cardiac cells [6–8] might have a impact.

Animal studies reported death for cardiac causes after administration of a sofosbuvir metabolite at blood concentrations much higher than the therapeutic index used in humans [9]. Currently there is a lack data on the effects of sofosbuvir on heart function. Such data are important to confirm safety of sofosbuvir because we are currently treating aging populations with a significant prevalence of heart diseases. On the other way round, it is possible that

* Correspondence: torti.carlo@libero.it
†Maria Mazzitelli and Carlo Torti contributed equally to this work.
[1]Unit of Infectious and Tropical Diseases, Department of Medical and Surgical Sciences, "Magna Graecia" University of Catanzaro, Viale Europa, 88100 Catanzaro, Italy
Full list of author information is available at the end of the article

clearance of HCV with interferon-free regimens would act favourably, as it was previously demonstrated that HCV eradication with interferon based regimens is able to reduce mortality for cardiovascular events [10, 11].

Left ventricular function (LVF) is routinely evaluated through the ejection fraction (EF), calculated by means of the modified Simpson method in current clinical practice, with the use of trans-thoracic echocardiography [12]. Trans-thoracic echocardiography based speckle tracking assessment is more reliable and precise for the assessment of myocardial function than trans-oesophageal ultrasound [13].

More recently, the global longitudinal strain (GLS) was developed as a more reliable index to measure left ventricular function [14]. Indeed, GLS was shown to be a valuable clinical parameter and a independent predictor of all cause mortality in patients with CVD [15]. Moreover, variations of GLS have been found in diverse conditions such as doxorubicin-induced cardiomyopathy, HIV infection in children and young adults, or viral myocarditis [16–19]. In these conditions, even minor variations of GLS were clinically meaningful, even when EF seemed to be preserved [18, 19]. For instance, data showed that GLS provides incremental diagnostic and prognostic information, that are correlated with histological findings in patients with viral myocarditis for whom conventional 2D echocardiography is unspecific, particularly in those with a preserved EF [18, 19]. This correlation was independent from conventional 2D echocardio-graphic parameters showing that strain rate and strain imaging are more sensitive in the detection of early changes or mild myocardial damage. Moreover, patients with impaired strain rate and strain at the acute phase of the disease showed worse short-time echocardiographic outcomes. For these patients, clinical history, physical examination, ECG, and serology were shown to be unreliable compared with GLS.

Methods
Aim
In the present study, we aimed at measuring possible changes of cardiovascular function in patients with chronic HCV infection before and after sofosbuvir-based regimens, using both left ventricular EF and GLS. The latter was chosen as advanced biomarker to measure the effect.

Population and data collection
We conducted a longitudinal study from March 2015 to January 2017, enrolling all HCV infected patients treated with sofosbuvir-based regimens at the outpatient clinic of "*Mater Domini*" teaching hospital in Catanzaro (Italy), according to the criteria set by the Italian Medicinal Agency (AIFA) (see Additional file 1: Table S1). For patients without clinical cirrhosis or extra-hepatic manifestations, transient elastography (FibroScan™) was performed in order to estimate liver fibrosis so as to ascertain indications for treatment.

Exclusion criteria were: age less than 18 years old, pregnancy, and severe chronic disease (estimated glomerular filtration rate, eGFR< 30 mL/min).

Patients were assessed at four time points: baseline (i.e., before treatment initiation), after one month, at the end of the treatment course (either month 3 or month 6), and after 6 months from the end of treatment (off treatment follow-up).

Cardiac ultrasound was performed at baseline and at each follow-up using trans-thoracic Vivid E9 ultrasound. Speckle tracking echocardiography analysis was performed from apical views. Standard grayscale 2D images were obtained at a frame rate of 70–90 frames/s during three cardiac cycles and software package (EchoPAC™, GE healthcare) was used for offline analysis. Two expert cardiologists (L.G.D.A. and J.S.) performed cardiac ultrasound blinded of previous examinations, type and length of prescribed treatments.

At baseline, risk factors for CVD (i.e., hypertension, diabetes mellitus, cigarette smoking, previous stroke or myocardial infarction were recorded), and heart diseases were carefully investigated. Patients were considered to be underweighted (BMI ≤ 18.4 Kg/m^2), normal (BMI = 18.5–24.9 Kg/m^2), over-weighted (BMI = 25–29.9 Kg/m^2) or obese (BMI ≥ 30 Kg/m^2) [20].

Complete blood count, AST, ALT, total and fractioned bilirubin, and HCV RNA were recorded at enrolment and each follow-up points. Indirect indices of fibrosis, such as Fibrosis 4 index (FIB-4) and AST to platelets ratio (APRI) score were calculated at baseline and at month 6 after the end of treatment [21–23]. At these time points, alpha-fetoprotein, cholesterol, creatinine, glucose, INR, triglycerides were also evaluated. Data were stored in an ad-hoc electronic database.

Drug interactions with other co-medications were carefully evaluated using the application HEP Drug Interaction [24]. Drugs with a significant risk of interaction with antivirals were substituted. For example, after cardiological consultation, amlodipine was reduced from 10 mg to 5 mg per day in patients who received daclatasvir or ledipasvir, if possible, or otherwise substituted.

This study was coordinated by the Infectious and Tropical Diseases Unit in collaboration with the Cardiology Unit of "*Mater Domini*" teaching hospital in Catanzaro (Italy) and was conducted in accordance with the guidelines of the Declaration of Helsinki and the principles of Good Clinical Practice [25–27]. The local Ethical Committee (Calabria Region) approved the study protocol and written informed consent was obtained from all subjects enrolled.

Statistical analysis

To adjust the analysis for treatment duration, the enrolled patients were ranked into two groups: group A, i.e. patients with indication for a 3 month treatment, and group B, i.e. patients with indication for a 6 month treatment with DAAs. Study parameters were expressed as means (standard deviation, SD) or proportions as appropriate. FIB-4, APRI score, alpha-fetoprotein, creatinine, cholesterol, glucose, haemoglobin, and triglycerides values at baseline were compared with those at last follow-up using Student's t-test for paired data. We evaluated the temporal trends of AST, ALT, platelet count, total bilirubin, EF and GLS using univariate mixed models for repeated measures. We also assessed the temporal trend of GLS using a multivariate mixed model adjusting for BMI, fibrosis and duration of treatment (3 or 6 months). Moreover, although in the analysis hypertension was not a confounder by definition, since it could have been associated with the outcome (GLS) but not with the exposure, we tested whether hypertension was a effect modifier.

Lastly we explored whether ribavirin could have a role on the change of GLS over time using a mixed model with an interaction term between ribavirin and time.

All statistical tests were two-sided, assuming a level of significance of 0.05 and were performed using Stata software version 12.0 (StataCorp, College Station, TX, USA).

Results

Patient flow and characteristics

Among 109 patients who started a DAA treatment during the study period, 87 subjects were eligible and 82 were enrolled (56% males, mean age of 66.1 years). Amongst these patients, 71/82 (86.6%) continued follow-up until the end of the study (Fig. 1).

Seventy-two (87.9%) patients met AIFA criterion 1 or 4. Nine patients had extra-hepatic manifestations (AIFA criterion 3), and one patient had a HCV RNA relapse after liver transplantation (AIFA criterion 2). Fifty-seven (69.5%) patients were prescribed a treatment lasting for three months, while 25 (30.5%) were prescribed a treatment for six months. The baseline characteristics of patients are described in Table 1. With regards to CV risk factors, 59.3% patients were overweighed, 4.7% had a previous major cardiovascular event (stroke or myocardial infarction), 17.4% were smokers, 62.8% had hypertension and 26.7% had diabetes mellitus. Overall, only 20% of subjects did not present any CV risk factors or comorbidities. About 70% patients had previous experience to interferon-based regimens.

Treatment course

Prescribed treatments and related outcomes are described in Table 2. Most patients (97.56%) reached the end of treatment; only one patient stopped prematurely for a psychotic syndrome and another for virological failure. Seventy-nine (96.4%) patients gained sustained virological response (SVR) at weeks 12 after the end of treatment. Two patients (2.4%) had virological failure. All patients tolerated treatments very well, without any severe adverse events recorded. Among 49 patients who received ribavirin, folic acid and/or erythropoietin were added for anaemia in 11 (22.4%) and in 1/49 (2.04%) ribavirin was stopped for the same reason. Table 3 shows temporal trends of selected parameters. Liver parameters improved, whereas cholesterol rose in both groups (treatment length of 3 or 6 months).

Evaluation of cardiac function

At baseline, mean EF and GLS were 56.7% and − 20.9%, respectively. Hence, 20/82 (24.1%) patients had abnormal EF (< 55%), while 3/82 (3.6%) had abnormal GLS (> − 16.5%) according to litereature standards [28, 29]. Compared to those with lower values, subjects with GLS ≥ median value of the study population (− 20.3%) had higher BMI (mean 27.9 vs. 26.0), higher haemoglobin (14.6 vs. 13.5 g/dL), higher triglycerides (123.5 vs. 98.3 mg/dL) and a greater proportion of current smokers was found (71.4% vs. 44.1%) (see, Additional file 1: Table S2). Moderate mitral and tricuspid insufficiencies were diagnosed in 2 patients.

As illustrated in Table 3, while there were not statistically significant variations of EF along the follow-up in both groups, a statistically significant worsening of GLS was found in the group of patients treated for three months (group A), while in patients treated for six months (group B) only a tendency towards a statistically significant worsening was found. Interestingly, GLS displayed a biphasic trend in the 3-month group, decreasing from − 20.8% at baseline to − 21.4% at month 1, before rising up to − 20.3% at the end of the follow-up ($p = 0.031$) (Fig. 2A). By contrast, GLS increased steadily from − 21.1% to − 20.1% in the six-month group ($p = 0.097$) (Fig. 2B). The rise of GLS over time was confirmed in a multivariate mixed model adjusted for BMI, liver fibrosis and treatment length with a mean GLS increase of 0.07 (0.01–0.13) per month ($p = 0.013$) (see, Additional file 1: Table S3).

Lastly, we explored whether hypertension was a effect modifier but we did not found any significant evidences (coefficient − 0.43, 95% CI: -1.42 to 0.55; $p = 0.388$). We also tested whether ribavirin could have a role on the change of GLS over time and in a mixed model with an interaction term between ribavirin and time but ribavirin exposure did not exert a statistically significant effect on GLS (absent ribavirin coefficient − 0.607, 95% CI: -1.608 to 0.395; $p < 0.235$) or a statistically significant role as effect modifier was not demonstrated (coefficient − 0.018, 95% CI: -1.69 to 0.39; $p = 0.749$).

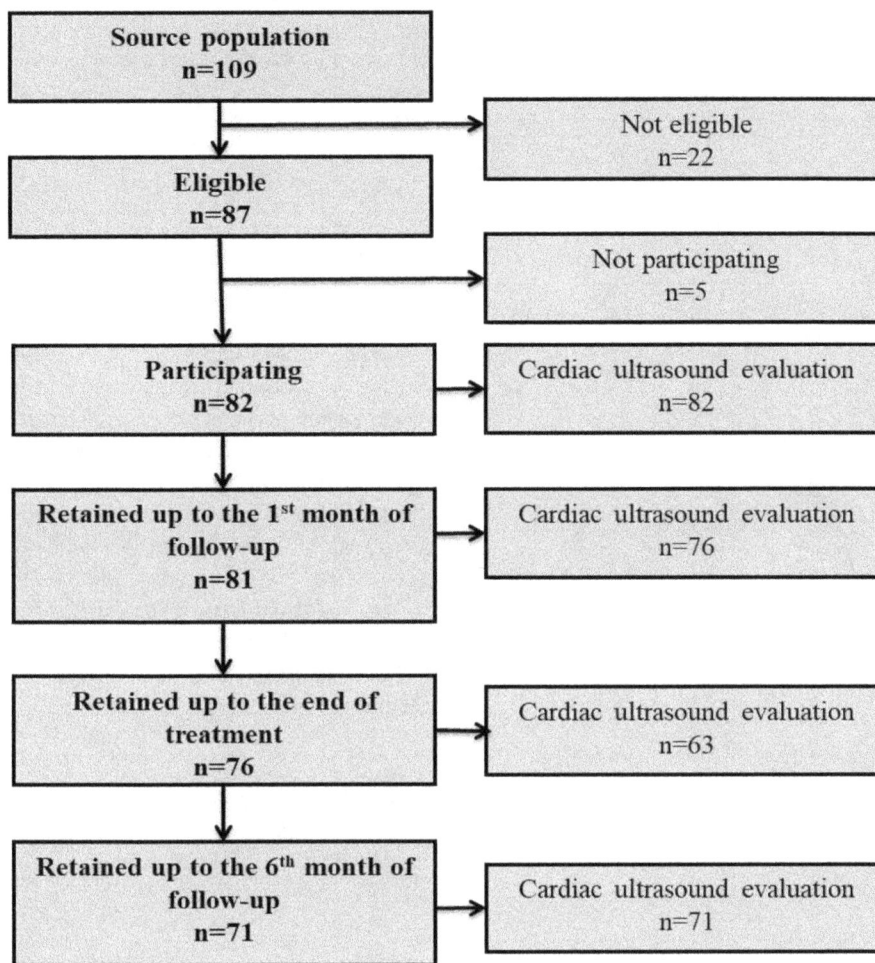

Fig. 1 Flow chart of the patients along the study time points. Eighty-two patients decided to participate and underwent cardiac ultrasound at baseline. Fifty-seven patients were prescribed a 3-month treatment (group A) while 25 patients underwent treatment for 6 months (group B). Among patients who showed up at clinical checks, 76/81 presented to perform cardiac ultrasound at first month, 63/76 at the end of treatment and 71/71 at the last follow-up point

Discussion

The main finding of our study is that cardiac function measured through GLS seemed to worsen in the overall population, while EF did not change significantly. This may indicate that sofosbuvir based treatment could exert a negative impact on cardiac function. Possible toxicity of sofosbuvir may be supported from data showing that development of another NS5B polymerase inhibitor (BMS5986094) was stopped after a safety signal of cardiotoxicity [30]. In this work a young male died for rapidly progressive heart failure and 41.2% (14/34) patients had some evidence of cardiac dysfunction (6/14 with EF < 30% and 8/14 from 30 to 50%). So, as far as cardiotoxicity is concerned, a class effect of NS5B polymerase inhibitors should be studied further. Interestingly, after stopping DAAs, GLS continued to worsen, possibly indicating a prolonged effect. In addition, since

EF remained stable, we may hypothesize that, similar to other conditions [14, 15], GLS is a more sensitive method to measure cardiac function.

However, the clinical significance and the long-term effects of the GLS variations in our patients are unknown. Correlations with other biomarkers of heart dysfunction (such as troponin, NT-pro-BNP, and micro-RNAs) [31–34] and long term studies with "hard" clinical end-points would be helpful. Also, it is difficult to explain why such an effect was demonstrated. In fact, besides a direct effect of sofosbuvir, other explanations may be found, including a random effect due to the small number of patients, an effect of concomitant drugs, or an indirect effect of HCV eradication mediated by inflammatory changes [4, 35]. So, the major difficulty that comes with the dataset studied herein is to dissect whether the effect can be ascribed entirely to sofosbuvir or to other factors. For this reason, more

Table 1 Characteristics of the enrolled patients overall and by length of treatment (group A: treatment lasting for 3 months and group B: treatment lasting for 6 months)

Variable	Total n (%)	Group A n (%)	Group B n (%)	p-value
Gender				
Male	46 (56.1)	35 (61.4)	11 (44)	
Female	36 (43.9)	22 (38.6)	14 (56)	0.144
Age (years)				
≤ 60	22 (26.8)	17 (29.8)	5 (20)	
61–68	22 (26.8)	16 (28.1)	6 (24)	
69–74	24 (29.3)	15 (26.3)	8 (32)	
≥ 75	14 (17.1)	9 (15.8)	6 (24)	0.666
Type of liver disease				
No cirrhosis or HCC	45 (54.9)	34 (59.6)	9 (36)	
Cirrhosis	35 (42.7)	23 (40.4)	14 (56)	
HCC with cirrhosis	2 (2.4)	0 (0)	2 (8)	0.025
Transient elastography				
None	7 (8.5)			
F0	0 (0)	0 (0)	0 (0)	
F1	2 (2.4)	2 (3.9)	0 (0)	
F2	3 (3.8)	3 (5.9)	0 (0)	
F3	33 (40.2)	29 (56.9)	3 (13)	
F4	37 (45.1)	17 (33.3)	20 (87)	< 0.01
HCV Genotype				
1a	2 (2.4)	1 (1.7)	1 (4)	
1b	60 (73.3)	42 (73.7)	17 (68)	
2	6 (7.3)	3 (5.3)	3 (12)	
2a/2c	5 (6.1)	6 (10.5)	0 (0)	
3	4 (4.8)	1 (1.7)	3 (12)	
4	5 (6.1)	4 (7.1)	1 (4)	0.148
Co-infections				
None	81 (98.8)	56 (98.3)	25 (100)	
HIV +	1 (1.2)	1 (1.7)	0 (0)	
HBsAg +/HIV -	0 (0)	0 (0)	(0)	0.505
BMI				
Normal	23 (28)	18 (31.6)	5 (20)	
Overweight/Obese	59 (71.0)	39 (68.4)	20 (80)	0.283
Risk factors for CV diseases[a]				
None	19 (23.2)	15 (26.3)	4 (16)	0.308
Hypertension	51 (62.2)	34 (59.6)	17 (68)	0.473
Diabetes mellitus	21 (25.6)	12 (21.1)	8 (32)	0.288
Smoking habits	14 (17.1)	11 (19.3)	3 (12)	0.419
Previous CV events	4 (4.8)	3 (5.3)	1 (4)	0.807
Comorbidities[a]				
None	19 (23.2)	15 (26.3)	4 (16)	0.308
eGFR < 90 ml/min	43 (52.4)	32 (39)	11 (13.4)	0.350

Table 1 Characteristics of the enrolled patients overall and by length of treatment (group A: treatment lasting for 3 months and group B: treatment lasting for 6 months) *(Continued)*

Variable	Total n (%)	Group A n (%)	Group B n (%)	p-value
Osteoporosis	15 (18.3)	10 (17.6)	5 (20)	0.791
Depression	14 (17.1)	11 (19.3)	3 (12)	0.419

[a]Each patient may have more than one risk factors and comorbidities
CV Cardiovascular, eGFR Estimated glomerular filtrate rate

powerful studies should adjust for possible confounders (including concomitant drugs and co-morbidities such as hypertension or cholesterol level and its variations), and using immune parameters to provide more specific and detailed information from the pathogenic point of view. Also, we need studies with a different design to assess whether sofosbuvir or HCV eradication (and possible immune effects related to this eradication) are implicated. For instance, one could compare cardiac function in patients with sustained virological response with respect to those without response, or cardiac function may be evaluated in healthy volunteers. Moreover, a group of control patients

Table 2 Prescribed treatment, supportive drugs and related outcome (n = 82)

Cate	n (%)
Prescribed DAAs	
SOF + RBV	10 (12.2)
SOF + SIM ± RBV	29 (35.4)
SOF + LDV ± RBV	31 (37.8)
SOF + DCV ± RBV	12 (14.6)
Ribavirin	
Yes	49 (59.7)
No	33 (40.3)
Ribavirin modification	
None	26 (53.1)
Reduction	22 (44.9)
Suspension	1 (2)
Adding support drug for anaemia in patients with ribavirin	
None	38 (77.6)
Folic acid	7 (14.2)
Erythropoietin	2 (4.1)
Folic acid + erythropoietin	2 (4.1)
Reason for stopping DAAs	
End of treatment	80 (97.6)
Patient decision	1 (1.2)
Virological failure	1 (1.2)

DAAs Direct antiviral agents, SOF Sofosbuvir, RBV Ribavirin, SIM Simeprevir, LDV Ledipasvir, DCV Daclatasvir

Table 3 Parameters at baseline and during follow-up

Parameters	Group A baseline mean (SD)	Month 1 mean (SD)	End of treatment mean (SD)	6th month of follow-up mean (SD)	p-value*	Group B baseline mean (SD)	Month 1 mean (SD)	End of treatment mean (SD)	6th month of follow-up mean (SD)	p-value*
FIB-4	3.8 (3.6)	–	–	2.7 (1.8)	0.003	5.5 (5.3)	–	–	3.7 (4.7)	< 0.001
APRI SCORE	1.2 (1.1)	–	–	0.6 (0.9)	< 0.001	1.7 (1.8)	–	–	0.9 (2.1)	0.002
INR	1.1 (0.2)	–	–	1.1 (0.1)	0.111	1.1 (0.2)	–	–	1.1 (0.1)	0.435
α-fetoprotein (ng/mL)	12.8 (20.9)	–	–	7.8 (19.3)	< 0.001	19.5 (28.9)	–	–	5.9 (3.1)	0.014
Creatinine (mg/dL)	0.8 (0.2)	–	–	0.9 (0.2)	0.031	0.7 (0.1)	–	–	0.8 (0.1)	0.032
Glucose (mg/dL)	112 (29)	–	–	110.5 (30.8)	0.266	128.6 (41.7)	–	–	119.3 (31.7)	0.337
Haemoglobin (g/dL)	14.2 (2.2)	–	–	14.1 (2.1)	0.551	13.6 (1.9)	–	–	13.9 (1.8)	0.625
Cholesterol (mg/dL)	155.2 (30.8)	–	–	163.5 (29.8)	0.070	149.9 (38.1)	–	–	179.3 (46.2)	0.003
Triglycerides (mg/dL)	111.25 (46.12)	–	–	110.96 (46.49)	0.155	112.12 (39.64)	–	–	100.8 (46.73)	0.295
AST (UI/L)	59.2 (40.9)	24.8 (13.3)	22.9 (9.1)	25.6 (13.4)	< 0.001	68.7 (40.6)	29.8 (19.7)	23.8 (8.3)	24.3 (8.3)	< 0.001
ALT (UI/L)	65 (41.3)	21.7 (11.4)	18.3 (6.8)	20.5 (9.4)	< 0.001	69.7 (52.3)	24 (15.1)	20.5 (8.5)	20.3 (10)	< 0.001
Platelet (×10 [3]/mL)	166.8 (65.8)	183.4 (78.5)	171.1 (77.5)	167.1 (61.5)	0.399	139.3 (62.1)	161.2 (72.3)	153.9 (65.4)	150.2 (58.9)	0.779
Total bilirubin (mg/dL)	0.9 (0.7)	1.1 (0.7)	0.9 (0.8)	0.7 (0.5)	< 0.001	1 (0.8)	1 (0.7)	0.7 (0.6)	0.8 (0.5)	< 0.001
Ejection Fraction (%)	56.5 (3.1)	56.9 (3.5)	56.6 (2.5)	56.7 (2.8)	0.499	56.9 (2.9)	57 (3)	57.2 (3.2)	57.4 (3.6)	0.535
GLS (%)	−20.8 (2.8)	−21.4 (2.4)	−20.9 (2.6)	−20.3 (2.6)	0.031	−21.1 (2.4)	−20.7 (2.7)	−20.3 (2.8)	−20.1 (2.5)	0.097

We compared baseline and 6th month of follow-up values of the two groups of treatment (group A = 3 months of treatment, group B = 6 months of treatment) with t-test for FIB-4, APRI SCORE, α-fetoprotein, creatinine, glucose, haemoglobin, cholesterol, and triglycerides. We use mixed-linear models to evaluate the linear trend of the other parameters

–: the parameter is not available at this follow-up point

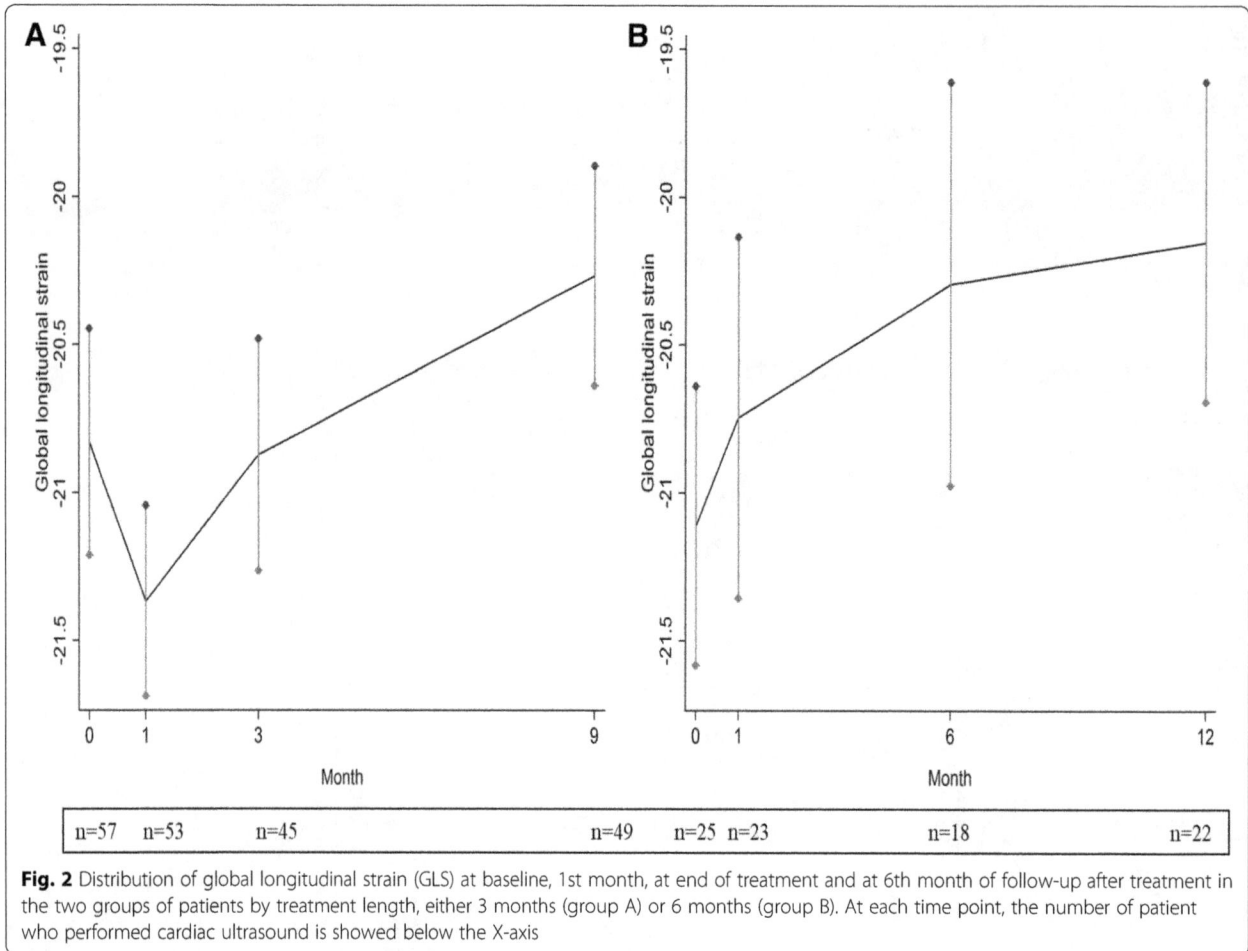

Fig. 2 Distribution of global longitudinal strain (GLS) at baseline, 1st month, at end of treatment and at 6th month of follow-up after treatment in the two groups of patients by treatment length, either 3 months (group A) or 6 months (group B). At each time point, the number of patient who performed cardiac ultrasound is showed below the X-axis

with other aetiologies presenting the same risk factors, but not treated with sofosbuvir-based treatments would be helpful. Unfortunately, however, this is difficult (or unethical) to be accepted for the legitimate desires of patients to be treated as soon as possible.

Since we did not find any significant correlations between GLS and ribavirin or anaemia (data not shown), we may hypothesize that these factors were not implicated. However, we have to take into account that the small sample size reduced the power to detect a smaller effect of ribavirin, significantly. Indeed, the evidence of a prolonged worsening of GLS after stopping treatment is more consistent with an effect of ribavirin (whose multiple dose half-life is around 12 days, persisting in non-plasma compartments for as long as 6 months) than with an effect of sofosbuvir (whose half life is only 0.4 h). For the same reason, the trend in GLS is more consistent with an immune-mediated phenomenon occurring after viral eradication, so consideration of immune markers could provide better insights on the phenomenon. With regard to hypertension, we did not find any significant evidences of a possible role at interaction model independently from time, but a complete assessment in a

multivariable model would require grater numbers and a time-dependent consideration of hypertension as a variable in future studies.

In patients treated for three months, we noted an initial improvement of GLS, followed by a progressive worsening. The first phase of improvement could be due to a beneficial reduction of HCV RNA [10] while apparent sofosbuvir toxicity or other negative phenomena may have become more evident afterwards. This biphasic trend was not evident in patients treated for 6 months. The fact that patients who received 6 months of treatment were older, more likely to present advanced liver fibrosis or cirrhosis and comorbidities (including cardiac ones) could explain the discordant trends of GLS in the two groups. In fact, healthier individuals could benefit more from HCV RNA clearance in the short-term, while more compromised patients may suffer from a more prompt cardiotoxicity of sofosbuvir. Thus, it is worth considering that extreme elderly patients are receiving DAA treatments, with a high SVR rate, but at the same time they may experience more frequent cardiovascular complications, therefore a close and accurate monitoring of heart function could be required [36–38].

The associations between worse GLS and smoking or high BMI at baseline was not unexpected, suggesting the importance to quit negative behaviours, such as smoking and unhealthy diet in patients chronically infected by HCV. This is even more relevant if one considers that cardiac function may worsen after treatment, concomitantly with an increase of cholesterol occurring after HCV eradication as demonstrated in our study and confirmed by others [39]. Appropriate time dependent analysis should be conducted to assess whether variations in cholesterol levels may lead to GLS changes during SOF-based regimens.

Conclusions

In conclusions, if confirmed by datasets from independent cohorts to replicate the data, our results are important because demonstrated for the first time the possible cardiotoxicity of DAA treatments. The same study protocol for patients who are eligible for DAAs treatment with sofosbuvir-free regimens should be applied, in order to evaluate whether worsening of GLS is a specific drug-related or a class effect. While these results should be confirmed in more powerful studies and pathogenic hypotheses should be tested in translational studies, in the meantime a cautious approach should include assessment of cardiac function during DAA treatment, particularly for the most fragile patients, who may benefit from interventions to reduce the risk of cardiovascular diseases both before and after treatment.

Abbreviations

AIFA: Italian medicinal agency; APRI: AST to platelets ratio; BMI: Body mass index; CVD: Cardiovascular diseases; DAAs: Direct antiviral agents; DCV: Daclatasvir; EF: Ejection fraction; eGFR: Estimated glomerular filtrate rate; FIB 4: Fibrosis 4 index; GLS: Global longitudinal strain; HCV: Hepatitis C virus; LDV: Ledipasvir; LVF: Left ventricular function; RBV: Ribavirin; SD: Standard deviation; SIM: Simeprevir; SOF: Sofosbuvir; SVR: Sustained virological response

Acknowledgements

We want to thank all the patients who accepted to participate in our study. The CARDIAC Study group at UMG includes: Giorgio Settimo Barreca, Francesco Saverio Costanzo, Daniela Foti, Giorgio Fuiano, Giuseppe Greco, Francesca Serapide, Elio Gulletta, Nadia Marascio, Maria Concetta Postorino, Maria Adelina Simeoni, Alfredo Focà, Maria Carla Liberto, Aida Giancotti. This work has been presented in part at the American Association for the Study of Liver Diseases (AASLD) - The Liver Meeting® 2017, October 20-24 2017, Washington DC (poster #1079).

Funding

CARDIAC Study (Cardiovascular Diseases in new Antiviral Therapies for HCV) did not receive specific grant from any funding agency in the public, commercial and non-profit sectors.

Authors' contributions

MM designed the study, wrote the protocol, acquired informed consent, collected and processed the data, and contributed to write the manuscript; CT coordinated the protocol, and contributed to write and revise the final version of the manuscript; JS contributed in clinical management of patients, performed cardiac ultrasound, and helped in data collection and in the revision of final version of the manuscript; GLDA performed cardiac ultrasound and helped in data collection; CC contributed in clinical management of patients and in data collection; VP contributed in clinical management of patients and in data collection; ER processed data and performed all statistical analysis; AS contributed in clinical management of patients and in data collection; SDR contributed to write the manuscript and helped in the revision of final version; AF coordinated microbiological tests, helped to revise the final version of the manuscript; MCL coordinated microbiological tests, helped to revise the final version of the manuscript; CI coordinated the protocol, contributed to write and to revise the final version of the manuscript. All the authors read and approved the final version of the manuscript

Competing interests

The authors declare that they have no competing interests..

Author details

[1]Unit of Infectious and Tropical Diseases, Department of Medical and Surgical Sciences, "Magna Graecia" University of Catanzaro, Viale Europa, 88100 Catanzaro, Italy. [2]Cardiovascular Institute, Department of Medical and Surgical Sciences, "Magna Graecia" University of Catanzaro, Viale Europa, 88100 Catanzaro, Italy. [3]Unit of Hygiene, Epidemiology and Public Health, Department of Medical and Surgical Specialities, Radiological Sciences and Public Health, Viale Europa, 25123 Brescia, Italy. [4]Institute of Microbiology, Department of Health Sciences, "Magna Graecia" University of Catanzaro, Viale Europa, 88100 Catanzaro, Italy.

References

1. Ferri C, Sebastiani M, Giuggioli D, et al. Hepatitis C virus syndrome: a constellation of organ- and non-organ specific autoimmune disorders, B-cell non-Hodgkin's lymphoma, and cancer. World J Hepatol. 2015;7(3):327–43.
2. Gill K, Ghazinian H, Manch R, Gish R. Hepatitis C virus as a systemic disease: reaching beyond the liver. Hepatol Int. 2016;10(3):415–23.
3. Ambrosino P, Lupoli R, Di Minno A, et al. The risk of coronary artery disease and cerebrovascular disease in patients with hepatitis C: a systematic review and meta-analysis. Int J Cardiol. 2016;221:746–54.
4. Zampino R, Marrone A, Restivo L, et al. Chronic HCV infection and inflammation: clinical impact on hepatic and extra-hepatic manifestations. World J Hepatol. 2013;5(10):528–40.
5. Adinolfi LE, Zampino R, Restivo L, et al. Chronic hepatitis C virus infection and atherosclerosis: clinical impact and mechanisms. World J Gastroenterol. 2014;20(13):3410–7.
6. Matsumori A. Role of hepatitis C virus in cardiomyopathies. Ernst Schering Res Found Workshop. 2006;55:99–120.
7. Matsumori A, Shimada T, Chapman NM, Tracy SM, Mason JW. Myocarditis and heart failure associated with hepatitis C virus infection. J Card Fail. 2006; 12(4):293–8.
8. Matsumori A, Yutani C, Ikeda Y, Kawai S, Sasayama S. Hepatitis C virus from the hearts of patients with myocarditis and cardiomyopathy. Lab Investig. 2000;80(7):1137–42.
9. SOVALDI ® (sofosbuvir) tablets, for oral use initial U.S. 2013. Published 2013. https://www.accessdata.fda.gov/drugsatfda_docs/label/2015/204671s004lbl.pdf. Accessed 7 Oct 2018.
10. Hsu YC, Lin JT, Ho HJ, et al. Antiviral treatment for hepatitis C virus infection is associated with improved renal and cardiovascular outcomes in diabetic patients. Hepatology. 2014;59(4):1293–302.
11. Nahon P, Bourcier V, Layese R, et al. Eradication of Hepatitis C Virus Infection in Patients With Cirrhosis Reduces Risk of Liver and Non-Liver Complications. Gastroenterology. 2017;152(1):142–156.e142.
12. Folland ED, Parisi AF, Moynihan PF, Jones DR, Feldman CL, Tow DE. Assessment of left ventricular ejection fraction and volumes by real-time, two-dimensional echocardiography. A comparison of cineangiographic and radionuclide techniques. Circulation. 1979;60(4):760–6.

13. Marcucci CE, Samad Z, Rivera J, et al. A comparative evaluation of transesophageal and transthoracic echocardiography for measurement of left ventricular systolic strain using speckle tracking. J Cardiothorac Vasc Anesth. 2012;26(1):17–25.

14. Reisner SA, Lysyansky P, Agmon Y, Mutlak D, Lessick J, Friedman Z. Global longitudinal strain: a novel index of left ventricular systolic function. J Am Soc Echocardiogr. 2004;17(6):630–3.

15. Sengeløv M, Jørgensen PG, Jensen JS, et al. Global longitudinal strain is a superior predictor of all-cause mortality in heart failure with reduced ejection fraction. JACC Cardiovasc Imaging. 2015;8(12):1351–9.

16. Piegari E, Di Salvo G, Castaldi B, et al. Myocardial strain analysis in a doxorubicin-induced cardiomyopathy model. Ultrasound Med Biol. 2008;34(3):370–8.

17. Thavendiranathan P, Poulin F, Lim KD, Plana JC, Woo A, Marwick TH. Use of myocardial strain imaging by echocardiography for the early detection of cardiotoxicity in patients during and after cancer chemotherapy: a systematic review. J Am Coll Cardiol. 2014;63(25 Pt A):2751–68.

18. Sims A, Frank L, Cross R, et al. Abnormal cardiac strain in children and young adults with HIV acquired in early life. J Am Soc Echocardiogr. 2012; 25(7):741–8.

19. Kasner M, Sinning D, Escher F, et al. The utility of speckle tracking imaging in the diagnostic of acute myocarditis, as proven by endomyocardial biopsy. Int J Cardiol. 2013;168(3):3023–4.

20. Khosla T, Lowe CR. Indices of obesity derived from body weight and height. Br J Prev Soc Med. 1967;21(3):122–8.

21. Adler M, Gulbis B, Moreno C, et al. The predictive value of FIB-4 versus FibroTest, APRI, FibroIndex and Forns index to noninvasively estimate fibrosis in hepatitis C and nonhepatitis C liver diseases. Hepatology. 2008; 47(2):762–3 author reply 763.

22. Bota S, Sirli R, Sporea I, et al. A new scoring system for prediction of fibrosis in chronic hepatitis C. Hepat Mon. 2011;11(7):548–55.

23. Vallet-Pichard A, Mallet V, Nalpas B, et al. FIB-4: an inexpensive and accurate marker of fibrosis in HCV infection. Comparison with liver biopsy and fibrotest. Hepatology. 2007;46(1):32–6.

24. http://www.hep-druginteractions.org. Accessed 8 Oct 2018.

25. Vijayananthan A, Nawawi O. The importance of good clinical practice guidelines and its role in clinical trials. Biomed Imaging Interv J. 2008;4(1):e5.

26. Ndebele P. The declaration of Helsinki, 50 years later. JAMA. 2013;310(20): 2145–6.

27. Association WM. World medical association declaration of Helsinki: ethical principles for medical research involving human subjects. JAMA. 2013; 310(20):2191–4.

28. Yingchoncharoen T, Agarwal S, Popović ZB, Marwick TH. Normal ranges of left ventricular strain: a meta-analysis. J Am Soc Echocardiogr. 2013;26(2):185–91.

29. Marwick TH, Leano RL, Brown J, et al. Myocardial strain measurement with 2-dimensional speckle-tracking echocardiography: definition of normal range. JACC Cardiovasc Imaging. 2009;2(1):80–4.

30. Ahmad T, Yin P, Saffitz J, et al. Cardiac dysfunction associated with a nucleotide polymerase inhibitor for treatment of hepatitis C. Hepatology. 2015;62(2):409–16.

31. Babuin L, Jaffe AS. Troponin: the biomarker of choice for the detection of cardiac injury. CMAJ. 2005;173(10):1191–202.

32. Vuolteenaho O, Ala-Kopsala M, Ruskoaho H. BNP as a biomarker in heart disease. Adv Clin Chem. 2005;40:1–36.

33. Divakaran V, Mann DL. The emerging role of microRNAs in cardiac remodeling and heart failure. Circ Res. 2008;103(10):1072–83.

34. Corsten MF, Dennert R, Jochems S, et al. Circulating MicroRNA-208b and MicroRNA-499 reflect myocardial damage in cardiovascular disease. Circ Cardiovasc Genet. 2010;3(6):499–506.

35. Burdette D, Haskett A, Presser L, McRae S, Iqbal J, Waris G. Hepatitis C virus activates interleukin-1β via caspase-1-inflammasome complex. J Gen Virol. 2012;93(Pt 2):235–46.

36. Toyoda H, Kumada T, Tada T, et al. Efficacy and tolerability of an IFN-free regimen with DCV/ASV for elderly patients infected with HCV genotype 1B. J Hepatol. 2017;66(3):521–7.

37. Ji F, Wei B, Yeo YH, et al. Systematic review with meta-analysis: effectiveness and tolerability of interferon-free direct-acting antiviral regimens for chronic hepatitis C genotype 1 in routine clinical practice in Asia. Aliment Pharmacol Ther. 2018;47(5):550–62.

38. Ji F, Tian C, Li Z, Deng H, Nguyen MH. Ledipasvir and sofosbuvir combination for hepatitis C virus infection in three patients aged 85 years and older. Eur J Gastroenterol Hepatol. 2017;29(8):977–9.

39. Mauss S, Berger F, Wehmeyer MH, et al. Effect of antiviral therapy for HCV on lipid levels. Antivir Ther. 2017;21(1):81–8.

4

Protocol, rationale and design of SELPHI: a randomised controlled trial assessing whether offering free HIV self-testing kits via the internet increases the rate of HIV diagnosis

Michelle M. Gabriel[1,8]* (iD), David T. Dunn[1], Andrew Speakman[2], Leanne McCabe[1], Denise Ward[1], T. Charles Witzel[3], Justin Harbottle[4], Simon Collins[5], Mitzy Gafos[1,6], Fiona M. Burns[7], Fiona C. Lampe[2], Peter Weatherburn[3], Andrew Phillips[2], Sheena McCormack[1] and Alison J. Rodger[2]

Abstract

Background: Among men who have sex with men (MSM) in the UK, an estimated 28% have never tested for HIV and only 27% of those at higher risk test at least every 6 months. HIV self-testing (HIVST), where the person takes their own blood/saliva sample and processes it themselves, offers the opportunity to remove many structural and social barriers to testing. Although several randomised controlled trials are assessing the impact of providing HIVST on rates of HIV testing, none are addressing whether this results in increased rates of HIV diagnoses that link to clinical care. Linking to care is the critical outcome because it is the only way to access antiretroviral treatment (ART). We describe here the design of a large, internet-based randomised controlled trial of HIVST, called SELPHI, which aims to inform this key question.

Methods/design: The SELPHI study, which is ongoing is promoted via social networking website and app advertising, and aims to enroll HIV negative men, trans men and trans women, aged over 16 years, who are living in England and Wales. Apart from the physical delivery of the test kits, all trial processes, including recruitment, take place online. In a two-stage randomisation, participants are first randomised (3:2) to receive a free baseline HIVST or no free baseline HIVST. At 3 months, participants allocated to receive a baseline HIVST (and meeting further eligibility criteria) are subsequently randomised (1:1) to receive the offer of regular (every 3 months) free HIVST, with testing reminders, versus no such offer. The primary outcome from both randomisations is a laboratory-confirmed HIV diagnosis, ascertained via linkage to a national HIV surveillance database.

Discussion: SELPHI will provide the first reliable evidence on whether offering free HIVST via the internet increases rates of confirmed HIV diagnoses and linkage to clinical care. The two randomisations reflect the dual objectives of detecting prevalent infections (possibly long-standing) and the more rapid diagnosis of incident HIV infections. It is anticipated that the results of SELPHI will inform future access to HIV self-testing provision in the UK.

Keywords: HIV, Self-testing, HIVST, MSM, Diagnosis, Prevalent, Incident

* Correspondence: m.gabriel@ucl.ac.uk
[1]MRC Clinical Trials Unit at UCL, London, UK
[8]Trial Sponsor – University College London via MRC Clinical Trials Unit at UCL, Institute of Clinical Trials & Methodology, 90 High Holborn, 2nd Floor, London WC1V 6LJ, UK
Full list of author information is available at the end of the article

Background

The United Nations (UN) 90–90-90 targets aim by 2020, that 90% of all people living with HIV (PLWH) are diagnosed, that 90% of people diagnosed with HIV are on ART, and that 90% of those on ART have a suppressed viral load [1]. The first target (90% diagnosis) remains the key challenge with global estimates of 47% of PLWH being unaware of their infection. Knowledge of one's own HIV status and accessing ART benefits health on both an individual and population level. People who are unaware of their status are estimated to contribute disproportionally to new transmissions (between 60 and 80%) [2]. In the 2017 PHE (Public Health England) report on HIV, it was estimated that 10% of gay/bisexual men who have sex with men (MSM) were unaware of their HIV status. Although this percentage has decreased since 2010, testing is often less frequent than current recommendations. For example, UK guidelines [3] currently recommend annual HIV testing for MSM, and three-monthly testing for those considered 'at higher risk' (a definition that includes condomless (CL) anal sex with a new partner, diagnosis of new STI or chemsex drug use). In UK MSM, an estimated 28% have never tested for HIV and only a quarter of men at 'higher risk' of HIV infection test even 6-monthly (27%) [4–6]. Late diagnosis of HIV also remains a problem in the UK; 32% of all MSM diagnosed with HIV in 2016 (663/2,096) had CD4 counts below 350 mm^3, which is associated with greater morbidity and mortality than those who are diagnosed earlier in the course of infection. All guidelines now recommend that PLWH commence ART at diagnosis as this has been shown to be beneficial to individual health even at high CD4 counts [7].

HIV diagnoses in MSM in London have fallen since 2016 and this is thought to be a combination of increased rates of HIV testing, rapid initiation of ART when HIV is diagnosed (which reduces transmission risk through sex to almost zero) and increasing use of pre-exposure prophylaxis (PrEP) [8]. Rates of HIV diagnosis in MSM outside London have also reduced but to a lesser degree [9]. Expanding ways for MSM to test for HIV outside of traditional settings (such as GUM clinics) has been a focus for over a decade and there is now a national self-sampling service. This involves an individual taking their own test sample which they post back to the relevant laboratory for testing and are subsequently contacted with the result.

A further approach is to offer HIV self-testing (HIVST) where the person not only takes their own blood/saliva sample but also processes it themselves using a self-testing kit, and obtains the results immediately. A potential advantage of HIVST is that, removing structural and social barriers to testing and increasing associated privacy and convenience, may lead to increased testing [10, 11].

HIVST is also an opportunity for prevention synergies with the availability of PrEP (which requires frequent testing), and for harm reduction strategies, such as sexual partner screening. The WHO now incorporate HIVST into its global HIV testing guidelines as a 'supplementary' or 'additional' option [12] and has described it as "an empowering and innovative way to help achieve the first of the United Nations 90–90–90 treatment targets" [13].

HIVST also has a number of potential challenges, although empirical data are lacking. Firstly, a person who has a reactive HIVST requires confirmatory HIV testing to link to care which relies on the individual seeking more traditional testing as a gateway to care and support. It remains unknown what proportion of individuals who obtain a reactive result on HIVST link to care in a timely manner [14]. A further issue may be the potential for social and emotional harms from a reactive test in the absence of counselling, or coercion to test from a partner. HIVST may also be a missed opportunity for STI screening and advice about risk management due to fewer visits to GUM clinic settings, which may put MSM at increased risk of other STIs. HIVST kit accuracy is also an area of concern, as the window period is prolonged in comparison to 4th generation tests (antibody and P24 antigen test) and the sensitivity is relatively low, particularly with oral fluid HIVST in early infection or in breakthrough infections on tenofovir-based PrEP as antibody levels may be low. This is particularly important during early infection, when the risk of onward transmission is markedly increased.

Existing evidence base

Evidence suggests that HIVST is acceptable to MSM and other key populations at risk of HIV globally both in high and low-income settings [10, 15, 16]. However, despite the theoretical benefits of HIVST, there are limited European data exploring potential HIVST acceptability, as well as the values and preferences of MSM or trans people at risk of HIV infection on the potential impacts of self-testing approaches in the UK [17–19]. There is also a lack of evidence on whether HIVST increases rates of HIV diagnosis in populations at risk of HIV. It is also unknown whether it is cost-effective for the NHS to provide free or subsidised HIVST kits. Observational studies, using follow-up surveys, have documented the number of self-reported reactive tests as a proportion of the number of HIVST kits sent out [20]. However, there is likely to be selection bias in those responding to surveys and it is not known how many individuals would have sought and obtained their HIV diagnosis through another testing modality.

There are four on-going or recently reported RCTs of HIVST in MSM in high resource settings (three in the US and one in Australia) [21–24]. All use self-reported frequency of testing as the primary outcome comparing HIVST to standard of care. These studies therefore do not address the key question of whether provision of HIVST can increase rates of HIV diagnoses that link to clinical care, which is the gateway to ART. We describe here the design of a large, internet-based randomised controlled trial of HIVST, which aims to inform this question.

Rationale

The primary aim of SELPHI is to measure the impact of HIVST on new confirmed HIV diagnoses linked to clinical care by addressing the following key questions:

- Is the online promotion and postal delivery of free HIV self-test kits (with testing reminders) feasible and acceptable?
- Will the offer of a single free HIV self-test at enrolment lead to the confirmed diagnosis of prevalent HIV infections and entry to standard HIV clinical care?
- Among seronegative individuals at high risk of acquiring HIV infection, will the offer of regular free self-tests with testing reminders result in more rapid confirmed diagnosis of an incident HIV infection and entry in to standard HIV clinical care?
- What data can be generated to inform key parameters for a cost effectiveness model?

Subsidiary objectives include: describing the usage and acceptability of HIVST; determining if the offer of free HIVST kits affects the overall frequency of HIV testing and testing options utilised; assessment of post-test linkage with counselling and treatment services; assessing whether free HIVST kits affects the frequency of STI screening or the frequency of condomless sex; investigating the impact of demographic, socio-economic, health-related factors, and sexual risk behaviours on testing behaviours.

Methods/design

Design

SELPHI is an ongoing open-label parallel group randomised controlled trial with a two-stage simple randomisation aiming to enrol 10,000 participants (Fig. 1). Randomisation A takes place at enrolment, with participants randomly allocated (in a 3:2 ratio) to the offer of a free baseline HIV self-test (BT) versus no offer of a free baseline HIV self-test (nBT). An unequal allocation ratio was chosen so that a majority of those agreeing to participate would receive a free self-test and to increase the number of participants eligible for Randomisation B. This second randomisation occurs at month 3 after

enrolment, and is more restrictive, being open only to participants who were initially allocated to the BT group in Randomisation A who complete the 3-month survey, and who meet additional eligibility criteria, including being at high risk of incident HIV infection, assessed at 3 months. Eligible participants are randomised (1:1) to receive the offer of regular (immediately and every 3 months thereafter) free HIV self-tests + testing reminders (RT) versus no such offer (nRT).

Primary outcome measure

The primary outcome for both randomisations is a laboratory-confirmed HIV diagnosis, with date of diagnosis defined as the date of the first confirmatory test at clinic. This key feature of SELPHI distinguishes it from other randomised trials of HIVST.

Inclusion criteria

The inclusion criteria for SELPHI are broad in order to maximise generalisability and are detailed in Table 1. The residency restriction was a requirement of the funding body. The consent for linkage to Public Health Databases was essential as this is the main mechanism for determining the trial primary endpoints. The criterion in Randomisation B of reporting at least one male condomless anal sex act in the previous 3 months is intended to identify individuals at higher risk of acquiring HIV infection.

Study procedures

Recruitment and enrolment

SELPHI is an internet-based study using advertising campaigns, placed on social networking websites and via mobile phone applications designed to facilitate sexual and social contact, to recruit participants for example Facebook, Grindr, Hornet and community webpages. Advertising is tailored to attract individuals from a broad spectrum of MSM and trans people. Depending on the advertising platform, messages take a number of forms: "Broadcast Message" (sent directly to an individual's "inbox" in a particular app), "Pop-up Message" (pop-up message which shows when an individual logs in to an app), "Banner Ad" (shown on screen within an app or website whilst a user is online). Examples of adverts are shown in Fig. 2.

Participants are directed to the study registration page where they are asked to complete a two-stage sign-up process. All data are collected in electronic surveys hosted by Demographix Ltd. The first stage provides information about the study, assesses eligibility, obtains informed consent, and requests an email address. An email is immediately sent to this address with a link to complete the second stage of the process. This serves to validate the email address provided by the participant, which is the means of all future communication throughout the trial.

RANDOMISATION A - INCLUSION
- Men (including trans men) and trans women
- Has ever had anal sex with a man
- Is not known to be HIV Positive
- Aged ≥16 years old
- Resident in England or Wales
- Willing to provide name, date of birth, and a valid email address
- Gives consent to linkage with surveillance and clinic databases.
- Has not been previously randomised to the study

Randomisation A
(n=10,000)

No baseline self-test [nBT]
n=4,000

Free baseline self-test [BT]
n=6,000

Primary Outcome A
confirmed HIV diagnosis within 3 months of enrolment, with date defined as the date of the first confirmatory test at clinic

3-Month Survey*

RANDOMISATION B - INCLUSION
- Allocated to baseline self-test (BT) in randomisation A
- Has completed 3-month survey and;
  - reports using self-test sent at baseline
  - remains HIV negative
  - expresses interest in using HIV self-test kits in the future
  - is considered to be at high-risk for HIV infection. Defined as reporting condomless anal sex with ≥1 male partners in previous 3 months.

Randomisation B
(n=3,000)

No regular test offer [nRT]
(n=1,500)

Regular test offer [RT]
(n=1,500)

Primary Outcome B: confirmed HIV diagnosis between the date of this randomisation and study closure, with date defined as the date of the first confirmatory test at clinic.

* Surveys include Questions on Sexual behaviour and HIV testing

*Regular Survey***

Test reminders + *Regular survey***

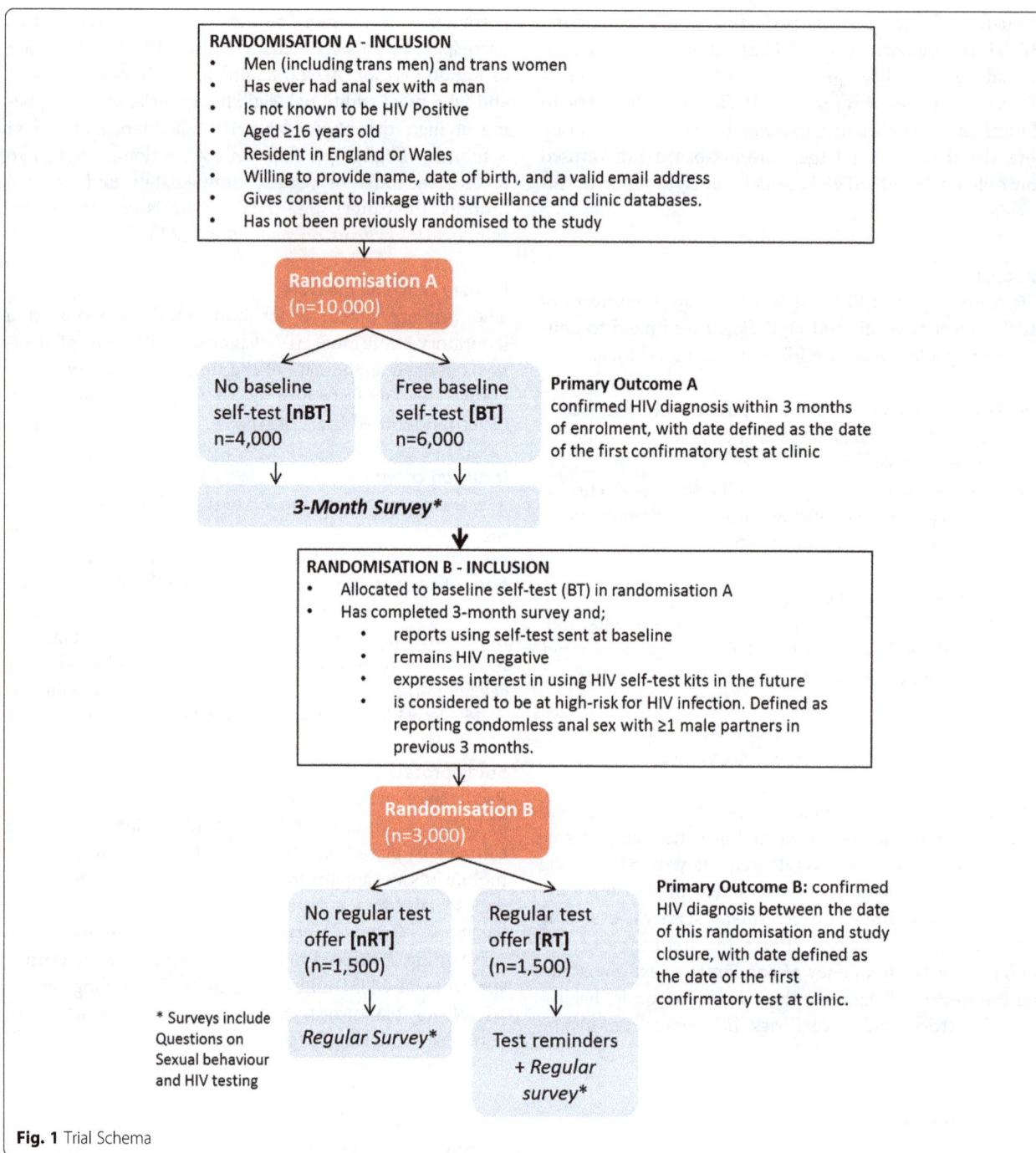

Fig. 1 Trial Schema

In the second stage, further demographic and behavioural characteristics are collected (summarised in Table 2). Once the second stage is completed, participants are randomised and allocated to receive a free baseline HIV self-test (BT) or no free baseline test (nBT). Those allocated to BT are directed to provide postal details for shipment of the test kit; those allocated to nBT are directed to an area on the study website (www.selphi.org) which provides information on how to obtain an HIV test in other ways (e.g. local GUM clinics).

HIV self-testing kits

In the UK, HIVST was legalised in April 2014, and the first CE marked kit (BioSURE® HIV Self Test, BioSURE, United Kingdom) was released to the UK market in April 2015. The BioSURE® HIV Self Test kit is classed as a 2nd generation test (an antibody immunoassay detecting HIV 1/2 antibodies from approximately 28 days after infection), uses a whole blood sample and retail at £30–£35. Further HIVST kits have subsequently obtained a CE mark, including the blood based INSTI HIV Self

Table 1 Inclusion criteria

Randomisation A	Randomisation B

• Male (including trans men) and trans women
• Aged ≥16 years old
• Resident in England or Wales
• Not known to be HIV-positive
• Has ever had anal sex with a man
• Willing to provide name, date of birth, and a valid email address
• Consent for linkage to surveillance and clinic databases held by Public Health England
• Not previously randomised to the study
	• Allocated to baseline self-test (BT) in Randomisation A
	• Completes the first survey after 3-months and:
	  o Reports using self-test sent at baseline
	  o Remains HIV-negative
	  o Reports condomless anal sex with ≥1 male partners in previous 3 months
	  o Interested in using HIV self-test kits in the future

Test (bioLytical Laboratories, Canada) which detects anti-HIV-1 IgM antibodies as well as anti-HIV-1 IgG (a 3rd generation assay) and can detect HIV infection from 21 days after infection.

The HIV self-testing kit used in the study is the BioSURE® HIV Self Test which is CE marked and licensed for use in the UK. The test comprises a paper test strip inside a plastic barrel, and is performed by mixing a small drop of blood with test reagents contained in the buffer pot where the liquid reagents are absorbed by the paper strip. When the test is completed, two lines can appear on the paper test strip. The upper line (the Control line) becomes visible if the test has been performed correctly. The lower line (the Test line) becomes visible if the applied sample contains sufficient antibodies to HIV. The BioSURE® HIV self-test product insert estimates its sensitivity to be 99.7% (95% CI 98.9–100).

In addition to written information provided with the test kit, an online video providing instructions on kit use (produced by BioSURE) is also promoted to participants on joining the study and is available on the study website (https://youtu.be/N4CAqsmN_6g).

Follow up

All follow-up in SELPHI is conducted via online surveys which are only accessible using a unique personalised URL sent to participants by email. The content of surveys depends on the randomised allocation and uses conditional

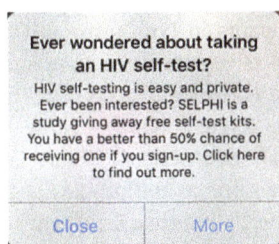

Pop-up Message

Broadcast Message

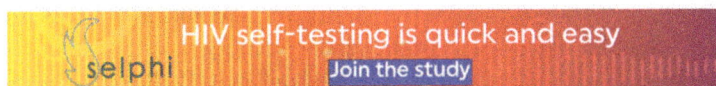

Banner Ad

Fig. 2 Advertising Samples

Table 2 Summary of variables collected on electronic surveys

Variable	Patient Group	Time point(s)
Age	ALL	Baseline
Soundex	ALL	Baseline
Postcode	ALL	Baseline
Country of Birth	ALL	Baseline
Length of residency in the UK	ALL	Baseline
Ethnicity	ALL	Baseline
Highest Educational Qualification	ALL	Baseline
Sexual Identity	ALL	Baseline
Timing of last HIV test	ALL	Baseline
Timing of last STI screen	ALL	Baseline
Number condomless anal intercourse partners (last 3 months)	ALL	Baseline
PrEP and PEP usage	ALL	Baseline
Confirmation of HIVST Kit receipt	BT/RT	2-weeks post kit shipment
	BT	3-month post baseline
	RT	3-monthly post Randomisation B entry
Confirmation of HIVST Kit usage	BT/RT	2-weeks post kit shipment
	BT	3-month post baseline
	RT	3-monthly post Randomisation B entry
Self-reported HIVST result	BT/RT	2-weeks post kit shipment
	BT	3-month post baseline
	RT	3-monthly post Randomisation B entry
Kits receipt & usage experiences	BT	3-month post baseline
	RT	3-monthly post Randomisation B entry
Timing of HIV tests in last 3 months (not including HIVST)	BT/NBT	3-month post baseline
	RT/NRT	3-monthly post Randomisation B entry
Self-reported HIV positive test result (from any other source)	BT/NBT	3-month post baseline
	RT/NRT	3-monthly post Randomisation B entry
Timing of STI tests in last 3 months	BT/NBT	3-month post baseline
	RT/NRT	3-monthly post Randomisation B entry
Number condomless anal intercourse partners (last 3 months)	BT/NBT	3-month post baseline
	RT/NRT	3-monthly post Randomisation B entry
Interest in future HIVST If available	BT/NBT	3-month post baseline
Offer of another free HIVST	RT	Randomisation B Entry
	RT	3-monthly post Randomisation B entry

branching to create a customised path through the survey based on responses to earlier questions.

Following entry to Randomisation A participants randomised to BT are asked to provide a postal address for shipment of their free HIVST (which arrives within 5–7 days). Participants in the BT arm receive an invite to complete a short follow-up 2 weeks later, primarily to confirm that they received the HIVST and to ascertain if they have used it. Participants in the control arm are provided with signposts to allow them to access other options for HIV testing. All participants in Randomisation A are followed up at 3 months in an online survey, asking about HIV tests (type and number) conducted since baseline and the results of these tests, STI testing and the number of sexual partners since baseline. Questions are identical in the two groups, except the BT group is also asked to rate their experiences in receiving and using the HIVST. This survey also includes questions which determine eligibility for Randomisation B (refer to Table 2). Participants who do not enter Randomisation B receive no further surveys apart from one at the end of the study. Participants randomised to RT are immediately informed that they can order a further free HIVST now and every 3 months subsequently.

Participants in both arms (nRT and RT) of Randomisation B receive an invite to complete a survey every 3 months until the end of the study. For those in the RT arm, both the invitation and survey include a reminder to test and the offer of another free HIVST kit. The process for obtaining a kit is the same as the process at baseline; kits are not sent automatically but the participant "orders" another kit if they wish to. Participants are not obliged to order a kit every 3 months, if they choose not to receive another kit they will continue to be offered kits three-monthly. Following every kit order the participant will receive a 2-week follow-up as with their first kit. Follow-up in Randomisation B will continue until the last participant randomised is followed-up for 2 years. All participants who have not tested positive during the study will be sent an email at the end of the study inviting them to complete a final survey and to thank them for their participation.

If a participant reports testing HIV positive at any point during the study they are directed to resources where they can access support (e.g. THT Direct 24-h Helpline) and are no longer invited to complete any further follow-up surveys.

Determination of primary outcomes

Primary outcomes will be identified by linking the personal identifiers collected in SELPHI to the national (England and Wales) HIV surveillance database maintained by PHE, who are collaborators on the trial. Linkage will be performed by a computer algorithm, primarily based on date of birth and patient surname (encoded to Soundex). Putative links will be confirmed manually by matching on common variables, including geographical region, ethnicity, gender, and initials. On confirmed matched cases, PHE will return information on date of diagnosis, region of diagnosis, CD4 count and viral load at diagnosis, whether participants have linked to care and initiated treatment, and GUM clinic attendance history. Furthermore, at each follow-up survey participants are asked about any HIV tests taken and any HIV-positive diagnoses. Consistency between this information and that recorded in PHE databases will be cross-checked. A self-reported diagnosis will not be accepted as a primary outcome if it cannot be matched to a confirmatory test in the PHE database or from a local clinic.

Patient and public involvement (PPI)
As per the NIHR INVOLVE guidelines, patient and public involvement (PPI) was sought during the trial development. PPI representatives from HIV i-Base, NAM and other organisations are included in programme management group and the trial management group. These community members led the establishment of a study specific Community Advisory Group (CAG) and developed other public involvement models. Patient and public involvement was integrated throughout the study and budgeted in the initial grant application. For example, it informed the development of the trial design, protocol, participant information and consent materials, surveys, recruitment strategy and advertising materials. This involvement notably expanded the entry criteria to include transgender women, even though the original grant was limited to gay and bisexual men. The change was driven by the lack of specific research and access for this population and the precedent of broader inclusion in other prevention studies (for example with PrEP).

Ethical considerations
The potential adverse psychological consequences of a reactive test result were considered during the process of obtaining CE-marking for the BioSURE® self-test kit, but the regulatory authorities were satisfied that benefit of an individual knowing that they had HIV outweighed the small risk of harm. A second potential adverse consequence is that people who obtain a reactive test result might not subsequently attend clinical services for confirmatory HIV testing and therefore might not engage with care. Consequently, participants who report a reactive HIV test result in the study are directed to appropriate resources through the study website. These include guidance on how to find local GUM clinics and links to the Terrance Higgins Trust (THT) Direct hotline and the NHS Direct service to assist them in dealing with a new diagnosis and accessing confirmatory testing and HIV care services. There was extensive discussion around whether the lower age limit should

be 18 years (standard age for consent for adult medical research) or 16 years (the legal age for consent for consensual sex). The latter age was chosen following consultation with the SELPHI CAB and then the Ethics Committee that approved the protocol.

Identifiable and sensitive data are collected within the trial, including questions on sexual behaviours, recreational drug use and HIV status. In compliance with all relevant legislation (including the Data Protection Act), data are stored securely within appropriate systems operated by Demographix Ltd. and University College London (Data Safe Haven) which meet the ISO27001 information security standard as a minimum. In datasets provided to PHE for the purposes of linkage, the minimum number of data fields are transferred, forenames are redacted to initials and surnames are encoded to Soundex, a phonetic algorithm which indexes names by sound as pronounced in English. All personal identifiers are stripped from datasets produced for statistical analyses.

Through patient and public involvement, it was decided that describing the full complexity of the trial design would result in information overload and could hinder recruitment. Potential participants are therefore simply informed that they will be randomised to one or more self-tests to which they are asked to consent, rather than explicit and separate consents for Randomisation A and Randomisation B.

Statistical analysis
The primary analyses will compare the randomised groups as allocated (intention to treat, ITT) in terms of a confirmed HIV diagnosis. Specifically, the primary outcome for Randomisation A is a confirmed HIV diagnosis within 3 months of the date of randomisation i.e. before the 3-month survey, which could influence testing behaviour in the nBT group, is sent out. The difference between randomised arms will be tested by a chi-squared test for comparison of proportions. Logistic regression analysis will be used to explore the effect of other covariates and potential interactions with randomisation arm. As the offer of a free test at enrolment could theoretically also affect future testing behaviour, a secondary survival analysis will examine the time to confirmed diagnosis.

The primary outcome for Randomisation B (RT versus nRT) is time to confirmed diagnosis of HIV from the date of randomisation. The analysis includes information on participants who do not experience the event, using time-to-event methods. Ideally, we would describe the interval from the time of acquisition of HIV infection rather than randomisation, but this is not generally observed. We note that the number and timing of endpoints is a function both of underlying HIV incidence and the interval between infection and diagnosis. If the self-testing intervention affects the former this will induce a difference between the randomised groups, even if there is no impact on diagnosis rates; although we cannot exclude the possibility of such a mechanism we consider it to be unlikely. The difference between randomised arms will be tested by a log rank test, supplemented by Cox regression models to examine the effect of covariates. The (administrative) censoring date for participants who do not experience the primary outcome will depend on the calendar date when linkage to PHE datasets is performed (see Determination of primary outcomes).

Sample size

The standard approach to sample size is to first pre-specify key parameters, including the desired statistical power, and then calculate the sample size. However, this approach was not practicable as we were constrained by the budget for the HIVST kits and as certain key parameters were highly uncertain. Instead, for the pre-determined sample size of 10,000 we have estimated the statistical power over plausible ranges of values for these parameters.

The power of the analysis of Randomisation A is a function of underlying HIV seroprevalence and the proportion of seropositive participants in the BT and nBT groups diagnosed within 3 months. We considered HIV seroprevalence values between 1.5 and 2.5%, based on HIV self-sampling in the UK, [25] and proportions diagnosed between 20 and 50% in the nBT group and between 50 and 80% in the BT group. Table 3 shows the statistical power for various combinations of these proportions when HIV seroprevalence is 2.0%. In general, power is acceptably high when the difference between the BT and nBT groups is at least 30% (in absolute terms).

We have assumed that 3,000 participants will enter Randomisation B i.e. 50% of those enrolled in the BT group meet the additional eligibility criteria. We used simulation to estimate the statistical power for this randomisation as an analytical approach was not tractable. As repeat HIV self-tests can only affect the time to diagnosis of participants who become infected during the study, a key parameter is the underlying HIV incidence rate. Values between 1.5 and 3.0 per 100 person-years (PY) were explored,

based on estimates among MSM attending GUM clinics in England. Another important parameter is the interval between infection and diagnosis in the nRT group: this was assumed to follow a Weibull distribution with a shape parameter of 0.4 (to produce a higher initial rate of detection of infection) and a median ranging from 1.0 to 2.5 years [26, 27]. The corresponding interval in the RT group was determined by the uptake of the offer of repeat tests and the proportion linking to care following a reactive self-test. Table 4 shows the statistical power and other analytical outputs as a function of key parameters.

Discussion

Globally, SELPHI is the largest RCT evaluating the offer of free HIVST kits via the internet, and has uniquely been designed to assess the impact of this intervention on HIV diagnosis with linkage to clinical care and thus access to early ART.

SELPHI was challenging to design and the results will also need to be interpreted carefully. First, any future offer of free HIVST kits within a health services context will be a direct offer rather than the possibility (determined by randomisation) of receiving a test and agreeing to complete regular follow-up questionnaires. This raises concerns about generalisability, particularly if some participants joined the trial for altruistic motives, and may

Table 3 Power (%) to detect a difference between BT and nBT groups in Randomisation A

Diagnosis rate in nBT group (%)	Diagnosis rate in BT group (%)			
	50	60	70	80
20	91	99	100	100
30	53	83	96	99
40	16	45	75	92
50	5	14	39	68

Power to detect a difference at $2\alpha = 0.05$ by chi-squared test
Assumes seroprevalence rate = 2%

Table 4 Power to detect a difference between RT and nRT groups in Randomisation B

HIV Incidence (per 100 PY)	Median time to diagnosis (years) in nRT group	Power (%)	Estimated HIV infections per group	Median number HIV diagnoses (nRT/RT)	Median hazard ratio (RT versus nRT)
1.5	1.0	56	53	24/40	1.73
	1.5	72	53	21/40	1.91
	2.0	82	53	19/40	2.08
	2.5	87	53	18/40	2.21
2.0	1.0	75	71	30/53	1.70
	1.5	83	71	28/52	1.94
	2.0	91	71	26/52	2.08
	2.5	93	71	24/51	2.20
2.5	1.0	83	89	38/66	1.73
	1.5	93	89	34/65	1.92
	2.0	96	89	32/65	2.09
	2.5	98	89	30/64	2.25
3.0	1.0	89	107	46/78	1.74
	1.5	96	107	41/77	1.92
	2.0	98	107	38/77	2.09
	2.5	99	107	36/77	2.23

Power to detect a difference at $2\alpha = 0.05$ by log-rank test affect recruitment to the trial, as a free HIV-test is not guaranteed. Secondly, results will need to be interpreted in the context of the current "standard of care". When the trial was initially being designed HIVST was illegal in the UK, whereas the BioSURE kits were commercially available when SELPHI launched in February 2017. The study objectives therefore needed to be defined carefully i.e. the effectiveness of offering *free* tests rather than offering tests per se. A related issue is the impact of other self-sampling and self-testing initiatives from other organisations in the UK.

Another moot design point was whether sending testing reminders should be an intrinsic part of the intervention or whether this should be considered as a separate intervention. We considered a factorial design but eventually decided that the HIVST kits and testing reminders should constitute a single "package", reflecting the likely promotion of HIVST kits during implementation and to maximise the chance of demonstrating an effect. A residual concern is that the regular 3-monthly questionnaires will act as a reminder for participants in the nRT group to seek an HIV test and reduce the difference between the groups. However, we expect that a large proportion of participants in this group will opt out of receiving emails or ignore the follow-up surveys. This highlights the importance of determining the study primary endpoint from an independent national surveillance database to mitigate potential selective survey completion bias. A similar linkage to the PHE national dataset has been conducted to identify additional infections in the long-term follow-up of participants in the PROUD trial of HIV pre-exposure prophylaxis [28]. Reassuringly, of the 32 participants who were diagnosed in one of the PROUD clinics, only 1 (3%) was not identified in the national surveillance database [29]. The sample size calculation for SELPHI factored in a linkage failure rate of 10%. Another consideration is the delay in the centralisation and reconciliation of reports of HIV diagnoses from clinics and laboratories across the country, and a finalised dataset for a given calendar year is usually not available until June of the following year.

SELPHI is expected to complete in 2020 although the results of Randomisation A should be available earlier than this. As well as the main randomised comparisons, we are undertaking qualitative sub-studies of SELPHI participants, process evaluation and developing cost-effectiveness models which will be informed by the results of the trial.

With expanded prevention and treatment options available for people living with HIV, the need for testing and diagnosis is more important than ever. The reality of shrinking NHS resources and radical cuts and changes to sexual health service provision will require increased innovation with cost saving services such as e-health and postal services. This shift will increase the relevance of results from this trial.

Abbreviations

ART: Antiretroviral Treatment; CAB: Community Advisory Board; CE Mark: "Conformité Européene" which literally means "European Conformity" Mark; GUM: Genitourinary Medicine; HIVST: HIV self-test; PLWH: People Living with HIV; PPI: Patient and public involvement; RCT: Randomised controlled trial; REC: Research Ethics Committee; SELPHI: An HIV Self-testing Public Health Intervention; STI: Sexually transmitted infection; UK: United Kingdom; UN: United Nations

Acknowledgements

We would like to acknowledge the involvement in the design of the trial of the Participant and Public Involvement Representatives (Roger Pebody and Roy Trevelion), the SELPHI Community Advisory Group (CAG), the UK HIV treatment advocates network Community Advisory Board (CAB) (http://www.ukcab.net) and members of the public recruited via the PROUD study and the PrEP update mailing lists. MRC CTU Clinical Trial Unit salaries are part funded through MRC core funding (MC_UU_12023/23).

Funding

SELPHI is funded by the NIHR under its Programme Grants for Applied Research Programme (Grant Reference Number RP-PG-1212-20006): A comprehensive assessment of the cost-effectiveness of HIV prevention and testing strategies, including HIV self-testing, among men who have sex with men (MSM) in the UK (PANTHEON). The views expressed are those of the authors and not necessarily those of the NHS, the NIHR or the Department of Health. The funding body had no input in to the study design, collection, analysis, and interpretation of data or in the writing of this the manuscript.

Authors' contributions

DD, SC, FB, FL, AP, SMc and AR obtained study funding. MMG, DD, SC, MG, TCW, FB, FL, PW, AP, SMc and AR were involved in the design of the study. MMG, DD, AS, LMcC, DW, TCW, JH, SC, MG, FB, FL, PW, AP, SMc and AR were involved in the implementation of the study. MMG, DD, and AR drafted and edited the manuscript. All authors made critical comments and approved the final draft of the manuscript.

Competing interests

BioSURE® HIV Self Tests were obtained from BioSURE (UK) Ltd., at a reduced cost. BioSURE will not have any influence on the study design, analysis, and reporting. The authors declare that they have no competing interests.

Author details

[1]MRC Clinical Trials Unit at UCL, London, UK. [2]Centre for Clinical Research, Epidemiology, Modelling and Evaluation, Institute for Global Health, UCL, London, UK. [3]Department of Social and Environmental Health Research, Sigma Research, Faculty of Public Health & Policy, London School of Hygiene and Tropical Medicine, London, UK. [4]Terrence Higgins Trust, London, UK. [5]HIV i-Base, London, UK. [6]Department of Global Health and Development, London School of Hygiene and Tropical Medicine, Faculty of Public Health and Policy, London, UK. [7]Royal Free London NHS Foundation Trust, London, UK. [8]Trial Sponsor – University College London via MRC Clinical Trials Unit at UCL, Institute of Clinical Trials & Methodology, 90 High Holborn, 2nd Floor, London WC1V 6LJ, UK.

References

1. Bezemer D, de Wolf F, Boerlijst MC, van Sighem A, Hollingsworth TD, Prins M, Geskus RB, Gras L, Coutinho RA, Fraser C. A resurgent HIV-1 epidemic

among men who have sex with men in the era of potent antiretroviral therapy. AIDS. 2008;22(9):1071–7.

2. Williamson LM, Dodds JP, Mercey DE, Hart GJ, Johnson AM. Sexual risk behaviour and knowledge of HIV status among community samples of gay men in the UK. AIDS. 2008;22(9):1063–70.

3. Clutterbuck DJ, Flowers P, Barber T, Wilson H, Nelson M, Hedge B, Kapp S, Fakoya A, Sullivan AK. UK national guideline on safer sex advice. Int J STD AIDS. 2012;23(6):381–8. https://doi.org/10.1258/ijsa.2012.200312.

4. Witzel T, Melendex-Torres G, Hickson F, Weatherburn P. HIV testing history and preferences for future tests among gay men, bisexual men and other MSM in England: results from a cross-sectional study. BMJ Open. 2016;6(9): e011372.

5. Hickson F, Melendez-Torres GJ, Reid D, Weatherburn P. HIV, sexual risk and ethnicity among gay and bisexual men in England: survey evidence for persisting health inequalities. Sex Transm Infect. 2017;93(7):508–13. https://doi.org/10.1136/sextrans-2016-052800 Epub052017 Mar 052827.

6. Knussen C, Flowers P, McDaid LM. Factors associated with recency of HIV testing amongst men residing in Scotland who have sex with men. AIDS Care. 2014;26(3):297–303.

7. Lundgren JD, Babiker AG, Gordin F, Emery S, Grund B, Sharma S, Avihingsanon A, Cooper DA, Fatkenheuer G, Llibre JM, et al. Initiation of Antiretroviral Therapy in Early Asymptomatic HIV Infection. N Engl J Med. 2015;373(9):795–807. https://doi.org/10.1056/NEJMoa1506816 Epub 1502015 Jul 1506820.

8. Nwokolo N, Whitlock G, McOwan A. Not just PrEP: other reasons for London's HIV decline. Lancet HIV. 2017;4(4):e153. https://doi.org/10.1016/S2352–3018(1017)30044–30049.

9. Brown AEKP, Chau C, Khawam J, Gill ON, Delpech VC. Towards elimination of HIV transmission, AIDS and HIV - related deaths in the UK – 2017 report. London: Public Health England; 2017.

10. Figueroa C, Johnson C, Verster A, Baggaley R. Attitudes and acceptability on HIV self-testing among key populations: a literature review. AIDS Behav. 2015;19(11):1949–65.

11. Witzel TC, Rodger AJ. New initiatives to develop self-testing for HIV. Curr Opin Infect Dis. 2016;15:15.

12. Guidelines on HIV Self-Testing and Partner Notification: Supplement to consolidated guidelines on HIV testing services. In. Edited by organisation WH. Geneva; 2016.

13. Fast-Track - Ending the AIDS epidemic by 2030. In. Edited by HIV/AIDS GJUNPo; 2014.

14. Johnson CC, Kennedy C, Fonner V, Siegfried N, Figueroa C, Dalal S, Sands A, Baggaley R. Examining the effects of HIV self-testing compared to standard HIV testing services: a systematic review and meta-analysis. J Int AIDS Soc. 2017;20(1):21594. https://doi.org/10.27448/IAS.21520.21591.21594.

15. Pant Pai N, Sharma J, Shivkumar S, Pillay S, Vadnais C, Joseph L, Dheda K, Peeling RW. Supervised and unsupervised self-testing for HIV in high- and low-risk populations: a systematic review. PLoS Med. 2013;10(4):e1001414.

16. Ibitoye M, Frasca T, Giguere R, Carballo-Dieguez A. Home testing past, present and future: lessons learned and implications for HIV home tests. AIDS Behav. 2014;18(5):933–49.

17. Witzel T, Rodger A, Burns F, Rhodes T, Weatherburn P: HIV self-testing among men who have sex with men (MSM) in the UK: a qualitative study of barriers and facilitators, intervention preferences and perceived impacts. PLoS One. 2016;11(9):e0162713.

18. Witzel TC, Weatherburn P, Rodger AJ, Bourne AH, Burns FM. Risk, reassurance and routine: a qualitative study of narrative understandings of the potential for HIV self-testing among men who have sex with men in England. BMC Public Health. 2017;17(1):491. https://doi.org/10.1186/s12889–12017–14370-12880.

19. Flowers P, Riddell J, Park C, Ahmed B, Young I, Frankis J, Davis M, Gilbert M, Estcourt C, Wallace L, et al. Preparedness for use of the rapid result HIV self-test by gay men and other men who have sex with men (MSM): a mixed methods exploratory study among MSM and those involved in HIV prevention and care. HIV Med. 2017;18(4):245–55. https://doi.org/10.1111/hiv12420 Epub 12016 Aug 12425.

20. Witzel TC, Rodger AJ. New initiatives to develop self-testing for HIV. Curr Opin Infect Dis. 2017;30(1):50–7. https://doi.org/10.1097/QCO.0000000000000336.

21. Jamil MS, Prestage G, Fairley CK, Grulich AE, Smith KS, Chen M, Holt M, McNulty AM, Bavinton BR, Conway DP, et al. Effect of availability of HIV self-testing on HIV testing frequency in gay and bisexual men at high risk of infection (FORTH): a waiting-list randomised controlled trial. Lancet HIV.

2017;4(6):e241–50. https://doi.org/10.1016/S2352–3018(1017)30023–30021 Epub 32017 Feb 30017.

22. MacGowan RJ, Chavez PR, Gravens L, Wesolowski LG, Sharma A, McNaghten AD, Freeman A, Sullivan PS, Borkowf CB, Michele Owen S. Pilot evaluation of the ability of men who have sex with men to self-administer rapid HIV tests, prepare dried blood spot cards, and interpret test results, Atlanta, Georgia, 2013. AIDS Behav. 2017;20(10):017–1932.

23. Stephenson R, Freeland R, Sullivan SP, Riley E, Johnson BA, Mitchell J, McFarland D, Sullivan PS. Home-Based HIV Testing and Counseling for Male Couples (Project Nexus): A Protocol for a Randomized Controlled Trial. JMIR Res Protoc. 2017;6(5):e101. https://doi.org/10.2196/resprot.7341.

24. Katz D GM, Hughes J, Farquhar C, Stekler J. : HIV self-testing increases HIV testing frequency among high-risk men who have sex with men: a randomized controlled trial. In: IAS 2015 8th Conference on HIV Pathogenesis, Treatment and Prevention July 19–22, 2015. Vancouver; 2015.

25. Elliot E, Rossi M, McCormack S, McOwan A: Identifying undiagnosed HIV in men who have sex with men (MSM) by offering HIV home sampling via online gay social media: a service evaluation. Sex Transm Infect 2016, 24(052090):2015–052090.

26. Phillips AN, Cambiano V, Miners A, Lampe FC, Rodger A, Nakagawa F, Brown A, Gill ON, De Angelis D, Elford J, et al. Potential impact on HIV incidence of higher HIV testing rates and earlier antiretroviral therapy initiation in MSM. AIDS. 2015;29(14):1855–62. https://doi.org/10.1097/QAD.0000000000000767.

27. Birrell PJ, Gill ON, Delpech VC, Brown AE, Desai S, Chadborn TR, Rice BD, De Angelis D. HIV incidence in men who have sex with men in England and Wales 2001-10: a nationwide population study. Lancet Infect Dis. 2013;13(4):313–8.

28. McCormack S, Dunn DT, Desai M, Dolling DI, Gafos M, Gilson R, Sullivan AK, Clarke A, Reeves I, Schembri G, et al. Pre-exposure prophylaxis to prevent the acquisition of HIV-1 infection (PROUD): effectiveness results from the pilot phase of a pragmatic open-label randomised trial. Lancet, doi: https://doi.org/10.1016/S0140-6736(1015)00056-00052. 2016;387(10013):53–60 Epub 02015 Sep 00059.

29. White ED, D Gilson, R Sullivan, A Reeves, I Schembri, G Mackie, N Dewsnapp, C Lacy, C Apea, C Brady, M Fox, J Taylor, S Rooney, J Gafos, M Gill, N McCormack, S Long term follow up of PROUD evidence for high continued HIV exposure and durable effectiveness of PrEP. In: IAS 2017: conference on HIV pathogenesis treatment and prevention July 23–26 2017. Paris, France; 2017.

5

Epidemiology of HIV, syphilis, and hepatitis B and C among manual cane cutters in low-income regions of Brazil

Déborah Ferreira Noronha de Castro Rocha[1], Luana Rocha da Cunha Rosa[1], Carla de Almeida Silva[1], Brunna Rodrigues de Oliveira[2], Thaynara Lorrane Silva Martins[1], Regina Maria Bringel Martins[2], Marcos André de Matos[1], Megmar Aparecida dos Santos Carneiro[2], Juliana Pontes Soares[3], Ana Cristina de Oliveira e Silva[3], Márcia Maria de Souza[1], Robert L. Cook[4], Karlla Antonieta Amorim Caetano[1] and Sheila Araujo Teles[1]*

Abstract

Background: In recent decades the epidemic of asymptomatic sexually transmitted infections has extended deep into Brazil, including small towns and rural areas. The purpose of this study was to investigate the epidemiology of HIV, syphilis, and hepatitis B (HBV) and hepatitis C viruses (HCV), and to evaluate immunization coverage against hepatitis B in a group of rural workers in Brazil.

Methods: In 2016, a cross-sectional study was conducted with 937 manual sugarcane cutters of the Midwest and Northeast Regions of Brazil. All individuals were interviewed and screened for HIV, syphilis, HBV and HCV. Correlating factors with lifetime HBV infection were investigated using logistic regression. Positive Predictive Values, Negative Predictive Values, sensitivity and specificity were also calculated relative to vaccination against Hepatitis B, comparing anti-HBs titers to vaccination reports.

Results: Most reported previous hospitalization (55%), occupational injuries (54%), sharing of personal items (45.8%), alcohol consumption (77.2%), multiple sexual partners in previous 12 months (39.8%), and no condom use during sexual intercourse in last 12 months (46.5%). Only 0.2% reported using injection drugs. Anti-HIV-1 was detected in three individuals (0.3%). Serological markers of lifetime syphilis (treponemal test) were detected in 2.5% (95% CI: 1.6–3.6) of participants, and active syphilis (treponemal test and VDRL) present in 1.2%. No samples were positive for anti-HCV. The prevalence of lifetime HBV infection (current or past infection) was 15.9%, and 0.7% (95% CI 0.4 to 1.5) were HBsAg-positive. Previous hospitalization (OR 1.53, CI 1.05–2.24, $p < 0.01$) and multiple sexual partners in the last 12 months (OR 1.80, CI 1.25–2.60, $p < 0.01$) were predictors for lifetime HBV infection. Although 46.7% (95% CI 43.4–49.9) of individuals reported having been vaccinated against hepatitis B, only 20.6% (95% CI 18.1–23.3) showed serological evidence of previous hepatitis B vaccination (positive for anti-HBs alone).

Conclusions: The high prevalence of syphilis and HBV compared to the general population and the high frequency of risk behaviors show the potential for sexual and parenteral dissemination of these agents in this rural population. In addition, the low frequency of hepatitis B vaccinated individuals suggests a need for improved vaccination services.

Keywords: Sexually transmitted diseases, Rural population, Poverty areas, Viral hepatitis vaccines

* Correspondence: sheila.fen@gmail.com
[1]Faculty of Nursing, Federal University of Goias/Universidade Federal de Goiás, Goiânia, GO, Brazil
Full list of author information is available at the end of the article

Background

Despite advancements in prevention and diagnosis, asymptomatic sexually transmitted infections are a major challenge for global infection control [1, 2]. Worldwide, 36.7 million people are living with HIV [3], while approximately 5.6 million new cases of syphilis occur each year [4]. Hepatitis B and C, in turn, are also a major public health challenge, and 325 million people are chronic carriers of these viruses [2]. Although globally the hepatitis B vaccine has decreased the burden of hepatitis B virus infection significantly, most adult individuals remain susceptible to HBV [2].

The distribution of asymptomatic sexually transmitted infections varies worldwide, and studies have shown that social, economic and behavioral conditions influence their epidemiology [4, 5]. Therefore, in general, higher prevalences of HIV, syphilis, and hepatitis B and C have been found in low- and middle-income countries compared to developed countries [4, 6].

In Brazil, the epidemic of HIV infection started in the industrialized regions of the southeast and south, and vulnerable urban groups have the highest burden of this infection [7–9]. However, in the last decade the HIV epidemic has reached inner cities and rural regions, far from the epicenter of the epidemic, where access to health services is limited and often low quality [10]. Further, HIV infection is often accompanied by other asymptomatic sexually transmitted infections such as syphilis and viral hepatitis, which, like HIV, have great potential for dissemination in impoverished vulnerable populations [1]. There are few studies in Brazil on the epidemiology of these infections in less populated regions of the country [8, 10].

Brazil is the largest producer of sugar cane in the world, and sugar cane-based industries are a significant economic activity. Brazil's sugar-alcohol industry employs around 500,000 workers linked exclusively to sugarcane [11] and almost 90% of production takes place in the Central and Southern regions of the country, followed by the Northeast region [12]. Although the mechanization of sugarcane cutting has been expanded in the last decade, this trend occurred predominantly in the Southern Region. In the Midwestern and Northeastern region, manual cane cutting remains the principal mode of cane harvesting. This activity is physically and mentally taxing, and despite advances in working conditions, these individuals still experience exploitation and dangerous working conditions as well as social marginalization [13].

Due the nature of sugar cane cutting, these workers are usually males, young adults, and sexually active [14]. The seasonality of sugarcane cultivation and the possibility of better income encourages the temporary inter-regional migration of workers, who live their lives isolated from their families and partners for months. Most of them live in large communal houses on sugarcane farms, where the sharing of personal care items is frequent. Further, on their days off they visit the cities or villages nearby sugarcane plantations to buy personal items and have fun, which can include binge drinking and unsafe sexual encounters [15].

This corollary of factors may put manual sugar cane cutters at high risk of asymptomatic sexually transmitted infections, and they could be potential disseminators of these infections in remote regions. However, data about the epidemiology of these vulnerable rural workers is virtually non-existent in Brazil. This study estimated HIV, viral hepatitis B and C, and syphilis prevalence, and analyzed risk factors for lifetime HBV infection, and evaluated immunization against hepatitis B in sugarcane cutters in Central and Northeastern Brazil.

Methods

This is a cross-sectional, multicenter study in Goiás (Midwest Region) and Paraíba (Northeast Region), Brazil. Goiás has an estimated population of 6,778,772, monthly nominal household income per capita of $348 and a Human Development Index (HDI) of 0.735. Paraíba has an estimated population of 4,025,558 inhabitants, monthly nominal household income per capita of $240 and HDI of 0.658. The agricultural industry that has been developed in both states has great significance to the national economic situation [16].

In Goiás there are 38 alcohol and sugar producing units distributed across different regions of the state, and in 14 of them manual cane harvesting is still used. Among them, four were in harvest activity during the period of the study, and they were included in the investigation. In Paraíba there are nine alcohol and sugar production plants, only one sugar producing unit was eligible, being that It used manual cutting and was active [17]. This is the largest sugar producing unit in the State.

The minimum required sample, considering a statistical power of 80% ($\beta = 20\%$), significance level of 95%, (< 0,05), precision of 0.5%, design effect of 1.5 and a global prevalence for anti-HIV for the general population at 0.39% [18] was 895 manual sugar cane cutters.

Inclusion criteria were: be a manual sugar cane cutter (by self-report) and be aged 18 years or older. Five alcohol and sugar producing units agreed to participate in the study, representing the manual sugar cane cutters from these regions (Fig. 1).

Data collection was carried out from February to September 2016. All participants signed a free and informed consent form, approved by the research ethics committee of the Federal University of Goiás and Paraíba, according to resolution CNS No. 466/12, under protocols 042796/2015 and 1,507,737/2016, respectively.

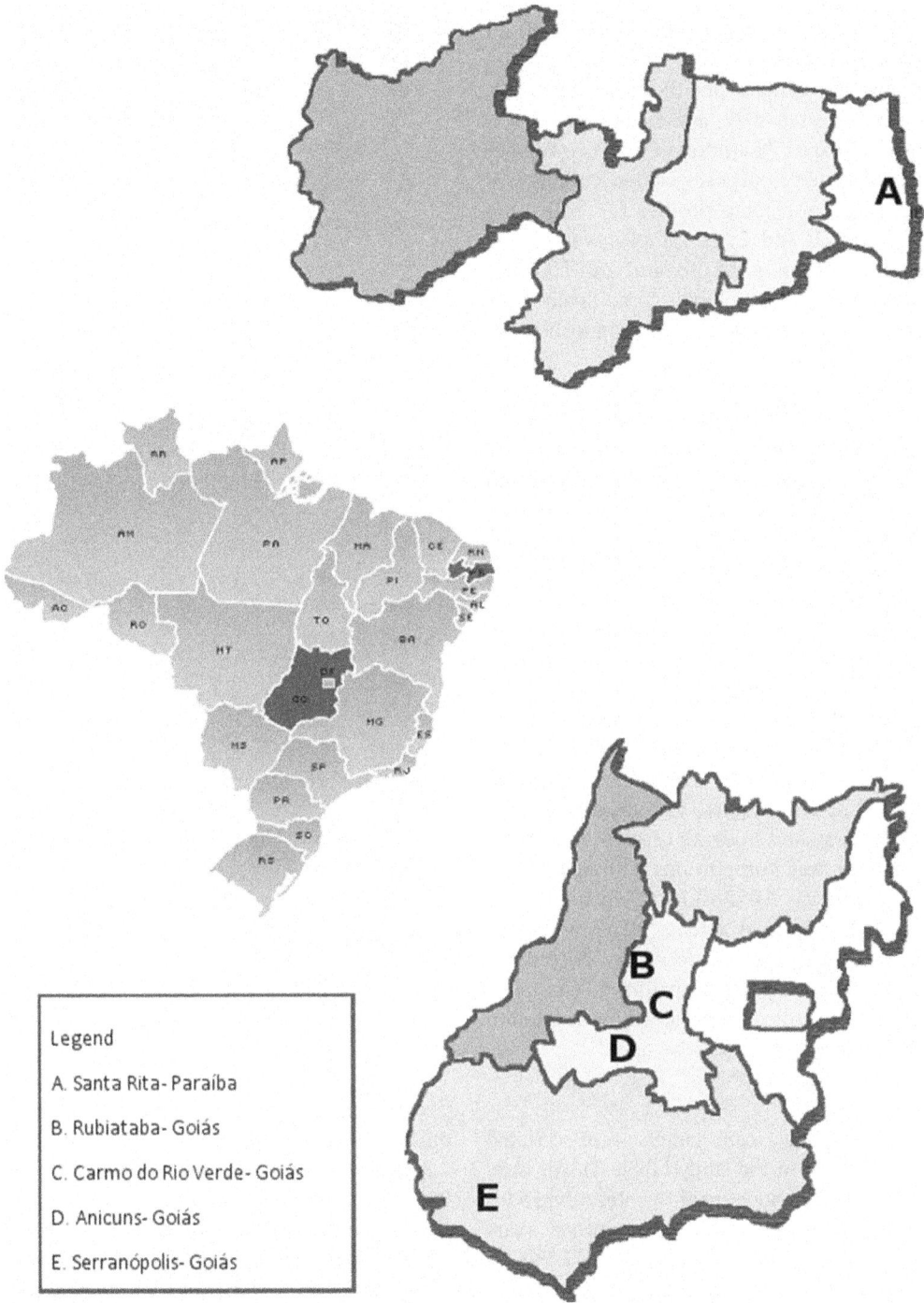

Fig. 1 Geographical location of the sampling sites in the states of Goiás (GO) and Paraíba (PB), Central-West and Northeast regions, respectively

Legend

A. Santa Rita- Paraíba

B. Rubiataba- Goiás

C. Carmo do Rio Verde- Goiás

D. Anicuns- Goiás

E. Serranópolis- Goiás

Participants were interviewed by trained research assistants using a structured script containing questions about sociodemographic characteristics, work characteristics, risk behaviors for sexually transmitted infections (STIs), also referred to as sexually transmitted diseases (STDs) and viral hepatitis, as well as vaccination status. "Reported Shared Accommodation" was defined as individuals who shared their living space with roommates or flatmates, or in shared employer-provided housing.

Rapid screening tests for HIV (Bioeasy HIV, Republic of Korea) and syphilis (Alere Syphilis, Republic of Korea) were performed on all participants, as well as confirmatory rapid tests for HIV (Abon™ HIV 1/2/O, China). For complementary serological tests for syphilis, hepatitis B, and C, 10 ml of blood were collected.

For syphilis, positive samples per the treponemal test (Rapid Test) were retested by a non-treponemal test - venereal disease research laboratory (VDRL) (Wiener Lab, Argentina). For study purposes, active syphilis was defined as the participant being positive for both tests [19, 20]. For hepatitis B and C, all samples were tested for HBsAg, anti-HBs, total anti-HBc, and anti-HCV by enzymatic immunoassay using Biokit S.A., Spain. Persons with positive tests were referred for diagnostic confirmation and/or treatment.

Interview data and serological test results were digitized and analyzed using the STATA statistical software version 13.0 (StataCorp, College Station, TX). Prevalences were calculated with 95% confidence intervals. Univariate and multivariate analyses were performed to identify factors associated with lifetime HBV infection. The term "lifetime HBV infection" refers to the presence of the HBsAg and/ or anti-HBc markers, indicating current or past HBV infection. Therefore, for the purposes of analysis, cases that showed isolated positivity for anti-HBs were excluded. Initially, risk factors for seropositivity to lifetime HBV infection were estimated. Those factors that presented a statistically significant association ($p < 0.20$) were subjected to multivariate Logistic regression analysis and controlled by "work region". The Chi-squared, Chi-squared test for trend, Fisher's exact test, and student's t tests were used to evaluate differences between proportions. The significance level used in the tests was 5%. Positive Predictive Values (PPV) and Negative Predictive Values (NPV) were also calculated for sensitivity and specificity related to self-reported vaccination against Hepatitis B (complete series), considering the serological profile of immunization as the gold standard (i.e. HBsAb positive only).

Results

A total of 937 manual sugar cane cutters were recruited and agreed to participate in the study (Table 1). All were male and 68.9% were under 40 years of age. Regarding education, almost half (47.4%) reported having 4 or fewer years of education. Most participants were married (77.5%). In terms of region, 85.7% were from the Northeast of the country; however, 67.9% worked in plants located in the Central region of Brazil. The average monthly salary was $554.10.

Table 2 shows risk factors for sexual and bloodborne pathogens reported by the sugar cane cutters in this study (Table 2). Most reported previous hospitalization (55%), occupational injuries (54%), sharing of personal items – such as razor blades, nail pliers, toothbrushes (45.8%), alcohol consumption (77.2%), age of first sexual intercourse before 16 years old (49.4%), multiple sexual

Table 1 Sociodemographic characteristics of manual sugar cane cutters in the Northeast and Central regions of Brazil, 2016 ($n = 937$)

Variables	Participants $n = 937$	%
Sex		
Male	937	100.0
Age[a] mean (standard deviation)	35.4 (9.2)	
= < 29	266	28.4
30–39	380	40.5
= > 40	291	31.1
Education[a] mean (standard deviation)	5.2 (3.6)	
< = 4	444	47.4
> 4	493	52.6
Civil Status		
Married	726	77.5
Single	211	22.5
Region of Origin		
Northeast	803	85.7
Midwest	129	13.8
North	4	0.4
Southeast	1	0.1
Work region		
Paraíba	301	32.1
Goiás	636	67.9
Income[b] mean (standard deviation)	554.1 (165.7)	
≤ 461	326	34.8
462–615	412	44
> 616	199	21.2

[a]Years; [b]US$/per month

partners (last 12 months) (39.8%), and no condom use during sexual intercourse (last 12 months) (46.5%).

Anti-HIV-1 was detected in three individuals (0.3%; 95% CI: 0.1–1.0). Serological markers of lifetime syphilis (Treponemal test) were detected in 2.5% (95% CI: 1.6–3.6) of sugar cane cutters, and of active syphilis (Treponemal test and VDRL) in 1.2% (95% CI: 0.6–2.1). The prevalence of lifetime HBV infection was 15.9% (95% CI: 13.7–18.4), where 0.7% (95% CI: 0.4–1.5) were HBsAg-positive, 9.8% (95% CI: 8.1–11.9) were for both anti-HBs and anti-HBc markers, and 5.3% (95% CI: 4.1–7.0) were positive for anti-HBc alone. No samples tested positive for anti-HCV (Table 3).

Among those sugar cane cutters positive for HBsAg and/or anti-HBc ($n = 149$), 4% (6/149) of the subjects were also positive by the Treponemal tests, 2% (3/149) for VDRL and one for anti-HIV-1 (0.7%).

Table 2 Risk factors for sexual and bloodborne pathogens in manual sugar cane cutters in the Northeast and Central regions of Brazil, 2016 (n = 937)

Variables	N	%
Knowledge of signs or symptoms of STI in women (no)	639	68.2
Knowledge of signs or symptoms of STI in men (no)	600	64
Tattoos or piercings on body (yes)	106	11.3
Previous transfusion (yes)	38	4.1
Previous hospitalization (yes)	515	55
Previous occupational injuries (yes)	505	54
Reported shared accommodation (yes)	277	29.6
Sharing sharp personal care items (yes)	429	45.8
History of incarceration (yes)	90	9.6
History of drug use (yes)	126	13.4
History of marijuana use (yes)	110	11.7
History of cocaine/crack use (yes)	43	4.6
History of injection drug use (yes)	2	0.2
Drinking alcohol (yes)	723	77.2
Age of first sexual intercourse = < 15 years (15.7; 2.7)[a]	463	49.4
History of STI (yes)	101	10.8
History of homosexual relations (yes)	52	5.5
History of sexual abuse (yes)	13	1.4
Sexual partner number = > 2 in the last 12 months (2.8; 4.6)[a]	373	39.8
No condom use at least once in the past 12 months	436	46.5
Report of genital ulcer/sore in the last 12 months (yes)	34	3.6
Report of genital discharge in the last 12 months (yes)	29	3.1

[a]Mean; standard deviation

Table 3 Prevalences of HBV, HCV, HIV, and Syphilis serological markers in manual sugar cane cutters in the Northeast and Central regions of Brazil, 2016 (n = 937)

Serological markers	Positive		(CI 95%)[a]
	n	%	
Isolated HBsAg	1	0.1	0.0–0.6
HBsAg + anti-HBc	6	0.6	0.3–1.4
Anti-HBs + anti-HBc	92	9.8	8.1–11.9
Anti-HBc alone	50	5.3	4.1–7.0
Lifetime HBV infection	149	15.9	13.7–18.4
Anti-HBs alone	193	20.6	18.1–23.3
Anti-HCV	0	–	
Lifetime Syphilis (TT)[b]	23	2.5	1.6–3.6
Active Syphilis (TT[b] and VDRL[c])	11	1.2	0.6–2.1
Anti-HIV	3	0.3	0.1–1.0

[a]CI: Confidence Interval [b]TT: treponemal test [c]VDRL Venereal disease research laboratory

In univariate analyses for lifetime HBV infection, six variables showed p value < 0.20 and were included in the multivariate model: civil status, history of incarceration, history of marijuana use, history of cocaine/crack, previous hospitalization, age at first sexual intercourse, history of STI, number of sexual partners and no condom use at least once in the past 12 months. The final model showed previous hospitalization (OR 1.53, CI 1.05–2.24, p = 0.027) and multiple sexual partners in the last 12 months (OR 1.8, CI 1.25–2.60, p < 0.01) were predictors for lifetime HBV infection among the sugar cane cutters investigated (Table 4).

Although 46.7% (95% CI: 43.4–49.9) of individuals reported having been vaccinated against hepatitis B, only 20.6% (95% CI: 18.1–23.3) showed serological profile of previous hepatitis B vaccination (positive for anti-HBs alone) and the mean age was 30.7 years (SD: 8.5). Therefore, self-reported previous HBV vaccination reports showed a positive predictive value and specificity to identify individuals immunized against hepatitis B of only 27.6% and 57.4%, respectively. The negative predictive value and sensitivity of the vaccination report were 85.6% and 62.7%, respectively.

Discussion

In Brazil, the epidemic of HIV/AIDS is moving from urban centers and reaching small cities and villages [10], and this investigation supports this dynamic. Most rural workers were poor seasonal migrants with low education, from small cities of the poorest regions of Brazil (North and Northeast). In fact, the anti-HIV-1 prevalence found among these sugar cane cutters was similar to that found in the general population in Brazil and worldwide. In 2016, the World Health Organization reported a prevalence of 0.8% [0.7–0.9%] in adults [21], and in Brazil, a rate of 0.39% among people aged 15 to 49 years is estimated [18].

The potential of HIV dissemination in the study population may be measured by the prevalence of other sexually transmitted infections. Unlike HIV, the lifetime syphilis prevalence found among study participants was higher than that estimated in the general population worldwide and in Brazil [18, 22]. A meta-analysis including data of 154 countries showed a global pooled mean prevalence of 1.11% (95% CI: 0.99–1.22). Further, when only studies carried out in American regions were considered, the prevalence decreased to 0.13 (95% CI: 0.09–0.19) [20]. In Brazil, a survey carried out among 35,460 Brazilian male conscripts found a lifetime syphilis prevalence of 0.55% (95% CI: 0.45–0.61) [23].

Concerning hepatitis B, though the prevalence of lifetime HBV infection suggests a low HBV endemicity among the sugarcane cutters investigated, it should be emphasized this prevalence was slightly higher than that

Table 4 Univariate and multivariate analyses of risk factors associated with HBV of sugar cane cutters, Northeast and Central regions of Brazil, 2016

Variable	Univariate analysis[a]				Multivariate analysis[a]	
	HBV		Pvalue	OR[b](95% CI)	HBV	
	Positive (n = 149)	Negative (595)			Pvalue	OR[b] (95% CI)
Age (years) (36.7; 8.9)[c]						
18–29	31 (19.4%)	129 (80.6%)		1		
30–39	65 (20.4%)	254 (79.6%)	0.796	1.06 (0.66–1.71)		
> =40	53 (20%)	212 (80%)	0.875	1.04 (0.63–1.70)		
Education (years) (4.7; 3.5)[c]						
< =4	74 (19.2%)	311 (80.8%)		1		
> 4	75 (20.9%)	284 (79.1%)	0.569	1.10 (0.77–1.59)		
Civil Status						
Married	110 (18.5%)	484 (81.5%)		1		1
Single	39 (26%)	111 (74%)	0.042	1.54 (1.02–2.35)	0.300	1.27 (0.81–1.98)
Reported shared accommodation						
No	112 (21%)	422 (79%)		1		
Yes	37 (17.6%)	173 (82.4%)	0.304	0.80 (0.53–1.22)		
Work region						
Northeast	44 (17.7%)	204 (82.3%)		1		
Midwest	105 (21.2%)	391 (78.8%)	0.271	1.24 (0.84–1.84)		
History of incarceration						
No	129 (19.3%)	541 (80.7%)		1		1
Yes	20 (27%)	54 (73%)	0.115	1.55 (0.89–2.69)	0.122	1.55 (0.89–2.70)
History of marijuana use						
No	136 (20.9%)	516 (79.1%)		1		1
Yes	13 (14.1%)	79 (85.9%)	0.134	0.62 (0.34–1.15)	0.084	0.58 (0.31–1.08)
History of cocaine/crack use						
No	147 (20.7%	564 (79.3%)		1		1
Yes	2 (6.1%)	31 (93.9%)	0.058	0.25 (0.6–1.05)	0.067	0.26 (0.06–1.10)
Tattoos or piercings on body						
No	131 (19.8%)	530 (80.2%)		1		
Yes	18 (21.7%)	65 (78.3%)	0.689	1.12 (0.64–1.95)		
Drinking alcohol						
No	29 (16.8%)	144 (83.2%)		1		
Yes	120 (21%)	451 (79%)	0.222	1.32 (0.84–2.06)		
Previous transfusion						
No	144 (20.1%)	574 (79.9%)		1		
Yes	5 (19.2%)	21 (80.8%)	0.918	0.95 (0.35–2.56)		
Previous hospitalization						
No	54 (16.2%)	280 (83.8%)		1		1
Yes	95 (23.2%)	315 (76.8%)	0.018	1.56 (1.07–2.26)	0.027	1.53 (1.05–2.24)
Previous work accident						
No	64 (18.5%)	281 (81.5%)		1		
Yes	85 (21.3%)	314 (78.7%)	0.350	1.18 (0.83–1.71)		

Table 4 Univariate and multivariate analyses of risk factors associated with HBV of sugar cane cutters, Northeast and Central regions of Brazil, 2016 (Continued)

Variable	Univariate analysis[a]		Pvalue	OR[b](95% CI)	Multivariate analysis[a]	
	HBV				HBV	
	Positive	Negative			Pvalue	OR[b] (95% CI)
	(n = 149)	(595)				
Sharing sharp personal care items						
No	78 (18.8%)	337 (81.2%)		1		
Yes	71 (21.6%)	258 (78.4%)	0.346	1.18 (0.83–1.70)		
Age at first sexual intercourse (years) (15.7; 2.7)[c]						
7–15	86 (22.9%)	289 (77.1%)		1		1
>=16	63 (17.1%)	306 (82.9%)	0.046	0.69 (0.48–0.99)	0.116	0.74 (0.51–1.07)
History of STI						
No	126 (18.9%)	539 (81.1%)		1		1
Yes	23 (29.1%)	56 (70.9%)	0.035	1.75 (1.04–2.96)	0.088	1.59 (0.93–2.72)
History of homosexual relations						
No	139 (19.8%)	564 (80.2%)		1		
Yes	10 (24.4%)	31 (75.6%)	0.474	1.30 (0.62–2.73)		
History of sexual abuse						
No	146 (19.9%)	589 (80.1%)		1		
Yes	3 (33.3%)	6 (66.7%)	0.325	2.02 (0.49–8.16)		
Number of sexual partners in the last 12 months (2.6; 3.4)[c]						
<=1	74 (16.2%)	383 (83.8%)		1		1
>=2	75 (26.1%)	212 (73.9%)	0.001	1.83 (1.27–2.63)	0.002	1.8 (1.25–2.60)
No condom use at least once in the past 12 months						
No	84 (22.2%)	295 (77.8%)		1		1
Yes	65 (17.8%)	300 (82.2%)	0.138	0.76 (0.53–1.09)	0.866	1.04 (0.67–1.61)
Report of genital ulcer/sore in the last 12 months						
No	140 (19.6%)	573 (80.4%)		1		
Yes	9 (29%)	22 (71%)	0.205	1.67 (0.75–3.72)		
Report of genital discharge in the last 12 months						
No	144 (20.1%)	574 (79.9%)		1		
Yes	5 (19.2%)	21 (80.8%)	0.918	0.95 (0.35–2.56)		

[a]Logistic Regression, adjusted by work region; [b]Odds Ratio; [c]Mean; standard deviation

estimated in the urban population (20 to 69 year) from the Midwest (12.4%; 95% CI: 11.1–14.3) and Northeast (12.1%; 95% CI: 10.5–13.9) regions of Brazil [24]. On the other hand, this prevalence was similar to that reported recently in populations at risk for STIs, such as sex workers (17.1%; 95% CI: 11.6–23.4) [25] and men who have sex with men (MSM) (15.4%; 95% CI: 8.7–25.8) in Goiás [26]. In addition, seven individuals were HBsAg positive, being therefore potential disseminators of HBV. Further, six individuals had been infected by HBV and *T. pallidum*, and three of them had active syphilis. One sugar cane cutter had been infected by HBV and HIV.

The asymptomatic characteristics of these infections favor their quiet dissemination. In the absence of knowledge of these diseases, diagnosis and treatment, they scatter efficiently in vulnerable populations that present risk behaviors, like manual sugarcane cutters [27, 28]. In this study, these conditions favorable to STI dissemination were present. The average education level reported was only 4 years of study and few had knowledge about STIs and access to public health services. Indeed, of the total, 40% had not sought health services in the last 12 months, and 30% had only sought health services one time (data not shown).

The analyses of potential risk factors for HBV identified two predictors: multiple partners and previous hospitalization. HBV sexual transmission is well established [2], and supports the potential of sugar cane cutters as disseminators of other STIs, including HIV. In fact, the use of condoms during sexual intercourse is not a regular practice and the consumption of alcohol is high in this population. These behaviors have encouraged the spread of STIs [1, 29].

In this investigation, the high frequency of previous hospitalization ($n = 520$) was a surprise, and we could speculate that this occurred due to workplace hazards including those that present multiple health-risk situations [30]. In this study, 509/943 individuals reported an occupational injury, and 156/943 suffered one in the last 12 months. These rural workers are exposed to long daily shifts and numerous injuries, including stress, dehydration, bites of venomous animals, accidents, burns by sunburn or by fire, poisoning by pesticide residues, etc. [30–32]. Sometimes these situations require health care and hospitalizations, which in low-income regions may be a cause of HBV infection [33]. This is often a consequence of a lack of resources to perform proper hygiene as well as staff trained in proper patient safety procedures. Brazil is a continental country with large economic and cultural diversity [34]. Therefore, the findings of previous hospitalization as a predictor of lifetime HBV infection among sugar cane cutters, suggest HBV dissemination in healthcare facilities where infection control measures may be a luxury where qualified human resources, equipment, and supplies are scarce, favoring parenteral transmission. In fact, previous studies conducted in Brazil have also shown an association between invasive medical procedures and HBV infection [35–37].

Hepatitis B vaccine is the main preventive measure against HBV infection [2]. In Brazil, currently, the HBV vaccine is available free of charge for the entire population [22]. Despite this policy, vaccine coverage is still low among adults, mainly men [38]. In this investigation, only 20.6% of sugarcane cutters had isolated anti-HBs protective titers, indicating previous immunization. Low education, low-income and lack of public health services very probably contributed to these findings. In fact, some authors have shown that individuals with a greater understanding of the disease and with a higher economic level tend to be vaccinated against hepatitis B compared to those who are unaware of hepatitis B vaccine [39].

The best information about an individual's previous vaccination is their vaccination card [40]. If it is not available, many health professionals trust in the verbal report of previous vaccination [41]. However, this study supports that a hepatitis B vaccination self-report is not an accurate indicator of previous vaccination status. In fact, our findings showed that a self-report of HBV vaccination had a sensitivity and specificity of 62.7% and 57.4% to identify individuals immunized against HBV, respectively. In a study conducted in the United States with 818 individuals of an integrated health care system, better results were found (sensitivity and specificity of 73% and 67%, respectively), but the social differences between these two populations are noteworthy, including education and income [42]. Therefore, a report of previous hepatitis B vaccination should not be considered an indicator of hepatitis B immunization, mainly in impoverished populations. For these populations, in the absence of the vaccination card, "Don't Ask, Vaccinate"! [43].

There were no cases of hepatitis C among the individuals investigated. HCV is predominantly transmitted by blood. Therefore, transfusion of unscreened blood and sharing of syringes and needles among drug addicts has been the major cause of HCV transmission [2]. However, these were uncommon among the individuals studied and should explain in part our findings.

This investigation has some limitations. Initially, due to financial restrictions the data collection was carried out in February and March in Paraíba, Northeast Region, which is the period at the end of the sugar cane harvest season. Therefore, only one mill was included in the study. However, this represents the biggest mill in the region. Further, the study was conducted in only two states, and may not represent all Brazilian manual sugar cane cutters, although these two states represent the most significant alcohol producing areas in Brazil. All interviews were performed face-to-face, therefore some personal and private questions may have biased responses, and therefore underestimate the prevalence of such sensitive variables as condom use, sex with men who have sex with men (MSM), illicit drug use, etc. Otherwise, some strategies were used to minimize potential biases: previously trained male interviewers, and private places for interviews.

Conclusion

This research presents the situation of poor, rural workers from non-industrialized areas of Brazil, a population often disregarded from a public health standpoint. The situation of these young men includes wide circulation of HIV and high prevalences of syphilis and HBV compared to the national population. In addition, the variables associated with HBV infection, multiple partners and previous hospitalization, showed the risk of dissemination of sexually and parenterally transmitted infections in this rural population. Finally, the low frequency of individuals vaccinated against hepatitis B suggests a need for improved vaccination services. It is therefore recommended that sugar and ethanol plants act to strengthen specific prevention and health promotion programs for rural sugarcane workers in Brazil.

Abbreviation

CI: Confidence Interval; HBV: Hepatitis B virus; HCV: Hepatitis C virus; HDI: Human development index; HIV: Human immunodeficiency virus; MSM: Men who have sex with men; NPV: Negative predictive values; PPV: Positive predictive values; STD: Sexually transmitted disease; STI: Sexually transmitted infection; TT: Treponemal test; VDRL: Venereal disease research laboratory

Acknowledgements

We would like to thank the members of the Center for Studies in Epidemiology and Care in Infectious Diseases, with emphasis on Viral Hepatitis/ *Núcleo de Estudos em Epidemiologia e Cuidados em Agravos Infecciosos, com ênfase em Hepatites Virais* (NECAIH) for their participation during the planning, execution, and evaluation of this study. Brian Ream edited this manuscript in English.

Funding

This study was made possible by the financial support of the National Counsel of Scientific and Technological Development in Brazil/*Conselho Nacional de Desenvolvimento Científico e Tecnológico do Brasil*, funding call: CNPq Universal/2014, and by the University Extension Program/*Programa de Extensão Universitária* (ProExt 2016/2017).

Authors' contributions

DFNCR study concept and design, data collection, literature search. LRCR study concept and design, data collection, literature search. CAS study concept and design, data collection, literature search. BRO data collection, literature search. TLSM data collection, literature search. RMBM study concept and design, data collection, literature search. MAM study concept and design, data collection, literature search. MASC study concept and design, data collection, literature search. JPS study concept and design, data collection, literature search. ACOS study concept and design, data collection, literature search. MMS study concept and design, data collection, literature search. KAAC study concept and design, literature search, data collection, statistical analyses, data interpretation and supervision, drafting of the manuscript. RLC critical revision of the manuscript for important intellectual content. SAT study concept and design, data collection, critical revision of the manuscript for important intellectual content and supervision. All authors read and approved the final manuscript.

Competing interests

The authors declare that they have no competing interests.

Author details

[1]Faculty of Nursing, Federal University of Goias/Universidade Federal de Goiás, Goiânia, GO, Brazil. [2]Institute of Tropical Pathology and Public Health, Federal University of Goias/Universidade Federal de Goiás, Goiânia, GO, Brazil. [3]Faculty of Nursing, Federal University of Paraiba/Universidade Federal da Paraíba, João Pessoa, PB, Brazil. [4]Department of Epidemiology, College of Public Health and Health Professions and College of Medicine, University of Florida, Gainesville, FL, USA.

References

1. Unemo M, Bradshaw CS, Hocking JS, de Vries HJC, Francis SC, Mabey D, Marrazzo JM, Sonder GJB, Schwebke JR, Hoornenborg E, Peeling RW, Philip SS, Low N, Fairley CK. Sexually transmitted infections: challenges ahead. Lancet Infect Dis. 2017;17(8)::e235–e279. https://doi.org/10.1016/S1473-3099(17)30310-9..

2. World Health Organization [WHO]. Global Hepatitis Report. (2017). http://apps.who.int/iris/bitstream/10665/255016/1/9789241565455-eng.pdf?ua=1. Accessed 19 Jan 2018.

3. World Health Organization [WHO]. HIV/AIDS Fact sheet Updated July 2017. (2017). http://www.who.int/mediacentre/factsheets/fs360/en/. Accessed 19 Jan 2018.

4. Peeling RW, Mabey D, Kamb ML, Chen XS, Radolf JD, Benzaken AS. Syphilis. Nat Rev Dis Primers. 2017;3:17073. https://doi.org/10.1038/nrdp.2017.73.

5. Frew PM, Parker K, Vo L, Haley D, O'Leary A, Diallo DD, Golin CE, Kuo I, Soto-Torres L, Wang J, Adimora AA, Randall LA, Del Rio C, Hodder S, HIV Prevention Trials Network 064 (HTPN) Study Team. Socioecological factors influencing women's HIV risk in the United States: qualitative findings from the women's HIV SeroIncidence study (HPTN 064). BMC Public Health. 2016; 16(1):803. https://doi.org/10.1186/s12889-016-3364-7.

6. Degenhardt L, Peacock A, Colledge S, Leung J, Grebely J, Vickerman P, Stone J, Cunningham EB, Trickey A, Dumchev K, Lynskey M, Griffiths P, Mattick RP, Hickman M, Larney S. Global prevalence of injecting drug use and sociodemographic characteristics and prevalence of HIV, HBV, and HCV in people who inject drugs: a multistage systematic review. Lancet Glob Health. 2017;5(12):e1192–e1207. https://doi.org/10.1016/S2214-109X(17)30375-3.

7. Saffier IP, Kawa H, Harling G. A scoping review of prevalence, incidence and risk factors for HIV infection amongst young people in Brazil. BMC Infect Dis. 2017;17(1):675. https://doi.org/10.1186/s12879-017-2795-9.

8. Souto FJ. Distribution of hepatitis B infection in Brazil: the epidemiological situation at the beginning of the 21 st century. Rev Soc Bras Med Trop. 2016;49(1):11–23. https://doi.org/10.1590/0037-8682-0176-2015.

9. Puga MA, Bandeira LM, Pompilio MA, Croda J, Rezende GR, Dorisbor LF, Tanaka TS, Cesar GA, Teles SA, Simionatto S, Novais AR, Nepomuceno B, Castro LS, Lago BV, Motta-Castro AR. Prevalence and incidence of HCV infection among prisoners in Central Brazil. PLoS One. 2017;12(1). https://doi.org/10.1371/journal.pone.0169195.

10. Komninakis SV, Mota ML, Hunter JR, Diaz RS. Late presentation HIV/AIDS is still a challenge in Brazil and worldwide. AIDS Res Hum Retrovir. 2017. https://doi.org/10.1089/AID.2015.0379.

11. União da Indústria de Cana-de-Açúcar [ÚNICA]. Avanço Da Mecanização Incentiva Adoção De Tecnologias De Última Geração Em Sp. (2013). http://www.unica.com.br/noticia/2981091792031019628/avancodamecanizacaoincentivaadocaodetecnologiasdeultimageracaoemsp. Accessed 19 Jan 2018.

12. Companhia Nacional de Abastecimento [CONAB]. Acompanhamento Da Safra Brasileira De Cana-De-Açúcar, Primeiro Levantamento, Abril 2017. Monitoramento agrícola – Cana-de-açúcar. 2017;4(1):1–57 http://www.conab.gov.br/OlalaCMS/uploads/arquivos/17_04_20_14_04_31_boletim_cana_portugues_-_1o_lev_-_17-18.pdf. Accessed 19 Jan 2018.

13. Morte CC. Por Exaustão No Trabalho. Universidade Federal da Bahia, Salvador. Caderno CRH. 2017;30(79):105–20 http://www.redalyc.org/articulo.oa?id=347651659007. Accessed 19 Jan 2018.

14. Costa PFF, Silva MS, Santos SL. O desenvolvimento (in)sustentável do agronegócio canavieiro. Ciênc saúde coletiva. 2014;19(10):3971–80. https://doi.org/10.1590/1413-812320141910.09472014.

15. Rosendo JS, Matos PF. Social impacts with the end of the manual sugarcane harvest: a case study in Brazil. Sociol Int J. 2017;1(4). https://doi.org/10.15406/sij.2017.01.00020.

16. Instituto Brasileiro de Geografia e Estatística[IBGE]. Conheça Cidades E Estados Do Brasil. (2017). https://cidades.ibge.gov.br/brasil. Accessed 19 Jan 2018.

17. Novacana. As usinas de Açúcar e Etanol do Brasil. (2017). https://www.novacana.com/usinas_brasil/. Accessed 19 Jan 2018.

18. Ministério da Saúde. Secretaria de Vigilância em Saúde. Boletim Epidemiológico HIV. Brasília. 2015;4(1).

19. Henao-Martínez AF, Johnson SC. Diagnostic tests for syphilis: new tests and new algorithms. Neurol Clin Pract. 2014;4(2):114–22. https://doi.org/10.1212/01.CPJ.0000435752.17621.48.

20. Smolak A, Rowley J, Nagelkerke N, Kassebaum NJ, Chico RM, Korenromp EL, Abu-Raddad LJ. Trends and predictors of syphilis prevalence in the general population: global pooled analyses of 1103 prevalence measures including 136 million syphilis tests. Clin Infect Dis. 2017. https://doi.org/10.1093/cid/cix975.

21. World Health Organization [WHO]. Data on the size of the HIV/AIDS epidemic. (2017). http://apps.who.int/gho/data/view.main.22500WHOREG?lang=en Acessed 19 Jan 2018.

22. Brasil. Ministério da Saúde. Secretaria de Vigilância em Saúde. Departamento de DST, Aids e Hepatites Virais. Protocolo Clínico e Diretrizes Terapêuticas para Atenção Integral às Pessoas com Infecções Sexualmente Transmissíveis / Ministério da Saúde, Secretaria de Vigilância em Saúde, Departamento de DST, Aids e Hepatites Virais. – Brasília: Ministério da Saúde. 2015. p. 120. ISBN 978-85-334-2352-7.

23. Ribeiro D, Rezende EF, Pinto VM, Pereira GF, Miranda AE. Prevalence of and risk factors for syphilis in Brazilian armed forces conscripts. Sex Transm Infect. 2012;88(1):32–4. https://doi.org/10.1136/sextrans-2011-050066.

24. Pereira LM, Martelli CM, Merchán-Hamann E, Montarroyos UR, Braga MC, de Lima ML, Cardoso MR, Turchi MD, Costa MA, de Alencar LC, Moreira RC, Figueiredo GM, Ximenes RA. Hepatitis study group. Population-based multicentric survey of hepatitis B infection and risk factor differences among three regions in Brazil. Am J Trop Med Hyg. 2009;81(2):240–7.

25. Matos MA, França DDDS, Carneiro MADS, Martins RMB, Kerr LRFS, Caetano KAA, Pinheiro RS, Araújo LA, Mota RMS, Matos MAD, Motta CARC, Teles SA. Viral hepatitis in female sex workers using the respondent-driven sampling. Rev Saude Publica. 2017;51:65. https://doi.org/10.1590/S1518-8787.2017051006540.

26. Oliveira MP, MA1 M, Silva AM, Lopes CL, Teles SA, Matos MA, Spitz N, Araujo NM, Mota RM, Kerr LR, Martins RM. Prevalence, risk behaviors, and Virological characteristics of hepatitis B virus infection in a Group of men who Have sex with men in Brazil: results from a respondent-driven sampling survey. PLoS One. 2016;11(8). https://doi.org/10.1371/journal.pone.0160916.

27. Mendoza C. Hot news: HIV epidemics - current burden and future prospects. AIDS Rev. 2017;19(4).

28. O'Hara GA, McNaughton AL, Maponga T, Jooste P, Ocama P, Chilengi R, Mokaya J, Liyayi MI, Wachira T, Gikungi DM, Burbridge L, O'Donnell D, Akiror CS, Sloan D, Torimiro J, Yindom LM, Walton R, Andersson M, Marsh K, Newton R, Matthews PC. Hepatitis B virus infection as a neglected tropical disease. PLoS Negl Trop Dis. 2017;11(10). https://doi.org/10.1371/journal.pntd.0005842.

29. Gamarel KE, Nichols S, Kahler CW, Westfall AO, Lally MA, Wilson CM. Adolescent medicine trials network for HIV/AIDS intervention. A cross-sectional study examining associations between substance use frequency, problematic use and STIs among youth living with HIV. Sex Transm Infect. 2017. https://doi.org/10.1136/sextrans-2017-053334.

30. Rocha FLS, Marziale MHP, Hong S. Work and health conditions of sugar cane workers in Brazil. Rev Esc Enferm USP. 2010;44(4):974–9.

31. Priuli RMA, Moraes MS, Chiaravalloti RM. The impact of stress on the health of sugar cane cutters. Rev Saude Publica. 2014;48(2):225–31.

32. Wesseling C, Aragón A, González M, Weiss I, Glaser J, Bobadilla NA, Roncal-Jiménez C, Correa-Rotter R, Johnson RJ, Barregard L. Kidney function in sugarcane cutters in Nicaragua - a longitudinal study of workers at risk of Mesoamerican nephropathy. Environ Res. 2016;147:125–32.

33. Umare A, Seyoum B, Gobena T, Haile Mariyam T. Hepatitis B virus infections and associated factors among pregnant women attending antenatal Care Clinic at Deder Hospital, eastern Ethiopia. PLoS One. 2016;11(11). https://doi.org/10.1371/journal.pone.0166936.

34. Szwarcwald CL, Junior PRBS, Marques AP, Almeida WS, Montilla DER. Inequalities in healthy life expectancy by Brazilian geographic regions: findings from the National Health Survey 2013. Int J Equity Health. 2016; 15(141). https://doi.org/10.1186/s12939-016-0432-7.

35. Arboleda M, Castilho MC, Fonseca JCF, Albuquerque BC, Saboia RC, Yoshida CFT. Epidemiological aspects of hepatitis B and D virus in the northern region of Amazonas, Brazil. Trans R Soc Trop Med Hyg. 1995;89:481–3.

36. Teles SA, Martins RMB, Silva SA, DMF G, DDP C, Vanderborght BOM, Yoshida CFT. Hepatitis B virus infection profile in central Brazilian hemodialysis population. Rev Inst Med Trop Sao Paulo. 1998;40(5):281–6.

37. Ximenes RA, Figueiredo GM, Cardoso MR, et al. Population-based multicentric survey of hepatitis B infection and risk factors in the north,

38. south, and southeast regions of Brazil, 10-20 years after the beginning of vaccination. Am J Trop Med Hyg. 2015;93(6):1341–8.

38. Nelson NP, Easterbrook PJ, McMahon BJ. Epidemiology of hepatitis B virus infection and impact of vaccination on disease. Clin Liver Dis. 2016;20(4): 607–28. https://doi.org/10.1016/j.cld.2016.06.006.

39. Zhu D, Guo N, Wang J, Nicholas S, Wang Z, Zhang G, Shi L, Wangen KR. Socioeconomic inequality in hepatitis B vaccination of rural adults in China. Hum Vaccin Immunother. 2017;26. https://doi.org/10.1080/21645515.2017.1396401.

40. Murray CJ, Shengelia B, Gupta N, Moussavi S, Tandon A, Thieren M. Validity of reported vaccination coverage in 45 countries. Lancet. 2003;362(9389): 1022–7. https://doi.org/10.1016/S0140-6736(03)14411-X.

41. Schweitze A, Akmatov MK, Krause G. Hepatitis B vaccination timing: results from demographic health surveys in 47 countries. Bull World Health Organ. 2017;95(3):199–209. https://doi.org/10.2471/BLT.16.178822.

42. Rolnick SJ, Parker ED, Nordin JD, Hedblom BD, Wei F, Kerby T, Jackson JM, Crain AL, Euler G. Self-report compared to electronic medical record across eight adult vaccines: do results vary by demographic factors? Vaccine. 2013; 37:3928–35. https://doi.org/10.1016/j.vaccine.2013.06.041.

43. Kuo I, Mudrick DW, Strathdee SA, Thomas DL, Sherman SG. Poor validity of self-reported hepatitis B virus infection and vaccination status among young drug users. Clin Infect Dis. 2004;38(4):587–90. https://doi.org/10.1086/381440.

6

Modified genome comparison method: a new approach for identification of specific targets in molecular diagnostic tests using *Mycobacterium tuberculosis* complex as an example

Alireza Neshani[1,2], Reza Kamali Kakhki[1], Mojtaba Sankian[3], Hosna Zare[1], Amin Hooshyar Chichaklu[1], Mahsa Sayyadi[1] and Kiarash Ghazvini[1,4*] (iD)

Abstract

Background: The first step of designing any genome-based molecular diagnostic test is to find a specific target sequence. The modified genome comparison method is one of the easiest and most comprehensive ways to achieve this goal. In this study, we aimed to explain this method with the example of *Mycobacterium tuberculosis* complex and investigate its efficacy in a diagnostic test.

Methods: A specific target was identified using modified genome comparison method and an in-house PCR test was designed. To determine the analytical sensitivity and specificity, 10 standard specimens were used. Also, 230 specimens were used to determine the clinical sensitivity and specificity.

Results: The identity and query cover of our new diagnostic target (5KST) were ≥ 90% with *M. tuberculosis* complex. The 5KST-PCR sensitivity was 100% for smear-positive, culture-positive and 85.7% for smear-negative, culture-positive specimens. All of 100 smear-negative, culture-negative specimens were negative in 5KST-PCR (100% clinical specificity). Analytical sensitivity of 5KST-PCR was approximately 1 copy of genomic DNA per microliter.

Conclusions: Modified genome comparison method is a confident way to find specific targets for use in diagnostic tests. Accordingly, the 5KST-PCR designed in this study has high sensitivity and specificity and can be replaced for conventional TB PCR tests.

Keywords: *Mycobacterium tuberculosis* complex, PCR, Genome comparison method, Specific target, 5KST

Background

One of the methods to find a specific target to use in diagnostic tests is genome comparison method. In this method, the full genome of the organism is compared with close organisms and the most specific sequences can be identified and used for the design of nucleic acid-based diagnostic tests [1]. Unfortunately, this method causes confusion due to the lack of transparency in the protocol, and use of the unfamiliar software. In this study, we applied some changes to the previous method such as defining an obvious pathway using on-line and available software and aimed to employ this method to find a new specific target for *Mycobacterium tuberculosis* complex. It is clear that this new approach to detect specific diagnostic targets is also appropriate in other microorganisms, and it makes the first step of designing any genome-based diagnostic test (finding a specific target) easier.

Tuberculosis (TB) has been among the 10 leading causes of human death since 2000 [2]. It causes more

* Correspondence: Ghazvinik@mums.ac.ir; kiarash_ghazvini@yahoo.com
[1]Antimicrobial Resistance Research Center, Mashhad University of Medical Sciences, Mashhad, Iran
[4]Department of Microbiology and Virology, School of Medicine, Mashhad University of Medical Sciences, Mashhad, Iran
Full list of author information is available at the end of the article

than 1.3 million deaths each year, which is even higher than road traffic accidents and HIV/AIDS [2].

WHO has planned for a 90% reduction in TB deaths by 2030. To achieve this, both parts of diagnosis and treatment must be strengthened. TB is a treatable infection, provided it is diagnosed promptly. The importance of the diagnostic part becomes clearer by knowing this fact that timely diagnosis and treatment from 2000 to 2016, saved the lives of over 53 million people with TB [2].

So far, many laboratory tests have been designed to diagnose TB, but some of these tests despite their high levels of performance, have not been used in high TB burden countries due to the costs [3]. The most common methods for TB diagnosis in low-income countries include acid-fast bacilli microscopy, culture and PCR [4].

PCR is the most important molecular diagnostic method used to detect TB during past two decades, and it has maintained its position despite the introduction of newer methods such as *loop*-mediated isothermal amplification (LAMP). Over the past years, various target sequences were used for TB PCR such as *IS6110*, *mpb64*, *devR*, *hsp65*, 38 KDa (*pstS1*), 30 KDa (*fbpB*), *esat6*, *cfp10*, 16S rDNA gene (*rrs*) and *rpoB* [5–9]. Diagnostic tests based on these targets have high sensitivity and specificity. Nevertheless, sensitivity of the test is greatly reduced on clinical specimens [10, 11]. This reduction of sensitivity can be attributed to the presence of inhibitors in clinical specimens. According to the results of some articles, there are unknown substances in the respiratory specimens (especially sputum) that have been shown to cause 10 to 26% false-negative results in PCR test and thereby reduce the sensitivity [12–14]. other items such as poorly designed primers [15], or partial loss of target DNA during purification [16] are also effective in the reduction of PCR sensitivity, especially on clinical specimens.

Each of the targets used to date has limitations. For example, about two widely used targets (*IS6110*, *mpb64*), it has been shown that in some parts of Southeast Asia, there are strains of *M. tuberculosis* which lack the *IS6110* sequence [17], and the nonspecifically positive result of *mpb64*-PCR was also seen in *M. scrofulaceum* [18].

Therefore, we still need to find a specific and long enough sequence that would allow us to design the best possible diagnostic primers with minimal mispairing, hairpin, and dimer, to enhance the PCR sensitivity.

In this study, by modifying the genome comparison method, we identified a 5 Kbp sequence which is specific for *M. tuberculosis* complex (MTBC) and named it 5KST (5 Kbp Specific Target). It was then used to design a sensitive and highly specific PCR test. Next, the efficacy of this target was evaluated on clinical specimens (true positives and negatives) and pure genomic DNA.

Methods

Employment of this method for the genome of *Mycobacterium tuberculosis* with about 4.4 million bp, required 45–50 h of continuous work. To reduce the errors, all dedicated work of finding the target was divided between 4 people and each part was performed separately. With this approach, 11–12 h were needed for them to investigate their fragments, which were included in three working days (4 h of continuous work per day).

Finding specific target by modified genome comparison method

At this stage, the complete genome sequences of MTBC members were compared with available genomic sequences on nucleotide collection database (a part of NCBI) and the most specific sequence was selected. It should be noted that this instruction can be accomplished for any other microorganisms. The steps are summarized as follows:

1. First, available genomic sequences of MTBC members on NCBI database were determined and one case, preferably RefSeq, was considered as the reference for each species (Table 1).
2. Then, one of these seven items should be selected as the initial basis. For this study, the sequence of *M. tuberculosis* H37Rv (NC_000962.3) was considered as the basis and its genomic sequence was downloaded from the NCBI and cut to about 5000 bp fragments, providing about 882 fragments.
3. Each fragment was compared separately with other NCBI available genomic sequences by blastn (https://blast.ncbi.nlm.nih.gov/Blast.cgi). The required time for each fragment was about 30 s.
4. Then, the blast search results were evaluated, and appropriate fragments were selected. Two criteria were considered for the result evaluation: 1. Presence of all 7 species of MTBC (Table 1) in Blast search results, with both identity and query cover ≥90%. To simplify, we used Ctrl+F of windows operating system. 2. No bacteria other than MTBC

Table 1 MTBC members with available complete genome on NCBI database (preferably RefSeq)

Species	Accession number
Mycobacterium tuberculosis H37Rv	NC_000962.3
Mycobacterium africanum GM041182	NC_015758.1
Mycobacterium bovis AF2122/97	NC_002945.4
Mycobacterium bovis BCG Pasteur 1173P2	NC_008769.1
Mycobacterium canettii CIPT 140010059	NC_015848.1
Mycobacterium caprae strain Allgaeu	NZ_CP016401.1
Mycobacterium microti strain 12	CP010333.1

members would appear with query cover > 10%. Blast search results are sorted by their query cover (by default) and are shown in descending order. So, the bacteria with a query cover > 10% can be easily found with a glance at the end of the list. The required average time for this step was about 2 min to check each fragment.

5. For the second screening, from selected sequences of previous step, the sequence which could identify the most of MTBC members was considered as the most specific sequence (Fig. 1).

Bioinformatics control

A) Comparison with *rpoB*: In this part the *rpoB* gene, an essential target sequence, was used as a positive control in bioinformatic investigations and *rpoB* sequence compared with all registered complete genomes in the nucleotide collection database (*https://www.ncbi.nlm.nih.gov/nuccore/?term=*), using blastn search. Then, all strains of *M. tuberculosis* (with complete genome) identified by this target, were extracted and compared with the strains identified by 5KST. The identity of these two groups showed that the 5KST is conserved among the all registered *M. tuberculosis* strains in nucleotide collection database.

B) Investigating the 5KST conservation with the help of *TB-ARC project* data:

The genomic sequence of 304 strains of *M. tuberculosis*, *M. africanum*, and *M. bovis* related to the TB Antibiotic Resistance Catalog project [19] around the world, were randomly downloaded from the site *(http://olive.broadinstitute.org/projects/tb_arc)* and the presence of 5KST sequence among these 304 strains was studied by blastn search. The geographic regions and the number of randomly studied strains for each region are listed in Table 2.

Primer design

Designing and analysis of primers for the 5 Kbp Specific Target (5KST) was performed with Oligo7 [20] and Oligoanalyzer 3.1 software (https://eu.idtdna.com/calc/analyzer). Primers and 128 bp amplicon sequence are shown in Table 3.

Polymerase chain reaction

PCR reaction was prepared in the total volume of 25 µl containing 1 µl of sample DNA, 2.5 µL of 10× PCR buffer (100 mM Tris-HCl [pH 8.3], 500 mM KCl), 1.5 µL of 25 mM $MgCl_2$, 0.5 µL of 200 µM (each) of the four dNTPs, 1 µL of each 10 µM forward and reverse primers, PCR grade water, and 0.625 U of *Taq DNA polymerase*. The positive control contained 1 ng of *M.*

<NC_000962.3:3127000-3132000 *Mycobacterium tuberculosis* H37Rv, complete genome

ATCTCGTTGAGCGTAAGCTTCTTTCGAGTCATGCGCCCGCCTCGACCACGAGATGCACGTCGCGGTTCGATCGACCCGATCTTCACCTCGTAACCTCGATGCTTAGCAGGATCCAGCTTGACCGCGTTTGGCTCTACCCACTCTTTGAGT
GGCGCCGTCGCCTGTGCCCCATCGGTGTTCATGACGAACGCTTCGAAAGACTTCCTCTTGTGAGCCGGAATGTCTGCGTAAAGAAGTTCCATGTCCGGGAAGTAGACCCGGTCGCCCTCCACGTGGTACTCCTTCGAGGTCCGCTTCT
CGCCGGATCCGATAAACACCGGCCCCAGGCACCGCAGCGTGAGTTCGAACGGCTTCAGGTAGGTGTTCATGCGGCGGACTCCGGGAGTGCGAGAAATAGCGGTCGCGCGTAGCTGTAGACCGGATGGTTTCCGCCCAGGCTGACG
TCGAGGATGCCTCCTTGGAAGGGTCGCGAGAAGACCGAGCCGGCGGCGAATTTGTAGATGTCGCGTTTGCGCAGGGGCATGTCAGCGTATGTGCTCGACGCGACGAATCCACTGCGCTTGACGAGGCGGTACGTCGCGCCGGCGA
GTGCGGCTTCGAGCTCGTCGTCCGTGGGTAGGGATGTCGTGAGCGTCATCAGACTGGCCGCGTCGACTGTCGGCGTGAGTGCGGCGGGTGCTTCTGACTCGGTAAGGTTAAACGCTCCGAACCCGCTTGTCCGTTCGCCGCCCAGCG
CGGAGATCCCTTTCAACAGCCTGGTGAGTAGGCCGAGCTCGGACTCGGATCCGGTCGCCAGCAACCACAGACCCGCGTCCAGCTCGAACCGGAAGTAGCCGACACGGTACGGGTCGGCGTCTTTCTTTCCGTTGTGGATCGCTGCCT
TCGCTGACACGGCGTGGACACCGATCTTGGTCTGCCGCGCCGCGAGTTCTTTCAGGTCGGCCGTGCCATCGAGGAAGCTGCCAAGCTGGGCAGCGGGAAGAAAGCCGATCTTCTTCGCCAGCTTCTTCTGCATACTTGAGCCGTCGG
ACCGAACGCTGTGCAGGGGCTTGGGAACCAGGTAATCGGGCCCCACATAGGGCAGCAGATCGGTCAACCGCAGCGTCGAGCACGCAACGAGTTCGCCAAGCAGCTGCTGGCCACCCATCCGTAGCGCTTCAACGCAAAGCGCAGA
GTAGAGGGTGTCCGCGGGGCAGCTAATCGTGGACGACTCGAGGCCGTGGTCGCCGAAGTGTGTGCGGTCGAAGTCGAACCTAAACAGCCGCGAGTTCATGGTTTAGCTTCTCCAGCAGAGAACCGTCGAGGGCGCCGACTGCGGC
GCGGGCTTTCAGGTTGCTGAACTTGACCTGCCCGTA**GCCACGGGTTCCGCTGCCGCCGAGGTAGTCGAGTTCGAGCAACTTCAGGCCGCGCGCGATGGCGTTGAAGTCCTCGATGATCTC**ATCGGAGGAAGGCAGAGACGCCTTC
TGTTCCTCGCCGGGGGTGCCGAAGGAGACCTCGTAGACAAGTGAGAACGCGAACTCGCTGCCGGGGATCACGCGTTCCATCTGGCGAAGGTTTGCCTTTGCGGTCACCCGGTTGATGGCGTTCTCGAATTTCACCTCGGTGAGAGTC
TTAGCGCCGCGGGCTTCGAGGTCGTCTTTGTTGGTGAGCTTCGTGTCGCGGAAGACGAGTCGGCCCGTCATGTACTCCTCGGTGTCGCCGAAAAGCCGACGGATATGGGCGTGGTCCTCATTCGGCTTCCTGTAAAACGTTTCTGTGT
CGGCGCCGTATTGGCGGGACAGCAAGGTGCGGACCTTGCCCTTCAGGCTGGTACCCGGAATCATCGGCAGCCTGCTCAGCGGATCACGAACGACAGGCTTGTCGACCGCGCCGATGGCGGAGAAGCCATCGCCGGCCCCGATCTGC
AGGCCCGTCAGGACGGTCAGTGTCCCGGTTATCTCGATCTTGGCGTAGCTCGTAGTCATTGGGTTGTCTCACTTGTCCTTCGGATCGAGGTACTTCTTGTATGCGGCTAGGGCTTCCATGTACCGGCAGAATCGCAGCAGCCCGTCGC
GGCTATCGCCTATCCCTTCCAGCGCTTCTAGGAGTTTCGCGTTTCGGACGAATGTCTTAACCGCGTCTTCACGCCCGGACTGGTAGACGAACCGGACCCGCAGGTACTGGACCTTCTCCTTCAGCTGACGCGGGAGCGTGGGGTTGGC
GCTCTGCTGCGCCTCGTCGAAGAGCTGTGCGGTCAGGCTGAGTAGCACCCGCAGCTGGGTTGTGGTCAGCTCGAAGCCGTTCTTTTTCTTTGGCAGGCCGCGAATTACTTCGGCCTGTTTCACATAGTCGTCTTGGATGACGCTCATTC
GGACTCCTCCTTGCGAGTGCGATAGATGTAGAGGTGCAGCGCGGTCTTGAGTTGCTTGGCGTCTGTCGGATCTTGGAACCATTGGTGTAGCCGGTTAGCAAACTGCTGAAAAGGCGCTGTGTCACCGGTGGGGTTACGCATGCGCGT
GAGGAAGTACACCCATCTGGCCTTTGTGATTCGATCGTCGCGTTCGGCGAGTAGTTCGAGCAGCTTGTAGATGAAGGCCATGCCGCGTTCTTCGTTGCCACTGAAATAGTCGGCGATGTGCCGGTACTTCTCCTCGATCACCTTGCTGA
GCAGCTCATCCCAGCCGAAGGTGAACTCGCGATCGAAGAGTGCAACCCCGTTCTTGCCGGGCAGCGACTTCGCCGCGTCTTCGAGATCTCCGACTTCGCGGGCCATCACGGAGATGGGGTACTTGTCGGGGAACATGCCGATGCCAG
CCGACACGGTGAGTTTGCCCTGGGTGAATTCGTGGAACCGCTCCCGAAGCTCGATCCCGAACTCGATGACGTCGTCCCACGCGCCCACGACGAAGACGTCATCGCCACCGGAGTAGATGATCGTGGCCTCGCGGGGCCGCGCCGGG
TCATCGCCGGTGATCGGGCGCAGTTTCGGGCGTGCCAACACGTAGTTGATGTGCTGCCGGAAGAACAACGACAGCATCCGGGAGAACGCGGCCGTGCGGCTAATCGTGTTGAACTTGCCGTTGCCTTGCTCCATGAAGCCGTGCGT
GAATGCCTGGCCCAGGTTATCGACGTCAAGGCGCAGAACCCCGAGGCGCGCGATTCCGCTCGCACGCTTCACGTAGTCACCGAACTCCATCTGTGCGACGTAGTCGCCCACCCAGAGCCCGGTGCCCAAACACTCGCCGGCGAAGAA
CTTGTTCTTCGCGTACCGCCTTCGGGTTTGGGGTTGCTGGAGTGCCTTATCGGCGTCGGCTCGGCTACAGAACGTGAGTGTGGCGCCGAACGGCAGGGGCAGACCTTTGGTGGCGCCGTCAGAGATGAGTAGGAAGCGGCGAGACT
CGGATTGAATCTGCGAAGACGCAGCGGTCAGCGCTTGGCACAGGCTGCACTTTGGCTCGTCGTCGGCGCTGACCGTGCGGTTGACCGTGTGGCACACGCTGCATTCCCGGTCACCTTTCTGACCGTCGTGATCGCGCGAGTTGAGTT
CCCGCAGTTGGTCAGCGCTGTATCGGGCGAGCTTCTTCGCGGAAAGTTGCTCGCTCAACTCACGGTAGAGCCCGCTGTAGCGGAGGGCGCGGTTACTTGCCTGGCTCGCACTCTCGTTCGGCCGACGCATCAGGTCGTTCGCGGCAA
GCGGTACGCTGCCCGTGGCGATGAAGAGCCGGGTTGCGAAGTTTTCCAGCAGCCAGTCGTTGGCCTCACGCTCGAACTGTTCGACGGATTTCCGCGCGGACTCCGTGTTGGGCAGCAGCAGGTACGCGTGCCCGCCGCCGGAGTAG
TTGAGATTCGCGCGGCTGAGACCCACCCGCGCAAGTAGCTCGTCGATGAGATGCTCGGTCAGCATCTCCAGGTAGAAGCTGCGGGCACGCAGCATCTTCGCGGCACCCGAGGAATGGATCGTGTAGATGAAGTCCTGGATGCCTGA
GACGTCGAAAGTTGTGAGCAGGAAGGCTTTTTCGTTGTAGAAGGTGTCCTGCTTGTCGAACAGCGCTGACTTGAAGTCGCTTTGTCCGGTGGCTTGTAGGTAGTGCCAGATGCAGGCGCCGAGCGCACCCGTCAGCTTCAGGTGGTC
GAAGAGTGAGACGTCGACGACCTCGGACGCGTCGGTCGAGGACGGCACGAACGACAGCGTCGCCTCGAGGACGTTGAGGAGGCTGGCGAGGTAGGTGTCGGAACGTTCGAGGTCGACCAGAATGGCTTTAAGTTTGTTGACGAT
GGCGGCGTAGCGGTCCTTGTCGAATTCGATCCGGCGTGGCGACGGTATATTGATCGGCTTGCGGTCGTCGAGCATCTCCGGGGCAAATGCCAGATTCGCTGTGCCGGAGCCGAATCGGTTGAACATCGAATACAGGGGCGTGTCCG
GATCCCAAGTGCTCGCACCATGGCCGTCGTCGGAGTCGGCCTTGCGGCGGTCGGTTCCGGCCGCGATATTGTAGGCGATGTAGGCCGGCGCATCGGCGGCAAGGCGGCCATTCTCGGCCGCCGTACGCAGCGCAGAACTGTGGTGA
TAGCTGATCGCGTCGAGAATGCGGCGGTCGGAGACCCCAATGTCAGCCTCATCCACCTCGTCGGTGAACTGCGACGGATTGCGGCTGTCGCGCAACCACACCTTCTTCATAAAAGCGCGGCCAATCGCACTGTGCCTGCCCGGGTAG
CCGAGCGCCGCGCGCTGGACCGGTTTGCCAATGTCGTGCAAGAGGCAGCCGATTATGGCCTCGATGAGTTGCGGGTTCATGGCTTCGGTACGCATTTTTCCCTCGGTGCCAGTGGCTGGACCCGGATCGCGCCCATCCCCATGGATG
CCTTTATTCCGCATCCCGAGAACTCCCCGAACCACAACAGCGCCGCGATATAGCTCGCAAAAGTATCCACACCGCGGACGGTGAACGTGGCCGAGCCGGTGAAGCCGGGAACACGCGCCGCGCCCACCGCGAACGGGGCCGACGCC
ACCCGGAACGCGGA

Fig. 1 The sequence of 5 Kb Specific Target (5KST). The 5KST primers are shown

Table 2 The number of randomly studied strains and their geographical regions, to prove the 5KST conservation

Location	Number of strains
India	53
Sweden	36
Iran	8
Uganda and South Korea	40
Moldova	16
South Africa(KwaZulu-Natal)	56
Africa	51
Mali	27
Romania	9
USA	8
Total	304

tuberculosis purified DNA, and the negative control contained no DNA.

The DNA amplification was performed by thermocycler (Atlas G Japan). Initial denaturation at 95 °C for 5 min, was proceeded by 40 cycles of (i) denaturation at 95 °C for 15 s, (ii) annealing at 60 °C for 20 s, (iii) extension at 72 °C for 30 s, followed by a final extension at 72 °C for 5 min.

Then, 5 µL of PCR product was electrophoresed on 2% agarose gel containing DNA green viewer and DNA bands were visualized under ultraviolet light from UV transilluminator (UVTEC). The presence of a 128 bp fragment indicated the positive result. 10% of positive specimens were selected randomly and sequencing was performed on their amplicons.

Analytical sensitivity (detection limit)

Purified genomic DNA of *M. tuberculosis* H37Rv was extracted from colonies by Dick Van Soolingen method [21]. DNA concentration was determined by spectrophotometer (Thermo Scientific). Then, serial dilution of genomic DNA was prepared using distilled water (10 pg, 1 pg, 100 fg, 10 fg, 5 fg, 1 fg) and 1 µL was used as template. This process was performed for three times, on three different days.

Analytical specificity

To determine the analytical specificity for 5KST-PCR, genomic DNA of two members of MTBC (*M. tuberculosis*

Table 3 Primers and the amplicon sequence of 5KST-PCR

Forward	5'-TTGCTGAACTTGACCTGCCCGTA
Reverse	5'-GCGTCTCTGCCTTCCTCCGAT
Amplicon	5'TTGCTGAACTTGACCTGCCCGTAGCCACGGGTTCCGCTGC CGCCGAGGTAGTCGAGTTCGAGCAACTTCAGGCCGCGCGCGA TGGCGTTGAAGTCCTCGATGATCTCATCGGAGGAAGGCAGA GACGC

H37Rv and *M. bovis* BCG) and four Non-tuberculosis mycobacteria (*M. smegmatis*, *M. chelonae*, *M. simiae*, *M. fortuitum*) and four non-Mycobacterium bacteria (*Corynebacterium diphteriae*, *Escherichia coli*, *Staphylococcus aureus* and *Streptococcus pneumoniae*) were used which purchased from Pasteur Institute (Tehran, Iran). The amount of 10 ng of genomic DNA was used in the reaction for each species.

Evaluation of clinical specimens
Specimen collection

A total of 100 smear-positive and culture-positive, and 100 smear-negative and culture-negative sputum specimens were obtained from tuberculosis laboratory of Qaem hospital in Mashhad. The ethical approval for performing this study was obtained from the Ethics Committee of the Mashhad University of Medical Sciences (Ethics code of IR.mums.fm.rec.1397.143). To confirm TB, *mpb64*-PCR and *IS6110*-PCR were performed on colonies of each specimen [22].

Specimen processing

To homogenize and concentrate the specimens, all clinical specimens examined in this study was processed using modified Petroff's method and cultured on LJ medium [23]. In brief, 5 ml of sputum was homogenized for 15 min in a shaker using an equal volume of 4% NaOH. After centrifugation at 6000 rpm for 15 min, the sediment was neutralized with 20 ml of sterile distilled water. The samples were again centrifuged. The supernatant was discarded and the precipitate was dissolved in the little residual liquid in the bottom of falcon to be used for the next steps.

Providing smear negative, culture-positive specimens

A total of 30 smear-positive and culture-positive processed samples were diluted with the processed negative specimen and two-fold serial dilutions were prepared (1/2, 1/4, 1/8, 1/16, 1/32, 1/64, 1/128). Then, all of the dilutions were subjected to ziehl-neelsen staining and smear-negative dilutions were cultured on Lowenstein Jensen medium (LJ). The lowest concentrations with a positive culture were considered as smear-negative, culture-positive specimens.

DNA extraction

Autoclave method with some modification was used to extract DNA [24]. The processed specimens were transferred to 1.5 ml microtubes. Then, microtube lids were sealed and the autoclave process was performed (121°c for 5 min). No other substance was added to the specimens. In order to remove the debris, microtubes were centrifuged at 12000 rpm for 5 min. Then, the supernatant was used as the template for 5KST-PCR test.

Investigating the inhibitory effect of clinical specimens on 5KST-PCR

To study the inhibitory effect of clinical specimens, 8 true negative processed sputum samples were pooled together. Then the pure genomic DNA provided in the previous step, was added to 50 µl of this pooled specimen up to the final concentration of 100 pg/µl of DNA. Then, two groups of six dilutions were prepared by the remained pooled specimen. The first group included 10 pg, 1 pg, 100 fg, 10 fg, 5 fg, and 1 fg dilutions and the second group included 5 pg, 0.5 pg, 50 fg, 5 fg, 2.5 fg, and 0.5 fg dilutions. Then, 1 µl of DNA for the first group and 2 µl of DNA for the second group were used for the 5KST-PCR test. So, the amount of DNA used in both groups was equal and the only difference was the amount of clinical specimen used in the reactions.

Results

Target finding

The 5000 bp fragment containing nucleotides 3,127,000 to 3,132,000 of *M. tuberculosis* H37Rv genome (NC_000962.3) was identified as the most specific possible sequence (Fig. 1). The blastn search showed that among the NCBI-registered complete genomes (nucleotide collection database), this sequence could specifically detect 237 strains of *M. tuberculosis* (Additional file 1: Table S1), 12 strains of *M. bovis* BCG, 8 strains of *M. bovis*, 3 strains of *M. africanum*, 2 strains of *M. canettii*, 1 strain of *M. caprae* and 1 strain of *M. microti*.

Results of bioinformatics control

Two hundred thirty-seven strains of *M. tuberculosis* (with complete genome registered in nucleotide collection database) could be identified by *rpoB* sequence, which was quite identical to the strains which could be identified by 5KST-PCR (Additional file 1: Table S1).

Furthermore, the study of 5KST presence in 304 strains of *M. tuberculosis* related to the TB-ARC project also showed that this sequence is present in the all 304 strains and is considered as a conserved sequence (Additional file 1: Table S2).

Analytical sensitivity (detection limit)

Analytical sensitivity is the lowest DNA concentration that a test can detect. Accordingly, the 5KST-PCR analytical sensitivity was 5 fg approximately equivalent to 1 copy of *M. tuberculosis* genomic DNA per µl (Fig. 2).

Analytical specificity

Both species of *M. tuberculosis* and *M. bovis* BCG which studied in this study were identified by 5KST-PCR, but no amplicon was produced for studied Non-tuberculosis mycobacteria (*M. smegmatis*, *M. chelonae*, *M. simiae*, *M. fortuitum*) and non-Mycobacterium bacteria

(*Corynebacterium diphteriae*, *Escherichia coli*, *Staphylococcus aureus* and *Streptococcus pneumoniae*) (Table 4).

Clinical specimen's result

Before beginning the study, all the specimens were cultured on the LJ medium. To select the true positive specimens, DNA extraction of the colonies was performed by simple boiling method and positive specimens were confirmed by *mpb64*-PCR and *IS6110*-PCR.

Only those specimens were included in the study as the true positives, which had clinical symptoms of the patient, and also simultaneous positive results of acid-fast bacilli smear, culture, and both PCR tests on the colonies. In addition, only those negative specimens were included in the study as true negatives, which had negative result of acid-fast bacilli smear and the culture, with the final clinical diagnosis of non-tuberculosis infection.

Clinical sensitivity and specificity

All 100 smear-positive, culture-positive specimens were positive for 5KST-PCR test (100% sensitivity) and 25 of 30 smear-negative, culture-positive samples were positive by the test (85.7% sensitivity). All 100 smear-negative and culture-negative specimens, were negative in 5KST-PCR test (100% clinical specificity). The 5KST-PCR results on clinical specimens are provided in Table 5.

Inhibitory effect of clinical specimens on 5KST-PCR

The results showed the sensitivity of 5 fg/µl and 10 fg/µl when using 1 µl and 2 µl of processed clinical specimen in our test, respectively. (Additional file 1: Figure S1).

Discussion

One of the most important parts of designing a nucleic acid amplification test (NAAT) such as PCR, is having a completely specific and long enough target. Specificity of the target would eliminate the false positive results. The long sequence would help the researcher to design efficient and sensitive primers. In this study, genome comparison method with few modifications was used to achieve completely specific and long sequence (1). In this method, using bioinformatic facilities provided by the NCBI database, genomic sequences of 7 members of MTBC were compared with complete genomes available on the database (up to 2018.08.20) and a 5000 bp sequence with high specificity was identified.

Based on in silico studies, the 5KST can specifically detect the most of NCBI-registered complete genomes of MTBC members including: 237 strains of *M. tuberculosis*, 12 strains of *M. bovis* BCG, 8 strains of *M. bovis*, 3 strains of *M. africanum*, 2 strains of *M. canettii*, 1 strain of *M. caprae* and 1 strain of *M. microti*.

Furthermore, the investigation of 5KST presence in 304 strains of *M. tuberculosis* from different parts of the

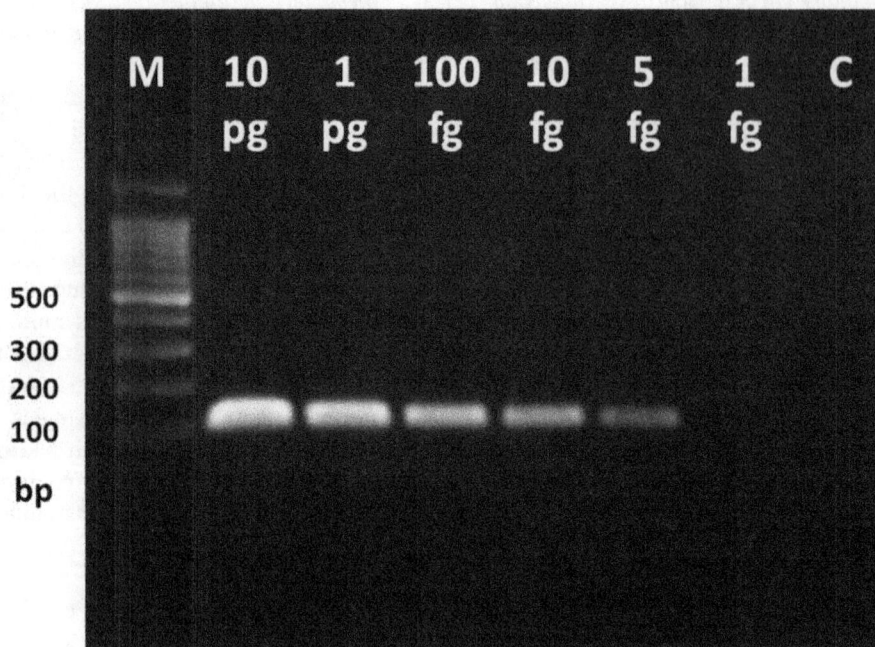

Fig. 2 Gel electrophoresis of 5KST-PCR products. It shows target amplicons at different concentrations of M. tuberculosis H37Rv genomic DNA as template. Lane M shows 100 bp DNA ladder and successive lanes show amplicons using 10 pg, 1 pg, 100 fg, 10 fg, 5 fg, 1 fg of M. tuberculosis genomic DNA. Lane C shows negative control

world (TB-ARC project) showed that this sequence is conserved among all these strains (Additional file 1: Table S2). It should be noted that few of these 304 strains had the query cover of less than 100% (about 81–85%). After evaluating the sequences of these strains, we found that the query cover of less than 100% was not due to the less similarity to our sequence, but also it resulted from the gaps of the sequence during the sequencing process that recorded NNN's instead of G, C, A, T bases.

Tuberculosis is a disease which has caused millions of deaths so far. Despite the advances in human science, it still puts millions of people at the risk of death every year. Therefore, extensive studies are being conducted in

many parts of the world to control it in prevention, diagnosis and treatment parts [2]. The aim of the present study was to improve the diagnostic part of TB. If the diagnosis is timely, TB can be controlled and treated with minimal side effects when the disease is not advanced [25].

Three tests that are routinely used in most TB laboratories include acid-fast bacilli microscopy, culture and PCR [26]. PCR is fast, sensitive and highly specific. In most studies on clinical specimens, it showed higher sensitivity than acid-fast bacilli microscopy, but lower or equal sensitivity than culture. PCR acts more specific than the two other tests [26–28].

The most important factors that reduce the sensitivity of the PCR test on clinical specimens include 1. Presence of inhibitors in clinical specimens 2. Partial loss of DNA during purification 3. Chemical inhibitors residue from the purification process 4. Poorly designed and inefficient primers [16, 28, 29].

In this study, to prevent the negative effects of inhibitors in clinical specimens, only 1 μL of the specimen was used in 25 μL of reaction. The results of this study, previous experiences of our team in molecular

Table 4 The results for analytical specificity of 5KST-PCR

Groups	Bacterial Species	5KST-PCR result
M. tuberculosis complex	M. tuberculosis H37Rv	+
	M. bovis BCG	+
Non-tuberculosis mycobacteria	M. smegmatis	-
	M. chelonae	-
	M. simiae	-
	M. fortuitum	-
Non-Mycobacterium bacteria	Corynebacterium diphteriae	-
	Escherichia coli	-
	Staphylococcus aureus	-
	Streptococcus pneumoniae	-

Table 5 5KST-PCR results on clinical specimens

	Clinical sensitivity (Smear +,culture +)	Clinical sensitivity (Smear -,culture +)	Clinical specificity (Smear -,culture -)
5KST-PCR result	100%	85.7%	100%

laboratory, as well as reviewing the studies of other researchers, showed that the sensitivity of PCR test is lower when using clinical specimens (either natural or artificial) than pure DNA in the reaction. We don't know exactly which inhibitor exists, but generally the substances of clinical specimens, especially sputum, cause the reduction in the sensitivity of test. As JE Clarridge et al. (1993), in a large study to evaluate the PCR test on clinical specimens, showed that the substances of clinical specimens, especially sputum, could cause up to 20% false-negative results and reduce the sensitivity [14]. In another study on sputum specimens, FS Nolte et al. reported that the sputum could produce 10 to 17% false-negative [12]. In a study on 76 respiratory specimens in Turkey, the inhibition rate of up to 26% was observed in the real-time PCR test and caused false-negative results [13]. Also in our study, the use of ≥2 μl clinical specimen in the 25 μl 5KST-PCR reaction worsened the sensitivity from 5 fg to 10 fg.

Also, to prevent DNA loss during purification, this step was removed and only autoclave extraction with few modifications was performed. Furthermore, since the 5KST sequence is long enough, we were able to design efficient primers with the best probable condition of not producing hairpin and dimer structures.

Our studies with blastn showed that all the important targets that have been used so far, have short length or contain long nonspecific regions. Unlike other targets, the 5KST target in addition to being long enough (5000 bp), does not have any statistically significant relationship to NTM bacteria. Some of the targets that have been used more than others or had better detection limit include: rpoB, IS6110, devR, mpb64, sdaA.

IS6110 has been used as one of the most widely used diagnostic targets for TB [8]. This 1361 bp sequence, is repeated multiple times in the genome of M. tuberculosis and thus is regarded as a sensitive diagnostic target. Up to now, various PCR tests are designed based on this sequence, and the reported detection limit usually equals 2 copy of M. tuberculosis genomic DNA per μl [18, 30–32]. Various studies showed that the PCR tests based on this target had a clinical sensitivity of 63–98% and clinical specificity of 82.1–100%. [18, 33–36] This sequence has limitations despite the high sensitivity. For example, some strains of M. tuberculosis have been found which lack the IS6110 sequence [17]. Furthermore, our in silico analysis with blastn showed that large fragments of this sequence have similarities with other NTM bacteria (M. rutilum, M. smegmatis, M. chimaera) and some Nocardia species such as N. brasiliensis. The 5KST sequence has only one copy in the genome of MTBC, nevertheless, it acts completely specific. In addition, unlike the IS6110, the 5KST is quite long which allows to design highly effective primers with minimal hairpin and dimer structures. Although the result of poorly designed primers may not appear in the test sensitivity of pure genomic DNA, it would quietly affect the clinical specimens and reduce the sensitivity [15].

Another diagnostic target sequence which many studies are based on, is mpb64 [28, 37, 38]. This sequence has 687 bp length [39]. Our in silico study by blastn showed that it also contains large regions with high similarity to NTM species such as M. kansasii, M. ulcerans, and M. hemophilum. These nonspecific regions as well as the short length of sequence, make it very difficult to design efficient primers. As in most cases, the sensitivity reported for mpb64 primers is lower than the IS6110 primers [35]. An analytical sensitivity that eventually reported for 5KST-PCR was 1 copy per μl, which according to previous studies is better than mpb64 -PCR (20 copies per μl) [18]. Also, mpb64-PCR had 88–91% specificity and 48–91% sensitivity on clinical specimens [18, 34, 35, 37].

rpoB diagnostic target has also been used to detect rifampicin-resistant TB in several studies [40]. Sensitivity and specificity of the PCR assays based on this target gene have been reported in two clinical trials about 93.3–95.8 and 100% respectively [41, 42]. However, our in silico analysis showed that this sequence has nonspecific similarities with some other mycobacteria. As the analytical specificity of this target in another study showed that the common primers designed for this sequence can also detect M. chelonae, M. kansasii, M. scrofulaceum, M. smegmatis and M. szulgai nonspecifically [18].

The devR sequence is another diagnostic target. In various studies, the detection limit of 200–500 copy per μl has been reported. This sequence has similarities with M. kansasii and may therefore results in false positives. In a clinical study of intraocular TB, same specificity and lower sensitivity compared to mpb64 were reported [18, 43, 44].

In a comparative study between common diagnostic target sequences of TB, the sensitivity of mpb64 was highest (84% in confirmed cases and 77.5% in clinically suspected cases). The clinical sensitivity of other targets was as follows: mpb64 > IS6110 > hsp65 > 38KDa (pstS1) > 30KDa (fbpB) > esat6 > cfp10 > devR [5].

sdaA is another target sequence with few studies. This 1383 bp sequence encodes a protein called serine dehydratase. Although the detection limit equivalent to 1 copy per μl has been reported for this target [18], but our blastn results showed the presence of many nonspecific regions. This sequence has 70–80% similarity to some non-tuberculosis mycobacteria (M. ulcerans, M. marinum, M. smegmatis, and M. fortuitum) and many non-Mycobacterium bacteria such as Rhodococcus and Nocardia.

Conclusions

In this study, we succeeded to introduce highly specific novel target using modified genome comparison method. We also designed highly specific primers, as they were able to detect even 1 copy of *M. tuberculosis* genomic DNA per μl. We think that the unique sensitivity of these primers is due to our long enough target which allows the software to give us the best possible primers.

Our recommendations for future studies include: 1. Using modified genome comparison method to identify diagnostic targets for other pathogens. 2. 5KST-PCR analysis on more and various clinical specimens. 3. Simultaneous comparison of 5KST-PCR with other PCR tests based on other targets to determine its efficiency. 4. Discovering the 5KST genes and their functions 5. Use of 5KST target in other diagnostic tests such as LAMP.

Abbreviations

LAMP: loop-mediated isothermal amplification;; MTBC: Mycobacterium tuberculosis complex; NCBI: National Center for Biotechnology Information; NTM: Nontuberculous Mycobacteria; PCR: Polymerase Chain Reaction; TB-ARC: Tuberculosis Antibiotic Resistance Catalog

Authors' contributions

AN, KG, RKK, MS contributed in the study design and target finding. AN designed the primers. AN, RKK, HZ, AH, Ma.S collected and evaluated the clinical specimens. AN, HZ wrote the manuscript. All authors approved the final version of the paper.

Competing interests

The authors declare that they have no competing interests.

Author details

[1]Antimicrobial Resistance Research Center, Mashhad University of Medical Sciences, Mashhad, Iran. [2]Student Research Committee, Mashhad University of Medical Sciences, Mashhad, Iran. [3]Immunology Research Center, School of Medicine, Mashhad University of Medical Sciences, Mashhad, Iran. [4]Department of Microbiology and Virology, School of Medicine, Mashhad University of Medical Sciences, Mashhad, Iran.

References

1. ZHU DS, Zhou M, FAN YL, SHI XM. Identification of new target sequences for PCR detection of Vibrio parahaemolyticus by genome comparison. J Rapid Methods Autom Microbiol. 2009;17(1):67–79.
2. The top 10 causes of death [Internet]. World Health Organization. 2017. Available from: http://www.who.int/mediacentre/factsheets/fs310/en/.
3. Bojang AL, Mendy FS, Tientcheu LD, Otu J, Antonio M, Kampmann B, et al. Comparison of TB-LAMP, GeneXpert MTB/RIF and culture for diagnosis of pulmonary tuberculosis in the Gambia. J Inf Secur. 2016;72(3):332–7.
4. Kivihya-Ndugga L, van Cleeff M, Juma E, Kimwomi J, Githui W, Oskam L, et al. Comparison of PCR with the routine procedure for diagnosis of tuberculosis in a population with high Prevalences of tuberculosis and human immunodeficiency virus. J Med Microbiol. 2004;42(3):1012–5.
5. Raj A, Singh N, Gupta KB, Chaudhary D, Yadav A, Chaudhary A, et al. Comparative evaluation of several gene targets for designing a multiplex-PCR for an early diagnosis of Extrapulmonary tuberculosis. Yonsei Med J. 2016;57(1):88–96.
6. Mehta PK, Raj A, Singh N, Khuller GK. Diagnosis of extrapulmonary tuberculosis by PCR. FEMS Immunol Med Microbiol. 2012;66(1):20–36.
7. Sharma K, Gupta N, Sharma A, Singh G, Gupta PK, Rajwanshi A, et al. Multiplex polymerase chain reaction using insertion sequence 6110 (IS6110) and mycobacterial protein fraction from BCG of Rm 0.64 in electrophoresis target genes for diagnosis of tuberculous lymphadenitis. Indian J Med Microbiol. 2013;31(1):24–8.
8. Eisenach KD, Donald Cave M, Bates JH, Crawford JT. Polymerase chain reaction amplification of a repetitive DNA sequence specific for Mycobacterium tuberculosis. J Infect Dis. 1990;161(5):977–81.
9. Haldar S, Bose M, Chakrabarti P, Daginawala HF, Harinath BC, Kashyap RS, et al. Improved laboratory diagnosis of tuberculosis--the Indian experience. Tuberculosis (Edinburgh, Scotland). 2011;91(5):414–26.
10. Bessetti J. An introduction to PCR inhibitors. J Microbiol Methods. 2007; 28:159–67.
11. Wilson IG. Inhibition and facilitation of nucleic acid amplification. Appl Environ Microbiol. 1997;63(10):3741.
12. Nolte FS, Metchock B, McGowan J, Edwards A, Okwumabua O, Thurmond C, et al. Direct detection of Mycobacterium tuberculosis in sputum by polymerase chain reaction and DNA hybridization. J Clin Microbiol. 1993; 31(7):1777–82.
13. Döşkaya M, Caner A, Değirmenci A, Wengenack NL, Yolasığmaz A, Turgay N, et al. Degree and frequency of inhibition in a routine real-time PCR detecting pneumocystis jirovecii for the diagnosis of pneumocystis pneumonia in Turkey. J Med Microbiol. 2011;60(7):937–44.
14. Jr C, Shawar RM, Shinnick TM, Plikaytis BB. Large-scale use of polymerase chain reaction for detection of Mycobacterium tuberculosis in a routine mycobacteriology laboratory. J Clin Microbiol. 1993;31(8):2049–56.
15. Chou Q, Russell M, Birch DE, Raymond J, Bloch W. Prevention of pre-PCR mis-priming and primer dimerization improves low-copy-number amplifications. Nucleic Acids Res. 1992;20(7):1717–23.
16. Afghani B, Stutman HR. Polymerase chain reaction for diagnosis ofM. Tuberculosis:comparison of simple boiling and a conventional method for DNA extraction. Biochem Mol Med. 1996;57(1):14–8.
17. Lok KH, Benjamin WH Jr, Kimerling ME, Pruitt V, Lathan M, Razeq J, et al. Molecular differentiation of Mycobacterium tuberculosis strains without IS6110 insertions. Emerg Infect Dis. 2002;8(11):1310.
18. Nimesh M, Joon D, Pathak AK, Saluja D. Comparative study of diagnostic accuracy of established PCR assays and in-house developed sdaA PCR method for detection of Mycobacterium tuberculosis in symptomatic patients with pulmonary tuberculosis. J Inf Secur. 2013;67(5):399–407.
19. Manson AL, Cohen KA, Abeel T, Desjardins CA, Armstrong DT, Barry CE III, et al. Genomic analysis of globally diverse Mycobacterium tuberculosis strains provides insights into the emergence and spread of multidrug resistance. Nat Genet. 2017;49(3):395.
20. Rychlik W. OLIGO 7 primer analysis software. Methods Mol Biol. 2007:35–59.
21. Parish T, Stoker NG. Mycobacterium tuberculosis protocols: Springer Science & Business Media; 2001.
22. Aziz MM, Khan AY, Hasan KN, Azad Khan AK, Hassan MS. Comparison between IS6110 and MPB64 primers for the diagnosis of Mycobacterium tuberculosis in Bangladesh by polymerase chain reaction (PCR). Bangladesh Med Res Counc Bull. 2004;30(3):87–94.
23. Tripathi K, Tripathi PC, Nema S, Shrivastava AK, Dwiwedi K, Dhanvijay AK. Modified Petroff's method: an excellent simplified decontamination technique in comparison with Petroff's method. Int J Recent Trends Sci Tech. 2014;10:461–4.
24. Simmon KE, Steadman DD, Durkin S, Baldwin A, Jeffrey WH, Sheridan P, et al. Autoclave method for rapid preparation of bacterial PCR-template DNA. J Microbiol Methods. 2004;56(2):143–9.
25. Lönnroth K, Migliori GB, Abubakar I, D'Ambrosio L, De Vries G, Diel R, et al. Towards tuberculosis elimination: an action framework for low-incidence countries. Eur Respir J. 2015;45(4):928–52.
26. Aslanzadeh J, de la Viuda M, Fille M, Smith WB, Namdari H. Comparison of culture and acid-fast bacilli stain to PCR for detection of Mycobacterium tuberculosis in clinical samples. Mol Cell Probes. 1998;12(4):207–11.
27. Organization WH. Definitions and reporting framework for tuberculosis–2013 revision. 2013.
28. Narotam S, Veena S, Ch NS, Raj SP, Kushwaha RS, Shivani S, et al. Conventional PCR usage for the detection of Mycobacterium Tuberculosis complex in Cerebrospinal Fluid by MPB64-Target PCR. Int J Drug Dev & Res. 2012;4(4):206–210.
29. Amita J, Vandana T, Guleria R, Verma R. Qualitative evaluation of mycobacterial DNA extraction protocols for polymerase chain reaction. Mol Biol Today. 2002;3(2):43–9.
30. Sankar S, Kuppanan S, Balakrishnan B, Nandagopal B. Analysis of sequence diversity among IS6110 sequence of Mycobacterium tuberculosis: possible implications for PCR based detection. Bioinformation. 2011;6(7):283–5.
31. Thierry D, Cave M, Eisenach K, Crawford J, Bates J, Gicquel B, et al. IS6110, an IS-like element of Mycobacterium tuberculosis complex. Nucleic Acids Res. 1990;18(1):188.

32. Tumwasorn S, Kwanlertjit S, Mokmued S, Charoenlap P. Comparison of DNA targets for amplification by polymerase chain reaction for detection of Mycobacterium tuberculosis in sputum. J Med Assoc Thai. 1996;79(Suppl 1):S113–8.

33. Haldar S, Sharma N, Gupta V, Tyagi JS. Efficient diagnosis of tuberculous meningitis by detection of Mycobacterium tuberculosis DNA in cerebrospinal fluid filtrates using PCR. J Med Microbiol. 2009;58(5):616–24.

34. Rafi W, Venkataswamy MM, Ravi V, Chandramuki A. Rapid diagnosis of tuberculous meningitis: a comparative evaluation of in-house PCR assays involving three mycobacterial DNA sequences, IS6110, MPB-64 and 65 kDa antigen. J Neurol Sci. 2007;252(2):163–8.

35. Asthana AK, Madan M. Study of target gene IS 6110 and MPB 64 in diagnosis of pulmonary tuberculosis. Int J Curr Microbiol Appl Sci. 2015; 4(8):856–63.

36. Haldar S, Chakravorty S, Bhalla M, De Majumdar S, Tyagi JS. Simplified detection of Mycobacterium tuberculosis in sputum using smear microscopy and PCR with molecular beacons. J Med Microbiol. 2007; 56(10):1356–62.

37. Martins LC, Paschoal IA, Von Nowakonski A, Silva SA, Costa FF, Ward LS. Nested-PCR using MPB64 fragment improves the diagnosis of pleural and meningeal tuberculosis. Rev Soc Bras Med Trop. 2000;33(3):253–7.

38. Aryal R, Sah AK, Paudel DS, Joshi B, Lekhak SP, Rajbhandari R, et al. Polymerase chain reaction using the MPB64 fragment for detection of Mycobacterium tuberculosis complex DNA in suspected TB cases. Int J Med Sci Public Heal. 2014;3:1.

39. Mycobacterium tuberculosis H37Rv complete genome [Internet]. The National Center for Biotechnology Information 2015. Available from: https://www.ncbi.nlm.nih.gov/nuccore/AL123456.3?from=2223343&to=2224029.

40. Kim B-J, Hong S-K, Lee K-H, Yun Y-J, Kim E-C, Park Y-G, et al. Differential identification of Mycobacterium tuberculosis complex and nontuberculous mycobacteria by duplex PCR assay using the RNA polymerase gene (rpoB). J Med Microbiol. 2004;42(3):1308–12.

41. Yang S, Zhong M, Zhang Y, Wang Y. Rapid detection of rpoB and katG genes from the sputum of multidrug-resistant Mycobacterium tuberculosis by polymerase chain reaction (PCR)-direct sequencing analysis. Afr J Microbiol Res. 2011;5(26):4519–23.

42. Li J, Xin J, Zhang L, Jiang L, Cao H, Li L. Rapid detection of rpoB mutations in rifampin resistant M. tuberculosis from sputum samples by denaturing gradient gel electrophoresis. Int J Med Sci. 2012;9(2):148.

43. Kataria P, Kumar A, Bansal R, Sharma A, Gupta V, Gupta A, et al. devR PCR for the diagnosis of intraocular tuberculosis. Ocul Immunol Inflamm. 2015; 23(1):47–52.

44. Dasgupta N, Kapur V, Singh K, Das T, Sachdeva S, Jyothisri K, et al. Characterization of a two-component system, devR-devS, of Mycobacterium tuberculosis. Tuber Lung Dis. 2000;80(3):141–59.

7

Urogenital pathogens, associated with *Trichomonas vaginalis*, among pregnant women in Kilifi, Kenya: a nested case-control study

Simon C. Masha[1,2,3*] , Piet Cools[2], Patrick Descheemaeker[4], Marijke Reynders[4], Eduard J. Sanders[1] and Mario Vaneechoutte[2]

Abstract

Background: Screening of curable sexually transmitted infections is frequently oriented towards the diagnosis of chlamydia, gonorrhea, syphilis and trichomoniasis, whereas other pathogens, sometimes associated with similar urogenital syndromes, remain undiagnosed and/or untreated. Some of these pathogens are associated with adverse pregnancy outcomes.

Methods: In a nested case-control study, vaginal swabs from 79 pregnant women, i.e., 28 *T. vaginalis*-positive (cases) and 51 *T. vaginalis*-negative (controls), were screened by quantitative PCR for Adenovirus 1 and 2, Cytomegalovirus, Herpes Simplex Virus 1 and 2, *Chlamydia trachomatis, Escherichia coli, Haemophilus ducreyi, Mycoplasma genitalium, M. hominis,* candidatus *M. girerdii, Neisseria gonorrhoeae, Streptococcus agalactiae, Treponema pallidum, Ureaplasma parvum, U. urealyticum,* and *Candida albicans*. Additionally, we determined whether women with pathogens highly associated with *T. vaginalis* had distinct clinical signs and symptoms compared to women with *T. vaginalis* mono-infection.

Results: *M. hominis* was independently associated with *T. vaginalis* (adjusted odds ratio = 6.8, 95% CI: 2.3–19.8). Moreover, *M. genitalium* and Ca *M. girerdii* were exclusively detected in women with *T. vaginalis* ($P = 0.002$ and $P = 0.001$, respectively). Four of the six women co-infected with *T. vaginalis* and Ca *M. girerdii* complained of vaginal itching, compared to only 4 out of the 22 women infected with *T. vaginalis* without Ca *M. girerdii* ($P = 0.020$).

Conclusion: We confirm *M. hominis* as a correlate of *T. vaginalis* in our population, and the exclusive association of both *M. genitalium* and Ca. *M. girerdii* with *T. vaginalis*. Screening and treatment of these pathogens should be considered.

Keywords: Trichomonas, Mycoplasma hominis, M. Genitalium, M. Girerdii, Kenya, Pregnant, STIs

Background

Sexually transmitted infections (STIs) constitute a huge proportion of the most prevalent acute infections globally [1]. The most prevalent curable sexually transmitted pathogens include *Chlamydia trachomatis, Neisseria gonorrhoeae, Treponema pallidum* subspecies *pallidum* (syphilis) and *Trichomonas vaginalis*. These four pathogens are associated with acute conditions like genital/anorectal/oral ulceration, cervicitis-endometritis, vaginal/urethral discharge, and urethritis. They can also cause critical complications and long term sequelae, which includes oophoritis, salpingitis, pelvic inflammatory disease, ectopic pregnancy, infertility, neurological disease, neonatal death, premature delivery and blindness [2]. Another public health concern is the association of STIs with the augmented possibility of HIV acquisition and transmission [3].

Of the four most prevalent curable STIs, *T. vaginalis* is globally the most prevalent pathogen [1], with a prevalence of up to 11.5% among women in sub-Sahara Africa [1]. Although there is a wealth of data regarding the

* Correspondence: schengo@kemri-wellcome.org
[1]Kenya Medical Research Institute, Centre for Geographic Medicine Research – Coast, Kenya Medical Research Institute, P.O. Box 230, Kilifi, Kenya
[2]Laboratory Bacteriology Research, Faculty of Medicine and Health Sciences, Ghent University, De Pintelaan, 185 Ghent, Belgium
Full list of author information is available at the end of the article

clinical presentation and global burden of *T. vaginalis* [4], studies assessing associations of *T. vaginalis* with other genital pathogens are scarce, although it has been intimated that *T. vaginalis* has a unique symbiotic relationship with *Mycoplasma hominis* (*M. hominis*) [5]. *T. vaginalis* is also associated with an increase in vaginal pH [6] which may influence the composition of the associated vaginal microbial community and is strongly associated with bacterial vaginosis (BV) [6]. Less appreciated pathogens like *M. hominis*, *M. genitalium*, *Ureaplasma parvum* and *U. urealyticum* are increasingly being associated with adverse pregnancy outcomes as well as respiratory infections in neonates [7].

STI screening programs and STI research mostly focus on the four most common curable STIs, whereas other pathogens, associated with similar urogenital syndromes, remain undiagnosed and/or untreated. Detection of urogenital pathogens that may be associated with *T. vaginalis* may be important as it might have an effect on the clinical presentation and management and the long-term outcome of those infections. Here, we assess the occurrence of specific urogenital species in *T. vaginalis*-positive (cases) and *T. vaginalis*-negative (controls) among pregnant women in Kilifi, Kenya.

Methods

Study setting

Kenya, an East African country, is divided administratively into 47 counties. Kilifi County, which lies along the Indian Ocean Coast, is one of the poorest and is typical of a rural equatorial Africa setting. Among pregnant women in Kilifi the HIV prevalence is estimated to be 6.4%, for chlamydia 14.9%, for gonorrhea 1.0 and 7.4% for trichomoniasis [8].

From July till September 2015, we carried out a curable STI study at the prenatal care clinic of Kilifi County Hospital, Kenya. The key objective of the curable STI study was to illustrate the prevalence and predictors of curable sexually transmitted infections (STIs) among 350 pregnant women attending the prenatal care clinic [8]. The eligibility criteria for the curable STI study included: residing in the Kilifi Health and Demographic Surveillance area, age 18–45 years, willingness to undergo free STI and bacterial vaginosis (BV) screening procedures, gestation ≥14 weeks, and willing to give written informed consent. This study presents a secondary aim of the curable STI study, which is to describe urogenital pathogen correlates of *T. vaginalis* among pregnant women in Kilifi, Kenya.

For the above-described curable STI study, a nurse at the prenatal care clinic collected vaginal secretions from the vaginal introitus using two sterile cotton swabs. The first vaginal swab was used for *T. vaginalis* detection using the InPouch system (BioMed Diagnostics, White City, Oregon, USA), a highly specific and sensitive device

containing a fluid medium supporting the growth of *T. vaginalis* and allowing microscopic observation of *T. vaginalis*. The inoculated InPouch was transported to the laboratory within 15 min for direct microscopy, and incubation at 37 °C ± 1 °C. Daily microscopic observation (at both × 10 and × 40 magnification, for six fields) of the InPouch system was performed by qualified technicians. Motile trichomonads within 5 days of culture were indicative of being positive for *T. vaginalis*.

Same day treatment was offered for women who were determined to be positive for *T. vaginalis* by means of direct microscopy. For women whose culture turned positive but were negative for *T. vaginalis* on direct microscopy, they were contacted to return to the clinic for treatment the moment the culture turned positive. Secnidazole 2 g statim was administered as treatment, and participants were also asked to refer their sexual partner(s) to the clinic for treatment or were given the same medication to take to their sexual partner(s).

The second swab had its shaft broken by bending the shaft against the neck of a sterile, labeled 2 ml Eppendorf tube, the tube containing the swab tip was closed and transferred to the laboratory where it was immediately stored at – 80 °C. No transport or freezing medium was added prior to storage.

Specimens for this case-control study are derived from the stored swabs from the curable STI study, published previously [7]. Because of financial and logistic constraints we could process only a subset of the 350 vaginal swabs from the main study. Vaginal swabs from 79 pregnant women were divided in two groups for analysis, i.e., those from women positive for *T. vaginalis* (cases) and those from women negative for *T. vaginalis* (controls) as determined by PCR. Controls were age-matched (+/– 5 years) and all were bacterial vaginosis (BV) negative by Nugent score, largely matching the cases because only 4 out of the 28 TV+ cases were BV+. Selection of controls was guided by being TV negative. The swabs of 51 women selected as controls were not significantly different from the swabs of the other 271 women not selected as controls (Additional file 1: Table S1).

DNA extraction

Before DNA extraction, which was performed in Kilifi, the frozen swabs were thawed at room temperature (approximately 25 °C) for 30 min. Extraction was performed using the QIAamp DNA Mini Kit (Qiagen, Hilden, Germany) according to manufacturer's instructions and 160 μl of eluted DNA was transferred to Eppendorf tubes and frozen at – 80 °C until shipment to the Laboratory of Bacteriology Research (LBR, Ghent University, Belgium). Shipment was performed using shipping boxes filled with dry ice (– 78.5 °C). Once at the LBR the Eppendorf tubes with DNA-extracts were transferred back to − 80 °C until molecular analysis was performed. No thawing and freezing occurred after freezing the DNA extract until the point of molecular testing in the laboratory in Belgium.

Quantitative PCR

Most quantitative PCRs were performed using a highly sensitive and specific TaqMan® Array Card (TAC), developed at AZ Sint-Jan Brugge-Oostende, Belgium. The array card was used for detecting Chlamydia trachomatis (including Lymphogranuloma venereum (LGV) serovars L1-L2-L3), Neisseria gonorrhoeae, Haemophilus ducreyi, Mycoplasma genitalium (including M. genitalium macrolide resistance-mediating mutations A2058G, A2059G, A2058T, A2058C in region V of the 23S rRNA gene), M. hominis, Ureaplasma parvum, U. urealyticum, Treponema pallidum, Herpes Simplex virus-1/− 2 (HSV 1/2), adenoviruses, Cytomegalovirus (CMV), and T. vaginalis. The assay has multiple genetic targets per pathogen in order to maximize both specificity and sensitivity [9]. Samples were determined to be positive for a particular species on the TaqMan® Array Card (TAC), only in case the assay was positive for two independent PCR targets of that species. Sample quality was assessed by amplification of human DNA, to evaluate the quantity of epithelial cells recovered by the swab.

Further individual qPCRs were performed at the LBR for Candida albicans [10], Escherichia coli [11] and Streptococcus agalactiae [11, 12]. The LightCycler 480 platform and the LightCycler 1480 Software Version 1.5 (Roche) were used for the amplification, detection and quantification. Each qPCR was performed in a final volume of 10 μl of which 2 μl of DNA extract or 2 μl of a negative control (HPLC water) or 2 μl of a positive control. All the specific primers and probes were synthesized by Eurogentec, Liège, Belgium. Specific qPCR details are provided in Additional file 1: Table S2.

The procedures as described by Cools et al. [10] were adopted for the construction of qPCR standard curves. Briefly, DNA was extracted from overnight cultures of C. albicans ATCC 90028 grown on Sabouraud agar (Becton Dickinson, Erembodegem, Belgium) and of E. coli ATCC 25922 or S. agalactiae LMG 14694^T grown on TSA + 5% sheep blood (Becton Dickinson). All colonies were collected from the plate and re-suspended in 1 ml of saline. The manufacturer's instructions of the High Pure PCR Template Preparation Kit (Roche Applied Science, Basel, Switzerland) were followed to extract DNA from this suspension. DNA-concentration was determined by means of Nanodrop and the number of genomes was calculated. A tenfold dilution series in HPLC-grade water was made to establish for each dilution the number of Cqs needed to pass the detection threshold. Using these data, a regression curve was constructed.

PCR for *T. vaginalis* and for Candidatus *Mycoplasma girerdii* (Ca. *M. girerdii*)

PCRs for T. vaginalis targeting the actin gene, using outer primers, previously used in a nested PCR [13] and yielding a fragment of 1100 bp and for Ca. M. girerdii, yielding a fragment of 594 bp [14], were carried out on the ABI Veriti thermocycler platform (ThermoFisher Scientific, Waltham, Massachusetts). The primers were synthesized by Eurogentec, Liège, Belgium. Amplified fragments were visualized under UV light after agarose gel electrophoresis and EtBr staining.

Details of these species-specific PCRs are summarized in Additional file 1: Table S2.

Sequencing

Sequencing of PCR amplicons was carried out by GATC Biotech (Constance, Germany) to confirm specificity of the PCR products. Sequencing was done using the forward PCR primers (Additional file 1: Table S2). Sequences were cleaned using Chromas Lite version 2.1 (Technelysium, Brisbane, Australia). BLAST was performed on the sequences to confirm the identity.

Data analysis

Epidemiological data were analyzed using StataCorp. 2013. Stata Statistical Software: Release 13 (College Station, TX: StataCorp LP). Prevalence of urogenital pathogens were computed with 95% confidence intervals (CIs). Associations between T. vaginalis positivity and socio-demographic, hygienic and behavioral characteristics were calculated using the χ2 test. To build a multivariate model of urogenital species associated with T. vaginalis, we first carried out univariate regression analysis. For computation of odds ratios (ORs), we replaced all zero values in cells by the value '0.5', as suggested by Deeks & Higgins [13].

Species that were significantly associated with T. vaginalis in univariate regression analysis P-value ≤0.1 were selected for multivariate logistic regression analysis. Associations in the final multivariate model were expressed as adjusted odds ratios (AORs) with p-values ≤0.05 considered significant. We further assessed whether pathogens, significantly associated with T. vaginalis infection, had an implication on the clinical presentation.

Results

A total of 23 out of 350 samples (6.5%) were positive by InPouch culture for Trichomonas vaginalis, of which eight (34.8%) were initially positive on direct microscopy. The T. vaginalis-specific PCR [13] detected one additional case of T. vaginalis from a sample that was negative by InPouch culture but positive by the TAC assay, which found four more positive samples. In summary, sensitivity of direct microscopy, of T. vaginalis

InPouch culture and of *T. vaginalis*-specific PCR were respectively 28.6, 82.1 and 85.7%, when compared to the TAC assay.

Distribution of age, religion, education level, marital status, parity, gestational age and number of lifetime sex partners were similar among cases and controls (Table 1). HIV and BV status was different between the two groups by our case-control study design (Table 2), but the resulting overall difference was minimal, i.e. 0 HIV and 0 BV cases in the control group compared to 3 HIV-positives (10.7%) and 4 BV-positives (14.3%) in the *Trichomonas* positive group. Moreover, we could show that these differences had no influence on the species associated with *T. vaginalis* (Additional file 1: Tables S3 and S4). Additionally, occupation was also significantly different (Table 1).

Prevalence of urogenital species

The prevalence of the co-infecting urogenital species is indicated in Table 2. Adenovirus, *Haemophilus ducreyi*, *Neisseria gonorrhoeae* and *Treponema pallidum* were

Table 1 Characteristics of *Trichomonas vaginalis* qPCR positive women (cases) and *T. vaginalis* qPCR negative women (controls)

Characteristic	Cases (%) N = 28	Controls (%) N = 51	χ2 x P-value
Age group (Years)			
18–24	42.9	31.4	0.307
≥ 25	57.1	68.6	
Religion			
Christian	64.3	68.6	0.383
Muslim	10.7	17.7	
Other/None	25.0	13.7	
Education			
None	21.4	23.5	0.946
Primary	60.7	56.9	
Secondary/Tertiary	17.9	19.6	
Employment status			
Employed/self-employed	50.0	72.6	**0.045**
Unemployed	50.0	27.5	
Parity			
0	25.0	35.3	0.234
1–2	46.4	25.4	
3+	28.6	37.3	
Gestational age (weeks)			
14–27	57.1	58.8	0.885
≥ 28	42.9	41.2	
Number of lifetime sex partners			
1	82.1	90.2	0.303
3+	21.7	9.8	

In bold: significantly associated, i.e., $P \leq 0.05$

not detected and are not reported in Table 1. *Ureaplasma parvum* was the most prevalent at 74.7% (95% Confidence interval (CI): 63.6–83.8), followed by *U. urealyticum* at 48.1% (CI: 36.7–59.6).

Univariate and multivariate association analysis

Although, *M. genitalium* and Ca. *M. girerdii*, had generally a low prevalences of respectively 6.3 and 7.6%, the two were exclusively detected in women with *T. vaginalis* (Chi-square test: $\chi^2 = 9.7$, df = 1, $P < 0.002$ and $\chi^2 = 11.8$, df = 1, $P < 0.001$, respectively). Both *M. genitalium* and Ca. *M. girerdii* were significantly associated with *T. vaginalis* on univariate analysis but not on multivariable analysis (Table 2). None of the samples for which *M. genitalium* could be detected showed macrolide resistance-associated mutations. In a univariate regression analysis, *M. hominis* and *U. urealyticum* were significantly associated with *T. vaginalis* (crude odds ratio (COR) = 7.3; 95% CI: 2.6–20.5 and COR = 2.2; 95% CI: 0.9–5.7, respectively). We detected *M. hominis* from the vaginal DNA extracts of approximately 70% of women with *T. vaginalis*. *M. hominis* was also independently associated with *T. vaginalis* in a multivariate regression analysis (adjusted odds ratio (AOR) = 6.8; 95% CI: 2.3–19.8).

Tables 3, 4 and 5 compare clinical signs and symptoms among *T. vaginalis*-infected women co-infected or not with *M. hominis* (Table 3), or with Ca *M. girerdii* (Table 4) or with *M. genitalium* (Table 5).

Women co-infected with *T. vaginalis* and Ca. *M. girerdii* were more likely to report vaginal itching compared to *T. vaginalis*-positive women not co-infected with Ca. *M. girerdii* (66.8% vs. 18.2% ($p = 0.020$)). There was no difference in clinical presentation of *T. vaginalis*-infected pregnant women co-infected with *M. hominis* or with *M. genitalium*, compared to those not co-infected with these species.

Of the five participants that had *M. genitalium* and the six that had Ca *M. girerdii*, only one participant had a co-infection with *M. genitalium* and Ca *M. girerdii*. However, *M. hominis* was always present in vaginal samples from which *M. genitalium* and Ca *M. girerdii* were detected. Due to the detection of CMV, HSV 1/ 2, *M. genitalium* and Ca. *M. girerdii* exclusively in cases or controls, the species were excluded from the regression model.

Discussion

Our results indicate that women with *Trichomonas vaginalis* (n = 28) have a high rate (71.4%) of co-infection with *Mycoplasma hominis* compared to only 25.5% of 51 women not infected with *T. vaginalis*. Comparable rates of co-infection have been reported by Becker et al. [15], i.e., 56.7% in Brazil and by Xiao et al. [16], i.e., 50.0% in China. Rappelli et al. [17] reported much higher rates

Table 2 Prevalence and co-occurrence of urogenital species among 28 *Trichomonas vaginalis*-positive and 51 *T. vaginalis*-negative women

Species	Overall prevalence (N = 79) (95% CI)	%TV +/%TV-	Univariate analysis		Multivariate analysis	
			COR (95% CI)	P-value	AOR (95% CI)	P-value
Candida albicans	24.1 (15.1–35.0)	32.1/19.6	1.9 (0.7–5.6)	0.216	–	–
Chlamydia trachomatis	13.9 (7.2–23.5)	21.4/9.8	2.5 (0.7–9.1)	0.163	–	–
Escherichia coli	27.8 (18.3–39.1)	35.7/23.5	1.8 (0.7–4.9)	0.251	–	–
Mycoplasma genitalium	6.3(2.1–14.2)	17.9/0.0	5.0 (0.3–94.3)*	**0.002**		
Ca. *Mycoplasma girerdii*	7.6 (2.8–15.8)	21.4/0.0	4.3 (0.2–78.4)*	**0.001**		
Mycoplasma hominis	41.8 (30.8–53.4)	71.4/25.5	7.3 (2.6–20.5)	**< 0.001**	6.8 (2.3–19.8)	**< 0.001**
Streptococcus agalactiae	11.4 (5.3–20.5)	7.1/13.7	0.5 (0.1–2.5)	0.386	–	–
Ureaplasma parvum	74.7 (63.6–83.8)	78.9/72.6	1.4 (0.5–4.1)	0.557	–	–
Ureaplasma urealyticum	48.1 (36.7–59.6)	60.7/41.2	2.2 (0.9–5.7)	0.099	1.3 (0.4–3.8)	0.624
Cytomegalovirus	1.3 (0–6.9)	0.0/2.0	1.7 (6.6–4210.4)*	0.456		
HIV	3.8 (0.7–10.7)	10.7/0.0	7.9 (0.4–158.5)*	**0.017**		
HSV 1, HSV 2	2.5 (0.3–8.8)	7.1/0.0	11.1 (0.5–238.6)*	0.053		
Bacterial vaginosis	5.1 (1.4–12.5)	14.3/0.0	6.2 (0.3–118.4)*	**0.006**		

TV Trichomonas vaginalis, HIV human immunodeficiency virus, HSV1 herpes simplex virus type 1; herpes simplex virus type 2, COR crude odds ratio, AOR adjusted odds ratio
in bold: significantly associated, i.e., $P \leq 0.05$* Separate computation not included in multivariable model

(94.3%) of co-infection among Italian, Mozambican, and Angolan women. *M. hominis* has been shown to have a symbiotic relationship with *T. vaginalis*. Owing to its small genome, this bacterial species is strongly dependent on host cell metabolism. *M. hominis* has the ability to enter trichomonad cells by endocytosis and to multiply in co-ordination with the protozoan [5]. We could not establish differences in clinical presentation of women co-infected with both *T. vaginalis* and *M. hominis* as compared to those infected with only *T. vaginalis*, in agreement with previous data [18]. As such, at present, co-infection of *T. vaginalis* with *M. hominis* seems to be of limited clinical relevance, also because antibiotic treatment of the former

will probably consecutively diminish the presence of the latter.

The pathogenic potential of *M. genitalium* among pregnant women in Kenya has not been extensively investigated probably because its prevalence is overshadowed by a higher prevalence of other STIs, as was the case in this study. Our results indicate that in our population *M. genitalium* was strongly associated with *T. vaginalis* ($p = 0.002$). Given the presence of *M. genitalium* exclusively in women with *T. vaginalis* infection, screening and treatment of women for *T. vaginalis* might also at once reduce the prevalence of *M. genitalium*. Although macrolide resistance associated mutations among *M. genitalium* strains are on

Table 3 Clinical signs/symptoms among women co-infected with *Trichomonas vaginalis* and *Mycoplasma hominis* versus *T. vaginalis* only

Clinical sign or symptom	TV with MH N = 20 (%)	TV without MH N = 8 (%)	χ2 P-value
Dyspareunia	40.0	37.5	0.903
Dysuria	30.0	37.5	0.701
Foul smelling vaginal odor	30.0	12.5	0.334
Genital ulcers	15.0	12.5	0.864
Genital warts	10.0	0.0	0.353
Lower abdominal pain	40.0	25.0	0.454
Vaginal discharge	75.0	62.5	0.508
Vaginal itching	30.0	25.0	0.791

MH Mycoplasma hominis, TV Trichomonas vaginalis

Table 4 Clinical signs/symptoms among women co-infected with *Trichomonas vaginalis* and Ca *Mycoplasma girerdii* versus *T. vaginalis* only

Clinical sign or symptom	TV with Ca MG N = 6 (%)	TV without Ca MG N = 22 (%)	χ2 P-value
Dyspareunia	50.0	36.4	0.544
Dysuria	50.0	27.3	0.291
Foul smelling vaginal odor	33.3	22.7	0.595
Genital ulcers	16.7	13.6	0.851
Genital warts	0.0	9.1	0.443
Lower abdominal pain	50.0	32.8	0.410
Vaginal discharge	100.0	63.6	0.081
Vaginal itching	66.7	18.2	**0.020**

Ca MG Candidatus Mycoplasma girerdii, TV Trichomonas vaginalis; in bold: significantly associated

Table 5 Clinical signs/symptoms among women co-infected with Trichomonas vaginalis and Mycoplasma genitalium versus T. vaginalis only

Clinical sign or symptom	TV with MG N = 5 (%)	TV without MG N = 23 (%)	(χ2).P-value
Dyspareunia	20.0	43.5	0.330
Dysuria	20.0	34.8	0.521
Foul smelling vaginal odor	40.0	21.7	0.393
Genital ulcers	0.0	17.4	0.314
Genital warts	0.0	8.7	0.494
Lower abdominal pain	40.0	34.8	0.825
Vaginal discharge	80.0	69.6	0.640
Vaginal itching	0.0	34.8	0.119

MG Mycoplasma genitalium, TV Trichomonas vaginalis

the rise, as was recently shown among female sex workers in Belgium [19], macrolide resistance-associated mutations could not be detected in any of the five samples positive for M. genitalium and therefore our results, although based on a very small sample, suggest that macrolides can still be used for treatment of M. genitalium in this population in Kilifi, Kenya.

To our knowledge, this is the first report of Ca. M. girerdii in Africa. In agreement with the two initial reports on the prevalence of Ca. M. girerdii [20, 21], we found it to be strongly associated with T. vaginalis (p = 0.001). Fettweis et al. [20], using a pyrosequencing approach, were the first to detect Ca. M. girerdii DNA in the vaginal swabs of a few women not infected with T. vaginalis, as assessed with qPCR, although in our study, Ca. M. girerdii was found only in T. vaginalis positive women. A recent report by Costello et al. [22] is in support of the close association of Ca. M. girerdii and T. vaginalis as they recovered Ca. M. girerdii and T. vaginalis genomes from the saliva of a premature infant.

Our data suggest that T. vaginalis-positive women, co-infected with Ca. M. girerdii, were more likely to report vaginal itching compared to T. vaginalis mono-infected women. Future studies should elucidate the nature of the interaction of these two pathogens and the effect that co-infection may have on clinical presentation.

U. parvum and U. urealyticum are commonly isolated from the vaginal microbiome of asymptomatic pregnant women [23], as was the case in our study. Although detection of U. parvum has been associated with preterm birth [24], opinions differ with regard to the need to screen and treat Ureaplasma spp. infection during pregnancy, since its presence often represents colonization rather than infection [25]. Our data did not show any association between T. vaginalis and either U. parvum or U. urealyticum.

C. trachomatis was highly prevalent (13.9%) in our study. All isolates were non-LGV strains, but were not associated with T. vaginalis infection. Our results on urogenital carriage of Candida, E. coli, and GBS indicate that the three were not associated with T. vaginalis infection, either. While the prevalence of Candida in our study was higher than that reported in a cross-sectional study by Cools et al. [11] among women in Kenya, Rwanda and South-Africa, our prevalence for E. coli and GBS is comparable to what they reported.

Our study had some limitations. First, it only included a relatively small sample size of pregnant women limiting the precision of our prevalence estimates. Furthermore, only BV negative samples were included in the control arm, which may represent a bias on the interpretation of the results. Among the 28 T. vaginalis-positive women, only four were positive for BV and excluding them in the analysis does not affect the results (Additional file 1: Table S3). It should be noted that our T. vaginalis/BV co-infection rate of 14% was comparable to that observed in a recent study, i.e. 17.5% among HIV + women [26]. Finally, no internal control was added during the DNA extraction process, so inefficient genome extraction or (partial) PCR inhibition could not be documented. However, sample adequacy was evaluated by detecting a minimal level of human DNA present in the sample, which was the case for all samples, moreover none of the samples that were culture-positive for T. vaginalis were missed by PCR.

Conclusion

We observed notable prevalence of urogenital micro-organisms, pathogens and colonizing germs among pregnant women which emphasizes the need for laboratory testing and treatment to avoid unfavorable pregnancy outcomes. We confirm M. hominis as a correlate of T. vaginalis in our population, but the most salient finding was the exclusive association of both M. genitalium and Ca. M. girerdii with T. vaginalis. The latter finding ought to be further addressed using a larger sample size.

Abbreviations
BV: Bacterial vaginosis; Ca. M. girerdii: Candidatus Mycoplasma girerdii; M. genitalium: Mycoplasma genitalium; M. hominis: Mycoplasma hominis; PCR: Polymerase chain reaction; STIs: Sexually transmitted infections; T. vaginalis: Trichomonas vaginalis; TAC: TaqMan® Array Card; U. parvum: Ureaplasma parvum; U. urealyticum: Ureaplsama urealyticum

Acknowledgements
We would like to thank the study participants. A special thanks to all nurses at the prenatal care clinic of the Kilifi County Hospital. We also wish to acknowledge Sarah Kioko who was a field worker in the curable STI study. This manuscript was submitted for publication with permission from the Director of the Kenya Medical Research Institute (KEMRI).

Funding
This research has been supported by a PhD Scholarship to Simon C. Masha from the Belgian Development Cooperation through VLIR-UOS. The funders had no role in the design of the study and collection, analysis, and interpretation of data and in writing the manuscript. The views expressed here are those of the authors and do not necessarily represent the views of the Belgian Development Cooperation.

Authors' contributions

SCM, PC, EJS and MV designed the study. SCM supervised the field data collections. SCM, PC, PD and MR conducted laboratory analysis. SCM performed data management, and analysis. All authors contributed to the interpretation of results. SCM wrote the initial manuscript draft, PC, PD, MR, EJS and MV critically reviewed the manuscript. MV gave overall supervision, and including on the manuscript preparation. All authors read and approved the final version of the manuscript and agree to be accountable for all aspects of the work.

Competing interests

The authors declare that they have no competing interests.

Author details

[1]Kenya Medical Research Institute, Centre for Geographic Medicine Research – Coast, Kenya Medical Research Institute, P.O. Box 230, Kilifi, Kenya. [2]Laboratory Bacteriology Research, Faculty of Medicine and Health Sciences, Ghent University, De Pintelaan, 185 Ghent, Belgium. [3]Faculty of Pure and Applied Sciences, Department of Biological Sciences, Pwani University, Kilifi, Kenya. [4]Department of Laboratory Medicine, Medical Microbiology, AZ St-Jan Brugge-Oostende, Bruges, Belgium.

References

1. Newman L, Rowley J, Vander Hoorn S, et al. Global estimates of the prevalence and incidence of four curable sexually transmitted infections in 2012 based on systematic review and global reporting. PLoS One. 2015;10: e0143304.

2. Vos T, Barber RM, Bell B, et al. Global, regional, and national incidence, prevalence, and years lived with disability for 301 acute and chronic diseases and injuries in 188 countries, 1990 -2013: a systematic analysis for the global burden of disease study 2013. Lancet. 2015;386:743–800.

3. McClelland RS, Sangare L, Hassan WM, et al. Infection with Trichomonas vaginalis increases the risk of HIV-1 acquisition. J Infect Dis. 2007;195: 698–702.

4. Petrin D, Delgaty K, Bhatt R, et al. Clinical and microbiological aspects of Trichomonas vaginalis. Clin Microbiol Rev. 1998;11:300–17.

5. Fichorova R, Fraga J, Rappelli P, et al. Trichomonas vaginalis infection in symbiosis with Trichomonasvirus and Mycoplasma. Res Microbiol. 2017; 168:882–91.

6. Azargoon A, Darvishzadeh S. Association of bacterial vaginosis, Trichomonas vaginalis, and vaginal acidity with outcome of pregnancy. Arch Iranian Med. 2006;9:213–7.

7. Donders GGG, Ruban K, Bellen G, et al. Mycoplasma/Ureaplasma infection in pregnancy: to screen or not to screen. J Perinat Med. 2017;45(5):505–15.

8. Masha SC, Wahome E, Vaneechoutte M, et al. High prevalence of curable sexually transmitted infections among pregnant women in a rural county hospital in Kilifi, Kenya. PloS One. 2017;12:e0175166.

9. Steensels D, Reynders M, Descheemaeker P, et al. Clinical evaluation of a multi-parameter customized respiratory TaqMan® array card compared to conventional methods in immunocompromised patients. J Clin Vir. 2015;72:36–41.

10. Duyvejonck H, Cools P, Decruyenaere J, et al. Validation of High Resolution Melting Analysis (HRM) of the amplified ITS2 region for the detection and identification of yeasts from clinical samples: Comparison with culture and MALDI-TOF based identification. PLoS ONE. 2015;10:e0132149 Erratum in: PLoS One 2015; 10:e0139501.

11. Cools P, Jespers V, Hardy L, et al. A multi-country cross-sectional study of vaginal carriage of group B streptococci (GBS) and Escherichia coli in resource-poor settings: prevalences and risk factors. PLoS One. 2016;11: e0148052.

12. El Aila NA, Cools P, Deschaght P, et al. Strong correspondence of the vaginal and rectal load of group B streptococci in pregnant women. J Clin Gynecol Obst. 2013;2:61–7.

13. Deeks JJ, Higgins JPT. Statistical algorithms in review. Manager. 2010;5 http://training.cochrane.org/handbook/statistical-methods-revman5. Accessed 6 Jun 2018.

14. Crucitti T, Abdellati S, Van Dyck E, Buve A. Molecular typing of the actin gene of Trichomonas vaginalis isolates by PCR-restriction fragment length polymorphism. Clin Microbiol Infect. 2008;14:844–52.

15. Becker DD, dos Santos O, Frasson AP, et al. High rates of double-stranded RNA viruses and Mycoplasma hominis in Trichomonas vaginalis clinical isolates in South Brazil. Infect Genet Evol. 2015;34:181–7.

16. Xiao JC, Xie LF, Fang SL, et al. Symbiosis of Mycoplasma hominis in Trichomonas vaginalis may link metronidazole resistance in vitro. Parasit Res. 2006;100:123–30.

17. Rappelli P, Addis MF, Carta F, et al. Mycoplasma hominis parasitism of Trichomonas vaginalis. Lancet. 1998;352:1286.

18. Van Belkum A, Van der Meijden WI, Verbrugh HA, et al. A clinical study on the association of Trichomonas vaginalis and Mycoplasma hominis infections in women attending a sexually transmitted disease (STD) outpatient clinic. Immun Med Microbiol. 2001;32:27–32.

19. Coorevits L, Traen A, Binge L, et al. Macrolide resistance in mycoplasma genitalium from female sex workers in Belgium. J Glob Antimicrob Resist. 2018;12:149–52.

20. Fettweis JM, Serrano MG, Huang B, et al. An emerging Mycoplasma associated with trichomoniasis, vaginal infection and disease. PloS One. 2014;9:e110943.

21. Martin DH, Zozaya M, Lillis RA, et al. Unique vaginal microbiota that includes an unknown Mycoplasma-like organism is associated with Trichomonas vaginalis infection. J Infect Dis. 2013;207:1922–31.

22. Costello EK, Sun CL, Carlisle EM, et al. Candidatus Mycoplasma girerdii replicates, diversifies, and co-occurs with Trichomonas vaginalis in the oral cavity of a premature infant. Sci Rep. 2017;7:3764.

23. Taylor-Robinson D. Mollicutes in vaginal microbiology: Mycoplasma hominis, Ureaplasma urealyticum, Ureaplasma parvum and Mycoplasma genitalium. Res Microbiol. 2017;168:875–81.

24. Payne MS, Ireland DJ, Watts R, et al. Ureaplasma parvum genotype, combined vaginal colonisation with Candida albicans, and spontaneous preterm birth in an Australian cohort of pregnant women. BMC Pregnancy Childbirth. 2016;16:312.

25. Donders GG, Ruban K, Bellen G, et al. Mycoplasma/Ureaplasma infection in pregnancy: to screen or not to screen. J Perinatal Med. 2017;45:505–15.

26. Gatski M, Martin DH, Clark RA, et al. Co-occurrence of Trichomonas vaginalis and bacterial vaginosis among HIV-positive women. Sex Transm Dis. 2011;38:163–6.

8

Total coliforms as an indicator of human enterovirus presence in surface water across Tianjin city, China

Jing Miao[1], Xuan Guo[1,2], Weili Liu[1], Dong Yang[1], Zhiqiang Shen[1], Zhigang Qiu[1], Xiang Chen[1], Kunming Zhang[1], Hui Hu[1], Jing Yin[1], Zhongwei Yang[1], Junwen Li[1*] and Min Jin[1*] (iD)

Abstract

Background: Enteric viruses in surface water pose considerable risk to morbidity in populations living around water catchments and promote outbreaks of waterborne diseases. However, due to poor understanding of the correlation between water quality and the presence of human enteric viruses, the failure to assess viral contamination through alternative viral indicators makes it difficult to control disease transmission.

Methods: We investigated the occurrence of Enteroviruses (EnVs), Rotaviruses (HRVs), Astroviruses (AstVs), Noroviruses GII (HuNoVs GII) and Adenoviruses (HAdVs) from Jinhe River over 4 years and analyzed their correlation with physicochemical and bacterial parameters in water samples.

Results: The findings showed that all target viruses were detected in water at frequencies of 91.7% for HAdVs, 81.3% for HuNoVs GII, 79.2% for EnVs and AstVs, and 70.8% for HRVs. These viruses had a seasonal pattern, which showed that EnVs were abundant in summer but rare in winter, while HAdVs, HRVs, AstVs, and HuNoVs GII exhibited opposite seasonal trends. Pearson correlation analysis showed that total coliforms (TC) was significantly positively correlated with EnVs concentrations while no consistent significant correlations were observed between bacterial indices and viruses that precipitate acute gastroenteritis.

Conclusions: Taken together, the findings provide insights into alternative viral indicators, suggesting that TC is a potentially promising candidate for assessment of EnVs contamination. However, it failed to predict the presence of HAdVs, HRVs, AstVs, and HuNoVs GII in surface water across the city of Tianjin.

Keywords: Surface water, Human enteric viruses, Total coliforms, Viral indicator

Background

Human enteric viruses are a diverse group of organisms including Enteroviruses (EnVs), Rotaviruses (HRVs), Astroviruses (AstVs), Noroviruses GII (HuNoVs GII), and Adenoviruses (HAdVs). These viruses are transmitted by the fecal-oral route, resulting in a wide range of waterborne diseases, such as gastroenteritis and hepatitis [1]. According to the World Health Organization (WHO), human enteric viruses infect billions of people every year and the resultant diarrheal disease accounts for the second leading cause of death in children under 5 years globally [2]. They pose an especially high risk of mortality in young children, immune-compromised patients, and the elderly [3].

The high infection rates and rapid transmission between humans contribute to the significant morbidity associated with enteric viruses [4]. The absence of specific vaccines for human enteric viruses (except HRVs) further enhances the risk of infection [5]. More importantly, exposure to enteric virus-contaminated environments and/or drinking water, are generally thought to be responsible for a large proportion of outbreaks of waterborne diseases [6]. In recent years, there have been significant efforts to investigate human enteric viruses in water sources. Almost all types of human enteric viruses,

---
* Correspondence: junwen9999@hotmail.com; jinminzh@126.com
[1]Tianjin Institute of Environmental & Operational Medcine, Key Laboratory of Risk Assessment and Control for Environment & Food Safety, Tianjin 300050, China
Full list of author information is available at the end of the article

including HAdVs, HRVs, AstVs, EnVs, and HuNoVs GII, have been found in surface water [7, 8], sewage [9], recreational water [10], raw water sources [11], and seawater [12].

The low viral removal efficiency of wastewater treatment and strong intrinsic resistance to the water disinfection processes [13], may aid viral survival in water [14], resulting in contamination of viruses in water. However, there are no ideal indicators that are typically correlated with or specific enough to predict the presence of human enteric viruses. This leads to the failure in assessing the occurrence of enteric viruses in surface water, which may be another important consideration for why viral contamination in water has been overlooked [15]. This is the case even where bacterial indicators are currently used in most countries around the world for assessment of fecal or pathogen contamination in surface water [16]. In such settings, it is essential to explore a sensitive indicator that sufficiently expedites an early warning system relating to the occurrence of enteric viruses, which enables corrective action to be applied in a timely manner in regions with enteric virus-contaminated waters.

Here, we investigated the prevalence of five enteric viruses, including HAdVs, HRVs, AstVs, EnVs, and HuNoVs GII, in the Jinhe River of Tianjin city over 4 years. By analyzing the correlations between viral prevalence in the river and bacterial indices e.g., heterotrophic plate counts (HPC), total coliforms (TC), and fecal coliforms (FC), viral indicator candidates were explored. Additionally, we also measured physicochemical parameters such as temperature, pH, conductivity, turbidity, chemical oxygen demand (COD_{Mn}) and ammonium content (NH_3-N) in water. We believed this would help reveal the relationship between human enteric viruses and some physicochemical parameters in surface waters. This study aimed to provide beneficial tools to assess the occurrence of enteric viruses in river water.

Methods

Sample collection

150 L of water was collected from a depth of 0.5 m below the surface of the sample site proximal to the Jinhe River in Tianjin located at 39°6′58.36″N, 117°13′20.66″E in the center of the city (Additional file 1: Figure S1). The Jinhe River is an important tributary of the Haihe River and is one of the most important rivers in Tianjin, with a full length of 18.5 km and a width of eight meters. It flows through the city center, which contains a large number of commercial, catering, cultural, and entertainment industries on both sides of the river, as well as a considerable residential area.

A total of 48 samples were collected once a month from March 2012 to February 2016 and they were transported in cold storage conditions to the laboratory in approximately 3 h. According to the Chinese Meteorological Administration, the period from March to May was defined as spring, June to August defined as summer, September to November defined as autumn, and December to February defined as winter.

Quality of surface water samples

All samples were assayed for HPC, TC, and FC on Luria-Bertani agar, M-Endo medium (BD Difco, USA) and M-FC medium (BD Difco, USA) according to the standard membrane filter procedure [17]. Turbidity and conductivity were measured with a HACH 1900C portable turbidity meter (HACH, USA) and a HACH sension5 conductivity meter (HACH, USA), respectively. Chemical oxygen demand (COD_{Mn}) and ammonium content (NH_3-N) were measured according to standard methods [17].

Virus concentration from water samples using a filter cartridge

Fifty L samples of the river water were filtered through a filter cartridge filled with electropositive granule media (EGM) according to Jin [18]. Then, 3 L of eluent (2% sodium hydroxide, 0.375% glycine, 1.5% sodium chloride, 3% tryptone, 1.5% beef powder) was passed through the column. Eluates were neutralized by the addition of 0.1 mol/L HCl immediately after collection and then 10% PEG was added to the eluates before overnight centrifugation (15,000×g for 30 min at 4 °C). Then, the pellets were resuspended in 40 mL PBS and stored at −70 °C until further analysis. To evaluate the efficiency of virus recovery, 10^5 PFU of bacteriophage MS2 was cultivated by confluent lysis on its host strain, E. coli (ATCC 15597), and then added to water samples as an indicator and detected using the double layer plaque assay. Virus recovery was calculated using the following eq. (1):

$$\text{Virus recovery } (\%) = (B{-}C)/A \times 100\% \qquad (1)$$

Where A is the number of seeded MS2 into the tested water samples before concentration; B is the number of MS2 measured in the final buffered concentrate; and C is the number of environmental/background MS2 measured in the final buffered concentrate.

Viral DNA/RNA extraction

According to the manufacturer's instructions, viral RNA was extracted from the concentrated viral suspensions using the QIAamp viral RNA mini kit (Qiagen, Hilden, Germany) to detect HRVs, HuNoVs GII, AstVs, and EnVs. UNIQ-10 viral DNA kit (Sangon Biotech) was used for DNA extraction of HAdVs. The purity and concentration of DNA/RNA were determined by a Gene

Quant1300 system (GE Healthcare), and samples meeting the purity standards (A260/A280, 1.8–2.0) were used for further analysis. The nucleic acid extraction recovery was evaluated by addition of internal control (IC) RNA to the lysis buffer according to the manufacturer's instructions (QIAamp Viral RNA Mini Handbook, Qiagen, Hilden, Germany).

Quantification of viruses by (RT-)qPCR

Reverse transcription was performed using a cDNA first-strand synthesis system (Thermo Fisher Scientific, Waltham, MA) for viruses. 15 μL of template RNA was added to 2 μL of Random Hexamer primer (0.2 μg/μL), incubated for 5 min at 65 °C, and chilled on ice. Then 23 μL of reaction mixture, which contained 8 μL of 5X Reaction Buffer, 2 μL of RevertAid M-MuLV Reverse Transcriptase (200 U/μL), 2 μL RiboLock RNase inhibitor (20 U/μL), 4 μL of 10 mM dNTP Mix, and 7 μL nuclease-free water, was added to the samples. The mixtures were incubated for 5 min at 25 °C, for 60 min at 45 °C, and the reaction was terminated by heating at 70 °C for 5 min in a 2720 thermocycler (Applied Biosystems, USA) to synthesize cDNA. The mixtures were then held at 4 °C for qPCR amplification.

A total volume of 20 μL was used for qPCR, including 2 μL of DNA from HAdVs or cDNA from EnVs, AstVs, HRVs, and HuNoVs GII; 10 μL PCR SuperMix-UDG (Platinum PCR SuperMix-UDG, Invitrogen, USA); 0.5 μL of each primer (10 μmol/L); 0.5 μL of TaqMan probe (5 μmol/L), and; 6.5 μL nuclease-free water. The reaction was performed in an ABI sequence detection system 7300 (Applied Biosystems, USA) under the following conditions: 95 °C for 30 s, followed by 40 cycles of 95 °C for 30 s and 60 °C for 1 min. All qPCR analyses were performed in triplicate with positive controls for each target and DEPC-treated water as the negative controls to ensure cycling efficiencies. All primers and probes (Invitrogen, Shanghai, China) labeled with FAM detector dyes and TAMRA quencher dyes are shown in Additional file 1: Table S1 [18–22].

The standard curves for the quantification of HRVs, HuNoVs GII, AstVs, EnVs, HAdVs, and HCVs (Hepatitis C virus) were obtained by analyzing 10-fold serial dilutions of viral RNA or DNA standards (SI Additional file 1: Figures S2 – S7) [18]. The detailed information pertaining to how viral RNA or DNA standards were prepared as shown in the SI for MM.

Inhibition control and calculations for virus concentration

To avoid inhibition occurring in the RT-qPCR reaction, 10^5 genome copies (GCs)/reaction of an HCV RNA IC was added to 2 μL nucleic acids (10- or 50-fold dilution or none) extracted from the samples or DEPC water (blank control) and then assayed using RT-qPCR. If the threshold cycle value (Ct) of the blank control was one cycle less than that of the HCV RNA IC mixed with the nucleic acid extracts from samples, inhibition of the reaction had occurred, and dilutions of the nucleic acid extracts were performed until no inhibition was observed [18]. As background controls, all samples should be verified for a lack of indigenous HCV using RT-qPCR prior to the inhibition check.

The quantification of HCV RNA IC was carried out using real-time procedures following the same conditions as for virus detection with Primer and TaqMan probe sequences listed in Additional file 1: Table S1. The equation for calculating the sample inhibition is:

$$\text{Virus recovery } (\%) = (A-B)/A \times 100\% \qquad (2)$$

Where A is the GCs of IC/reaction in the blank control, B is the measured GCs of IC/reaction mixed with the nucleic acid extracts in the tested water samples.

Calculations for virus concentration

HRVs, HuNoVs GII, AstVs, and EnVs concentrations in all water samples were quantified using the following eq. (3) and HAdVs concentration were quantified using the following eq. (4):

$$\text{Virus (GCs)} = \text{GCs}/reaction \times 80 \text{ μL}/2 \text{ μL}$$
$$\times \text{Ve}/140 \text{ μL} \times \text{N} \qquad (3)$$

$$\text{Virus (GCs)} = \text{GCs}/reaction \times 50 \text{ μL}/2 \text{ μL}$$
$$\times \text{Ve}/200 \text{μL} \times \text{N} \qquad (4)$$

Where 2 μL was the volume of sample per reaction tube, and the 140 and 80 μL are the volume of sample extracted and the RNA extract volume of HRVs, HuNoVs GII, AstVs and EnVs, respectively. The 200 and 50 μL are the volumes of sample extracted and the DNA extract volume of HAdVs, respectively. The Ve is the volume of final buffered concentrate (μL). N represents dilution of the nucleic acid extract.

Statistical analysis

Statistical analyses were performed using SAS9.2 and R language. Viral distributions were compared using the non-parametric Kruskal-Wallis test. Correlations between the virus positive rate and season were analyzed using Fisher's Exact Test. The run-length testing method was used to analyze the differences in viral concentrations between seasons. Virus concentrations within the same month of different years were analyzed using a Friedman test. Pearson test was calculated using R Studio to measure the strength of associations between enteric virus concentrations and detection indices. This was followed by a Student-Newman-Keuls-q test to analyze the correlation between these variables.

Results and discussion

The characteristics of water quality in Jinhe River

Table 1 summarizes the physicochemical and bacterial parameters of water samples from the Jinhe River during the periods from March 2012 to February 2016. It showed that all the parameters fluctuated continuously through the year, exhibiting periodic variation in a seasonal pattern (Additional file 1: Figures S8 and S9). Physicochemical parameters e.g., turbidity, water temperature, COD_{Mn}, NH_3-N, and bacterial parameters e.g., HPC, TC, and FC reached the maximal value during warm months (May–September) while the maximal pH and conductivity occurred in the cold months (November–February).

Fecal indicator TC and FC were detected in all samples collected across the four-year survey and 23 of 48 (47.9%) samples exceeded the regulations provided by the Pennsylvania Department of Environmental Protection (PA DEP) for TC (5000 CFU/100 mL) [23] at concentrations ranging from 5.3×10^3 to 1.1×10^5 CFU/100 mL, which were observed mainly between May and September. Concentrations of the FC in all samples ranged between 2.7×10^2 to 6.7×10^4 CFU/100 mL in May–September, which exceeded the PA DEP regulations for fecal coliforms (200 CFU/100 mL) during the season (May 1 through September 30) [23]. For this reason, high concentrations of TC and FC are likely indicative of high levels of human fecal contamination in warm months.

Detection of enteric viruses in Jinhe River

Figure 1a illustrated the occurrence and the abundances of enteric viruses in water samples from the Jinhe River between March 2012 and February 2016. It showed that all types of enteric viruses can be found in the Jinhe River and at least one of the target viruses could be detected positively every month. In particular, all targeted viruses were positive simultaneously in 22 of 48 (45.8%) samples, which were mainly in the periods between March–May and October–November. Among all the observed viruses (Fig. 1b), HAdVs were the most prevalent with a detection frequency of 91.7% (44/48). Its geometric mean concentration in positive samples was 4.96 $log_{10}GC/L$. For HuNoVs GII, the mean concentration of 4.32 log_{10} GC/L was the next most common with a detection frequency of 81.3% (39/48). AstVs and EnVs were detected in 79.2% (38/48) of samples with the highest mean concentrations of 5.10 $log_{10}GC/L$ and 4.86 log_{10} GC/L, respectively. HRVs were the least prevalent virus and were detected in 34 of 48 (70.8%) samples. They also had the lowest viral level of 4.21 $log_{10}GC/L$. There was a significant difference in the average concentrations of various viruses (Kruskal-Wallis, $P < 0.05$).

Generally, high concentrations of enteric viruses are found in the feces of infected patients [24]. Due to the their resistance to unfavorable circumstances and wastewater treatment, enteric viruses can persist in the wastewater treatment process (WWTP) effluent and retain survivability in the environment in recipient rivers for long periods [25]. Considering the Jinhe River as a river, which spans across Tianjin city, the frequent presence of these enteric viruses in water, even at low concentrations, may pose a public health threat to those in surrounding residences.

Figure 1a also exhibited the total load of observed enteric viruses in the Jinhe River, fluctuating from 4.42 to 7.20 log_{10} GC/L with the maximal value around November annually and minimally around May of the following year. There were no significant differences in the total viral loads between the same months during the four-year sampling period (Friedman test, $P > 0.05$). During the four-year sampling period, individual enteric viruses in water samples also exhibited seasonal patterns in their occurrence and concentrations, similar to the physicochemical and microbial parameters of water samples (Table 2, Run-length testing method, $P < 0.05$). Significant correlations were found between viral occurrence and season types for all five target viruses (Fisher's Exact Test, $P < 0.01$). For acute gastroenteritis viruses, including HAdVs, HRVs, HuNoVs GII and AstVs, their concentrations in the river were higher during cold weather rather than the warm weather months. They were positively detected every month in the seasons of spring and winter at concentrations ranging from 3.39 to 7.00, 2.83 to 6.02, 3.01 to 5.56, and 4.01 to 6.47 log_{10} GC/L for HAdVs, HRVs, HuNoVs GII, and AstVs, respectively. Only 16.7% of HRVs and 33.3% of HuNoVs were detected in summer at concentrations ranging from 0 to 3.29 and 0 to 2.95 log_{10} GC/L, respectively. In contrast, EnVs concentrations in the river were higher during the warm weather rather than the cold weather months. A detection rate of 100% every month in summer at concentrations ranging from 4.04 to 6.91 log_{10} GC/L but was only 33.3% in winter at concentrations ranging from 0 to 4.06 log_{10} GC/L.

Although high concentrations of acute gastroenteritis viruses were identified in cold weather (November–February), this may suggest that the river has high concentrations of human fecal contamination but concentrations of TC at the sampling site were generally low (maximum of 5.4×10^3 CFU/100 mL). This phenomenon may be a result of the high incidence of acute infectious gastroenteritis or diarrhea cases in clinics over the same timeframe. High infection rates of HRVs, HuNoVs GII, and AstVs among children in the

Table 1 Characteristics of bacterial indices and physicochemical parameters of water samples from Jinhe River

Season	Variation range			T (°C)	pH	Turbidity (NTU)	COD_{Mn} (mg/L)	NH_3-N (mg/L)	Conductivity (µs/cm)
	HPC (CFU/ml)	TC (CFU/100 ml)	FC (CFU/100 ml)						
Spring	4.0×10^2 –1.56×10^4	7.5×10^2 –1.6×10^4	1.0×10^2 -3.5×10^3	8.7–21	6.00–6.70	2.42–15.77	4.54–14.61	0.54–5.43	550–643
Summer	3.5×10^3 –2.8×10^5	1.0×10^2 –5.5×10^4	2.7×10^2 -3.8×10^4	26.5–32	6.00–6.90	6.55–29.23	8.93–22.40	0.80–9.54	514–647
Autumn	6.5×10^2 –4.5×10^5	2.5×10^2 -1.1×10^5	1.8×10^3 -6.7×10^4	6.3–27	6.00–7.40	4.07–24.23	9.53–22.30	1.54–7.53	605–828
Winter	5.5×10^1 –2.9×10^3	5.0×10^2 -1.7×10^4	2×10^4 -2.0×10^4	2–6.4	6.40–7.40	2.63–7.93	2.50–10.98	0.54–3.56	624–868
PA DEP reference values		5.0×10^3	2.0×10^2						

Abbreviations: *HPC* heterotrophic plate counts, *TC* total coliforms, *FC* fecal coliform, *T* water temperature, *NTU* nephelometric turbidity unit, *COD_{Mn}* chemical oxygen demand, *NH_3-N* ammonium content

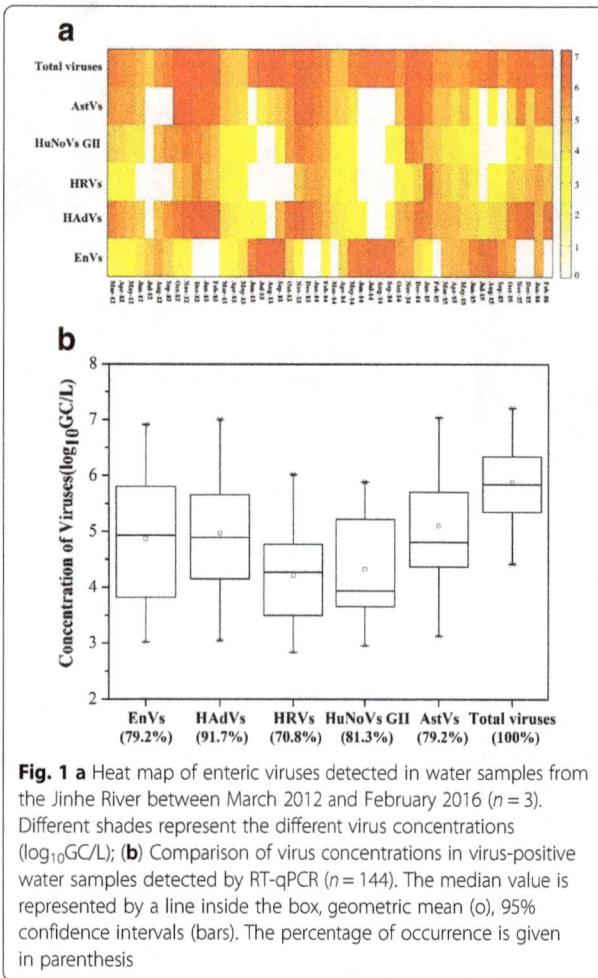

Fig. 1 a Heat map of enteric viruses detected in water samples from the Jinhe River between March 2012 and February 2016 ($n = 3$). Different shades represent the different virus concentrations ($\log_{10}$GC/L); (**b**) Comparison of virus concentrations in virus-positive water samples detected by RT-qPCR ($n = 144$). The median value is represented by a line inside the box, geometric mean (o), 95% confidence intervals (bars). The percentage of occurrence is given in parenthesis

Correlation between virus concentrations and physicochemical parameters in the Jinhe River

Enteric viruses were significantly correlated with all of the measured physicochemical indices (Fig. 2). EnVs showed the strongest positive correlation with temperature, turbidity, COD_{Mn}, and NH_3-N while they were negatively correlated with conductivity. In contrast, HAdVs, HRVs, AstVs, and HuNoVs GII were significantly correlated with temperature (negatively) or conductivity (positively). Above all, conductivity was the only physicochemical index that was positively correlated with total viral concentration ($P < 0.05$, Kendall's Tau-b).

Among all the physicochemical parameters, enteric viruses had the strongest correlation with water temperature with the exception of AstVs (Fig. 2 and Additional file 1: Figure S10; Pearson, $P < 0.01$). For acute gastroenteritis viruses, there was a significant negative correlation between their concentration and temperature. Viral concentrations remained the highest when temperatures ranged from 2 °C to 6 °C, while viral concentrations declined to the lowest when temperature was between 27 °C and 32 °C. This is likely due to their high clinical prevalence in winter as well as the lower temperatures, as higher viral persistence has been reported in vitro at lower temperatures [28, 29]. In contrast, EnVs were positively correlated with temperature, and EnVs concentrations increased to the highest value when temperature exceeded 16 °C. There were significant differences between viral concentrations under

autumn and winter have been observed in Tianjin, the river basin of the sampling site [26]. Also, a high incidence of diarrhea associated with EnVs occurred in the summer in China [27]. Therefore, all of these results suggest that enteric viruses in the river are strongly associated with the clinical epidemiology of the river catchment area. Correspondingly, TC could not predict the total enteric virus presence but was more specific to acute gastroenteritis viruses.

Table 2 Occurrence of enteric viruses in seasons ($n = 36$)

Season[a]	Detection rate (%)				
	EnVs	HAdVs	HRVs	HuNoVs GII	AstVs
Spring	91.7 ± 16.7	100 ± 0	100 ± 0	100 ± 0	100 ± 0
Summer	100 ± 0	66.7 ± 27.2	16.7 ± 33.3	33.3 ± 27.2	41.7 ± 31.9
Autumn	91.7 ± 16.7	100 ± 0	66.7 ± 27.2	91.7 ± 16.7	75 ± 16.7
Winter	33.3 ± 27.2	100 ± 0	100 ± 0	100 ± 0	100 ± 0

[a]Defined according to the Chinese Meteorological Institute: spring, from March to May; summer, from June to August; autumn, from September to November; winter, from December to February

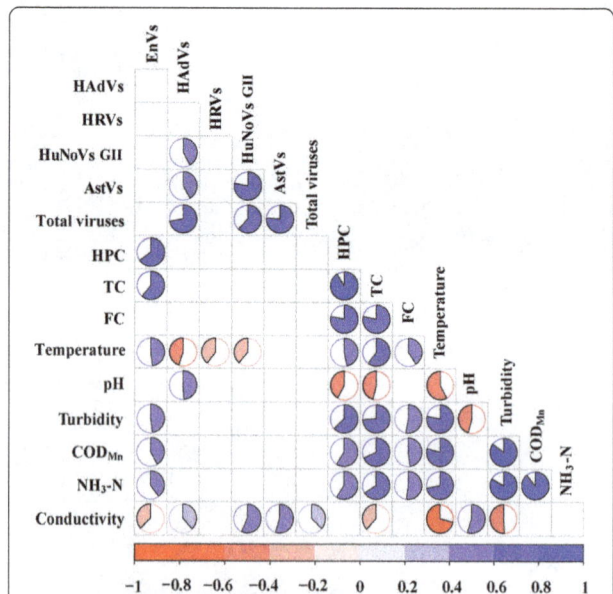

Fig. 2 Correlation matrix between virus concentration and water parameters analyzed by Pearson correlation analysis ($p < 0.01$). The range of the coefficients is from − 1 to 1, where − 1 indicates a direct negative correlation, 0 indicates no correlation, and 1 indicates a direct positive correlation

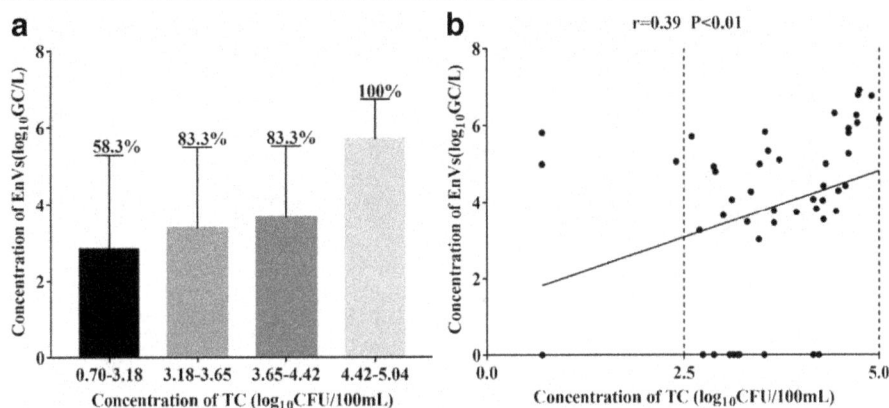

Fig. 3 Relationships between EnVs and total coliforms, which were selected from the quartiles of ranked observations. The percentage of EnVs occurrence is given in (**a**), the linearity between EnVs and total coliforms is shown in (**b**)

different temperature conditions (Student-Newman-Keuls-q test), which was consistent with the differences in viral concentrations under different seasonal conditions.

Correlation between virus concentrations and bacterial indices in the Jinhe River

Through Pearson analysis, only EnVs concentration in the Jinhe River showed a significant positive correlation with TC (Fig. 2; Pearson, P < 0.01). Meanwhile, only 58.3% (7/12) of the samples with TC levels that were lower than 3.18 $\log_{10}$CFU/100/mL was positive for EnVs but for the samples whose TC levels exceeded 4.42$\log_{10}$CFU/100 mL, we found that EnVs were significantly positive and there was a significant increase observed in the EnVs concentration (Fig. 3, Student-Newman-Keuls-q test). These data indicate that EnVs were more likely to be detected when the concentration of TC increased (Fig. 3, χ^2 test; P < 0.05). Therefore, TC may be a potentially promising candidate to assess the degree of EnVs contamination in the surface water across the city due to its stability and ability to identify origin of enteric viruses. This is true even if the results of several studies [30, 31] on drinking water demonstrated that TC did not reflect the occurrence of EnVs due to the frequent occurrence of EnVs in water which met current bacteriological standards. In effect, EnVs may be suggested as an alternative viral indicator of fecal pollution.

Significant positive correlations between the concentrations of HuNoVs GII, HAdVs, and AstVs can be observed. Furthermore, there were significant decreases in acute gastroenteritis virus concentrations when HPC exceeded 6.07 $\log_{10}$CFU/100 mL (Additional file 1: Figure S10, Student-Newman-Keuls-q test) and also in HRVs concentration when the TC exceeded 4.42 $\log_{10}$CFU/100 mL. However, no significant correlation was observed between concentrations of acute

gastroenteritis viruses with EnVs, TC, HPC, or FC (Fig. 2; Pearson, P < 0.01), indicating failure to predict the presence of non-EnVs enteric viruses in surface water using bacterial indices. It also meant acute gastroenteritis viruses should not be an alternative indicator of fecal or EnVs pollution even if there is prolonged virus persistence in the environment. Some previous studies [32, 33] have also suggested that bacteriological indicators e.g., TC concentrations do not accurately reflect human viral (HRVs, HuNoVs GII, and HAdVs) dispersal in marine waters, individual groundwater, and contamination of shellfish by sewage-derived viral pathogens.

Conclusions

A high occurrence of enteric viruses in a specific seasonal pattern were observed in the Jinhe River over a four-year survey. TC were significantly positively correlated with EnVs concentrations while bacterial indices and acute gastroenteritis viruses did not show any consistent significant correlations. These data indicate that TC seems to be a potentially promising candidate to assess the degree of EnVs contamination but fails to predict the presence of HAdVs, HRVs, AstVs, and HuNoVs GII in the surface water across the city of Tianjin. Furthermore, any one of HAdVs, HRVs, AstVs, and HuNoVs GII cannot be used as an alternative indicator of fecal or EnVs pollution in the environment.

Abbreviations
AstVs: Astroviruses; COD$_{Mn}$: Chemical oxygen demand; EnVs: Enteroviruses; FC: Fecal coliform; HAdVs: Adenoviruses; HCVs: Hepatitis C virus; HPC: Heterotrophic plate counts; HRVs: Rotaviruses; HuNoVs GII: Noroviruses GII; NH$_3$-N: Ammonium content; T: Water temperature; TC: Total coliforms

Acknowledgements
The authors would like to acknowledge the contribution from Xinwei Wang for sharing his valuable experience. This study was supported by grants from Tianjin Science and Technology Support Program (16YFZCSF00340) and Natural Science Foundation of Tianjin, China (15JCQNJC44100).

Authors' contributions

MJ conceived and designed the study, supervised data collection, contributed to data analysis and manuscript preparation. JM, XG, KMZ, HH and ZWY made substantial contributions to experimental operation, acquisition of data and contributed to manuscript preparation. JM completed the analysis of data and drafted the main manuscript. WLL, DY, ZQS, ZGQ, XC, JY and JWL supervised data entry, contributed to data analysis and manuscript preparation. All authors read and approved the final manuscript.

Competing interests

The authors declare that they have no competing interests.

Author details

[1]Tianjin Institute of Environmental & Operational Medcine, Key Laboratory of Risk Assessment and Control for Environment & Food Safety, Tianjin 300050, China. [2]Research Institution of Chemical Defense, Beijing 102205, China.

References

1. Husman AMDR, Bartram J. Chapter 7 global supply of virus-safe drinking water. Persp Med Virol. 2007;17:127–62.
2. WHO. http://www.who.int/zh/news-room/fact-sheets/detail/diarrhoeal-disease. Accessed 20 May 2018.
3. Gerba CP, Rose JB, Haas CN. Sensitive populations: who is at the greatest risk? Int J Food Microbiol. 1996;30(1–2):113.
4. Fong TT, Lipp EK. Enteric viruses of humans and animals in aquatic environments: health risks, detection, and potential water quality assessment tools. Microbiol Mol Biol Rev. 2005;69(2):357–71.
5. Clemens J. Evaluation of vaccines against enteric infections: a clinical and public health research agenda for developing countries. Philos Trans R Soc Lond Ser B Biol Sci. 2011;366(1579):2799–805.
6. Iaconelli M, Muscillo M, Della LS, Fratini M, Meucci L, De CM, Giacosa D, La RG. One-year surveillance of human enteric viruses in raw and treated wastewaters, Downstream River waters, and drinking waters. Food Environ Virol. 2016;9(1):1–10.
7. He X, Wei Y, Cheng L, Zhang D, Wang Z. Molecular detection of three gastroenteritis viruses in urban surface waters in Beijing and correlation with levels of fecal indicator bacteria. Environ Monit Assess. 2012;184(9):5563.
8. Prevost B, Lucas FS, Goncalves A, Richard F, Moulin L, Wurtzer S. Large scale survey of enteric viruses in river and waste water underlines the health status of the local population. Environ Int. 2015;79:42–50.
9. Kiulia NM, Netshikweta R, Page NA, Van Zyl WB, Kiraithe MM, Nyachieo A, Mwenda JM, Taylor MB. The detection of enteric viruses in selected urban and rural river water and sewage in Kenya, with special reference to rotaviruses. J Appl Microbiol. 2010;109(3):818–28.
10. Wynjones AP, Carducci A, Cook N, D'Agostino M, Divizia M, Fleischer J, Gantzer C, Gawler A, Girones R, Höller C. Surveillance of adenoviruses and noroviruses in European recreational waters. Water Res. 2011;45(3):1025–38.
11. Gibson KE, Schwab KJ. Detection of bacterial indicators and human and bovine enteric viruses in surface water and groundwater sources potentially impacted by animal and human wastes in lower Yakima Valley, Washington. Appl Environ Microbiol. 2011;77(1):355.
12. Yang N, Qi H, Wong MM, Wu RS, Kong RY. Prevalence and diversity of norovirus genogroups I and II in Hong Kong marine waters and detection by real-time PCR. Mar Pollut Bull. 2012;64(1):164–8.
13. Montazeri N, Goettert D, Achberger EC, Johnson CN, Prinyawiwatkul W, Janes ME. Pathogenic enteric viruses and microbial indicators during secondary treatment of municipal wastewater. Appl Environ Microbiol. 2015;81(18):6436–45.
14. Yezli S, Otter JA. Minimum infective dose of the major human respiratory and enteric viruses transmitted through food and the environment. Food Environ Virol. 2011;3(1):1–30.
15. Jurzik L, Hamza IA, Puchert W, Überla K, Wilhelm M. Chemical and microbiological parameters as possible indicators for human enteric viruses in surface water. Int J Hyg Envir Heal. 2010;213(3):210–6.
16. Zhu H, Yuan F, Yuan Z, Liu R, Xie F, Huang L, Liu X, Jiang X, Wang J, Xu Q. Monitoring of Poyang lake water for sewage contamination using human enteric viruses as an indicator. Virol J. 2018;15(1):3.
17. Walter WG. APHA standard methods for the examination of water and wastewater. Health Lab Sci. 1998;4(3):137.
18. Jin M, Guo X, Wang XW, Yang D, Shen ZQ, Qiu ZG, Chen ZL, Li JW. Development of a novel filter cartridge system with electropositive granule media to concentrate viruses from large volumes of natural surface water. Environ Sci Technol. 2014;48(12):6947.
19. Kageyama T, Kojima S, Shinohara M, Uchida K, Fukushi S, Hoshino FB, Takeda N, Katayama K. Broadly reactive and highly sensitive assay for Norwalk-like viruses based on real-time quantitative reverse transcription-PCR. J Clin Microbiol. 2003;41(4):1548–57.
20. Xagoraraki I, Kuo DH, Wong K, Wong M, Rose JB. Occurrence of human adenoviruses at two recreational beaches of the Great Lakes. Appl Environ Microbiol. 2007;73(24):7874.
21. Le CP, Ranarijaona S, Monpoeho S, Le GF, Ferré V. Quantification of human astroviruses in sewage using real-time RT-PCR. Res Microbiol. 2004;155(1):11–5.
22. Guo X, Wang S, Qiu ZG, Dou YL, Liu WL, Yang D, Shen ZQ, Chen ZL, Wang JF, Zhang B. Efficient replication of blood-borne hepatitis C virus in human fetal liver stem cells. Hepatology. 2017;66(4):1045–57.
23. Pennsylvania Department of Environmental Protection (PA DEP). https://www.pacode.com/secure/data/025/chapter93/s93.7.html. Accessed 20 May 2018.
24. Wong K, Fong TT, Bibby K, Molina M. Application of enteric viruses for fecal pollution source tracking in environmental waters. Environ Int. 2012;45(1):151–64.
25. Espinosa AC, Mazari-Hiriart M, Espinosa R, Maruri-Avidal L, Méndez E, Arias CF. Infectivity and genome persistence of rotavirus and astrovirus in groundwater and surface water. Water Res. 2008;42(10–11):2618–28.
26. Ouyang Y, Ma H, Jin M, Wang X, Wang J, Xu L, Lin S, Shen Z, Chen Z, Qiu Z. Etiology and epidemiology of viral diarrhea in children under the age of five hospitalized in Tianjin, China. Arch Virol. 2012;157(5):881–7.
27. Li W, Gao H, Zhang Q, Liu Y, Tao R, Cheng Y, Shu Q, Shang S. Large outbreak of herpangina in children caused by enterovirus in summer of 2015 in Hangzhou, China. Sci Rep. 2016;6:35388.
28. Am DRH, Lodder WJ, Rutjes SA, Schijven JF, Teunis PF. Long-term inactivation study of three enteroviruses in artificial surface and groundwaters, using PCR and cell culture. Appl Environ Microbiol. 2009;75(4):1050–7.
29. Lodder WJ, HHJLvd B, Rutjes SA, Husman AMDR. Presence of enteric viruses in source waters for drinking water production in the Netherlands. Appl Environ Microbiol. 2010;76(17):5965–71.
30. Gerba CP, Goyal SM, Labelle RL, Cech I, Bodgan GF. Failure of indicator bacteria to reflect the occurrence of enteroviruses in marine waters. Am J Public Health. 1979;69(11):1116–9.
31. Berg G. Indicators of viruses in water and food. Michigan: Ann Arbor Science; 1978.
32. Winterbourn JB, Clements K, Lowther JA, Malham SK, Mcdonald JE, Jones DL. Use of Mytilus edulis biosentinels to investigate spatial patterns of norovirus and faecal indicator organism contamination around coastal sewage discharges. Water Res. 2016;105:241.
33. Gamazo P, Victoria M, Schijven JF, Alvareda E, Tort LFL, Ramos J, Burutaran L, Olivera M, Lizasoain A, Sapriza G, et al. Evaluation of bacterial contamination as an Indicator of viral contamination in a sedimentary aquifer in Uruguay. Food Environ Virol. 2018;10(2):1867–0342.

9

Improvement in tuberculosis infection control practice via technical support in two regions of Ethiopia

Asfaw Ayalew[1][*] , Zewdu Gashu[1], Tadesse Anteneh[1], Nebiyu Hiruy[1], Dereje Habte[1], Degu Jerene[1], Genetu Alem[2], Ilili Jemal[3], Muluken Melese[1] and Pedro G. Suarez[4]

Abstract

Background: Globally recommended measures for comprehensive tuberculosis (TB) infection control (IC) are inadequately practiced in most health care facilities in Ethiopia. The aim of this study was to assess the extent of implementation of TB IC measures before and after introducing a comprehensive technical support package in two regions of Ethiopia.

Methods: We used a quasi-experimental design, whereby a baseline assessment of TB IC practices in 719 health care facilities was conducted between August and October 2013. Based on the assessment findings, we supported implementation of a comprehensive package of interventions. Monitoring was done on a quarterly basis, and one-year follow-up data were collected on September 30, 2014. We used the Student's *t*-test and chi-squared tests, respectively, to examine differences before and after the interventions and to test for inter-regional and inter-facility associations.

Results: At baseline, most of the health facilities (69%) were reported to have separate TB clinics. In 55.2% of the facilities, it was also reported that window opening was practiced. Nevertheless, triaging was practiced in only 19.3% of the facilities. Availability of an IC committee and IC plan was observed in 29.11 and 4.65% of facilities, respectively. Health care workers were nearly three times as likely to develop active TB as the general population. After 12 months of implementation, availability of a separate TB room, TB IC committee, triage, and TB IC plan had increased, respectively, by 18, 32, 44, and 51% ($p < 0.001$).

Conclusions: After 1 year of intervention, the TB IC practices of the health facilities have significantly improved. However, availability of separate TB rooms and existence of TB IC committees remain suboptimal. The burden of TB among health care workers is higher than in the general population. TB IC measures must be strengthened to reduce TB transmission among health workers.

Keywords: TB infection control, TB transmission, TB prevention, Health care workers, Ethiopia

Background

Tuberculosis (TB) is one of the major infectious diseases that have tested the knowledge and wisdom of mankind. Innovations related to TB diagnosis, prevention, and treatment have lagged behind other technological advancements. After isolation of the tubercle bacillus, it took 38 years to invent a preventive vaccine and 61 years to discover the first anti-TB drug [1, 2]. The death toll from TB is enormous, and it continues to claim millions of lives throughout the world, even though simple preventive measures exist. Through airborne transmission, its favored mode of dissemination, TB has managed to sustain itself for millennia [3, 4].

Against all odds, remarkable progress has been made in recent times through formulation and implementation of effective strategies like the Directly Observed Treatment, Short course (DOTS) and Stop TB strategies,

* Correspondence: aayalew@msh.org; asfonium2000@yahoo.com
[1]Management Sciences for Health, Help Ethiopia Address the Low Performance of Tuberculosis (HEAL TB) Project, Bole Sub City, Kebele 02, House Number 708, PO Box 1157, Code 1250 Addis Ababa, Ethiopia
Full list of author information is available at the end of the article

which greatly contributed to meeting the TB-related target of the Millennium Development Goals (MDGs) of halting and beginning to reverse the TB epidemic [5]. On one hand, between 2000 and 2015, TB mortality declined by 34% and the number of deaths averted as a result of TB treatment was estimated at 49 million. On the other hand, TB remained one of the top 10 killer diseases in 2015. Moreover, increasing TB mortality was seen in Congo and the Democratic People's Republic of Korea [6].

Ethiopia is one of the 30 high-TB-burden countries that have shown a substantial reduction in TB incidence and mortality since 2000. The estimated decline in the incidence rate as of 2010 was 6.7%. In 2015, the estimated TB incidence was 191,000, while the actual notified TB cases were 137,960. In the same year, 599 cases of drug-resistant TB (DR-TB) were notified. Of the notified TB cases, 8% were people living with the human immunodeficiency virus (HIV) [6].

In low-income countries such as Ethiopia, patients and visitors tend to congregate in health facilities' corridors and waiting areas. This congestion is due to uncontrolled population growth and an increasing number of health care seekers, on one hand, and a shortage of health care workers (HCWs) and limited number of health care facilities (HCFs), on the other hand [7]. This overcrowding, in turn, supports airborne nosocomial transmission of TB to HCWs, patients, and even visitors [8]. Highly vulnerable people, such as children, undernourished people, and immunocompromised people, are among the health service seekers in HCFs, which is an opportunity for TB to continue its spread. The emergence and rapid spread of drug-resistant mycobacterial strains, as well as its interaction with HIV, have heightened the demand for effective infection control (IC) interventions at all levels [9–11].

IC, in the TB context, aims at reducing the transmission of TB within populations and relies on a set of managerial, administrative, environmental, and personal protective interventions. When such measures are not implemented, the risk of TB (both drug susceptible and drug resistant) dramatically increases, in some circumstances to epidemic proportions. Inpatient outbreaks of DR-TB among people living with HIV have been reported in Africa and Europe [12, 13]. Implementing IC measures, however, is known to reverse the airborne threat [9]. The TB IC hierarchy of measures is so crucial that the World Health Organization (WHO) has issued a standalone policy document and implementation guidelines for member countries' action. TB IC has also been recommended in important global documents [8, 14–16].

Ethiopia developed its first national TB IC guidelines based on international recommendations in 2009—in the same year that the relevant WHO documents were published [5, 9]. The Federal Ministry of Health has trained a number of health care workers using a TB IC curriculum. Still others were trained in comprehensive TB/HIV services as well as programmatic management of DR-TB, both of which have incorporated TB IC topics [17, 18].

The Help Ethiopia Address the Low Performance of TB (HEAL TB) project led by Management Sciences for Health (MSH) implemented a comprehensive TB control program, one of the components being TB IC. Capacity building for health managers and health workers, supportive supervision, and technical and material support were among the interventions geared toward improving TB IC in HCFs. It is evident that there is little research, particularly intervention studies, about TB IC in low-income settings. The objective of this study was to compare the implementation of TB IC measures before and after introduction of a comprehensive technical support package in two regions of Ethiopia.

Methods

Setting

Ethiopia is the second most populous nation in Africa, with a population close to 99 million. It is administratively composed of nine regional states and two city administrations. Under each regional state there are a number of zonal administrations (also called zones), and under each zone are several *woredas* (districts) [19].

In 2017, there were 22,807 TB notified cases out of the 21.1 million population in Amhara, and 43,321 notified TB cases out of 35.8 million population in Oromia Region [20].

The study employed a pre- and post-intervention design built upon project implementation. All of the project HCFs were included in the study.

Funded by the United States Agency for International Development (USAID), the HEAL TB project supported the government of Ethiopia in addressing many of the major challenges posed by TB. The project began in July 2011 in two of the most populous regional states in the country: Oromia and Amhara, with a total population of 57 million. Before the intervention, HEAL TB conducted a baseline assessment in all HCFs of the selected 11 zones. Twenty-two hospitals and 697 health centers were included in the assessment, which ran from August through October 2013. Basic information on TB IC measures was collected.

Intervention

The intervention package consisted of capacity building, provision of standard operating procedures (SOPs), regular supportive supervision, and program review meetings. The project initially trained woreda TB focal persons on the basics of TB IC and on supervisory skills so that they could provide technical support to HCWs. The woreda TB focal person supervises, on average, five HCFs under his/her catchment once every three months, using supervision checklists and TB SOC indicators. Both templates address TB IC issues. Based on the findings of the supervision, the woreda TB focal person gives on-site feedback and subsequently follows the implementation status of the action plan developed during the last visit. In addition to the woreda TB focal persons, HCWs were also trained using a TB IC curriculum. Different SOPs appropriate to the service delivery points were developed and posted on the wall, starting with the triage room continuing all the way to the laboratory. TB program review meetings were held biannually; during the meetings, woreda TB focal points presented the performance of the HCFs in their respective woredas over the previous six months. In such meetings, TB IC is a major topic that is thoroughly discussed, and improvement plans are formulated.

Data collection instruments

Two types of checklists were used, one for baseline assessment and another for quarterly monitoring. The baseline checklist is a comprehensive tool of eight pages with 171 items structured into different thematic areas, including TB IC. The TB IC questionnaire asks about the (1) availability of a separate TB room, (2) opening of windows during consultation hours, (3) presence of cough triage, (4) TB IC committee, (5) TB IC plan, and (6) number of HCWs who developed active TB in the previous year. The quarterly monitoring instrument also contains a subsection on TB IC specifically referring to the presence of a functional multidisciplinary team/infection prevention committee, revised IC plan, triage/cougher prioritization, and separate TB room. Both tools were developed based on consultation with stakeholders and adaptation of international TB standards [21, 22]. Taking into account the large number of HCFs under project support, it was decided that the number of TB IC indicators should be kept to the minimum, while ensuring robustness, for the sake of efficient resource utilization.

Data collectors and data collection procedures

For the baseline assessment, the data collectors were HEAL TB employees who were medical doctors, health officers, and specialist laboratory professionals, all with public health experience. Training on the baseline assessment tools was provided for two days, before their departure to the field. Observation, review of documents, and interviews were the approaches used to collect the baseline data. Information about the number of HCWs who developed active TB was obtained from the TB registers kept in TB rooms. For this purpose, HCWs were defined as all people working in HCFs.

For quarterly monitoring, the trained woreda TB focal persons were in charge of data collection from their respective catchment HCFs. During the visits, they used the SOC tool, which required them to interview HCF TB focal persons about the status of TB IC activities, to review documents (minutes of infection prevention/IC committees), and to observe practices (prioritization of people with cough; status of the TB room). They spent on average half a day in each HCF to collect relevant TB program data. The following four TB IC indicators were monitored every three months: existence of (1) TB IC committee, (2) triage, (3) separate TB room, and (4) revised/updated TB IC plan. Data were collected from all 719 health facilities at baseline and every quarter thereafter.

Data management and analysis

A data entry template in the Census and Survey Processing System (CSPro), version 4.1 (US Census Bureau, ORC Macro International, and Serpro SA), was prepared, and data were entered into the template immediately after data collection. We checked the data for consistency and completeness by running frequency tables and cross-tabulations.

The data entered into CSPro 4.1 were exported to Stata 11 (College Station, TX: StataCorp., LP), where data cleaning, editing, and consistency checking were performed. Frequencies and percentages were computed to describe the data and compare TB IC practices before and after the program was implemented. We used the Student's t-test to determine significant differences between baseline and post-intervention data. The chi-squared test (Table 1) was also utilized to test for associations between the two regions as well as between hospitals and health centers (Tables 2 and 3).

Ethical considerations

We received ethical approval from the ethics committees of Amhara and Oromia Regional Health Bureaus to analyze the routine data and disseminate the findings. We used health facility level reports for this analysis with the consent of the reporting institutions. No patient identifiers were included in the routine reports.

Table 1 Comparison of the TB IC performance before and after intervention

Variables	Before intervention % ($N = 719$)	After intervention % ($N = 719$)	P-value (Before after t-test)
Separate TB room	69.1	87.1	$P < 0.001$
Cough triage	19.3	63.0	$P < 0.001$
IP/TB IC committee	29.1	61.1	$P < 0.001$
TB IC Plan	4.7	56.1	$P < 0.001$

Table 2 TB IC performance at baseline and after intervention by region

Characteristics	Baseline			After Intervention		
	Region		P-value (Chi-square)	Region		P-value (Chi-square)
	Amhara (n = 306)	Oromia (n = 413)		Amhara (n = 306)	Oromia (n = 413)	
% Cough triage	17.4	21.8	0.31	84.2	46.7	< 0.01
% IP/TB IC committee	57	14.7	< 0.01	71.2	53.6	< 0.01
% TB IC Plan	2.9	6.3	0.16	67.3	48.0	< 0.01

Results

At baseline, separate TB clinics existed in the majority of health facilities (69.1%). HCWs assigned to outpatient departments were reported to be working with open windows in 55.2% of the HCFs. However, coughing patients were prioritized for TB services in only 19.41% of the health facilities. Infection prevention committees and TB IC plans existed in only 29.11 and 4.65% of the assessed HCFs, respectively. There were no statistically significant differences between Amhara and Oromia regions regarding the practice of cough triage ($p = 0.31$) and existence of a TB IC plan ($p = 0.16$).However, regional differences in existence of TB IC committees ($p < 0.01$) did attain statistical significance (Table 2). Furthermore, hospitals differed from health centers significantly in terms of cough triage, TB IC committees, and TB IC plan availability ($p < 0.01$) (Table 3).

Sixty-one of the 8667 HCWs had developed active TB in the year preceding this assessment, making the annual incidence rate 704/100,000. Using WHO's 2012 TB incidence estimation for Ethiopia, which was 247/100,000, we calculated the incidence rate ratio to be 2.85 (for all forms of drug-susceptible TB, not only new cases). The incidence risk ratio was not age standardized; the rates were compared to the general population based on the WHO estimate, which is not age standardized.

Health care workers with TB were identified according to the national diagnostic algorithms, which consisted of sputum smear microscopy (the algorithm was recently revised, so that HCWs are tested with GeneXpert assay), radiography, and cytology—as indicated.

After 12 months of implementation, the number of HCFs with TB IC committees increased to 61%, and prioritized service for coughers had been put in place in

63% of the HCFs ($p < 0.001$). Furthermore, 56% of HFs had written TB IC plans, and 87% had designated separate TB rooms, which was significantly higher than the situation before intervention (p < 0.001) (Table 1).

Post-intervention, statistically significant differences occurred between Amhara and Oromia regions pertaining to availability of all the TB IC measures ($p < 0.01$). Moreover, with the exception of existence of TB IC committees ($p = 0.10$), hospitals differed from health centers significantly in terms of cough triage (p < 0.01) and availability of TB IC plans ($p = 0.01$).

Discussion

Before the technical support and comprehensive package of interventions, the majority of the health facilities lacked basic work procedures and policies to facilitate smooth implementation of TB IC. After intervention, availability of TB IC plans and use of triage showed marked improvement, while existence of TB IC committees and separate TB rooms improved modestly.

When comparing HCFs in Amhara with those of Oromia Region, the former did well post-intervention in availability of TB IC plans and triage, whereas the latter performed better in existence of TB IC committees. In addition, hospitals performed better than health centers in all the TB IC indicators, which can be explained by a relatively good start at baseline, presence of trained HCWs in sufficient number, and extra supervisory support from different stakeholders due to hospitals' physical accessibility.

According to the WHO directive, facility-level TB IC implementation begins with assignment of a coordinating body. Health facility risk assessment, formulation of a TB IC plan, and implementation of the plan should

Table 3 TB IC performance at baseline and after intervention by type of health facility

Characteristics	Baseline			After Intervention		
	Type of Health Facility		P-value (Chi-square)	Type of Health Facility		P-value (Chi-square)
	Health Center (n = 697)	Hospital (n = 22)		Health Center (n = 697)	Hospital (n = 22)	
% Cough triage	18.8	47.8	< 0.01	61.5	91.7	< 0.01
% IP/TB IC committee	28.6	56.5	< 0.01	60.4	79.2	0.10
% TB IC Plan	3.6	34.8	< 0.01	55.2	83.3	0.01

follow in that order [9]. In our baseline assessment, however, this logical order was not evident. Only 29% of the facilities had functional IP committees, meaning that the great majority of the facilities lacked a responsible body to combat TB transmission. Without this committee, it is not possible to do facility assessments and to plan TB IC activities, in line with the guidelines. The literature is scanty regarding availability of infection prevention/TB IC committees. Ogbonnaya et al. reported that 16.7% of the assessed TB/HIV implementing health facilities in Nigeria had IC committees [23]. This figure is lower than what we found at baseline in Ethiopia. A 32% improvement was seen post-intervention.

The least-implemented TB IC measure was the facility-level IC plan, which was found in only 4.7% of the HCFs. This also brings to light that 24.3% of the HCFs reported as having IC committees failed to develop plans, bringing into question their functionality. In sub-Saharan Africa, availability of TB IC plans in health facilities ranges from none to 77% [24, 25]. In Mozambique, it was 48% [26] and in Uganda, 31% [27]. Our baseline finding lies in between and was increased to 56% after intervention. Unavailability of a TB IC plan implies poor managerial activity and attention. It is very difficult to implement what has not been planned.

Close to 80% of the assessed facilities did not provide prioritized services for presumptive TB patients. Functional triage availability is reported from Nigeria [23] and South Africa [28] as 16.7, and 26%, respectively. In a 2012 study involving nine countries in sub-Saharan Africa, it ranged from 5 to 93% [25]. At baseline, triage availability in Ethiopia was a bit higher than the reported figure from Nigeria but modestly lower than in South Africa and within the range of figures in sub-Saharan Africa. In such a situation, generation of infectious droplet nuclei and contamination of the environment are facilitated; HCWs, visitors, and other patients become highly exposed.

Screening of all health facility care-seekers for TB symptoms, with subsequent isolation and/or fast tracking for services are triage functions and an essential component of administrative control. It is generally agreed that triage is the first defense mechanism against TB transmission in HCFs. Rapid diagnosis and effective TB treatment are the hallmarks of TB IC. Establishment of triaging had increased to 63% of the HCFs by the end of the intervention year.

At baseline, HCWs in half of the assessed facilities opened window(s) during consultation hours and thereafter. This practice was indicative of individuals' precautions rather than a concerted IC effort, given the low level of availability of TB IC committees and plans. Moreover, awareness among HCWs has been raised by their attending trainings related to TB, HIV, and DR-TB. Reports of increased awareness of HCWs (clinicians)

about IC were recently demonstrated in Addis Ababa and in northwest Ethiopia in a survey of knowledge, attitudes, and practices [29, 30].

In nearly 70% of the health facilities, TB rooms were standalone. This should not be counted as a strength, however, since all service delivery points are required to have separate rooms as a matter of health service standards. It also implies that the remaining one-third of HCFs are providing TB service together with other services, compromising space and ventilation. In South Africa, dedicated TB rooms were available in only 31% of HCFs [25]. Through project support in Ethiopia, it was possible to increase the level from the baseline of 69 to 87%.

Poor implementation of IC measures is reflected in HCWs' acquisition of TB disease, as this study showed. Sixty-one HCWs acquired TB in 1 year. They were about 2.85 times more likely to acquire active TB disease than the general population. Reports of TB among HCWs from sub-Saharan African countries [24] and resource-rich countries [31] show disparities. The TB case notification rate in HCWs of Malawi was 3.2% as compared to 1.8% for primary schoolteachers [32]. In South Africa, Claassens et al. stated that the standardized incidence ratio of smear-positive pulmonary TB in primary health care workers was more than double that of the general population [28]. A study in 2013 in the same country showed a 10% DR-TB rate among physicians with pulmonary TB diagnosis, which the researchers attributed to lack of effective IC work practices combined with negative attitudes of administrators [33]. A recent meta-analysis by Baussano et al. indicated that the stratified pooled estimates for annual TB incidence risk ratio for countries with high TB incidence (> 100 cases/100,000) is 3.68, whereas it is 2.42 for low-incidence (< 50 cases/100,000) and intermediate-incidence (50–99 cases/100,000) countries. The overall estimate of annual TB incidence risk ratio was 2.97, which is comparable to our finding of 2.85. They concluded that HCWs' risk of acquiring TB was higher than that of the general population across the globe and that effective TB IC measures could decrease annual TB incidence among HCWs by as much 81, 27, and 49% in countries with high, intermediate, and low TB incidence, respectively [34]. Most, if not all, countries have long recognized TB as an occupational disease [9, 35].

It is worth noting the following limitations of the study. We were not able to present data regarding the cross-ventilation status of outpatient departments and active TB disease among HCWs to make comparison with the baseline findings, since our quarterly data source did not capture these items. Furthermore, lack of randomization in quasi-experimental design makes it difficult to control for confounding variables, and hence statistical association may not necessarily imply causal association. Similarly, we used Student's *t*- and chi-squared tests, which do not allow adjustment for confounders. Moreover, we relied on facility-level registers to collect data about the number of HCWs with TB, which might miss those being treated outside the HCF; hence there is a possibility of underreporting.

Conclusions

Building the capacity of district TB focal persons to provide supportive supervision to health facilities, together with the other comprehensive TB program support, was instrumental in improving the TB IC situation of health facilities. Huge gaps in implementation of the recommended TB IC practices at health facility level can be narrowed, if systematized basic capacity building can be provided. The burden of TB among HCWs is higher than the prevalence in the general population. There is a need to further strengthen infection prevention/TB IC committees in order to plan and implement the hierarchy of TB IC activities and reduce TB transmission among patients and HCWs.

Abbreviations

DR-TB: Drug-resistant tuberculosis; HCF: Health care facility; HCW: Health care worker; HIV: Human immunodeficiency virus; IP: Infection prevention; SOC: Standard of care; TB IC: Tuberculosis infection control; TB: Tuberculosis; USAID: United States Agency for International Development; WHO: World Health Organization

Acknowledgements

We would like to thank all the data collectors, as well as the Amhara and Oromia Regional Health Bureaus, for facilitating the implementation of the project. We thank the administrative and clinical staff of the health facilities for their cooperation. Dr. Barbara K. Timmons edited the final manuscript, for whom we are very grateful.

Funding

The United States Agency for International Development (USAID) supported this work through Management Sciences for Health – the Help Ethiopia Address Low Tuberculosis Performance Project (HEAL TB), under cooperative agreement number AID-663 -A-11-00011. The contents of the article are the responsibility of the authors alone and do not necessarily reflect the views of USAID or the United States government.

Authors' contributions

AA conceived and designed the study; NH, DH, & AA participated in the acquisition, analysis, and interpretation of data; AA, DJ, and DH drafted the article; ZG, MM, TA, and PS have contributed to inception, design and implementation of the interventions. They also critically reviewed the first and subsequent drafts of the manuscript and provided critical inputs to the interpretation of the findings. IJ and GA have actively participated in the roll out and implementation of the TB IC in the study regions. Moreover, they have contributed to the drafting and subsequent revision of the manuscript. All authors read and approved the final manuscript.

Competing interests

The authors declare that they have no competing interests.

Author details

[1]Management Sciences for Health, Help Ethiopia Address the Low Performance of Tuberculosis (HEAL TB) Project, Bole Sub City, Kebele 02, House Number 708, PO Box 1157, Code 1250 Addis Ababa, Ethiopia. [2]Amhara Regional Health Bureau, PO Box 495, Bahir Dar, Ethiopia. [3]Oromia Regional Health Bureau, PO Box 24341, Addis Ababa, Ethiopia. [4]Management Sciences for Health, Health Programs Group, 4301 North Fairfax Drive, Suite 400, Arlington, VA 22203, USA.

References

1. Mandal A. History of tuberculosis. In: News medical. AZoNetwork. 2017. https://www.news-medical.net/health/History-of-Tuberculosis.aspx. Accessed 30 Nov 2017.
2. Rothman S. The white death: a history of tuberculosis. Med Hist. 2001;45(1): 140–1.
3. Daniel TM. The history of tuberculosis. Respir Med. 2006;100(11):1862–70.
4. Schaaf HS, Zumla AI, editors. Tuberculosis: a comprehensive clinical reference. London: Elsevier; 2009.
5. World Health Organization (WHO). Implementing the end TB strategy: the essentials. Geneva: WHO; 2015.
6. World Health Organization (WHO). 2016 global tuberculosis report. Geneva: WHO; 2016.
7. Federal Minstry of Health (FMOH). Guidelines for prevention of transmission of tuberculosis in health care facilities,congregate and community settings in Ethiopia. 1st ed. Addis Ababa: FMOH; 2009.
8. Jensen PA, Lambert LA, Iademarco MF, Ridzon R, Centers for Disease Control and Prevention. Guidelines for preventing the transmission of *Mycobacterium tuberculosis* in health-care settings. MMWR Recomm Rep. 2005;54(RR-17):1–141.
9. World Health Organization (WHO). WHO policy on TB infection control in health-care facilities, congregate settings and households. Geneva: WHO; 2009.
10. World Health Organization (WHO). Implementing the WHO policy on TB infection control in health-care facilities, congregate settings and households: a framework to plan, implement and scale-up TB infection control activities at country, facility and community level. Geneva: WHO; 2009.
11. Nardell E, Dharmadhikari A. Turning off the spigot: reducing drug-resistant tuberculosis transmission in resource-limited settings. Int J Tuberc Lung Dis. 2010;14(10):1233–43.
12. Gandhi NR, Weissman D, Moodley P, Ramathal M, Elson I, Kreiswirth BN, et al. Nosocomial transmission of extensively drug-resistant tuberculosis in a rural hospital in South Africa. J Infect Dis. 2013;207(1):9–17. https://doi.org/10.1093/infdis/jis631.
13. Moro ML, Gori A, Errante I, Infuso A, Franzetti F, Sodano L, et al. An outbreak of multidrug-resistant tuberculosis involving HIV-infected patients of two hospitals in Milan, Italy. AIDS. 1998;12(9):1095–102.
14. World Health Organization (WHO). The stop TB strategy: building on and enhancing DOTS to meet the TB-related millennium development goals. Geneva: WHO; 2006.
15. World Health Organization (WHO). WHO policy on collaborative TB/HIV activities: guidelines for national programmes and other stakeholders. Geneva: WHO; 2012.
16. World Health Organization (WHO). The global task force on XDR-TB: update. Geneva: WHO; 2007.
17. Federal Ministry of Health (FMOH). Guidelines for clinical and programmatic management of TB, TB/HIV and leprosy in Ethiopia. 5th ed. Addis Ababa: FMOH; 2012. https://www.medbox.org/ethiopia/guidelines-for-clinical-and-programmatic-management-of-tb-tbhiv-and-leprosy-in-ethiopia/preview. Accessed 30 Nov 2017.

18. Federal Ministry of Health (FMOH). Guidelines on programmatic management of drug resistant tuberculosis in Ethiopia. 2nd ed. Addis Ababa: FMOH; 2013. https://www.medbox.org/et-guidelines-hiv-tb/guidelines-on-programmatic-management-of-drug-resistant-tuberculosis-in-ethiopia/preview. Accessed 30 Nov 2017.

19. Federal Ministry of Health (FMOH). Health Sector Transformation Plan.2015/16–2019/20. Addis Ababa: FMOH; 2015. https://www.globalfinancingfacility.org/sites/gff_new/files/Ethiopia-health-system-transformation-plan.pdf. Accessed 30 Nov 2017.

20. US Agency for International Development (USAID), KNCV Tuberculosis Foundation, and Challenge TB. Challenge TB year 2 annual report, October 1st 2015-September 30th 2016. The Hague: KNCV Tuberculosis Foundation; 2017. http://www.challengetb.org/reportfiles/Challenge_TB_Annual_Report_Year_2.pdf. Accessed 30 Nov 2017.

21. World Health Organization (WHO). International standards for tuberculosis care. 3rd ed. Geneva: WHO; 2014. http://www.who.int/tb/publications/ISTC_3rdEd.pdf. Accessed 30 Nov 2017.

22. World Health Organization (WHO). Checklist for periodic evaluation of TB infection control in health-care facilities. Geneva: WHO; 2015. http://www.who.int/tb/areas-of-work/preventive-care/checklist_for_periodic_evaluation_of_tb_infection_control_in_health_facilities.pdf. Accessed 30 Nov 2017.

23. Ogbonnaya LU, Chukwu JN, Uwakwe KA, Oyibo PG, Ndukwe CD. The status of tuberculosis infection control measures in health care facilities rendering joint TB/HIV services in "German leprosy and tuberculosis relief association" supported states in Nigeria. Niger J Clin Pract. 2011;14(3):270–5. https://doi.org/10.4103/1119-3077.86765.

24. Robert J, Affolabi D, Awokou F, Nolna D, Manouan BA, Acho YB, et al. Assessment of organizational measures to prevent nosocomial tuberculosis in health facilities of 4 sub-Saharan countries in 2010. Infect Control Hosp Epidemiol. 2013;34(2):190–5. https://doi.org/10.1086/669085.

25. Reid MJA, Saito S, Nash D, Scardigli A, Casalini C, Howard AA. Implementation of tuberculosis infection control measures at HIV care and treatment sites in sub-Saharan Africa. Int J Tuberc Lung Dis. 2012;16(12):1605–12. https://doi.org/10.5588/ijtld.12.0033.

26. Brouwer M, Coelho E, das Dores Mosse C, Van Leth F. Implementation of tuberculosis infection prevention and control in Mozambican health care facilities. Int J Tuberc Lung Dis. 2015;19(1):44–9. https://doi.org/10.5588/ijtld.14.0337.

27. Buregyeya E, Nuwaha F, Verver S, Criel B, Colebunders R, Wanyenze R, et al. Implementation of tuberculosis infection control in health facilities in Mukono and Wakiso districts, Uganda. BMC Infect Dis. 2013;13:360. https://doi.org/10.1186/1471-2334-13-360.

28. Claassens MM, van Schalkwyk C, du Toit E, Roest E, Lombard CJ, Enarson DA, et al. Tuberculosis in healthcare workers and infection control measures at primary healthcare facilities in South Africa. PLoS One. 2013;8(10):e76272. https://doi.org/10.1371/journal.pone.0076272.

29. Tenna A, Stenehjem EA, Margoles L, Kacha E, Blumberg HM, Kempker RR. Infection control knowledge, attitudes, and practices among healthcare workers in Addis Ababa, Ethiopia. Infect Control Hosp Epidemiol. 2013;34(12):1289–96. https://doi.org/10.1086/673979.

30. Temesgen C, Demissie M. Knowledge and practice of tuberculosis infection control among health professionals in Northwest Ethiopia; 2011. BMC Health Serv Res. 2014;14:593. https://doi.org/10.1186/s12913-014-0593-2.

31. Lambert LA, Pratt RH, Armstrong LR, Haddad MB. Tuberculosis among healthcare workers, United States, 1995-2007. Infect Control Hosp Epidemiol. 2012;33(11):1126–32. https://doi.org/10.1086/668016.

32. Harries AD, Hargreaves NJ, Gausi F, Kwanjana JH, Salaniponi FM. Preventing tuberculosis among health workers in Malawi. Bull World Health Organ. 2002;80(7):526–31.

33. Naidoo A, Naidoo SS, Gathiram P, Lalloo UG. Tuberculosis in medical doctors: a study of personal experiences and attitudes. S Afr Med J. 2013;103(3):176–80. https://doi.org/10.7196/samj.6266.

34. Baussano I, Nunn P, Williams B, Pivetta E, Bugiani M, Scano F. Tuberculosis among health care workers. Emerg Infect Dis. 2011;17(3):488–94. https://doi.org/10.3201/eid1703.100947.

35. Chai SJ, Mattingly DC, Varma JK. Protecting health care workers from tuberculosis in China: a review of policy and practice in China and the United States. Health Policy Plan. 2013;28(1):100–9. https://doi.org/10.1093/heapol/czs029.

10

The role of socioeconomic and climatic factors in the spatio-temporal variation of human rabies in China

Danhuai Guo[1,2*], Wenwu Yin[3], Hongjie Yu[3], Jean-Claude Thill[4], Weishi Yang[5,6], Feng Chen[7] and Deqiang Wang[1,2]

Abstract

Background: Rabies is a significant public health problem in China. Previous spatial epidemiological studies have helped understand the epidemiology of animal and human rabies in China. However, quantification of effects derived from relevant factors was insufficient and complex spatial interactions were not well articulated, which may lead to non-negligible bias. In this study, we aimed to quantify the role of socio-economic and climate factors in the spatial distribution of human rabies to support decision making pertaining to rabies control in China.

Methods: We conducted a multivariate analysis of human rabies in China with explicit consideration for spatial heterogeneity and spatial dependence effects. The panel of 20,368 cases reported between 2005 and 2013 and their socio-economic and climate factors was implemented in regression models. Several significant covariates were extracted, including the longitude, the average temperature, the distance to county center, the distance to the road network and the distance to the nearest rabies case. The GMM was adopted to provide unbiased estimation with respect to heterogeneity and spatial autocorrelation.

Results: The analysis explained the inferred relationships between the counts of cases aggregated to 271 spatially-defined cells and the explanatory variables. The results suggested that temperature, longitude, the distance to county centers and the distance to the road network are positively associated with the local incidence of human rabies while the distance to newly occurred rabies cases has a negative correlation. With heterogeneity and spatial autocorrelation taken into consideration, the estimation of regression models performed better.

Conclusions: It was found that climatic and socioeconomic factors have significant influence on the spread of human rabies in China as they continuously affect the living environments of humans and animals, which critically impacts on how timely local citizens can gain access to post-exposure prophylactic services. Moreover, through comparisons between traditional regression models and the aggregation model that allows for heterogeneity and spatial effects, we demonstrated the validity and advantage of the aggregation model. It outperformed the existing models and decreased the estimation bias brought by omission of the spatial heterogeneity and spatial dependence effects. Statistical results are readily translated into public health policy takeaways.

Keywords: Human rabies, Socioeconomic and climate factors, Regression model, Heterogeneity, Spatial dependence, China

* Correspondence: guodanhuai@cnic.cn
[1]Computer Network Information Center, Chinese Academy of Sciences, 4th South Fourth Road Zhongguancun, Beijing 100190, China
[2]University of Chinese Academy of Sciences, 19th Yuquan Road, Beijing 100049, China
Full list of author information is available at the end of the article

Background

Rabies is a widely distributed zoonotic infectious disease. The latest estimates indicate that a total of 55,000 human fatalities occur each year worldwide as a result of rabies infection [1–3]. After India, China is the country with the second highest annual incidence of human rabies cases, where humans contract the infection from rabid animals. The rabies virus mainly spreads from animal to animal or animal to human through bites and scratches [4]. Among reservoirs animals, dogs play a pivotal role as a transmitter of rabies to humans in China [5] and it is estimated that more than four fifths of all human rabies infections in China are due to dogs [4]. Although the number of cases has decreased over the past decade, the epidemic situation remains serious and numerous cases have been reported in recent years: 924 cases in 2014 and 801 cases in 2015 [3, 6]. Unsuccessful control of rabid animals and inadequate post-exposure prophylaxis (PEP) of patients are thought to be the main factors leading to the high incidence of human rabies in China [7, 8].

Multiple studies have dug into the epidemiology and transmission dynamics of rabies to humans in China across various temporal and geographic scales [4, 7–14]. Phylogenetic analysis of Chinese rabies viruses from 1969 to 2009 illustrated that due to human-related activities infection transmission had been intra-provincial and extra-provincial [9]. Time-series analysis of human rabies has shown seasonal trends: the number of cases in summer and autumn is higher than in spring and winter [4, 12, 15]. In the only spatial epidemiological study of rabies in dogs, it can be seen that the spatial and temporal distribution of cases is not even across the country [16]. Cases of rabies infection in areas where there was no prior history of infection are reported yearly [16]. Investigation of spatial patterns of rabies in animals such as raccoons and skunks have shown obvious variations because of the diversity in geographic, climatic and environmental attributes: distance from major roads, presence of river, lake and land cover including deciduous forest, average temperature and nearness to enzootic zones have all been found to be covariates [17–19]. More recently, surveillance data have been exploited in spatial models to forecast the emergence of rabies in raccoons [20, 21]. However, the impact of risk factors on observed spatial distributions has so far not been studied quantitatively.

The quantification of risk factors associated with the occurrence of human rabies is critical for the epidemiologic analysis of rabies, as this knowledge crucially supports decision making for controlling and ultimately preventing the disease. A significant goal of the analysis is to predict the incidence of rabies or possibilities of rabies cases for specific regions. In order to predict feasibly and reliably, quantification of the risk factors is vital. A number of international studies have investigated the contribution of risk factors in the spatial distribution of rabies in humans [20, 22–24]. Some studies have looked for a correlation between rabies exposure risk and socioeconomic status using measurements derived from the records of patient PEP [25, 26]. However, these studies did not consider the spatio-temporal variation in environmental factors. The heterogeneity of local regions was also neglected. In addition, variations derived from spatially lagged geographical variables was inadequately accounted for in these models. Similarly designed studies have also been conducted for other infectious diseases [27–29].

In China, the spatial analysis of human rabies has shown that, while the overall number of rabies cases in humans decreased from 2007 to 2011, the scope of infection is still expanding [4]. It has been reported by numerous studies that the transmission of rabies was not restricted by administrative boundaries and the history of occurrence of the disease, but was impacted by surrounding environments, economic conditions and human habits, which all exhibit spatial heterogeneity [7, 30]. However, it remains unclear what the socioeconomic and environmental cause of human rabies are.

It is necessary to analyze rabies risk at the case level in order to accurately identify the influence of the geographic environment and of socioeconomic determinants on rabies distribution. The spatial pattern of human rabies has strong relations with the distribution and movement of animals like untied dogs and roaming dogs [24]. In this paper, we analyze the space-time distribution of rabies among humans, and conduct a large-scale study based on cases of human rabies.

Besides the possibilities of risk factors mentioned above, spatial heterogeneity and spatial dependence are also important issues to account for. Spatial heterogeneity refers to the variability of environmental and social factors across a study region, while spatial dependence refers to attributes of a spatial entity or region being correlated to attributes of another nearby entity, and vice versa. Few studies of human rabies have so far explicitly considered these effects. Heterogeneity is present and considerable, especially for a large country comprised of numerous regions that may exhibit totally different natural environments and socioeconomic complexions from one another. Heterogeneity is the result of the complicated aggregation of local factors, which may not be noted accurately or completely recognized, and thus may be overlooked in the inferential analysis. In addition, when the spatial arrangement of regions is not neutral and when their neighborhood relations interfere with epidemiologic processes, an effective analysis has to consider the spatial autocorrelation in the process under study, which reveals the interactions and interdependencies between events and attributes based on their geographic proximity. A biased estimation of effects of risk factors can result from the omission of neighborhood-based spatial dependence effects.

In this study, we aim to quantify the role of socioeconomic and environmental factors of human rabies risk in China. To this end, various regression models are used to capture the relations between normalized annual counts of rabies cases and relevant explanatory variables, which are extracted from the quantitative measurement of risk factors. To account for spatial heterogeneity and spatial dependence, panel data that encompass cross-sectional information and longitudinal variation are needed for the regression estimation. A spatially autoregressive error process is integrated to handle the spatial dependence effects [31]. Spatial heterogeneity can be handled through the specification of the error component. Then, seemingly unrelated regression (SUR) estimators are used for the computation of effects on the panel data. The estimation of effects from risk factors is expected to contribute to the design of better interventions in the context of public health decision making, which is aimed at reducing cases of rabies.

In Section "Methods", the theoretical model and econometric specifications are introduced. Section "Modeling Results" describes the data for the regression and relevant processing. Estimation results of different regression models are represented in Section "Discussion". Section "Conclusions" provides more detailed discussions of the estimation results in relation to the epidemiology of rabies infection. The last section summarizes the analysis and presents our conclusions.

Methods

Our analysis aims to build a model that provides explanation of the count of rabies cases and quantifies the respective effects of explanatory variables. The count of cases is used to present the degree of the incidence in geographically referenced territories across time. The model is built on panel data, which can output views through the spatial dimension and the temporal dimension. As mentioned above, we incorporate spatial heterogeneity and spatial dependence effects into the model. Before designing an appropriate model, the presence of spatial autocorrelation in the distribution of rabies cases is validated through Moran's I statistic. When the spatial autocorrelation is determined to be significant, we start with a reduced form of rabies regression and proceed to extend the model with the heterogeneity and spatial correlations taken into consideration. Moreover, the incidence may be influenced by unobserved variables and random factors. Therefore, a random effects model is adopted in the following analysis.

Moran's I statistic

In order to test for the presence of spatial autocorrelation, Moran's I statistic [32] is implemented. Moran's I is widely applied in evaluating spatial autocorrelation in univariate areal data series. The index is defined as:

$$Moran's\ I = \frac{\sum_{i=1}^{n}\sum_{j=1}^{n}W_{ij}(y_i-\bar{y})\left(y_j-\bar{y}\right)}{S^2\sum_{i=1}^{n}\sum_{j=1}^{n}W_{ij}}$$

$$S^2 = \frac{\sum_{i=1}^{n}(y_i-\bar{y})^2}{n}, \bar{y} = \frac{\sum_{i=1}^{n}y_i}{n}$$

where y_i denotes the recorded number of rabies cases in area i, n is the number of areas, and W is the so-called spatial weights matrix, whose element W_{ij} records the spatial relation between area i and area j. When the spatial relations are described by a binary matrix, the element W_{ij} is set to one whenever area i is a neighbor of area j, and zero otherwise. If the I statistic is greater than 0, the spatial relationship exhibits positive correlation; correlation is negative when I is negative. The larger the I statistic, the higher the correlation is; in other words, a region close to regions of observed rabies cases is more likely to experience rabies outbreaks, and vice versa.

Model specifications

When dealing with panel data collected over a large territory, the variance among different sub-regions cannot be ignored. Regions far away from each other can have drastically different socioeconomic or physical environments and consequently fall into different patterns. The effects originating from different patterns can hardly be fully narrated only by explanatory variables. Additionally, components of the effects may derive from some unknown or incidental factors so that the effects turn to be arbitrary. To incorporate spatial heterogeneity and control its unobserved shifting effects, the equation is enhanced with variable intercepts:

$$R_{it} = \beta^T X_{it} + \alpha_i + \eta_i, \eta_i \sim N\left(0, \sigma_i^2\right)$$

where R_{it} is the normalization numbers of rabies cases for area i at time t; X_{it} is the vector of predictors; α_i denotes a corresponding intercept for area i, which implies a specific level of disease incidence for this area, and thus reflects the spatial heterogeneity of rabies's impact factors. η_i represents the factors specific to region i that are not taken into account by the observed and intrinsic independent variables of rabies' onset; η_i is a Gaussian random variable with zero mean and controlled by variance σ_i^2.

Spatial dependence is handled explicitly in our analysis. Spatial autocorrelation measures the dependence between geographic objects, which is often depicted as a spatial dependence or spillover effect. Positive autocorrelation indicates that variable values similarity appears in the neighborhood, whereas negative autocorrelation involves considerable discrepancy in values assumed by nearby areas. Positive correlation among disease incidences in adjacent areas can be anticipated. Indeed, adjacent areas often share environmental conditions. With similar natural factors such as humidity, temperature, and slope, the rabies virus and animal vectors tend to have analogous survival and diffusion capacities. As a compounding consideration, similar socioeconomic factors such as traffic conditions, household incomes, educational attainments, and public health policies bring out similar post-exposure handling situations, while the proximity of areas also translates into more regular and intensive communication, such as the periodic movement of the animals that carry the virus.

To measure these neighborhood-based effects, we assume that the count of cases follows a spatial autoregressive process. Both substantive and error spatial dependences are concerned [33]. A Spatial Lag Model (SLM) is suitable for spatial substantive dependence, which is the interaction between the dependent variable and explanatory variables in their geographic vicinity through spillover across region boundaries. A Spatial Error Model (SEM) is suitable to handle spatial error dependence, which is also known as the spatial autocorrelation model; this model can simulate the spatial dissemination of random effects from factors that are not covered by the set of explanatory variables.

Then we attempt to treat both spatial effects simultaneous in a unified model. Therefore, a model that considers spatial dependence both in substantive attributes and in errors is a combination of SLM and SEM. This model consists of a complete SLM model supplemented by a component of simulated spatial random effect from the SEM model, as follows [34]:

$$R = \beta^T X + I_T \otimes \alpha + (I_T \otimes \rho_l W_N)R + u$$

with $\beta^T X + I_T \otimes \alpha + \eta + (I_T \otimes \rho_l W_N)$ as the expression of the SLM. The SLM, also known as the spatial autoregressive model, is employed to represent a system comprised of N areas and T time periods. In this model, $\otimes$ denotes the Kronecker product; R is an $NT \times 1$ space-time panel matrix of stored and normalized rabies cases; X is a $NT \times k$ matrix of explanatory variables; I_T is a time matrix that reflects the changes in the level of rabies outbreak over time; α is a $N \times 1$ vector of intercepts identifying the unobserved regression factors of rabies at various periods, whose value is not related to spatial relationships. Also, ρ_l is the scalar parameter for the autoregressive process and W_N is a $N \times N$ spatial weights matrix. In our work, a binary matrix is used and each

element $[W_N]_{ij} = 1$ signifies that regions i and j are adjacent; otherwise, it is 0. The diagonal elements of W_N are set to zero, and the scalar ρ_l limited to $|\rho_l| < 1$; hence $I_N - \rho_l W_N$ is nonsingular.

In our model, u is associated with the SEM model and simulates the spatial random spillover effect. This model component cannot be expressed as a function of the explanatory variables. It is given by:

$$u = (I_T \otimes \rho_e W_N)u + v$$

where u is a $NT \times 1$ space-time panel matrix of error terms that follow a spatial autoregressive process; ρ_e is the scalar parameter for this autocorrelation process and $|\rho_e| < 1$; $I_N - \rho_e W_N$ is also nonsingular. The disturbance term v is expressed as follows:

$$v = (e_T \otimes I_N)\mu_N + \vartheta_N$$

where e_T is a $T \times 1$ vector of ones. It encompasses two error terms. μ_N is a $N \times 1$ vector of unit specific error components, while ϑ_N is a $TN \times 1$ vector that contains error components that vary over areas and time periods. μ_N and ϑ_N are random vectors with zero means and their covariance matrices are $E(\mu_N \mu_N^T) = \sigma_{\mu_N}^2 I_N$ and $E(\vartheta_N \vartheta_N^T) = \sigma_{\vartheta_N}^2 I_{TN}$. Adopting the assumptions proposed by Kapoor et al. [31], the elements of μ_N are identically distributed and so are the elements of ϑ_N.

Estimation approach

We resort to several possible estimators to provide comparisons between classical regression models and models that allow for spatial heterogeneity and spatial dependence effects.

The estimation starts with a baseline OLS estimator derived from pooled OLS equations and ignoring spatial heterogeneity and spatial autocorrelation. The OLS model concentrates on measuring the associations between the dependent variable and explanatory variables.

Second, a random effects-generalized least squares (RE-GLS) estimator is used to represent the gains brought out by spatial heterogeneity. The RE-GLS estimator does not consider spatial dependence.

In order to identify gains derived from spatial effects, a SLM estimator and a SEM estimator must be exploited. Given the presence of spatial autocorrelation, the least-squares estimator is biased and the General Method of Moments (GMM) is employed as an estimation tool to obtain consistent estimates for unknown parameters. The estimators for SLM and SEM here do not consider spatial heterogeneity.

Finally, with heterogeneity and spatial effects both allowed for, an estimator for the aggregation model is built using GMM. The estimator is defined on the basis of the BP-FGLS system estimator proposed by Baltagi and Pirotte [35]. The estimated parameters are obtained through an iteration of two steps. In the first step, $\tilde{\beta}$ and $\tilde{\alpha}$, which denote parameters corresponding to explanatory variables and intercepts, respectively, are calculated using a feasible general least-squares (FGLS) method. An OLS estimator can supply the initial parameters. In the second step, with $\tilde{\beta}$ and $\tilde{\alpha}$ fixed, $\tilde{\rho}_l$ and $\tilde{\rho}_e$ can be estimated by GM estimators proposed by Kapoor. Several different moments are adopted to output unbiased estimators for the scalars. Furthermore, residuals can be calculated with the parameters fixed, and then the variance matrices are estimated using the residuals. The estimated variance matrices are used in the FGLS estimation in the first step in the next iteration. When the estimator converges, we can get an approximate result for the required parameters.

Comparison of model performances

To estimate the goodness of fit (GOF) of models, the sum of squared residuals and the standard error of regression are used as indicators of model performance. Generally, GOF of regression models can be measured by classical statistics like R-squared or F-statistic. However, the classical statistics are not suitable for GMM estimators. In order to verify the validity of models using GMM, J-statistic and corresponding probabilities are adopted. To provide a general measurement, the sum of squared residuals and the standard error serve as the reference. Furthermore, scatterplots of observations against predictions and residual graphs are illustrated to describe the regression results.

Data presentation
Human rabies data

The data on human rabies cases used in this study are from the National Notifiable Disease Reporting System (NDRS), the national information system of infectious disease mandatory notification of mainland China. Human rabies is classified as a B notifiable disease by the Law of the People's Republic of China on Prevention and Treatment of Infectious Diseases. All related information is provided by NDRS.

The data set contains 20,368 reported cases of human rabies, spanning from 2005 to 2013. The cases pertain to humans infected by dogs, cats, rats, bats and other transmitters. Among them, dogs are believed to be the most important transmitter and cause over 80 % of cases of human rabies in China. Although the detailed proportion of all transmitters of human rabies cases was not available for this study because of the insufficiency of the information (demographic and clinical data) for part of the cases, we can acquire information on the virus transmitters through analyses of a sample of all cases. Analysis

of human rabies cases in Guangdong province in 2003 and 2004 suggested that 85.7% of all cases were infected by dogs, followed by cats (3.7%) and rats (2.5%) [36].

Each suspected human case would be mandatorily reported to public health authorities. All reported cases with geocodes (i.e. longitude and latitude of the household home address) were included in our study. Four suspicious cases (found in 2005, 2008, 2011 and 2011, respectively) in Xinjiang Province were dropped from our analysis. The China Centers for Disease Control (CDC) ethical committee approved our research on these data and the data were anonymized.

Figure 1 [40] displays the numbers of rabies notification cases from 2005 to 2013. A downward trend of the count of cases, which first manifested itself in 2008, is depicted in the figure. However, the annual number of cases has remained high and the corresponding burden cannot be simply ignored. Therefore, it is fitting to seek to identify the factors that led to the downward trend of rabies cases in China during this nine-year timespan. Figure 2 represents the spatial distribution of human rabies cases in China. According to these maps, cases are more frequent in the eastern and southern parts of China, with a spatial pattern that has shifted over time.

For statistical analysis, each case was assigned to an administrative village, which served as the primary sampling unit. The number of administrative villages in China is so large that the result of this assignment turned out to be extremely sparse. Therefore, the primary unit for the regression analysis was set to be a cell instead of an administrative village. The cells were obtained through spatial clustering: villages that are adjacent or have direct geographical connections with each other and share the same or similar environmental conditions, were aggregated. Each cell consisted of several villages. The

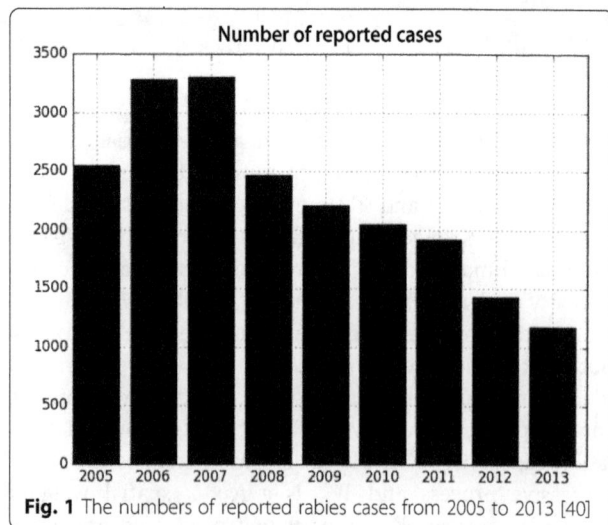

Fig. 1 The numbers of reported rabies cases from 2005 to 2013 [40]

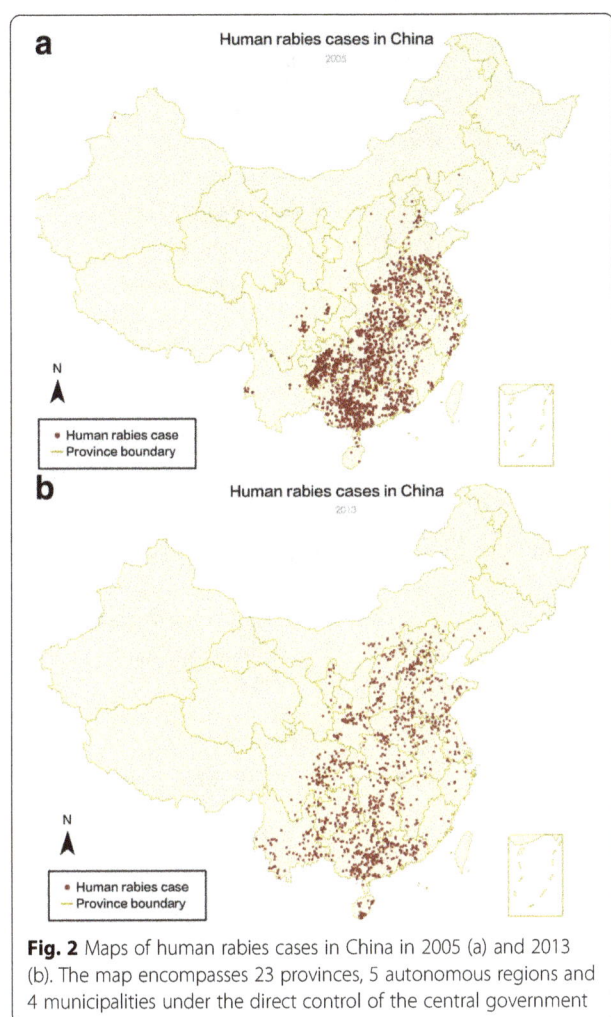

Fig. 2 Maps of human rabies cases in China in 2005 (a) and 2013 (b). The map encompasses 23 provinces, 5 autonomous regions and 4 municipalities under the direct control of the central government

number of villages contained in a cell and the spatial extent of a cell vary according to the size and condition of relevant administrative villages. Some rivers and (mountain) watersheds are not only natural unit boundaries but they are also the administrative boundaries, so there is a greater possibility that our cell boundaries overlap with the administrative boundaries in these instances. Due to the variability in the geographic characteristics of the statistical units that are grouped into the same cell, aggregation errors may be generated. However, because the aggregation was conducted so as to minimize information loss, aggregation errors should be small and rather uniform, thus mitigation impacts on the national scale analysis. Through this process, we obtained 271 spatially defined cells for the subsequent regression analysis.

Environmental and socioeconomic data

Explanatory variables were selected from a set of features that denote the geographic, climatic and socioeconomic conditions of a specific region. The environmental and geographic features included: the longitude and the latitude, the average annual land surface temperature (LST), the slope and the average elevation. To get the average value for a specific year, an adaptive Savitzky-Golay smoothing filter, implemented using the TIMESAT package [37], was employed. The socioeconomic features pertained to the human population density, yearly gross domestic product (GDP), per capita GDP, ratio of middle school graduates (RMS), and ratio of illiteracy (ROI). Data on human population were obtained from three national censuses (2000, 2005 and 2010) released by the National Statistics Bureau of China. The values of population for intervening years were estimated using a linear interpolation method. Furthermore, a spatial trend analysis methodology [38] was used to smooth data on several neighboring villages and provide equivalent values for the corresponding cell.

Also, the set of covariates was extended with transportation and spatial accessibility features, which included the Euclidean distances from a village to the road network, to the nearest downtown of a county or a city, to the nearest hospital, and to the nearest clinic. The smallest offset to the road network was used to describe the distance to the road network. Public health measures, including various programs for the prevention and control of the disease, are in effect restricted by the local traffic and accessibility conditions.

Finally, spatial epidemiology variables were incorporated. The epidemiologic features included the minimum spatial distance to the nearest case, the minimum temporal distance to the latest case, and the minimum spatio-temporal distance to the nearest case. Epidemiology variables may reveal correlations between infected zones. Moreover, the distance from nearest or latest case represented the degree of potential risk revealed by existing cases. Explicit information on the full set of variables is listed in Table 1.

Variable selection

Multiple backward stepwise regressions were carried out to select meaningful explanatory variables. The stepwise process was repeated 1000 times applying different training subsets. The 20 regression models with the best fit were picked, while the variables yielding non-significant effects (mean P-value > 0.05) were removed.

At the end of this process, the variables that were retained included the longitude, the average temperature, the distance to county center, the distance to road network and the minimum spatial distance to the nearest case. More detailed results are presented hereunder for this specification.

Table 1 List of explanatory variables

Category	Description of dataset	Abbreviation	Unit	Data source
Environmental variables	digital elevation	DEM	m	USGS
	digital slope	SLOPE	degree	USGS
	Average temperature	AT	°C	MODIS
	Human population density 2000	POPDENS	p/km²	National Statistics Bureau
Socioeconomic variables	Human population density 2005	POPDENS	p/km²	National Statistics Bureau
	Human population density 2010	POPDENS	p/km²	National Statistics Bureau
	Ratio of illiteracy	ROI	p/million	National Statistics Bureau of China
	Ratio of middle school and above	RMS	p/million	National Statistics Bureau of China
	Yearly GDP	GDP	10⁴RMB	National Statistics Bureau of China
	Yearly per Capita GDP	PCGDP	10⁴RMB	National Statistics Bureau of China
	Distance to road network	DTRN	km	National Administration of Surveying, Mapping and Geoinformation
Transportation variables	Distance to city center	DTCC	km	National Administration of Surveying, Mapping and Geoinformation
	Distance to county center	DTCNC	km	National Administration of Surveying, Mapping and Geoinformation
	Distance to nearest hospital	DTHSP	km	China's Health and Family Planning Commission
Epidemiologic variables	Distance to nearest clinic	DTCLC	km	China's Health and Family Planning Commission
	Minimum spatio-temporal distance to nearest case	MSTDNC	Km/day	China CDC Rabies Surveillance data
	Minimum spatial distance to nearest case	MSDNC	km	China CDC Rabies Surveillance data
	Minimum temporal distance to nearest case	MTDNC	day	China CDC Rabies Surveillance data

Modeling results

Spatial autocorrelation

The Moran's I computed on the normalized case count for 2005 to 2013 is illustrated in Fig. 3 [40]. The global index is statistically significant and positive; it provides evidence of positive spatial autocorrelation in rabies incidence in China. The graph also depicts the longitudinal downward trend of Moran's I, which may be a consequence of the continuous drop of rabies cases in China from 2008.

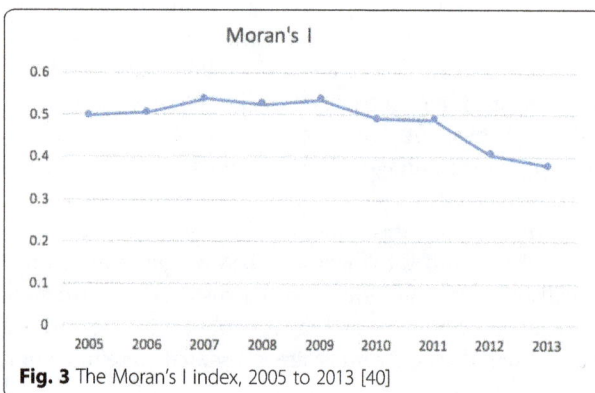

Fig. 3 The Moran's I index, 2005 to 2013 [40]

Estimation results

The input of the regression models is a balanced panel that contains 271 cross-sections with 9 time periods. Thus, 2439 samples are generated, each of which consists of the normalized rabies incidence and explanatory variables of an individual cell in a specific year. The estimation results are reported in Table 2. AM stands for the aggregation model that allows for both the heterogeneity effect and the spatial dependence effect. The results of the variable selection process show that the variables can be accepted as significant predictors of the normalized number of rabies cases. The J-statistic implies that the SLM, the SEM, and the aggregation model are all valid.

Table 2 provides reference for comparisons between different regression models. As is shown in the table, the use of variable intercepts improves the performance of the model by a wide margin. On the other hand, the residual and standard error of regression obviously decrease once spatial autocorrelation is taken into account. The SLM and the SEM provide better performance. The results imply that both the spatial heterogeneity and spatial dependence effects provide a meaningful contribution to understanding rabies risk. When the model combines estimators from SEM and SLM, it reaches the

Table 2 Estimation results

	OLS		SLM		SEM		RE-GLS		AM	
	Parameter Estimate	Standard Error	Parameter Estimate	Standard Error	Parameter Estimate	Standard Error	Parameter Estimate	Standard Error	Parameter Estimate	Standard Error
Longitude	0.03256	0	0.001901	0.0486	0.002056	0.0331	0.001603	0	0.00222	0
Temperature	0.03812	0.0001	0.011207	0.0004	0.012794	0.0001	0.013616	0	0.007505	0
DTCNC	0.005884	0.0102	0.002337	0.0319	0.002302	0.0360	0.000906	0	0.001898	0
DTRN	0.049686	0.0021	0.011251	0.0093	0.012252	0.0043	0.005268	0.0002	0.006013	0.0005
MSDNC	−0.002092	0.1651	−0.002264	0	−0.002466	0	−0.001311	0	−0.001691	0
C	0.047878	0	0.47645	0	0.455308	0	0.681607	0	0.4073	0.0019
ρ_l			0.008774	0					0.005153	0
ρ_e					0.117826	0			0.013151	0.0254
$\sigma_{\vartheta_N}^2$			0.866774		0.874635		1.043152		0.684197	
$\sigma_{\mu_N}^2$			0.903172		0.876109		0.934437		0.881217	
R-squared	0.3775						0.6691			
J-statistic			74.4461	0	71.3784	0			103.6390	0
sum-resid	5191.23		1311.323		1298.777		2060.687		756.4909	
S.E.	1.461011		0.832959		0.829185		0.976063		0.684197	

best performance of all models. This may suggest that both spatial substantive dependence and spatial error dependence have a significant influence on the prevalence of rabies cases.

Figure 4 shows the scatterplots of observed counts against predicted counts. Each dot denotes a pair of observed and predicted values for any given cell. We find that a preponderance of dots assemble near the diagonal line of the plot when spatial heterogeneity and spatial dependence are explicitly incorporated in the model. The plots prove that measurements for spatial heterogeneity and spatial dependence effects bring effective

improvements to the model, which is consistent with the analysis on the result of goodness of fit measures.

In Fig. 5, the residual for each sample case is depicted along with their actual and fitted values. The blue lines denote the residuals, while the red lines denote the actual observations. The green lines show the fitted values. The overlap between actual and fitted values grows with spatial heterogeneity and spatial dependence incorporated explicitly in the model. The OLS estimator fails to fit the observations well, especially in the areas with high incidence of rabies. The SLM estimator and the SEM estimator provide improved results, but it is hard to tell

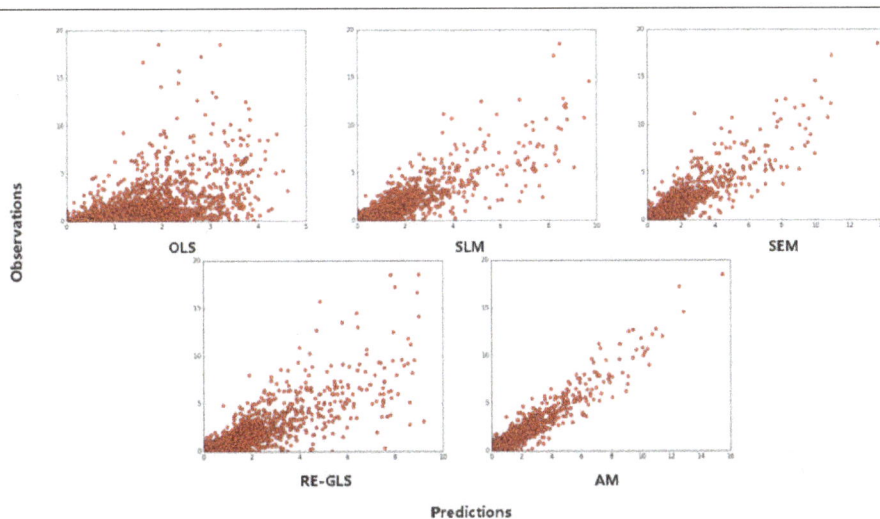

Fig. 4 Scatterplots of observed counts (vertical axis) and predicted counts (horizontal axis) of different regression models [40]

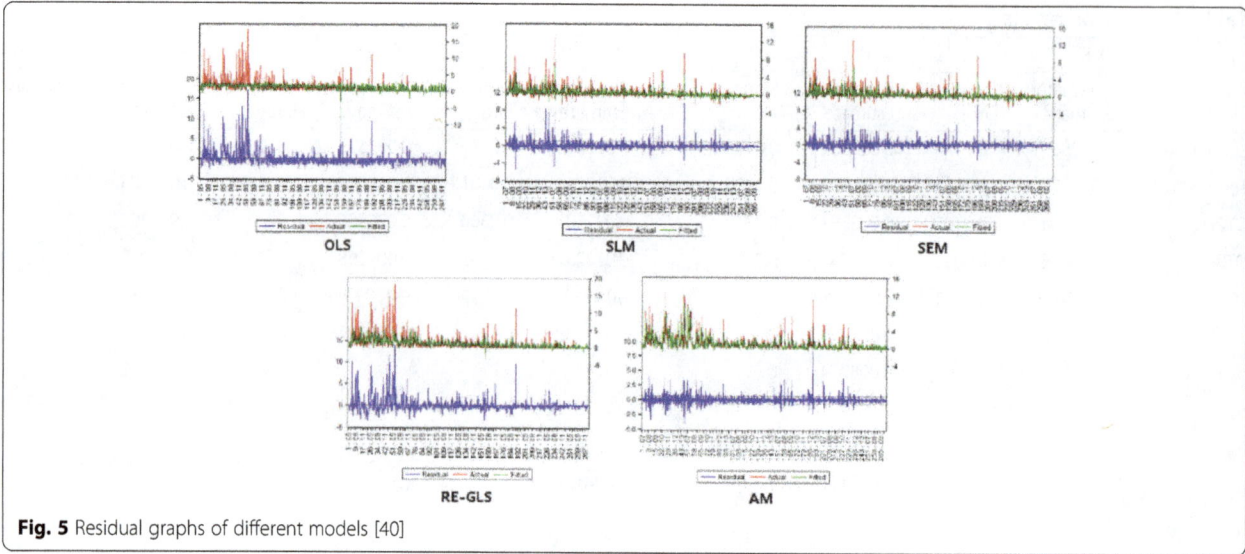

Fig. 5 Residual graphs of different models [40]

the difference between the two spatial dependence processes through the residual graphs. The RE-GLS estimator also gives better performance than the OLS estimator. The graphs suggest that accounting for spatial dependence leads to more improvements than spatial heterogeneity in this case. Furthermore, when spatial heterogeneity and spatial dependence effects are both considered, the aggregation model provides the best fit to the observations.

Figure 6 shows the distribution of actual human rabies cases in 2014 while Fig. 7 shows the prediction of human rabies cases in the same year according to the AM. The color depth in Fig. 7 denotes the possible extent of the disease; darker colors suggest more anticipated cases in the corresponding regions. Generally speaking, in comparison with the map of observed cases in 2014, the model simulation is good. However, the accuracy of simulation in the two regions of eastern Anhui and

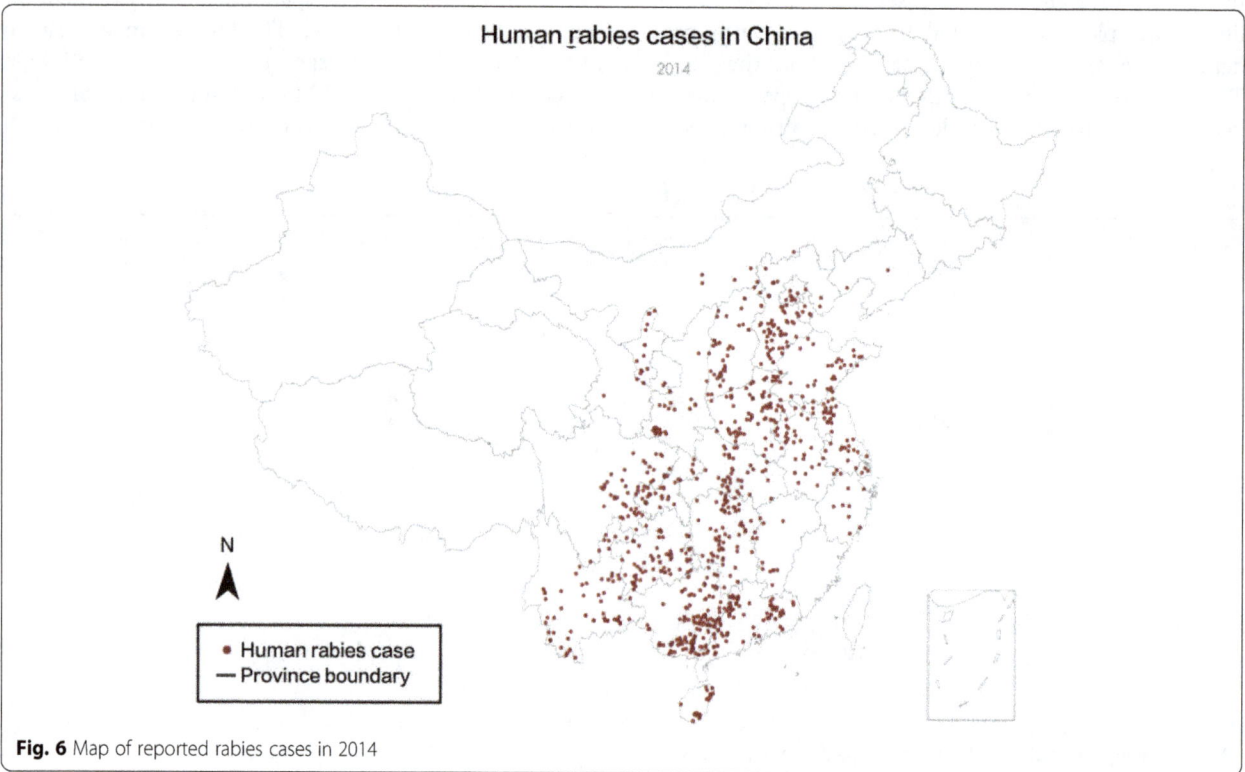

Fig. 6 Map of reported rabies cases in 2014

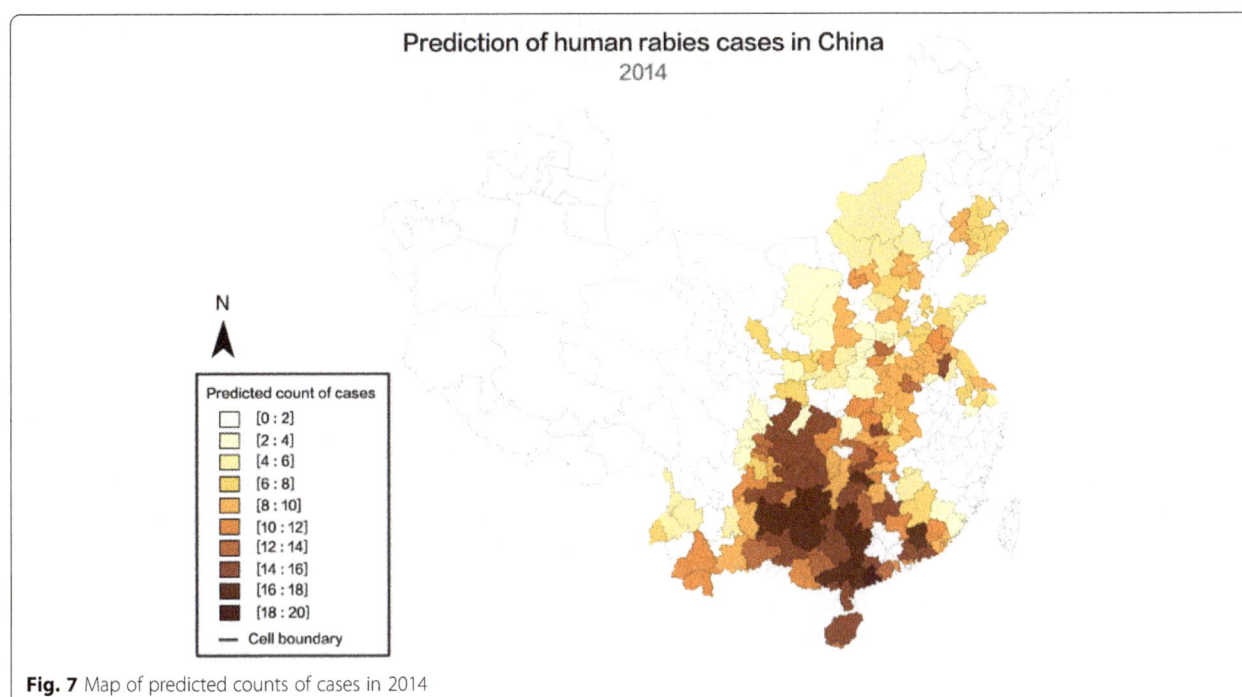

Fig. 7 Map of predicted counts of cases in 2014

Zhejiang Provinces is relatively low. This may be due to the following reasons: (1) rabies in Anhui is mainly concentrated in the northwestern part of the province; (2) Zhejiang and Anhui Provinces are not areas of high incidence of rabies. The two provinces have flat terrain, and the road traffic connectivity is relatively good, so that rabies simulation accuracy is relatively low. It can be concluded that the prediction fits the observations well in most regions of China.

Discussion

In section "Discussion", we compared the performance of different regression models and verified the validity of the models that incorporated spatial heterogeneity and spatial dependence effects. In this section an interpretation of the estimates is provided.

According to the *P*-values in Table 2, the selected variables can be accepted as effective independent variables for the regression of normalized rabies counts. The longitude and the average temperature both show positive correlation with the count of rabies. The longitude of an area is significant in the regression, as it reflects the environmental attributes across China on a relatively macro level. Physiographically, China can be separated into three divisions: the eastern part with low altitude and a long coastline; the middle part with numerous mountains and basins; the western part with high altitude and plateaus. The climatic environment varies according to the longitude and the differences between the eastern part and the western part can be enormous.

Generally, from west to east, as the longitude increases, rainfall and vegetation tend to be relatively higher, and the environment is more suitable for the survival and reproduction of animals, including rabies virus carriers. Moreover, the middle-western part consists of many plateaus and rugged mountainous regions, which is not fit for animals, like stray dogs, to roam. In contrast, in the plain areas, if the distance separating villages is larger than the range of roaming dogs, rabies can hardly spread through stray dogs. This suggests that different prevention and control measurements should be adopted in mountain regions and plain regions. For mountain regions, the key means is to control the movement and propagation of stray dogs inside the area, especially in rugged and forested landscapes. In the plains, however, the target is to control the connectivity between the infected villages, where human rabies cases have been recorded, and un-infected villages.

The incidence of rabies also increases as ambient temperature rises. A warmer climate means that animals are more active in their surroundings and track over greater distances, which contributes to the spread of rabies. In addition, higher temperatures often result in humans wearing lighter clothes and in exposing more skin, which increase the opportunity of being bitten by dogs.

Table 2 also suggests that the incidence is affected by transportation accessibility and spatial epidemiology considerations. The Euclidean distance to the road network and the distance to the nearest county center have positive coefficients in the regression. Distances can reflect the traffic conditions of an area and the intensity of connections with socioeconomic resources. The longer the distance is, the more isolated a region may be with respect to other communities. As a result of this isolation, the area receives less support for disease prevention and other public health interventions. Moreover, restricted by the limitations of local resources, the area would only have a slower response to rabies cases and thus be even more afflicted. According to WHO guidelines for post-exposure prophylaxis [39], it is critical to receive PEP in a rabies center as soon as possible after exposure. Although 98% of all patients were living in rural areas, great differences were recorded in the speed of seeking medical assistance: 64.19% of patients visited the rabies center within 4 h of exposure, 27.93% of patients visited the rabies center between 4 and 24 h of exposure and 7.88% of patients visited the rabies center over 1 day later [24]. These differences may be largely imputed to accessibility discrepancies. Although we did not collect information on PEP hospitals and rabies centers, the accessibility to these facilities can be revealed by the distances mentioned above. The distance to the nearest county center translates into the convenience of access to receive rabies PEP and immunoglobulin services.

The count of rabies has a negative correlation with the spatial distance to the nearest case. A negative coefficient implies that when the distance from existing cases becomes shorter, the risk of infection rises correspondingly. When one human case occurs, the rabies virus has spread among hosts in the regions near this case. Strict control and protection measures should be adopted in these regions. In current human rabies control and prevention plans issued by the Ministry of Agriculture of China, control areas include two buffer areas centered on the location of rabies cases, namely the infected areas (within a radius of 3 km) and the risk areas (within a radius of 5 km, excluding the infected areas). In the infected areas, the local CDC and the government will cull infected dogs and restrict others' movements. To control the rabies transmission, mandatory vaccination of dogs should be enforced in both the infected areas and the risk areas.

patial heterogeneity has been demonstrated to contribute to the improvement of the fit of the regression. The RE-GLS estimator provided a base constant and each area was fitted with an adjusted constant as its intercept. The incorporation of spatial heterogeneity greatly reduced the residuals of the regression. With spatial dependence accounted for, the constant was updated to fit the new model. The SLM and SEM also led to a further drop in the residuals. The corresponding P-values of ρ_l and ρ_e have proven the significance of spatial heterogeneity

and spatial dependence effects. The results showed that the variance of the random effects ($\sigma_{\vartheta_N}^2$ and $\sigma_{\mu_N}^2$) are also significant at 1% for all models. Furthermore, the aggregation model evidenced the successful combination of the two factors. The spatial heterogeneity and dependence effects are both actually recognized to play important roles in the spread of the disease in China. Consideration for differences across areas and for interactions between areas suggests the wisdom of some degree of local and decentralized decision making on the part of government agencies and medical institutions. As discussed above, effective strategies for controlling the disease are supposed to fit the specific conditions of the socioeconomic and physical environments in the localities. The adjacency relationships between localities need extra attention, for it may reveal the spread source of rabies in neighboring areas and it can be exploited to interrupt the path of the transmission.

Conclusions

In this research, we analyze human rabies in China using regression models with consideration for spatial heterogeneity and spatial dependence effects. We studied rabies cases recorded in China from 2005 to 2013 and applied regression models based on normalized case data. The regression estimates provide a reference for measuring effects concluded from explanatory variables whose significance were then extracted including the longitude, the average temperature, the distance to town center, the distance to the road network and the spatial distance to the nearest rabies case. The analysis explained inferred relationships between the case counts and relevant explanatory variables. For instance, the survival chance of stray dogs is higher when temperature is higher and less clothes are worn to protect from biting dogs. In rural areas, longer average distances between villages and town centers and greater distance to road network mean that it is more difficult to have timely PEP treatment. Given the variables identified as strong predictors, recommendations on how to prevent and control human rabies were presented.

Moreover, spatial heterogeneity and spatial dependence were explicitly considered in our analysis. Spatial autocorrelation is confirmed by Moran's I statistic. For a specific area, the incidence of rabies is affected by both its constant and inherent attributes, and the status of neighboring areas. The omission of the heterogeneity and spatial dependence effects can bring biased estimations, which has been proven by the results of pooled OLS estimation. Through comparisons between traditional models and the aggregation model that allows for the two types of effects simultaneously, we demonstrated the validity and advantage of the aggregation model. The aggregation model outperformed the existing models and fitted the observations well. The comparisons suggested that both spatial heterogeneity and spatial dependence effects can contribute to the model and that they can be combined in a single model without any interferences, thus effectively reducing the possibility of bias.

However, challenges remain for the spatial epidemiologic modeling of rabies. Although our approach obtained promising results on the dataset of rabies cases in China, it still needs to be verified on other datasets. While the approach that is advocated here recognizes the role of heterogeneity to reveal new insights in terms of missing variables and inherent characteristics of different regions, the aggregation of areas leads to the loss of fine-resolution information on villages assigned to a larger cell. Therefore, how to better account for the conditions within a cell and how to map the individual effects may be interesting issues to tackle in future extensions of this work. In addition, in this study, the time increment was set to a year and seasonal effects were not taken into consideration. Alternatively, it is possible to compute the monthly count of rabies cases and conduct relevant analysis according to the rhythm of seasons. In future work, we will enhance the specification of the aggregation model and test it on various datasets.

Abbreviations
AM: The aggregation model that allows for both the heterogeneity effect and the spatial autocorrelation effect; CDC: Centers for disease control; FGLS: Feasible general least-squares; GDP: Gross domestic product; GMM: General method of moments; GOF: Goodness of fit; LST: Land surface temperature; MODIS: Moderate Resolution Imaging Spectroradiometer; NDRS: Notifiable disease reporting system; OLS: Ordinary least squares; PEP: Post-exposure prophylaxis; RE-GLS: Random effects-generalized least squares; RMS: Ratio of middle school graduates; ROI: Ratio of illiteracy; SEM: Spatial error model; SLM: Spatial lag model; SUR: Seemingly unrelated regression; TIMESAT: A program package for extracting seasonal parameters from remotely sensed time-series data of vegetation; USGS: United States Geological Survey

Acknowledgements
The authors thank the National and provincial CDC, local hospitals and laboratories of China for their contributions of human rabies surveillance data.

Funding
This work is partly supported by Natural Science Foundation of China under Grant No. 41371386 and Beijing Natural Science Foundation under Grant No. 9172023. The funders had no role in study design, data collection and analysis, decision to publish, or preparation of the manuscript.

Authors' contributions
DG conceived and designed this study. WYin and HY collected the data and performed statistical analysis based on the data. DG conducted experiments and wrote the manuscript. JCT made significant contributions by proposing the spatial econometric approach of the research design and the polishing of various versions of the manuscript. WYang dealt with the spatial data processing of variables used in this article. FC and DW edited the article. All authors read and approved the final manuscript.

Competing interests
The authors declare that they have no competing interests.

Author details
[1]Computer Network Information Center, Chinese Academy of Sciences, 4th South Fourth Road Zhongguancun, Beijing 100190, China. [2]University of Chinese Academy of Sciences, 19th Yuquan Road, Beijing 100049, China. [3]Chinese Center for Disease Control and Prevention, 155 Changbai Road Changping District, Beijing 102206, China. [4]Department of Geography & Earth Sciences, The University of North Carolina at Charlotte, 9201 University City Blvd, Charlotte, NC 28223, USA. [5]School of Geography and Planning, Sun Yat-sen University, Guangzhou 510275, China. [6]Key Laboratory of Land Surface Pattern and Simulation, Institute of Geographic Sciences and Natural Resources Research, Chinese Academy of Sciences, Beijing 100101, China. [7]Department of East Asian Studies, The University of Arizona, 1512 E. First Street, Tucson, AZ 85719, USA.

References
1. Warrell DA, Davidson NM, Pope HM, Bailie WE, Lawrie JH, Ormerod LD, Kertesz A, Lewis P. Pathophysiologic studies in human rabies. Am J Med. 1976;60(2):180–90.
2. Organization WH: Weekly epidemiological record (WHO). 1999.
3. Jönsson P, Eklundh L. TIMESAT—a program for analyzing time-series of satellite sensor data. Comput Geosci. 2004;30(8):833–45.
4. C-p Y, Zhou H, Wu H, X-y T, Rayner S, S-m W, Tang Q, G-d L. Analysis on factors related to rabies epidemic in China from 2007–2011. Virol Sin. 2012; 27(2):132–43.
5. Tang X, Luo M, Zhang S, Fooks AR, Hu R, Tu C. Pivotal role of dogs in rabies transmission, China. Emerg Infect Dis. 2005;11(12):1970.
6. In 2014 the national statutory epidemic situation of infectious diseases [http://www.nhfpc.gov.cn/jkj/s3578/201502/847c041a3bac4c3e844f17309be0cabd.shtml].
7. Song M, Tang Q, Wang D-M, Mo Z-J, Guo S-H, Li H, Tao X-Y, Rupprecht CE, Feng Z-J, Liang G-D. Epidemiological investigations of human rabies in China. BMC Infect Dis. 2009;9(1):210.
8. Zhang J, Jin Z, Sun G-Q, Zhou T, Ruan S. Analysis of rabies in China: transmission dynamics and control. PLoS One. 2011;6(7):e20891.
9. Meng S, Xu G, Wu X, Lei Y, Yan J, Nadin-Davis SA, Liu H, Wu J, Wang D, Dong G. Transmission dynamics of rabies in China over the last 40 years: 1969–2009. J Clin Virol. 2010;49(1):47–52.
10. Gong W, Jiang Y, Za Y, Zeng Z, Shao M, Fan J, Sun Y, Xiong Z, Yu X, Tu C. Temporal and spatial dynamics of rabies viruses in China and Southeast Asia. Virus Res. 2010;150(1):111–8.
11. Yu J, Li H, Tang Q, Rayner S, Han N, Guo Z, Liu H, Adams J, Fang W, Tao X. The spatial and temporal dynamics of rabies in China. PLoS Negl Trop Dis. 2012;6(5):e1640.
12. Zhang J, Jin Z, Sun G-Q, Sun X-D, Ruan S. Modeling seasonal rabies epidemics in China. Bull Math Biol. 2012;74(5):1226–51.
13. Yin W, Dong J, Tu C, Edwards J, Guo F, Zhou H, Yu H, Vong S. Challenges and needs for China to eliminate rabies. Infect Dis Poverty. 2013;2(1):23.
14. Guo D, Zhou H, Zou Y, Yin W, Yu H, Si Y, Li J, Zhou Y, Zhou X, Magalhães RJS. Geographical analysis of the distribution and spread of human rabies in China from 2005 to 2011. PLoS One. 2013;8(8):e72352.
15. Wilson ML, Bretsky PM, Jr CG, Egbertson SH, Van Kruiningen HJ, Cartter ML. Emergence of raccoon rabies in Connecticut, 1991-1994: spatial and temporal characteristics of animal infection and human contact. Am J Trop Med Hyg. 1997;57(4):457.
16. Yao H-W, Yang Y, Liu K, Li X-L, Zuo S-Q, Sun R-X, Fang L-Q, Cao W-C. The spatiotemporal expansion of human rabies and its probable explanation in mainland China, 2004-2013. PLoS Negl Trop Dis. 2015; 9(2):e0003502.
17. Smith DL, Lucey B, Waller LA, Childs JE, Real LA. Predicting the spatial dynamics of rabies epidemics on heterogeneous landscapes. Proc Natl Acad Sci. 2002;99(6):3668–72.
18. Lucey B, Russell C, Smith D, Wilson M, Long A, Waller L, Childs J, Real L. Spatiotemporal analysis of epizootic raccoon rabies propagation in Connecticut, 1991–1995. Vector Borne Zoonotic Dis. 2002;2(2):77–86.
19. Guerra MA, Curns AT, Rupprecht CE, Hanlon CA, Krebs JW, Childs JE. Skunk and raccoon rabies in the eastern United States: temporal and spatial analysis. Emerg Infect Dis. 2003;9(9):1143.

20. Recuenco S, Blanton JD, Rupprecht CE. A spatial model to forecast raccoon rabies emergence. Vector Borne Zoonotic Dis. 2012;12(2):126–37.

21. Song M, Tang Q, Rayner S, Tao X, Li H, Guo Z, Shen X, Jiao W, Fang W, Wang J. Human rabies surveillance and control in China, 2005–2012. BMC Infect Dis 14,1(2014-04-18). 2014;14(1):212.

22. Wilde H, Khawplod P, Khamoltham T, Hemachudha T, Tepsumethanon V, Lumlerdacha B, Mitmoonpitak C, Sitprija V. Rabies control in south and Southeast Asia. Vaccine. 2005;23(17):2284–9.

23. Cliquet F, Picard-Meyer E. Rabies and rabies-related viruses: a modern perspective on an ancient disease. Rev Sci Tech. 2004;23(2):625–42.

24. Fang LX, Ping F, Hui BG, Yan YX. Socioeconomic status is a critical risk factor for human rabies post-exposure prophylaxis. Vaccine. 2010;28(42):6847–51.

25. Haupt W. Rabies–risk of exposure and current trends in prevention of human cases. Vaccine. 1999;17(13):1742–9.

26. Gautret P, Shaw M, Gazin P, Soula G, Delmont J, Parola P, Soavi MJ, Brouqui P, Matchett DE, Torresi J. Rabies postexposure prophylaxis in returned injured travelers from France, Australia, and New Zealand: a retrospective study. J Travel Med. 2008;15(1):25–30.

27. Si Y, Wang T, Skidmore A, de Boer W, Li L, Prins H. Environmental factors influencing the spread of the highly pathogenic avian influenza H5N1 virus in wild birds in Europe. Ecol Soc. 2010;15(3).26–26.

28. Martin V, Pfeiffer DU, Zhou X, Xiao X, Prosser DJ, Guo F, Gilbert M. Spatial distribution and risk factors of highly pathogenic avian influenza (HPAI) H5N1 in China. PLoS Pathog. 2011;7(3):e1001308.

29. Wang L, Hu W, Magalhaes RJS, Bi P, Ding F, Sun H, Li S, Yin W, Wei L, Liu Q. The role of environmental factors in the spatial distribution of Japanese encephalitis in mainland China. Environ Int. 2014;73:1–9.

30. Guo Z, Tao X, Yin C, Han N, Yu J, Li H, Liu H, Fang W, Adams J, Wang J, et al. National borders effectively halt the spread of rabies: the current rabies epidemic in China is dislocated from cases in neighboring countries. PLoS Negl Trop Dis. 2013;7(1):e2039.

31. Kapoor M, Kelejian HH, Prucha IR. Panel data models with spatially correlated error components. J Econ. 2007;140(1):97–130.

32. Moran PA. Notes on continuous stochastic phenomena. Biometrika. 1950; 37(1/2):17–23.

33. Anselin L, Rey S. Properties of tests for spatial dependence in linear regression models. Geogr Anal. 1991;23(2):112–31.

34. Elhorst JP. Spatial Panel Data Models. Spatial Econometrics: From Cross-Sectional Data to Spatial Panels. J. P. Elhorst. Berlin, Heidelberg, Springer Berlin Heidelberg. 2014. p. 37–93.

35. Baltagi BH, Fingleton B, Pirotte A. Estimating and forecasting with a dynamic spatial panel data model. Oxf Bull Econ Stat. 2014;76(1):112–38.

36. Si H, Guo Z-M, Hao Y-T, Liu Y-G, Zhang D-M, Rao S-Q, Lu J-H. Rabies trend in China (1990–2007) and post-exposure prophylaxis in the Guangdong province. BMC Infect Dis. 2008;8(1):113.

37. Eklundh L, Jönsson PT. 3.0 software manual. Lund: Lund University; 2010.

38. Douglas E, Vogel R, Kroll C. Trends in floods and low flows in the United States: impact of spatial correlation. J Hydrol. 2000;240(1):90–105.

39. WHO. WHO recommendations on rabies post-exposure treatment and the correct technique of intradermal immunization against rabies. Geneva: WHO/EMC/Zoo.96.6. http://www.who.int/iris/handle/10665/63396.

40. Zhu Y, Guo D, Wang D, Li J. How to find environmental risk factors of zoonotic infectious disease quickly. In: Proceedings of the Second ACM SIGSPATIALInternational Workshop on the Use of GIS in Emergency Management. New York: ACM; 2016. p. 2:1–7. https://doi.org/10.1145/3017611.3017613.

Rising rates of injection drug use associated infective endocarditis in Virginia with missed opportunities for addiction treatment referral: a retrospective cohort study

Megan E. Gray[*] [ID], Elizabeth T. Rogawski McQuade, W. Michael Scheld and Rebecca A. Dillingham[*]

Abstract

Background: Injection drug use (IDU) is a growing public health threat in Virginia, though there is limited knowledge of related morbidity. The purpose of this study was to describe the temporal, geographic and clinical trends and characteristics of infective endocarditis associated with IDU (IDU-IE) and to identify opportunities for better-quality care of people who inject drugs (PWID).

Methods: We reviewed charts for all admissions coded for both IE and drug use disorders at the University of Virginia Medical Center (UVA) from January 2000 to July 2016. A random sample of 30 admissions coded for IE per year were reviewed to evaluate temporal trends in the proportion of IDU associated IE cases.

Results: There were a total of 76 patients with IDU-IE during the study period, 7.54-fold increase (prevalence ratio: 8.54, 95% CI 3.70–19.72) from 2000 to 2016. The proportion of IE that was IDU-associated increased by nearly 10% each year (prevalence ratio of IDU per year: 1.09, 95% CI: 1.05–1.14). Patients with IDU-IE had longer hospital stays [median days (interquartile range); IDU-IE, 17 (10–29); non-IDU-IE, 10 (6–18); p-value = 0.001] with almost twice the cost of admission as those without IDU [median (interquartile range); IDU-IE, \$47,899 (\$24,578-78,144); non-IDU-IE, \$26,460 (\$10,220-60,059); p-value = 0.001]. In 52% of cases there was no documentation of any discussion regarding addiction treatment.

Conclusion: IDU-IE is a severe infection that leads to significant morbidity and healthcare related costs. IDU-IE rates are increasing and will likely continue to do so without targeted interventions to help PWID. The diagnosis and treatment of IDU-IE provides an opportunity for the delivery of addiction treatment, counseling, and harm reduction strategies.

Keywords: Infective endocarditis, Injection drug use, Opioid use disorder

Background

Injection drug use (IDU) is a serious public health threat due to the risk for transmission of Human Immunodeficiency Virus (HIV), Hepatitis C Virus (HCV), and overdose related deaths [1, 2]. Bacterial infections caused by IDU are common, the most severe form being infective endocarditis (IE). Though the mortality of IDU has been a major research focus [3], the extent of associated morbidity from other complications, such as IE, has been less extensively characterized.

IDU has increased significantly since the year 2000 in conjunction with a national opioid epidemic, with total opioid overdose related deaths increasing by two-hundred percent in 14 years [3]. This drug epidemic is distinctive in that it primarily affects socioeconomically depressed, rural, and predominantly non-Hispanic white populations [4–6]. Sharing injection equipment in social networks of individuals with HIV or HCV infections can lead to viral outbreaks [5, 7]. In addition, using dirty equipment to inject drugs that contain particulate matter and diluents can

* Correspondence: meg5cs@virginia.edu; RD8V@virginia.edu
Division of Infectious Diseases and International Health, University of Virginia Health System, PO Box 801379, Charlottesville, Virginia 22908-1391, USA

provoke endothelial damage to heart valves and introduce pathogens into the bloodstream that cause IDU-IE and other localized infections [8].

The incidence of IE in people with IDU is 150–200 per 100,000 person years, approximately 100 times higher than the incidence of IE in the general population [9]. IDU-IE is more likely to affect the right side of the heart and is more frequently caused by Staphylococcal species or polymicrobial infections [9]. Treatment of IE requires long courses of intravenous antibiotics often administered through peripherally inserted central venous catheters. Despite appropriate treatment, recurrence of IE is more common in people who inject drugs (PWID) [10]. The mortality of IDU-IE has been reported to be 10% compared to 20–35% in IE due to other causes (non-IDU-IE) [9]. However, the mortality after valve replacement surgeries is higher in IDU-IE and more than half of those who undergo valve replacement surgeries will require repeated surgical intervention due to persistent injection of drugs [11, 12].

Virginia has one of the fastest growing rates of drug overdose related deaths in the United States [3] and is home to eight of the projected top 5% most vulnerable counties across the United States for viral outbreaks related to IDU [4]. In 2015, emergency department visits for heroin overdose during a nine month period had increased by 89% compared to the same nine month period in 2014, and fatal drug overdoses were the most common cause of unnatural death in 2013 [13]. This led to the declaration of a public health emergency by Virginia's State Commissioner in October 2016 whereby a statewide standing order was issued that authorized pharmacists to dispense naloxone, an opioid antagonist that reverses the effects of opioids [13]. Several studies have described increasing rates of IDU-IE in the context of increasing IDU [14–18], though no studies have evaluated IDU-IE in Virginia. Few studies have evaluated how IDU is being addressed in the context of a diagnosis of IDU-IE.

Needle and syringe sharing, reuse, and injecting drugs through uncleaned skin are highly implicated in the development of IE, and these practices are common among PWID [19, 20]. Evidence supports the efficacy of several underutilized harm reduction strategies for PWID, such as supervised injection facilities, needle-syringe exchange programs, medication-assisted treatment, and opioid antagonists for overdose treatment [19, 21–26]. Unfortunately, there remains substantial stigma in relation to substance use disorders, which is a barrier to establishing public policies that benefit PWID, such as government funding for abstinence or maintenance-based treatment programs or regulations regarding insurance parity [27]. In order for beneficial policy and social change to take place, more needs to be known about patterns of IDU related morbidity. The purpose of this study was to describe the temporal, geographic and clinical trends and characteristics of IDU-IE in Virginia and to identify opportunities for better-quality care of PWID.

Methods
Study design and patient population
A single-center, retrospective cohort study was performed at the University of Virginia Medical Center in Charlottesville, Virginia (UVA). The study site is an 800 bed tertiary care medical center that serves a large rural catchment area extending into West Virginia and far southwest Virginia. The study period ranged from January 1, 2000 to July 1, 2016. Patients were included if they were treated during an inpatient admission at UVA with additional criteria noted below. Patients over the age of 89 were excluded as this age range is considered a patient identifier by the Health Insurance Portability and Accountability Act. Patients under the age of 12 were excluded, similar to other studies evaluating IDU trends [5]. This study was approved by the UVA Institutional Review Board.

The UVA Clinical Data Repository was searched using *International Classification of Diseases, Ninth Revision* and *Tenth Revision* (ICD) diagnosis codes for acute and subacute IE (421, 421.1, 421.9, 424.9, 424.99, 242.91, 112.81, B37.6, I33, I33.0, I33.9, I38, I39). ICD diagnosis codes pertaining to substance abuse, substance abuse counseling and HCV were used to search for patients who inject drugs. Diagnosis codes for cannabinoids were not used. HCV diagnosis codes were used as HCV has often been used as a surrogate marker for IDU [4, 17]. Patient admissions with any of these 453 codes (see Additional file 1) within one year of or at the time of the admission for IE were then selected for chart review. Chart reviews were completed to confirm active IDU and the diagnosis of IE. IDU was conservatively defined as any documentation of injecting drugs within six months of admission for IE. Patients that were suspected of injecting drugs by healthcare staff or family but who denied IDU themselves were not considered to be actively injecting drugs. IE was defined using the modified Duke criteria [28], with inclusion of only definite IE. Patient readmissions for the same episode of IDU-IE related illness were not included.

In order to evaluate the relative trend in total number of cases of IDU-IE compared to other causes of IE, an additional chart review was completed. A stratified random sample of 510 patient admissions for IE, 30 per year, were collected by use of pseudo-random number generator from the 3115 patient admissions ICD coded for IE in the clinical data repository. Admissions with any of the 453 substance use related codes were excluded from the pool used for random sampling. Each chart from the stratified random sample was reviewed to confirm the diagnosis of IE by the modified Duke criteria.

Data collection

A comprehensive chart review was completed for all patient admissions with IDU-IE in order to collect demographic, clinical and outcomes data. The chart review of the randomly sampled non-IDU-IE patient admissions was limited to verification of IE diagnosis and the causative pathogen. The counties of residence were categorized as rural or urban based on 2010 census data from the Office of Management and Budget [29]. Patients' health district was also noted.

Statistical analysis

We compared clinical and demographic characteristics between IDU-IE cases and non-IDU-IE using chi-square and Mann-Whitney tests. We used Poisson regression to model the temporal trend in total IDU-IE admissions over the study period. Year was included in the model as a quadratic variable based on optimal model fit as assessed by Akaike information criteria. We used log-binomial regression to model the temporal trend in the proportion of IDU-IE admissions compared to non-IDU-IE admissions over the study period. All analyses were adjusted for sampling weights.

Results

Temporal and geographic trends

Observed admissions for IDU-IE trended up over time and predictive modeling showed a 7.54-fold increase (prevalence ratio: 8.54, 95% CI 3.70–19.72) from 2000 to 2016 (Fig. 1). Based on this model, 44.6 (95% CI 21–95) IDU-IE admissions would be expected in 2018, which is a 125.8% increase from 2016. The proportion of all IE that was IDU-IE increased by nearly 10% each year

(prevalence ratio of IDU-IE per year: 1.09, 95% CI: 1.05–1.14). See Fig. 2.

We estimated that 63 % of all cases of IE in the Southwest region of Virginia were IDU-IE, while 29.4% of the cases were IDU-IE in the remaining regions of Virginia, West Virginia and other states. See Fig. 3.

IDU-IE and non-IDU-IE

There were a total of 3115 admissions coded for IE from January 2000 to July 2016 at UVA. Of these, 311 admissions also had some type of substance abuse code and these charts were therefore reviewed. A total of 76 admissions were IDU-IE, 235 were excluded for lack of active IDU in the six months prior to admission and/or definitive IE. Of the 510 admissions from the stratified sample of admissions coded for IE, 143 admissions had definite IE. Both populations were predominantly non-Hispanic white race, though patients with IDU-IE were more likely to be non-Hispanic white (96.1% vs 84.7%; p-value = 0.02). Patients with IDU-IE were more likely to be younger than non-IDU-IE with a mean age of 35 compared to 61 (p-value < 0.001). See Table 1.

Patients with IDU-IE had longer hospital stays [median days (interquartile range); IDU-IE, 17 (10–29); non-IDU-IE, 10 (6–18); p-value = 0.001] with almost twice the cost of admission as those without IDU [median (interquartile range); IDD-IE, $47,899 ($24,578-78,144); non-IDU-IE, $26,460 ($10,220-60,059); p-value = 0.001]. Forty-five percent of IDU-IE patients were uninsured and 29% were on Medicaid, while 7% of patients without IDU were uninsured and 7.7% were on Medicaid. Thirty-day and ninety-day mortality data were available for 189 (86%) and 178 (81%) patients respectively; there was no significant difference in mortality between patients with and without IDU.

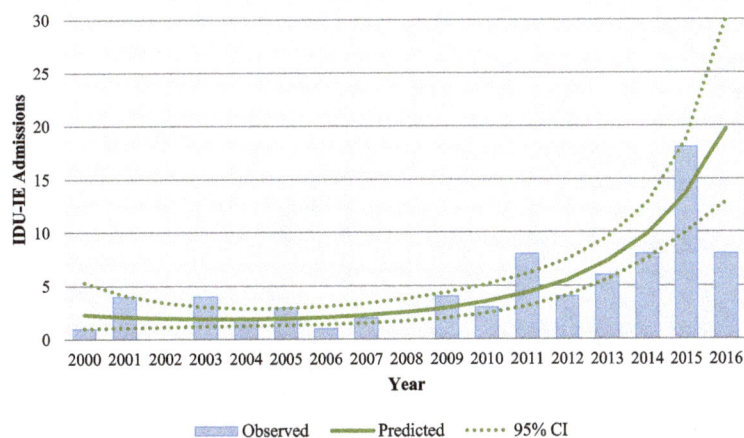

Fig. 1 Observed and predicted IDU-IE admissions over time. *In 2016 the observed cases are from only the first 6 months

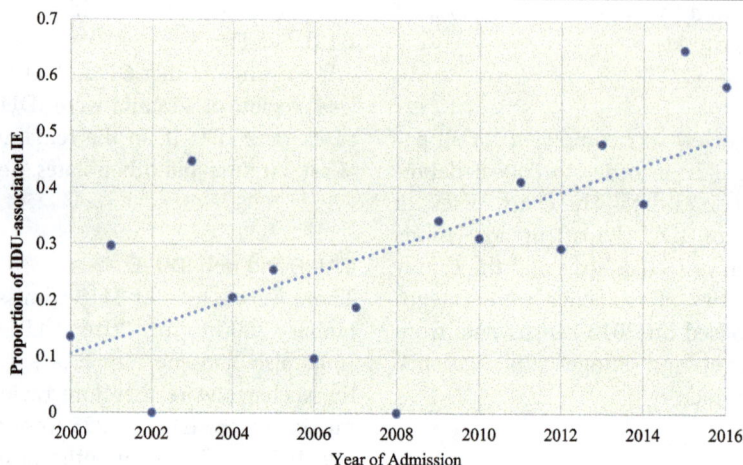

Fig. 2 Proportion of IDU-associated IE admissions per year. *Proportions were adjusted for sampling weights

Clinical and demographic results for IDU-IE
Clinical features and comorbid conditions

Documented fever at the time of admission was present in 36 (47.4%) patients with IDU-IE. Fifteen patients (19.7%) presented with septic shock and five patients (6.6%) presented with severe congestive heart failure. Twenty-four (31.6%) patients had a history of IE. Alcohol use disorder was present in 15 (19.7%) patients. Only five (6.6%) patients were infected with HIV. However, 50 (66%) of patients had been exposed to HCV based on a positive Hepatitis C antibody and negative viral load, with 33 (42.5%) patients having acute or chronic HCV infections with detectable viral loads. Not all patients were screened for HIV or HCV, those without available test results were presumed negative. The majority of IDU-IE patients were injecting some form of opioid (n = 51, 67%). See Table 2.

Substance use disorder treatment and patient disposition

The predominant post-hospital disposition among IDU-IE patients was to home with a home health agency to assist with intravenous antibiotic treatment (n = 35, 44.7%). Twenty-six percent of patients went to some type of health care facility including: skilled nursing facilities (n = 10), transitional care hospitals (n = 4), or acute rehabilitation centers (n = 6). Six patients (6.6%) died in the hospital. Cause of death was related to IE in all cases, including one death due to a brain abscess, one death due to an aortic root abscess, and two deaths from septic shock. Three patients (4%) left against medical advice and three patients (4%) were sent back to jail. Seven patients (8%) were able to go home without any intravenous catheter as they completed their treatment in the hospital. All other patients left the hospital with a peripherally inserted central venous catheter or other type of central venous catheter or port.

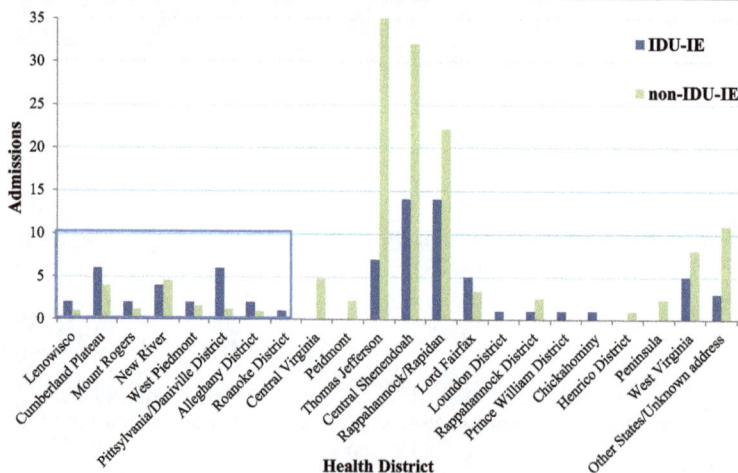

Fig. 3 Admissions for IDD-IE and non-IDU-IE by location of residence from January 2000 to July 2016. Blue box is surrounding health districts in Southwest Virginia. Non-IDU-IE cases weighted by year

Rising rates of injection drug use associated infective endocarditis in Virginia with missed...

99

Table 1 Characteristics of IDU-IE and non-IDU-IE at UVA from January 2000 to July 2016

Demographic factors	IDU-IE, N = 76	Non-IDU-IE N = 143	p-value
	N (%)	N (%)	
Sex			0.7
Male	86 (60.8)	44 (57.9)	
Female	55 (39.2)	32 (42.1)	
Race			0.02
Caucasian	73 (96.1)	120 (84.7)	
Black	2 (2.6)	21 (14.8)	
Hispanic	1 (1.3)	1 (0.5)	
Mean Age (range)	35 (19–63)	61 (12–89)	< 0.001
Residents of rural counties	24 (31.6)	45 (32.1)	0.9
In-hospital mortality	6 (7.9)	23 (16.6)	0.08
30 day mortality[a]	9 (14.5)	31 (24.4)	0.1
90 day mortality[a]	12 (21.8)	36 (29.3)	0.3
Insurance			< 0.0005
Medicaid	22 (28.9)	11 (7.7)	
Medicare	10 (13.2)	87 (60.8)	
Private	7 (9.2)	28 (19.6)	
Uninsured	34 (44.7)	10 (7)	
Tricare (Federally funded)	0 (0)	1 (0.7)	
State and Local Hospitalization Program	2 (2.6)	2 (1.4)	
Other	1 (1.3)	4 (1.8)	
Pathogen			< 0.0005
MRSA	29 (38.2)	33 (23.5)	
MSSA	17 (22.4)	18 (12.5)	
Other staphylococci	0	7 (4.6)	
Enteroccus faecalis	4 (5.3)	19 (13.1)	
Other enterococci	0	5 (3.8)	
Streptococci	7 (9.2)	35 (24.8)	
Candida species	3 (3.9)	6 (4.1)	
Polymicrobial infection	8 (10.5)	0	
Other	4 (5.3)	12 (8.3)	
No pathogen identified	4 (5.3)	7 (5.2)	
	Median (IQR)	Median (IQR)	p-value[b]
Length of stay in days	17 (10–29)	10 (6–18)	0.001
ICU length of stay in days (n = 44)[c]	6 (2–12)	5 (2–8)	0.8
Hospital cost in dollars	47,899 (24,578–78,144)	26,460 (10,220–60,059)	0.001

MSSA methicillin susceptible *Staphylococcus aureus*, *MRSA* methicillin resistant *Staphylococcus aureus*, *ICU* intensive care unit

All data were adjusted for sampling weights

[a]Excluding patients with missing mortality data: 14 patients with IDU-IE and 16 patients with non-I DU-IE for 30 day mortality and 21 patients with IDU-IE and 20 with non-IDU-IE for 90 day mortality

[b]p-value from Mann-Whitney non-parametric test, other p-values from chi-squared test

[c]Excluding 80% of patients with no ICU stay (IDU-IE = 58, non-IDU-IE = 117)

Thirteen percent of individuals were receiving long-acting opioid agonists (buprenorphine or methadone) for treatment of their substance use disorder at the time of their admission, while 8% had documentation of long-acting opioid agonist treatment in the past. Forty-eight (63%) of individuals had an opioid listed on their discharge medication list. From the first five years to the last five years of our study period this proportion

Table 2 Clinical characteristics of patients admitted for IDU-IE treatment from January 2000 to July 2016

Clinical Characteristics	N (%)
Right-sided endocarditis	36 (47)
Tricuspid valve	35 (46)
Pulmonic valve	0
Tricuspid and pulmonic valves	1 (1.3)
Left-sided endocarditis	24 (31.6)
Mitral valve	10 (13.2)
Aortic valve	12 (15.8)
Mitral and aortic valves	2 (2.6)
Unknown	2 (2.6)
Mixed (right and left) endocarditis	10 (13.2)
Cardiac device lead	1 (1.3)
No endocardial disease seen	3 (4)
Heart disease history	
Bicuspid aortic valve	1 (1.3)
Congenital heart disease	1 (1.3)
Myxomatous mitral valve	1 (1.3)
Prosthetic valve	11 (14.5)
History of endocarditis	24 (31.6)
Clinical Features	
Fever on presentation	36 (47.4)
Septic shock	15 (19.7)
Severe congestive heart failure	5 (6.6)
Indolent symptoms[a]	56 (73.7)
Indwelling catheter on admission	18 (23.7)
Need for CRRT during admission	12 (15.8)
Co-infections	
Human Immunodeficiency Virus	5 (6.6)
Hepatitis C Virus	
Acute and chronic	33 (42.5)
Past exposure	17 (22.4)
Hepatitis B Virus	
Acute	1 (1.3)
Past exposure	6 (8)
Co-morbid conditions	
Cirrhosis	2 (2.6)
Diabetes	5 (6.6)
End-stage renal disease	1 (1.3)
COPD/Active malignancy	0
Vascular/ Immunologic Phenomenon	
Janeway lesions	7 (9.2)
Splinter hemorrhages	4 (5.3)
Roth spots	2 (2.6)
Osler nodes	6 (8)

Table 2 Clinical characteristics of patients admitted for IDU-IE treatment from January 2000 to July 2016 *(Continued)*

Clinical Characteristics	N (%)
Glomerulonephritis	1 (1.3)
Septic pulmonary emboli/infarction	42 (55.3)
Cerebrovascular related events	19 (25)
Emboli to spleen	3 (3.9)
Emboli to bone	4 (5.3)
Septic arthritis	2 (2.6)
Type of injection drug	
Opioids, all[b]	51 (67)
Heroin	22 (29)
Morphine	22 (29)
Hydromorphone	4 (5.3)
Oxymorphone	2 (2.6)
Oxycodone hydrochloride XL	1 (1.3)
Buprenorphine	2 (2.6)
Not specified	16 (21)
Methamphetamines	20 (26.3)
Bath Salts	4 (5.3)
Cocaine	12 (16)
Unknown type	9 (11.2)
Valve surgery performed	31 (41)
Readmissions within 6 months	
One readmission	17 (22.4)
Two readmissions	7 (9.2)
Three readmissions	1 (1.3)

CRRT continuous renal replacement therapy, *COPD* chronic obstructive pulmonary disease
[a]Indolent symptoms defined as: fatigue, weight loss, night sweats, reported fevers
[b]Opioid injection type and substance type counts do not add up to total opioid users as some individuals reported injecting several types of substances

increased from 8/17 (47.1%) to 41/59 (69.5%) (p-value = 0.09). However, only 53% of discharge summaries documented IDU or substance use disorder as a problem. In 52% of cases there was no documentation of any discussion regarding substance use disorder treatment or available resources. In 28 (36.8%) patients there was documentation from a social worker regarding resources for substance use disorder being offered to the patient. Six (8%) patients had in-patient consultations from pain management, psychiatry or chronic-pain services in regards to their IDU. One patient had inpatient addiction rehabilitation arranged, but the patient was not able to go. The facility would not allow the patient's admission with a peripherally inserted central venous catheter. One patient was allowed to leave the hospital to go to Alcoholics Anonymous meetings on furlough during their hospital admission.

Discussion

A dramatic increase in the number of admissions for IDU-IE was seen at UVA from 2000 to 2016. Individuals with IDU-IE were more likely to be non-Hispanic white race and were younger than those without IDU. Median hospital length of stay was 70% longer and the median hospital cost was nearly two times the cost for those without IDU. A larger percentage of patients IDU-IE were uninsured (55%) compared to patients with non-IDU-IE (7%). Evaluation of the clinical characteristics of IDU-IE found that many patients presented to the hospital acutely ill with high rates of septic shock (19.7%). This is more than double what was seen in a one-year French cohort study (9%) of IE cases [30]. There were additionally high requirements for chronic renal replacement therapy (15.8%). IDU-IE is associated with right heart involvement, our results showed that a significant number of patients 24 (36%) patients actually had left heart involvement. There were also noteworthy embolic complications with septic pulmonary emboli seen in 42 (55.3%) patients and cerebrovascular related events in 19 (25%) patients. IDU-IE did have less in-patient mortality (7.9% IDU-IE, 16.6% non-IDU-IE), however, censored 90-day mortality in those with IDU-IE approached the mortality of the non-IDU-IE group (21.8% IDU-IE vs 29.3% non-IDU-IE, p-value = 0.3). The number of patients with previous IE (31.6%) and readmissions (22.4%) highlights the need for further prevention strategies. The high acuity at the time of hospital admission may be affected by delayed patient presentation. This could be partially driven by anticipatory fear of legal repercussions, uninsured status, or concern for withdrawal symptoms.

Increasing rates of IDU-IE in Virginia are consistent with statewide data showing an over 350% increase in rates of acute HCV, which is highly correlated with IDU, during a similar time period [5]. The causes of increasing rates of IDU in Virginia and nationally over this period are at least in part due to increases in opioid prescribing. Prescriptions for opioids have increased nationally from 2007 to 2012 [31] and the southwest region of Virginia prescribes considerably more than the rest of the state [32]. Indeed, in our study the number of patients discharged with an opioid medication on their medication list increased by 22.4%.

IDU-IE and other acute bacterial infections associated with high morbidity, mortality, and costs, may be important metrics to define regions in need of funding for additional addiction treatment and harm reduction services. Policy-makers often allocate public funds for substance use disorder treatment or harm reduction strategies based on rates of HIV and viral hepatitis since there is infrastructure to measure these rates. In our study, known prevalence of HIV (6.6%) and acute and chronic HCV (42.5%) were relatively low. However, increasing rates of IDU-IE may herald potential viral outbreaks, and IDU-IE's high morbidity and extensive healthcare costs are growing. Tracking of IDU-IE should be considered as an earlier warning sign of unsafe injection practices and the potential for blood-borne viral outbreaks. With this additional surveillance, regions with known increases in IDU-IE or other IDU-related bacterial infections could be targeted as priority areas for the development, authorization, and implementation of evidence-based substance use disorder treatment programs and harm reduction packages. This is especially important to consider in the context of Virginia's Bill 2317, which allows for syringe service programs as of January 12, 2017 and was passed with a main goal of reducing the transmission of blood borne pathogens [33]. Unfortunately, infrastructure for tracking IDU-IE is not currently available. State level surveillance of IDU-IE could be possible with strategies such as mandatory reporting of inpatient admissions for this condition. National level surveillance could be streamlined with the addition of ICD codes to address IDU and both infectious and non-infectious complications of IDU.

In our study a minority of patients were offered resources for substance use disorder treatment by a social worker or seen by consulting physician teams regarding their IDU. Several factors contribute to these low levels of substance use disorder treatment discussion and initiation. The capacity of available maintenance therapy programs, abstinence therapy programs, and harm reduction strategies do not meet national or the state of Virginia's demands. In 2014 the rate of opioid dependence in Virginia was 6.5–9.2 per 1000 person years, while the capacity for medication assisted treatment was 0.7–3 per 1000 person years [34]. Some rural areas in the United States have an average two year wait time for medication assisted treatment [35], in part due to insufficient physicians with the required expertise. Many addiction treatment programs are unable to bill insurance and do not receive needed state funding [36]. Deficiencies of available resources and the perception of recidivism by health care providers may make efforts to initiate treatment discussions feel futile. Lastly, stigmatization of IDU and substance use disorders may lead to the perception that the condition represents a moral failing rather than a medical illness [27].

Absence of addiction treatment is not unique to our study site. A similar study evaluating substance use disorder treatment among persons with IDU-IE showed high readmission rates for IDU-related infections, recurrent IDU-IE and high mortality. Only a quarter of patients were offered addiction consultations or psychiatry consultations for IDU [37]. Factors contributing to IDU, such as substance use disorder, must not be overlooked while the complications of IDU are treated in the hospital setting. In addition to enhancing availability of medication assisted treatment and treatment services, including treatment of withdrawal, a multidisciplinary approach with counseling by trained therapists is useful to address underlying factors such as childhood trauma [38]. An inpatient hospitalization is an opportunity to offer these services, link patients to care, and to offer harm reduction strategies. Specifically, education on safe injecting practices, the prescribing of naloxone to empower individuals to treat unintentional overdoses and the prescribing of HIV pre-exposure prophylaxis with adjunct HIV education and counseling [37, 39]. Relationships between healthcare staff and patients with IDU may be challenging due to many factors, not limited to real and perceived stigma [40]. Concerted efforts to better educate healthcare workers and the community regarding IDU-associated substance use disorders as curable diseases may reduce stigma and improve the care of PWID both inside and outside of the hospital setting [41].

The median 17 day hospital stay and six week intravenous antibiotic treatment course required for each case of IDU-IE is an additional opportunity for multidisciplinary addiction treatment. Almost half of all IDU-IE patients were discharged from the hospital with home health agencies and an additional quarter of patients were sent to some type of nursing facility. Residential addiction treatment services that offer antibiotic infusions for IE treatment have been shown to be cost effective in reducing hospital length of stay. There are concerns related to sending PWID home with peripherally inserted central catheters, largely related to risk for catheter infections from catheter misuse. In rural areas, this is often the only option due to lack of insurance and/or lack of facilities near patients' residence. Therefore, in these settings, engaging home health agencies to assist in providing addiction treatment services in conjunction with antibiotic infusions could be helpful [21].

This study was limited by potential errors associated with coding, specifically the lack of an ICD code for IDU. The chart review process was done in part to account for these errors. The conservative criteria use to define both IDU and IE may have led to missed cases of IDU-IE. The study did not determine the total number of admissions for IE, therefore the true proportion of IE due to IDU could not be determined. Finally, our institution implemented a new electronic medical record in 2011, which resulted in some changes in documentation practices.

Conclusion

IDU-IE is a severe infection that leads to significant morbidity and healthcare related costs. IDU-IE rates are increasing and will likely continue to do so without targeted interventions to help PWID. The diagnosis and treatment of IDU-IE provides an opportunity for the delivery of addiction treatment, counseling, and harm reduction strategies.

Summary

Numbers of infective endocarditis cases related to injection drug use (IDU) have increased significantly in Virginia. While infective endocarditis is treated medically, opportunities for addiction treatment referral are missed.

Abbreviations

HCV: Hepatitis C Virus; HIV: human immunodeficiency virus; ICD: International Classification of Diseases; IDU: injection drug use; IDU-IE: injection drug use associated infective endocarditis; IE: infective endocarditis; non-IDU-IE: infective endocarditis not related to injection drug use; PWID: people who inject drugs; UVA: University of Virginia

Acknowledgements

We thank UVA's Clinical Data Repository staff, Ken Scully, for his contribution.

Funding

This research was supported in part by Award Number 5 T32 AI007046–40 from the National Institutes of Health. The content is solely the responsibility of the authors and does not necessarily represent the official views of the National Institutes of Health. The National Institutes of Health had no role in the collection, analysis, or interpretation of the data or in the writing of the manuscript.

Authors' contributions

ETR contributed to the study design, statistical analysis, and manuscript revisions. WMS contributed to the study design and manuscript revisions. RAD contributed to the study design and manuscript preparation and revisions. MEG contributed to the study design, obtaining ethics board approval, data collection, statistical analyses, creation of figures and tables, and composition of the manuscript. All authors read and approved of the final manuscript.

Competing interests

The authors declare that they have no competing interests.

References

1. Altice FL, Azbel L, Stone J, Brooks-Pollock E, Smyrnov P, Dvoriak S, Taxman FS, El-Bassel N, Martin NK, Booth R, Stover H, Dolan K, Vickerman P. The perfect storm: incarceration and the high-risk environment perpetuating transmission of HIV, hepatitis C virus, and tuberculosis in Eastern Europe and Central Asia. Lancet. 2016;388(10050):1228–48.
2. Wejnert C, Hess KL, Hall HI, Van Handel M, Hayes D, Fulton P Jr, An Q, Koenig LJ, Prejean J, Valleroy LA. Vital signs: trends in HIV diagnoses, risk behaviors, and prevention among persons who inject drugs - United States. MMWR Morb Mortal Wkly Rep. 2016;65(47):1336–42.
3. Rudd RA, Aleshire N, Zibbell JE, Gladden RM. Increases in drug and opioid overdose deaths — United States, 2000–2014. Morbidity and Mortality Weekly Report (MMWR). 2016;64(50):1378–82.
4. Van Handel MM, Rose CE, Hallisey EJ, Kolling JL, Zibbell JE, Lewis B, Bohm MK, Jones CM, Flanagan BE, Siddiqi AE, Iqbal K, Dent AL, Mermin JH, McCray E, Ward JW, Brooks JT. County-level vulnerability assessment for rapid dissemination of HIV or HCV infections among persons who inject drugs, United States. J Acquir Immune Defic Syndr. 2016;73(3):323–31.
5. Zibbell JE, Iqbal K, Patel RC, Suryaprasad A, Sanders KJ, Moore-Moravian L, Serrecchia J, Blankenship S, Ward JW, Holtzman D, Centers for Disease Control and Prevention (CDC). Increases in hepatitis C virus infection related to injection drug use among persons aged. MMWR Morb Mortal Wkly Rep. 2015;64(17):453–8.

6. Fleischauer AT, Ruhl L, Rhea S, Barnes E. Hospitalizations for endocarditis and associated health care costs among persons with diagnosed drug dependence - North Carolina, 2010-2015. MMWR Morb Mortal Wkly Rep. 2017;66(22):569–73.

7. Janowicz DM. HIV transmission and injection drug use: lessons from the Indiana outbreak. Top Antivir Med. 2016;24(2):90–2.

8. Frontera JA, Gradon JD. Right-side endocarditis in injection drug users: review of proposed mechanisms of pathogenesis. Clin Infect Dis. 2000;30(2):374–9.

9. Mylonakis E, Calderwood SB. Infective endocarditis in adults. N Engl J Med. 2001;345(18):1318–30.

10. Miro JM, del Rio A, Mestres CA. Infective endocarditis and cardiac surgery in intravenous drug abusers and HIV-1 infected patients. Cardiol Clin. 2003; 21(2):167–84 v-vi.

11. Rabkin DG, Mokadam NA, Miller DW, Goetz RR, Verrier ED, Aldea GS. Long-term outcome for the surgical treatment of infective endocarditis with a focus on intravenous drug users. Ann Thorac Surg. 2012;93(1):51–7.

12. Osterdal OB, Salminen PR, Jordal S, Sjursen H, Wendelbo O, Haaverstad R. Cardiac surgery for infective endocarditis in patients with intravenous drug use. Interact Cardiovasc Thorac Surg. 2016;22(5):633–40.

13. Virginia Department of Health [http://www.vdh.virginia.gov/home/the-opioid-addiction-crisis-is-a-public-health-emergency-in-virginia/#a1]. Accessed 14 Apr 2017.

14. Hartman L, Barnes E, Bachmann L, Schafer K, Lovato J, Files DC. Opiate injection-associated infective endocarditis in the southeastern United States. Am J Med Sci. 2016;352(6):603–8.

15. Tung MK, Light M, Giri R, Lane S, Appelbe A, Harvey C, Athan E. Evolving epidemiology of injecting drug use-associated infective endocarditis: a regional Centre experience. Drug Alcohol Rev. 2015;34(4):412–7.

16. Keeshin SW, Feinberg J. Endocarditis as a marker for new epidemics of injection drug use. Am J Med Sci. 2016;352(6):609–14.

17. Wurcel AG, Anderson JE, Chui KK, Skinner S, Knox TA, Snydman DR, Stopka TJ. Increasing infectious endocarditis admissions among young people who inject drugs. Open Forum Infect Dis. 2016;3(3):ofw157.

18. Wright A, Otome O, Harvey C, Bowe S, Athan E. The current epidemiology of injecting drug use-associated infective endocarditis in Victoria, Australia in the midst of increasing crystal methamphetamine use. Heart Lung Circ. 2018;27(4):484–8.

19. Adamson K, Jackson L, Gahagan J. Young people and injection drug use: is there a need to expand harm reduction services and support? Int J Drug Policy. 2017;39:14–20.

20. Unger JB, Kipke MD, De Rosa CJ, Hyde J, Ritt-Olson A, Montgomery S. Needle-sharing among young IV drug users and their social network members: the influence of the injection partner's characteristics on HIV risk behavior. Addict Behav. 2006;31(9):1607–18.

21. Jewell C, Weaver M, Sgroi C, Anderson K, Sayeed Z. Residential addiction treatment for injection drug users requiring intravenous antibiotics: a cost-reduction strategy. J Addict Med. 2013;7(4):271–6.

22. Suzuki J. Medication-assisted treatment for hospitalized patients with intravenous-drug-use related infective endocarditis. Am J Addict. 2016; 25(3):191–4.

23. Weinmeyer R. Needle exchange Programs' status in US politics. AMA J Ethics. 2016;18(3):252–7.

24. Jozaghi E, Reid AA, Andresen MA, Juneau A. A cost-benefit/cost-effectiveness analysis of proposed supervised injection facilities in Ottawa, Canada. Subst Abuse Treat Prev Policy. 2014;9:31 597X-9-31.

25. Kwon JA, Anderson J, Kerr CC, Thein HH, Zhang L, Iversen J, Dore GJ, Kaldor JM, Law MG, Maher L, Wilson DP. Estimating the cost-effectiveness of needle-syringe programs in Australia. AIDS. 2012;26(17):2201–10.

26. Nguyen TQ, Weir BW, Des Jarlais DC, Pinkerton SD, Holtgrave DR. Syringe exchange in the United States: a national level economic evaluation of hypothetical increases in investment. AIDS Behav. 2014;18(11):2144–55.

27. Barry CL, McGinty EE, Pescosolido BA, Goldman HH. Stigma, discrimination, treatment effectiveness, and policy: public views about drug addiction and mental illness. Psychiatr Serv. 2014;65(10):1269–72.

28. Li JS, Sexton DJ, Mick N, Nettles R, Fowler VG Jr, Ryan T, Bashore T, Corey GR. Proposed modifications to the Duke criteria for the diagnosis of infective endocarditis. Clin Infect Dis. 2000;30(4):633–8.

29. Virginia Department of Health [http://www.vdh.virginia.gov/health-equity/division-of-rural-health/]. Accessed 28 May 2018.

30. Hoen B, Alla F, Selton-Suty C, Beguinot I, Bouvet A, Briancon S, Casalta JP, Danchin N, Delahaye F, Etienne J, Le Moing V, Leport C, Mainardi JL, Ruimy R, Vandenesch F, Association pour l'Etude et la prevention de l'Endocardite Infectieuse (AEPEI) study group: Changing profile of infective endocarditis: results of a 1-year survey in France. JAMA 2002, 288(1):75–81.

31. Center for Disease Control and Prevention [https://www.cdc.gov/drugoverdose/data/prescribing.html].

32. Virginia Department of Health [http://www.vdh.virginia.gov/content/uploads/sites/10/2016/06/Virginia-Hepatitis-C-Epidemiologic-Profile-2016.pdf]. Accessed 14 Apr 2017.

33. Virginia's Legislative Information System [https://lis.virginia.gov/cgi-bin/legp604.exe?171+ful+HB2317]. Accessed 28 Sept 2018.

34. Jones CM, Campopiano M, Baldwin G, McCance-Katz E. National and State Treatment Need and Capacity for Opioid Agonist Medication-Assisted Treatment. Am J Public Health. 2015;105(8):e55–63.

35. Sigmon SC. Access to treatment for opioid dependence in rural America: challenges and future directions. JAMA Psychiatry. 2014;71(4):359–60.

36. Andrews C, Abraham A, Grogan CM, Pollack HA, Bersamira C, Humphreys K, Friedmann P. Despite resources from the ACA, Most states do little to help addiction treatment programs implement health care reform. Health Aff (Millwood). 2015;34(5):828–35.

37. Rosenthal ES, Karchmer AW, Theisen-Toupal J, Castillo RA, Rowley CF. Suboptimal addiction interventions for patients hospitalized with injection drug use-associated infective endocarditis. Am J Med. 2016;129(5):481–5.

38. Taplin C, Saddichha S, Li K, Krausz MR. Family history of alcohol and drug abuse, childhood trauma, and age of first drug injection. Subst Use Misuse. 2014;49(10):1311–6.

39. Centers for Disease Control and Prevention [https://www.cdc.gov/hiv/pdf/guidelines/PrEPguidelines2014.pdf]. Accessed 15 Feb 2017.

40. Ford R, Bammer G, Becker N. The determinants of nurses' therapeutic attitude to patients who use illicit drugs and implications for workforce development. J Clin Nurs. 2008;17(18):2452–62.

41. McGinty EE, Goldman HH, Pescosolido B, Barry CL. Portraying mental illness and drug addiction as treatable health conditions: effects of a randomized experiment on stigma and discrimination. Soc Sci Med. 2015;126:73–85.

12

A systematic review of adherence to oral pre-exposure prophylaxis for HIV – how can we improve uptake and adherence?

David Sidebottom[1]* ⓘ, Anna Mia Ekström[1,3] and Susanne Strömdahl[1,2]

Abstract

Introduction: Oral pre-exposure prophylaxis (PrEP) is an effective strategy to reduce the risk of HIV transmission in high risk individuals. However, the effectiveness of oral pre-exposure prophylaxis is highly dependent on user adherence, which some previous trials have struggled to optimise particularly in low and middle income settings. This systematic review aims to ascertain the reasons for non-adherence to pre-exposure prophylaxis to guide future implementation.

Methods: We performed structured literature searches of online databases and conference archives between August 8, 2016 and September 16, 2017. In total, 18 prospective randomized control trials and implementation studies investigating oral pre-exposure prophylaxis were reviewed. A structured form was used for data extraction and findings summarized regarding efficacy, effectiveness, adherence and possible reasons for non-adherence.

Results: Adherence varied between differing populations both geographically and socioeconomically. Common reasons for non-adherence reported over multiple studies were; social factors such as stigma, low risk perception, low decision making power, an unacceptable dosing regimen, side effects, and the logistics of daily life. Oral pre-exposure prophylaxis with included antiviral regimens was not associated with a high risk of antiviral resistance development in the reviewed studies.

Conclusion: Our findings indicate that oral pre-exposure prophylaxis should be delivered within a holistic intervention, acknowledging the other needs of the targeted demographic in order to maximise acceptability. Socioeconomic factors and poor governmental policy remain major barriers to widespread implementation of pre-exposure prophylaxis.

Keywords: HIV, Pre-exposure prophylaxis, HIV prevention, Systematic review, Medication adherence, Antiviral drug resistance

Background

In the face of barriers due to policy, stigma, and culture, progress is being made in the struggle against HIV. Antiretroviral therapy (ART) is undergoing rapid global scale-up with the 90–90–90 2020 United Nations (UN) target in sight, reaching 46% global coverage in 2015 compared to less than 10% the decade before [1]. This translates into a 26% reduction in global AIDS-related deaths since 2010. Additionally, with the efficacy of treatment as prevention demonstrated in 2011 [2], ART holds the potential to reduce HIV incidence beyond the 36.7 million people already infected. However, despite these advances, the Joint United Nations Programme on HIV/AIDS (UNAIDS) notes that recent headway in HIV incidence reduction has slowed "alarmingly", and that disparities in progress are widening for certain key populations such as young women, sex workers, people who inject drugs (PWID) and men who have sex with men (MSM) [1].

It is within these key populations that the burden of HIV is disproportionately carried. The risk of HIV acquisition versus the general population is 10 times greater in sex workers and 24 times greater in PWID and MSM [3], although analysis reveals large diversity between regions. In Western Europe and North America, 49% of new infections occur within the MSM population and 15% in PWID, whereas in Eastern Europe and Central

---
* Correspondence: dbsidebottom@gmail.com
[1]Department of Public Health Sciences, Karolinska Institutet, Stockholm, Sweden
Full list of author information is available at the end of the article

Asia the figures are 6 and 51% respectively [1]. This variation reflects the diverse burden of stigma and discrimination borne by these populations [4]. Same-sex acts are illegal in 72 (37%) UN states, and punishable by the death penalty in 13 (6%) [4], just one example of the many additional challenges faced by individuals and organisations battling HIV. Effective prevention strategies to combat HIV are desperately needed by these hidden populations, none more so than transgender women (TGW), who have nearly 49 times greater odds of HIV acquisition than the general population [5].

In 2010 iPrEx became the first randomised controlled trial (RCT) to demonstrate the efficacy of pre-exposure prophylaxis (PrEP) in MSM, finding a 44% risk reduction in the experimental group receiving daily oral tenofovir-emtricitabine (TDF-FTC) as compared to placebo [6]. This success has since been replicated in several further studies encompassing both daily [7–9] and on-demand regimens [10], fuelling global excitement over this novel strategy. Following this data, PrEP is recommended for implementation among MSM by the World Health Organisation (WHO) and the Centres for Disease Prevention and Control (CDC) [11, 12]. However, failures have been observed in some at-risk groups, most notably heterosexual women [13, 14].

Previous literature notes that adherence is a critical link in the wider PrEP continuum, and that the success of PrEP intervention rides on its ability to maintain good adherence within the cohort under investigation [15, 16]. In 2013, a nested sub-study of the Partners trial found that high (> 80%) PrEP adherence was associated with 100% PrEP efficacy (95% CI 83.7 to 100%) [17]. Conversely, in 2015 the VOICE trial failed to demonstrate PrEP clinical effectiveness in young African women [14], where only 30% of quarterly plasma samples contained a detectable level of TDF. Whilst a number of reviews exist concerning various aspects of PrEP we conducted this global systematic review to assess adherence to oral PrEP in the context of the reported efficacy. We also aimed to discuss the reasons for non-adherence in detail to guide comprehensive PrEP implementation programming in the future.

Methods

Search strategy and inclusion criteria

The Population, Intervention, Comparison, Outcome (PICO) framework was used to develop the search strategy. The population was defined as all individuals 'at risk' of HIV acquisition that have been studied regarding PrEP. Eligible studies comprised of prospective RCTs and implementation studies that examined efficacy, effectiveness or adherence. Both studies reporting oral TDF and TDF-FTC as the intervention were included as this distinction has not been shown to be clinically

important [7, 18]. Daily, event and time driven regimens were all eligible (Fig. 1). The outcomes assessed were efficacy and adherence. For adherence all measurements were included. All comparison and no-comparison trials were included. In practice the 'at risk' population is reflected in trial recruitment criteria, so was not specified in our search. No restrictions were imposed regarding geographical location, sex or gender, sexual preference, or dosing regimen. Only English language trials discussing oral PrEP efficacy, effectiveness or adherence in detail were included.

We performed online searches in Ovid Medline (without revisions, 1996 to current), Web of Science, EMBASE and the Cochrane Library. An initial search was conducted in August 2016, and repeated in September 2017. In addition, we searched conference abstracts from the AIDS Conference, International AIDS Society Conference and the Conference on Retroviruses and Opportunistic Infections via their online archives.

Our search utilised a combination of medical subject heading terms (denoted by appended '/') and keywords as follows; (Pre-Exposure Prophylaxis/ OR PrEP OR chemoprophyla* OR antiretroviral prophyla*) AND (HIV/ OR HIV-1/ OR Anti-HIV Agents/). Results were limited to 'human' and 'clinical trial', from 2010 to 'current' as the first PrEP RCT was published in 2010.

Screening and data extraction

Published studies were identified through the search strategy described above, and titles were screened for relevance. Abstracts were further screened for eligibility and downloaded for further analysis when inclusion criteria were met. Identified articles were critically appraised using a checklist [19] to assess methodology prior to inclusion into the systematic review. Attention was paid to randomisation and blinding adequacy, allocation concealment and loss to follow up.

An initial online search on August 8, 2016 located 87 potentially relevant papers, and one conference abstract. A repeated search on September 15, 2017 located an additional 35 papers, and 12 conference abstracts. In total, 18 papers and 10 conference abstracts were found. DS extracted the data using a structured form regarding study design and population, geographical location and time, sample size, follow-up time, drug regimen, efficacy measurement, and adherence measurements. An additional 5 papers reported on qualitative exploration of factors affecting PrEP adherence. Authors were contacted by email if clarification was required.

All adherence measurements used were included, as defined in cited literature. Detection of TDF and/or FTC in plasma is highly concordant with the presence of TDF/FTC active metabolites within HIV-1 target cells, which provides protection from HIV [6, 20]. Tenofovir

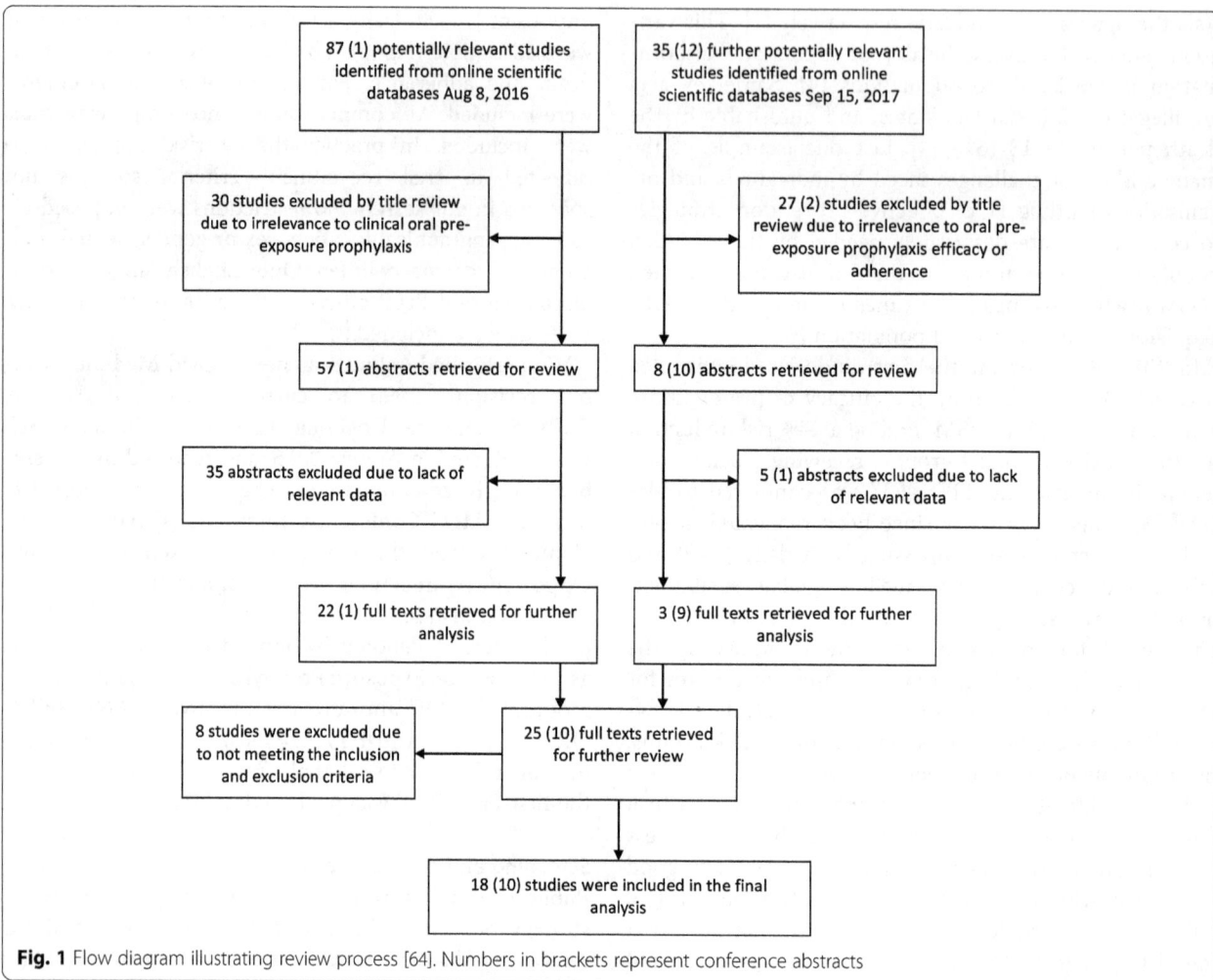

Fig. 1 Flow diagram illustrating review process [64]. Numbers in brackets represent conference abstracts

diphosphate levels, measured through dried blood spot testing, is increasingly used as an intrusive biomarker of long-term PrEP adherence, due to its long half-life of 17 days [15, 21]. However, a variety of soft adherence measures are also used (pill count, self-report, medication event monitoring systems (MEMS). Where adherence at multiple time points was available, the latest measurement was taken, as maintaining prolonged adherence to PrEP throughout the duration of possible exposure to HIV is arguably of most clinical interest. Efficacy data was also extracted from the literature, as this important outcome is best understood in the context of reported adherence.

Results

Study design is illustrated in Fig. 1. Randomised controlled trials have evaluated oral PrEP in a variety of geographical and sociological settings. The characteristics of included trials are displayed in Table 1.

Adherence

Table 2 describes reported study adherence by various measures. Wide disparity exists between soft (self-report, pill count, medication event monitoring system) and intrusive (levels of TDF and/or FTC in plasma samples, or tenofovir diphosphate measured in dried blood spots) measures of adherence. In all measured cases, a higher proportion of non-seroconverters have detectable plasma TDF than seroconverters. Two trials which failed in young African women are associated with poor adherence. Only 24% of non-seroconverters had detectable TDF in FEM-PrEP [13], and 29% in VOICE [14]. In contrast, results from a series of recent open label papers and abstracts suggest high adherence in a variety of real-world settings [22–30].

Reported reasons for poor adherence are described in Fig. 3. Start-up symptoms, including nausea, vomiting, and dizziness, that lessen after the first month of medication, have been explicitly reported by several trials [6, 8, 13, 31]. Low risk perception is also

Table 1 Overview of included studies examining the efficacy, effectiveness, and adherence of oral PrEP

	Characteristics								Number of incident HIV infections		
Year	Study name	Geographical location	Population	Sample size	Total follow-up time (person-years)	Design	Regimen	Drug	Study drug	Placebo/ comparator	Total
2010	iPrEx [6]	Global	MSM/TGW	2499	3324	RDBPCT	Daily	TDF-FTC	36	64	100
2012	Partners study [7]	Kenya and Uganda	Heterosexual HIV-discordant couples	4758	7820	RDBPCT	Daily	TDF-FTC	13	52	82
								TDF	17		
2012	TDF2 [8]	Botswana	Heterosexual	1219	1563	RDBPCT	Daily	TDF-FTC	9	24	33
2012	FEM-PrEP [13]	Kenya, Tanzania and South Africa	Heterosexual females	2120	–	RDBPCT	Daily	TDF-FTC	33	35	68
2012	Kenya safety and adherence study [38]	Kenya	MSM and Female sex workers	72	–	RDBPCT	Daily	TDF-FTC	0	1	1
							Time-driven		0		
2013	Partners adherence substudy [17]	Kenya and Uganda	Heterosexual HIV-discordant couples	1147	807	Convenience sub-cohort of a RDBPCT	Daily	TDF-FTC	0	14	14
								TDF	0		
2013	Bangkok tenofovir study [31]	Bangkok	PWID	2413	9665	RDBPCT	Daily	TDF	17	33	50
2013	Uganda safety and adherence study [35]	Uganda	Heterosexual HIV-discordant couples	72	–	RDBPCT	Daily	TDF-FTC	0	0	0
							Time-driven		0	0	
2013	ATN 082 (Project PrEPARE) [54]	United States	Young MSM	58	–	RBPCT	Daily	TDF-FTC	0	0	0
							No pill		0		
2014	iPrEx extension [15]	Global	MSM/TGW	1603 (1225 received)	–	Open Label	Daily	TDF-FTC	28	13	41
2015	VOICE [14]	South Africa, Uganda, Zimbabwe	Heterosexual females	3019	4253	RCT	Daily	TDF-FTC	61	60	173
								TDF	52		
2015	HPTN 067/ ADAPT[a] [36]	South Africa	Heterosexual females	191	–	RCT with different regimens as comparators	Daily	TDF-FTC	1	N/A	5
							Time-driven		2		
							Event-driven		2		
2015	Generating adherence Philadelphia [50]	United States	Young MSM of colour	23	7.5	Observational	Daily	TDF-FTC	0	N/A	0
2015	PROUD [9]	United Kingdom	MSM	544	465	RCT with a 1 year deferred group as comparator	Daily	TDF-FTC	3	20	23
2015	IPERGAY [10]	France and Canada	MSM/TGW	400	431	RDBPCT	Event-driven	TDF-FTC	2	14	16
2016	Bangkok MSM[a] [55]	Thailand	MSM /TGW	168	–	Observational	Daily	TDF-FTC	0	N/A	0
2016	Permanente Cohort [24]	USA	At-risk	972	850	Open label	Daily	TDF-FTC	0	2 Off-PrEP	2
2016	The Demo Project [23]	USA	MSM/TGW	557	481	Open label	Daily	TDF-FTC	1	1 Off-PrEP	2
2017	SPARK[a] [57]	United States	MSM	301	–	Open Label	Daily	TDF-FTC	–	–	–
2017	IPERGAY extension [22]	France/ Canada	MSM/TGW	361	518	Open label	Event-driven	TDF-FTC	0	1 Off-PrEP	1

Table 1 Overview of included studies examining the efficacy, effectiveness, and adherence of oral PrEP *(Continued)*

	Characteristics								Number of incident HIV infections		
Year	Study name	Geographical location	Population	Sample size	Total follow-up time (person-years)	Design	Regimen	Drug	Study drug	Placebo/comparator	Total
2017	Short term PrEP Mozambique[a] [25]	Mozambique	Heterosexual females	74	7.4	Open label	Daily	TDF-FTC	0	N/A	1
2017	Parisian MSM[a] [26]	France	MSM	785	215	Open label	Daily & Event-driven	TDF-FTC	3	N/A	3
2017	PRELUDE[a] [27, 28]	Australia	Gay/bisexual males	317	381	Open label	Daily	TDF-FTC	0	N/A	0
2017	PROUD adherence[a] [29]	UK	MSM	544 enrolled (481 initiated)	1253	Open label	Daily	TDF-FTC	10	N/A	10
2017	Pluspills[a] [30]	South Africa	Adolescents	148	131	Open label	Daily	TDF-FTC	0	1 Off-PrEP	1
2017	Brazil Demo[a] [65]	Brasil	MSM/TGW	450	389	Open label	Daily	TDF-FTC	0	2 Off-PrEP	2

[a] Abstract available only. *MSM* men who have sex with men, *TGW* transgender women, *PWID* people who inject drugs, *RCT* randomised controlled trial, *RDBPCT* randomised, double blinded, placebo controlled trial, *TDF* tenofovir, *FTC* emtricitabine

reported to be a common issue. Many studies report challenges aligning perceived risk with actual risk [13, 14, 32–34]. Participants described concern regarding perceived long term side effects in two studies [32, 33] and poor adherence was partly attributed to dosing regimen in five studies [32, 33, 35–37]. However, a recent study of MSM in Toronto found that high versus low actual HIV risk were more willing to take PrEP (OR 27.11; 95% CI, 1.33 to 554.43) [33].

Societal factors were repeatedly stated as major challenges to maintaining adherence. Governmental and policy factors were mentioned in several contexts, and stigma was reported by many participants in both quantitative and qualitative studies as a barrier to success [17, 38].

Efficacy

Reported efficacy is highly variable (Table 3), with overall HIV incidence relative risk reduction (RRR) ranging from −49 to 86% [9, 10, 14]. Both RCTs reporting non-significant RRRs were conducted in the population of young African women [13, 14]. Efficacy among MSM has been consistently high, with recent implementation studies in the UK and Canada both reporting a RRR of 86% in real-life clinical deployment [9, 10]. Heterosexual couples have also achieved high PrEP efficacy with the 2012 Partners study reporting a 75% RRR over 7820 person-years of follow up. Within the single trial in PWID, overall RRR was found to be 48.9 (95% CI, 9.6 to 72.2%).

Three main oral dosing regimen options have been investigated (Fig. 2). Daily dosing is the most frequently tested regimen, with 9 of 11 independent RCTs choosing this route. In event-driven dosing, individuals take two tablets prior to intercourse, followed by single doses 24

and 48 h after the first [10]. Only 1 independent randomised controlled trial, IPERGAY, has evaluated the efficacy of the event-driven regimen so far. Despite only 43% of participants meeting optimum adherence criteria, IPERGAY found an on-treatment RRR of 86%, on par with the daily regimen. Furthermore, mean pill use was halved with participants only using 15 pills per month, versus 30 per month with daily dosing. Time driven dosing, where individuals take pills twice weekly with a post-intercourse boost, has also been evaluated for safety and adherence [35, 36, 38]. This success was replicated in an open label extension, which found 97% (95% CI 81 to 100) effectiveness [22].

When analysis is limited to participants with detectable study-drug serum concentrations, efficacy is higher without exception [6–8, 10, 31] reaching 92% in the iPrEx study subgroup. In an open label extension of iPrEx, no participants with plasma TDF concentrations consistent with 4 or more pills per week underwent seroconversion [15]. The two trial arm participants to undergo HIV seroconversion returned 60 and 58 pills out of 60 for pill count, so were seemingly non-adherent.

Emergence of resistance in patients

Several trials report individuals who were infected between enrolment and randomisation [7, 9, 14], or had missed diagnoses of pre-existing HIV infection [8], and were later randomised to receive PrEP [Table 4]. Fem-PrEP reported 4 cases of resistance to FTC (3 cases of the M184 V mutation, 1 case of the M184I mutation) in trial-arm participants. VOICE reported FTC resistance in 2 women infected between enrolment and randomisation (2 cases of M184 V/I), and 1 woman

Table 2 Adherence to oral PrEP by different measures used

Characteristics					Adherence				
					Any detectable plasma drug (TDF or FTC) (%)		Self-report (%)	Pill count (%)	MEMS (%)
Year	Study name	Geographical location	Population	Regimen	HIV – (non-seroconverters)	HIV + (seroconverters)			
2010	iPrEx [6]	Global	MSM/TGW	Daily	51	9	95	> 90	–
2012	Partners study [7]	Kenya and Uganda	Heterosexual HIV-discordant couples	Daily	82	31	–	92	–
2012	TDF2 [8]	Botswana	Heterosexual	Daily	80	50	94	84	–
2012	FEM-PrEP [13]	Kenya, Tanzania, South Africa	Heterosexual females	Daily	24	15	95	88	–
2012	Kenya safety and adherence study [38]	Kenya	MSM and female sex workers	Daily	–	–	–	–	83% (IQR 63 to 92)
				Time-driven			100		55 (pre-coital), 26 (post-coital)
2013	Partners adherence substudy [17]	Kenya and Uganda	Heterosexual HIV-discordant couples	Daily	–	–	–	99	97
2013	Bangkok tenofovir study [31]	Bangkok	PWID	Daily	67	39	94	–	–
2013	Uganda safety and adherence study [35]	Uganda	Heterosexual HIV-discordant couples	Daily	–		–	–	97
				Time-driven			100		91 (pre-coital) 45 (post-coital)
2013	ATN 082 (Project PrEPARE) [54]	United States	Young MSM	Daily	20		62	–	–
2014	iPrEx extension [15]	Global	MSM/TGW	Daily	71		85 [c]	–	–
2015	VOICE [14]	South Africa, Uganda, Zimbabwe	Heterosexual females	Daily	29supp		87 (via computer), 90 (face to face)	88	–
					30		87 (via computer), 91 (face to face)	84	
2015	Generating adherence Philadelphia [50]	United States	Young MSM of colour	Daily	–		–	72	–
2015	HPTN 067/ ADAPT[a] [36]	South Africa	Heterosexual females	Daily	68		–	–	76
				Time-driven	56				65
				Event-driven	53				53
2015	PROUD [9]	United Kingdom	MSM	Daily	100 [c]		–	–	–
2015	IPERGAY [10]	France and Canada	MSM/TGW	Event-driven	87	0	29 (suboptimal), 43 (optimal) [b]	–	–
2016	Bangkok MSM[a] [55]	Thailand	MSM/TGW	Daily	–		9.8 (complete adherence)	–	–
2016	Permanente Cohort [24]	USA	At-risk	Daily	–		–	92	–
2016	The Demo Project [23]	USA	MSM/TGW	Daily	80 [d]		–	82	–
2017	SPARK[a] [57]	United States	MSM	Daily	90		–	–	–

Table 2 Adherence to oral PrEP by different measures used *(Continued)*

Characteristics					Adherence				
Year	Study name	Geographical location	Population	Regimen	Any detectable plasma drug (TDF or FTC) (%)		Self-report (%)	Pill count (%)	MEMS (%)
					HIV − (non-seroconverters)	HIV + (seroconverters)			
2017	IPERGAY extension [22]	France/ Canada	MSM/TGW	Event-driven	71 [e]	0	24 (suboptimal), 50 (optimal)	–	–
2017	Short term PrEP Mozambique[a] [25]	Mozambique	Heterosexual females	Daily	76				–
2017	Parisian MSM[a] [26]	France	MSM	Daily & Event-driven	83		–	–	–
2017	PRELUDE[a] [27, 28]	Australia	Gay/bisexual males	Daily	51 [d]		–	–	–
2017	PROUD adherence[a] [29]	UK	MSM	Daily	–		98	–	–
2017	Pluspills[a] [30]	South Africa	Adolescents	Daily	38		–	92	–
2017	Brazil Demo[a] [65]	Brasil	MSM/TGW	Daily	74		–	–	–

[a] Abstract available only, [b] At most recent sexual encounter, [c] Of participants reporting good adherence, [d] Dried blood spot concentration, [e]Only 33% of participants had plasma TDF concentrations consistent with taking > 4 tablets per week

infected post-randomisation (M184 V mutation), all in the trial arm. The 2012 TDF2 trial reported the K65R, M184 V, and A62V mutations in 1 of 10 trial-arm participants infected with HIV. That individual had an unrecognised HIV infection at baseline. The PROUD trial reported FTC resistance in 2 individuals assigned to the immediate arm who were infected with HIV at baseline or 4-weeks (66.6%), but no resistance in either of the 2 participants infected later on. Only 2 cases of resistance have been reported in HIV infected individuals assigned to placebo/comparator groups.

Discussion
Efficacy and effectiveness
This review discusses adherence to oral PrEP in the context of efficacy data from previous studies. We found that oral TDF and TDF-FTC PrEP for the prevention of HIV in humans is efficacious and effective in a variety of scenarios. Two recent trials within MSM populations in the UK and France/Canada report 86% effectiveness (90% CI, 64 to 96%) [9], and 86% efficacy (95% CI, 40 to 98%) [10] in daily and event-driven regimens respectively. Additionally, PrEP

Table 3 Modified Intention to Treat efficacy and effectiveness of studies examining oral PrEP

Characteristics					Outcome
Year	Study name	Population	Regimen	Drug	Efficacy (%, 95 CI)
2010	iPrEx [6]	MSM/TGW	Daily	TDF-FTC	44% (15 to 63)
2012	Partners study [7]	Heterosexual HIV-discordant couples	Daily	TDF-FTC	75% (55 to 87)
				TDF	67% (44 to 81)
2012	TDF2 [8]	Heterosexual	Daily	FTC- TDF	62.2% (21.5 to 83.4)
2012	FEM-PrEP [13]	Heterosexual Females	Daily	TDF-FTC	6% (−52 to 41%)
2013	Bangkok tenofovir study [31]	PWID	Daily	TDF	48.9% (9.6 to 72.2)
2014	iPrEx extension [15]	MSM/TGW	Daily	TDF-FTC	36% (−24 to 67)[a]
2015	VOICE [14]	Heterosexual Females	Daily	TDF-FTC	−4% (−49 to 27)
				TDF	−49% (− 129 to 3)
2015	PROUD [9]	MSM	Daily	TDF-FTC	86% (90% CI 64 to 96)
2015	IPERGAY [10]	MSM/TGW	Event-driven	TDF-FTC	86% (40 to 98)

[a] Unknown if intention to treat or modified intention to treat. *MSM* men who have sex with men, *TGW* transgender women, *PWID* people who inject drugs, *TDF* tenofovir, *FTC* emtricitabine

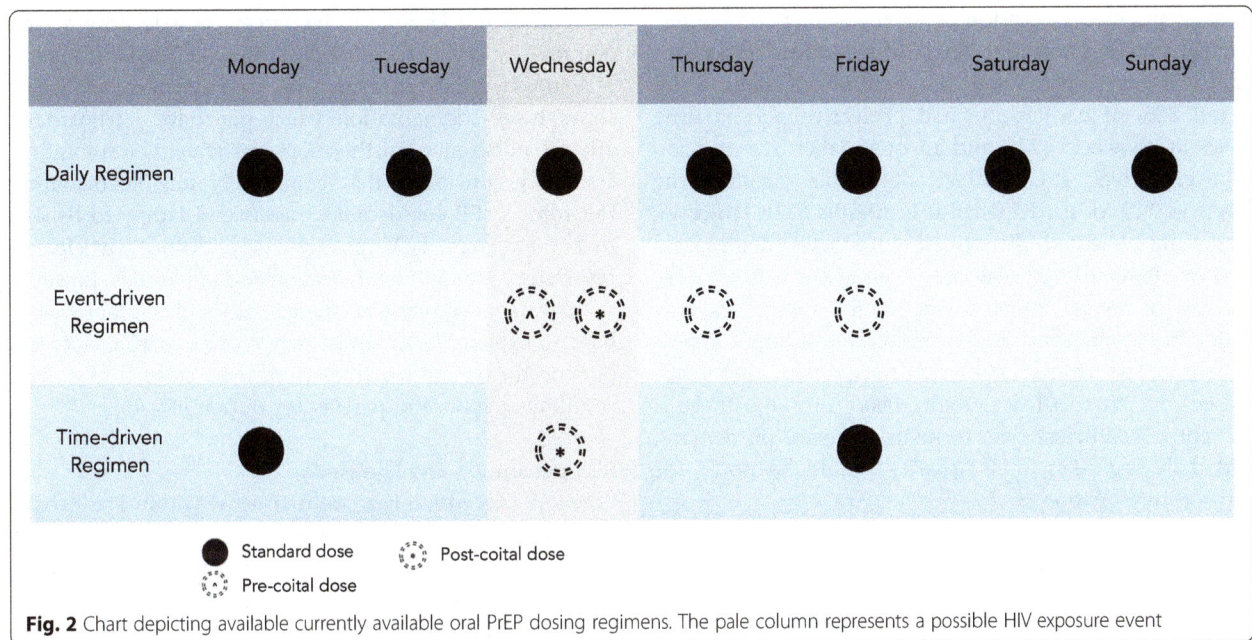

Fig. 2 Chart depicting available currently available oral PrEP dosing regimens. The pale column represents a possible HIV exposure event

is efficacious in serodiscordant heterosexual couples [7] (efficacy 75%; 95% CI, 55 to 87%).

However, two large trials in heterosexual women failed to demonstrate efficacy [13, 14]. Whilst adherence was low in both studies, as inferred from plasma drug levels, concerns have been previously raised regarding the differential distribution of antiretroviral (ARV) components within rectal and cervical mucosae [20]. Rectal tissue concentrations of TDF are two orders of magnitude greater than in cervical tissue at the same dose, suggesting that equal dosing for men and women may result in insufficient mucosal concentrations to prevent HIV infection in females. Atypical vaginal microbiota have been proposed to decrease the effectiveness of PrEP and increase the risk of HIV acquisition, possibly by increasing ARV metabolism or by weakening the cervicovaginal barrier [39]. However, a post-hoc analysis of the Partners study found that oral PrEP was equally efficacious among woman with bacterial vaginosis as without, and furthermore was not significantly different with the detection of *G. vaginalis* or *Bacteroides* spp. morphotypes [40]. This suggests that oral PrEP formulations do not require testing for bacterial vaginosis or treatment to ensure protection from HIV acquisition.

Adherence

Adherence to oral PrEP varies greatly between trials and study populations. We found that adherence was consistently high when measured via self-report, pill count and electronic methods, but generally lower when assessed via plasma drug concentrations of TDF and/or FTC. Furthermore, 'detectable plasma TDF' rates are frequently reported, however the lower limit of plasma drug detection corresponds to fewer than two pills per week (very poor adherence), making interpretation challenging. While many participants over-report adherence to PrEP, it is unclear whether this is intentional or not. This may be due to social desirability bias as participants in the trials frequently receive adherence counselling, and therefore are well aware of the importance of compliance to PrEP. Comparison of adherence between trials is further complicated by the large variety of adherence measures available, with different methods used within measures themselves. For example, self-report methodology varies from daily SMS reports to monthly interviews, whilst pill count methodology includes unannounced home visits, MEMS, and pharmacy counts amongst other strategies. Therefore, comparability is limited between studies and study populations.

Table 4 Cases of resistance have been reported in several oral PrEP studies

Study Name	Trial arm			Placebo/comparator arm		
	Total HIV infections	Cases of resistance	%	Total HIV infections	Cases of resistance	%
Fem-PrEP [13]	34	4	11.7	39	1	2.56
TDF2 [8]	10	1	10	26	1	3.85
VOICE (TDF-FTC arm) [14]	61	3	4.92			0
PROUD [9]	5	2	40	0	0	0

Promisingly, a succession of recent papers and conference abstracts report high levels of real-world adherence [22–24]. One open label intervention of daily PrEP found 80% of participants had protective plasma drug levels at 48 weeks [23], and an open label investigation of event-driven PrEP yielded detectable plasma drug levels in 71% of participants at 6 months [22]. However, Computer Assisted Structured Interviews determined that on-demand PrEP was only used at the correct dose in 50% of sexual intercourses. Whilst interviews may suffer from self-report and recall bias, one might expect adherence to be overestimated, rather than underestimated, due to social desirability bias. Although there is currently insufficient data to justly compare on-demand and daily regimens, this disparity should be noted for further investigation.

Reasons for non-adherence

The reasons reported for non-adherence (Fig. 3) are broad, reflecting the wide variety of populations and settings in which trials have been performed. Common qualitative reasons for poor adherence included participant low risk perception, side-effects, perceived stigma and dosing regimen incompatibility. These findings are consistent with reports from individual trials, which note that start-up side effects are frequent [6, 8] and may have influenced adherence. However, the Bangkok Tenofovir Study reported that nausea and vomiting were start-up symptoms which abated after the first couple of months [31]. However, of trials reporting dosing regimen as a reason for low adherence, three used a daily regimen and two used an on-demand regimen, implying limited acceptability regardless of daily or on-demand dosing regimen. However, comparatively little research has been performed using on-demand regimens, therefore further research is required to explore the differences in acceptability between daily and on-demand regimen. Recent modelling suggests weekly oral dosing with controlled release formulations may lead to improved adherence [41], implying that long-acting PrEP formulations may provide some solutions to poor acceptability of current dosing regimens.

Stigma

"Stigma remains the single most important barrier to public action [against HIV]", wrote ex-UN Secretary General Ban Kai-Moon in 2008 [42]. This statement is unfortunately still just as relevant in both low- and high-income settings, and has important implications for PrEP initiatives worldwide [43]. Qualitative investigation of PrEP trials has elicited both social and self-stigmatisation as instrumental challenges for participant adherence. Interviews with participants from the failed VOICE trial found that it was important for women from South Africa,

Zimbabwe and Uganda to be perceived as healthy by the community [44]. Taking medication associated with being HIV positive did not align with their narrative of health through self-stigmatisation, which may have detrimentally affected adherence. Furthermore, participants were understandably concerned that community misunderstanding regarding PrEP could cause friends and family to believe that they were HIV positive [45]. Some participants resorted to hiding the medication and pill bottles, however the conspicuous physical characteristics of the tablet were hard to explain. In the most severe cases, participants experienced extreme reactions from their close family, even resulting in spouse or partner separation [44, 45].

Risk perception and knowledge

Low risk perception is a common issue within PrEP trials. Despite adherence counselling, a large proportion of women (> 70%) from Kenya, Tanzania and South Africa reported themselves as at low or no risk of HIV in the failed FEM-PrEP trial [13]. Low risk perception was also a common reason for MSM declining PrEP in the United States PrEPARE trial [32], despite all eligible individuals belonging to a population at actual high risk. Reasons for low risk perception are unclear, although may relate to generally poor HIV education, which is often neglected in sex education [46–48]. PrEP will need to be delivered within a comprehensive package, including regular HIV awareness and PrEP adherence counselling if sufficient adherence for success is to be maintained.

Decision making power

PrEP is often prescribed to individuals who live in difficult circumstances. MSM, transgender, sex worker and PWID populations carry burdens of HIV disproportional to their size, and are at risk of being left behind in HIV prevention [49]. Stigma and criminalisation further marginalises these groups in many countries [3, 4]. The prospect of social ostracism and prosecution introduces further structural barriers to accessing healthcare services, reducing PrEP uptake and adherence. In a study of young MSM of colour in the USA, 39% had been kicked out of their home due to their sexual orientation and 43% had spent at least one night on the street [50]. These factors, combined with the prevalence of transactional sex, mean that young women and MSM, particularly transgender women, are often subject to abuse [5, 50] and frequently lack decision-making power over their bodies when it comes to sexual encounters [51]. These structural and social barriers, which reduce agency, can generate considerable difficulty in maintaining sufficient adherence to the dosing regimen and in accessing health services [3]. Despite this data previous trials within MSM populations have been surprisingly successful compared with young heterosexual women. This review cannot resolve this difference, but considering gender perspectives

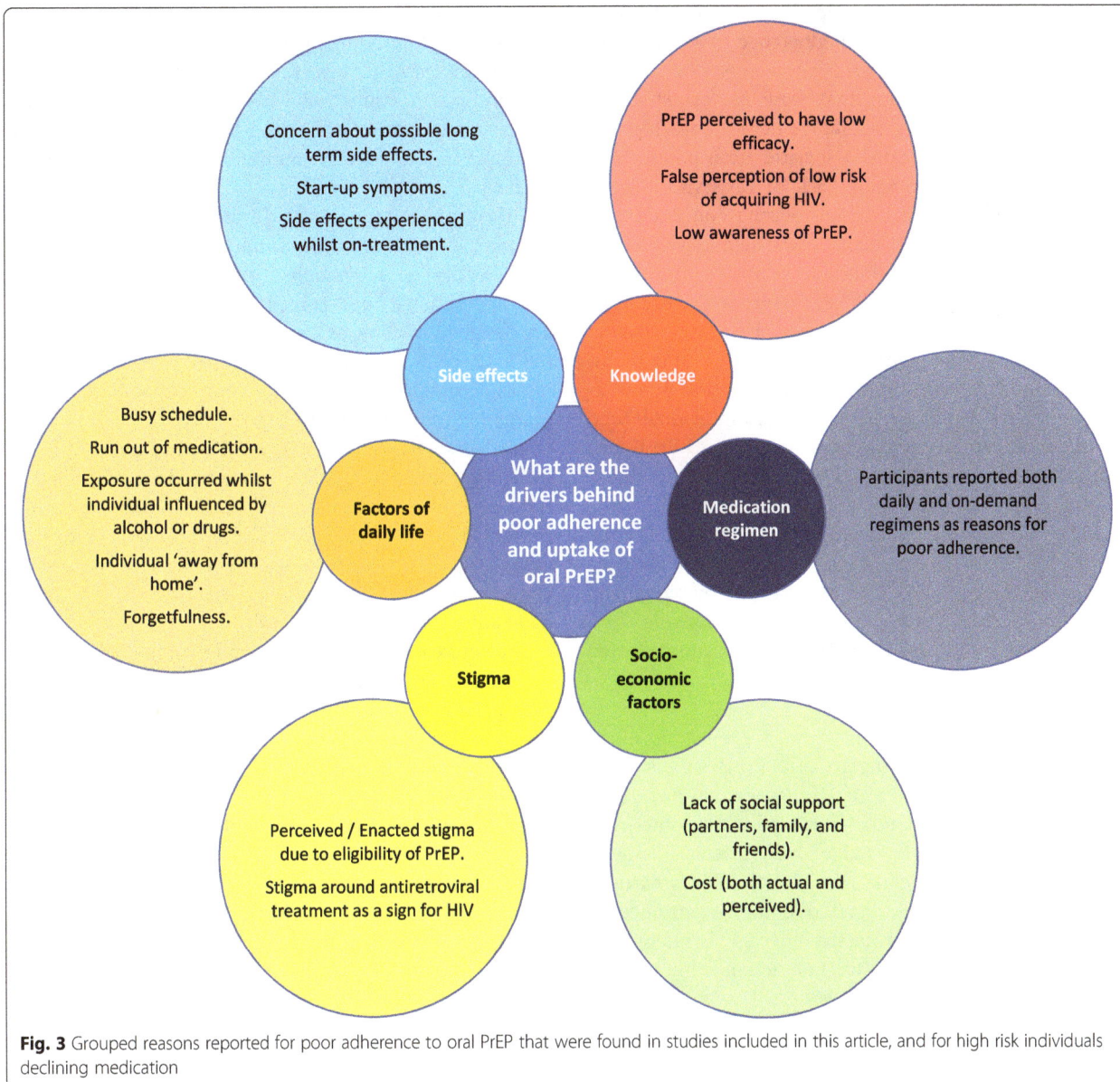

Fig. 3 Grouped reasons reported for poor adherence to oral PrEP that were found in studies included in this article, and for high risk individuals declining medication

within differing populations may offer some insight, particularly by considering the relation of cultural gender roles to decision-making power.

Drug resistance

With poor adherence a frequent issue in PrEP users, the question of drug resistance is of elevated concern. A full review of drug resistance in PrEP lies beyond this review, but most published RCTs report drug resistance as a rare outcome. Due to the rarity of resistance, it is also currently difficult to quantify the risk. However, it does appear to be more frequent among individuals receiving PrEP.

The infection of individuals between enrolment and randomisation [7, 9, 14], or missed diagnoses of pre-existing HIV infection [8], meant that these participants were likely exposed to high drug concentrations whilst in the acute phase of HIV infection. This was, however, very rare in the RCTs. As HIV serology assays that are often used cannot detect HIV infection during the acute phase, this remains a challenge for PrEP programmes in low income settings. HIV-RNA detection can be performed at enrolment to ensure that PrEP is not prescribed to any individual who recently acquired HIV, which may be cost effective and even cost-saving in higher prevalence populations [52]. Regardless, it is difficult to know whether mutations are due to prescribed medication, or due to previous exposure without healthcare worker consultation. We also note an MSM individual who was fully adherent to TDF-FTC PrEP was recently reported to have been infected with a resistant strain of HIV

[53]. This provided the first compelling evidence of break-through infection despite good adherence to oral PrEP by drug-resistant HIV-1.

From this data, it seems that PrEP is not associated with a large risk of drug-resistance developing. The low drug plasma concentrations associated with poor adherence appear to confer a low risk of resistance should HIV infection occur, whilst high plasma concentrations in adherent individuals make resistance development unlikely through successful inhibition of viral replication. However, with wide scale PrEP use around the corner, resistance may soon become a greater issue, especially in developing countries where follow-up and routine monitoring is more difficult. Furthermore, infection by resistant strains remains a rare possibility and individuals who are infected with HIV whilst truly adherent to PrEP may propagate resistant strains. Thorough disease history and clinical examination could help to detect acute phase HIV. When acute phase HIV is suspected, PrEP can be delayed to ensure a reliable negative HIV serology before initiation or HIV-RNA analysis can be performed in settings where this is available. Reasonable care should be taken to ensure participants are not infected with HIV prior to PrEP initiation.

Challenges in clinical practice

Current knowledge relating to oral PrEP suffers from knowledge gaps. There are few long-term studies relating to effectiveness and adherence, and while some trials report that adherence is stable over time [15], others suggest a long-term decline [17, 18, 54]. This is particularly important for oral PrEP due the importance of good adherence for its protective effect. It is often challenging to trace and maintain interaction with populations most at risk of HIV acquisition. This is critical for the success of PrEP due to the necessity of regular pill distribution and HIV/STI testing. To further complicate matters, a recent study in Bangkok found little association between participants *intending* to take PrEP and *actual* adherence at 1 month [55]. It is important to demonstrate that PrEP adherence can be maintained in key populations over time for it to be effective.

Effective methods of encouraging adherence are likely to be as varied as the populations themselves. Success was reported in a US community based programme [50] through four key strategies. First, PrEP was delivered as a key component within a comprehensive prevention package, from a place often visited by the population (e.g. young MSM). Secondly, high contact frequency (weekly) was maintained. Thirdly, the package promoted all aspects of a healthy lifestyle., and finally aimed to further empower individuals through optional weekly workshops focussing on life-skills. Linked with a comprehensive strategy, peer navigators, who aim to solve

individual barriers to PrEP, are being evaluated as an option to maintain adherence and retention [56]. One recent study (SPARK) also found high adherence rates at 3 months in conjunction with a comprehensive sexual health intervention, supporting the feasibility of incorporating PrEP adherence counselling into existing frameworks [57].

This promising model could feasibly be adapted for use in other populations. Multi-modal intervention models are effective in maintaining medication adherence for other conditions, but it is recommended that programmes are designed to allow evaluation of individual components [58]. There is already evidence that text messaging is highly acceptable and may improve retention in PrEP programs [59]. Smartphone penetration is also high in many countries, such as the UK where 91% of 18 to 34 year olds own a device [60], and Sub-Saharan Africa where penetrance is expected to exceed 50% by 2020 [61]. This could present an opportunity for innovative adherence solutions. Apps could be designed to display medication reminders, allow adherence self-reporting, and even to incentivise good adherence through reward.

The increasing online availability of generic PrEP, which is accessed and used by individuals without a doctor's prescription and without proper prior HIV screening, presents a real challenge. If the user cost of accessing PrEP on prescription exceeds the cost of purchasing generic versions online, then individuals are likely to take PrEP acquisition into their own hands. In France, the first and only European country to offer PrEP through public health services, over 60% of on-PrEP MSM access medication via their physician as opposed to less than 30% in other countries [62]. Correspondingly, less than 10% of on-PrEP French MSM access medication online as opposed to over 40% in other European countries [62]. Unmonitored PrEP usage could result in risk to users from adverse effects due to excessive dosing, and HIV infection due to insufficient dosing, whilst simultaneously accelerating the development of resistance if new infections are undiagnosed. It may also present a public health risk if high-risk individuals using unmonitored PrEP perceive themselves at lower risk of HIV, and subsequently do not attend HIV testing services as frequently. However, 31 European countries still identify cost of medication and service delivery as a major barrier to PrEP implementation, despite this unique opportunity to target HIV transmission in the most high-risk groups [62]. Despite this, recent modelling research in the UK suggests cost-effectiveness and long term cost-saving benefits across a wide range of PrEP introduction scenarios for the MSM population [63]. Cost savings depended on both the eligible population and the risk of HIV acquisition, so long term cost-effectiveness is likely to be even greater in locations with higher HIV prevalence. Notably, cost-effectiveness was highly time sensitive, suggesting that policy makers must consider PrEP over lifetimes, and not merely the political cycle.

Limitations

Despite best efforts to ensure a comprehensive search, there may be eligible studies that we failed to include. We made efforts to contact authors of soon to be released trials, but not all authors were contactable. Secondly, the conclusions we draw are only as good as the data provided. There is reason for concern over the use of pill counts and current electronic monitoring methods as measures of PrEP adherence due to the varying concordance with blood plasma drug concentrations. Furthermore, this review is limited to discussion of oral PrEP adherence in the context of efficacy. Long-term safety, cost effectiveness, HIV drug resistance and sexual behaviour trends are not evaluated or discussed in detail. Finally, whilst this paper discussed adherence in detail, it must be noted that adherence is just one step in the broader PrEP retention continuum [16].

Conclusions

Oral PrEP can be effective for the prevention of HIV. Some interventions have achieved high adherence and clinical effectiveness among MSM. However, further exploration of the biological and sociocultural reasons for poor adherence in other populations such as women is required. Cheap and accurate methods of long term adherence monitoring, such as urine testing, require development and validation. Interventions must be designed with user-appropriateness in mind, considering the sometimes unpredictable lives of at-risk individuals at the fringe of society in addition to those in the centre. Flexible medication delivery models and extended release PrEP formulations will likely play an important role in catering to these needs, and further research will be needed to design and prove these methods. Moreover, efforts should be taken to challenge the stigma, marginalisation and prosecution of minority groups, such as sex workers, PWID, and MSM, both within the community and at governmental level. Drug resistance to PrEP is still rare, but sufficient data to fully quantify the risk of resistance is likely to only be available once widespread use in lower income settings and at larger scale is achieved. Finally, the cost-issues for using preventive ARVs must be dealt with at national level in many countries.

Abbreviations

ART: Antiretroviral Therapy; ARV: Antiretroviral; CDC: Centres for Disease prevention and Control; FTC: Emtricitabine; MEMS: Medication Event Monitoring System; MSM: Men who have Sex with Men; PrEP: Pre-Exposure Prophylaxis; PWID: People Who Inject Drugs; RCT: Randomised Controlled Trial; RDBPCT: Randomised Double Blind Placebo Controlled Trial; TDF: Tenofovir disoproxil fumarate; TGW: Transgender Women; UN: United Nations; WHO: World Health Organisation

Acknowledgements

The authors thank the participants in the individual studies included in this systematic review for their contribution to evidence for PrEP.

Funding

DS provided support for this article in kind. AME was funded by Karolinska Institutet. SS was funded by Uppsala University. Funding institutions had no role in designing the review, the collection, analysis, or interpretation of the data, nor the writing of the manuscript.

Authors' contributions

All authors made significant contributions to the design of the review. DS and SS performed the systematic search. DS performed data extraction; DS, SS, and AME jointly performed analysis and interpretation. DS, SS and AME all contributed to writing the manuscript. All authors approved the manuscript and submission and agree to be accountable for the content.

Authors' information

Not applicable.

Competing interests

The authors declare that they have no competing interests.

Author details

[1]Department of Public Health Sciences, Karolinska Institutet, Stockholm, Sweden. [2]Department of Medical Sciences, Section of Infectious Diseases, Uppsala University, Uppsala, Sweden. [3]Department of Infectious Diseases, Karolinska University Hospital, Stockholm, Sweden.

References

1. UNAIDS. Global AIDS Update 2016. Geneva: UNAIDS; 2016.
2. Cohen MS, Chen YQ, McCauley M, Gamble T, Hosseinipour MC, Kumarasamy N, Hakim JG, Kumwenda J, Grinsztejn B, Pilotto JH, et al. Prevention of HIV-1 infection with early antiretroviral therapy. N Engl J Med. 2011;365(6):493–505.
3. Joint United Nations Programme on HIV/AIDS. Prevention Gap Report. Geneva: Joint United Nations Programme on HIV/AIDS; 2016.
4. Carroll A. State sponsored homophobia 2016: a world survey of sexual orientation laws: criminalisation, protection and recognition. 11th ed. Geneva: International Lesbian, Gay, Bisexual, Trans and Intersex Association; 2016.
5. Baral SD, Poteat T, Strömdahl S, Wirtz AL, Guadamuz TE, Beyrer C. Worldwide burden of HIV in transgender women: a systematic review and meta-analysis. Lancet Infect Dis. 2013;13(3):214–22.
6. Grant RM, Lama JR, Anderson PL, McMahan V, Liu AY, Vargas L, Goicochea P, Casapía M, Guanira-Carranza JV, Ramirez-Cardich ME, et al. Preexposure chemoprophylaxis for HIV prevention in men who have sex with men. N Engl J Med. 2010;363(27):2587–99.
7. Baeten JM, Donnell D, Ndase P, Mugo NR, Campbell JD, Wangisi J, Tappero JW, Bukusi EA, Cohen CR, Katabira E, et al. Antiretroviral prophylaxis for HIV prevention in heterosexual men and women. N Engl J Med. 2012;367(5): 399–410.
8. Thigpen MC, Kebaabetswe PM, Paxton LA, Smith DK, Rose CE, Segolodi TM, Henderson FL, Pathak SR, Soud FA, Chillag KL, et al. Antiretroviral preexposure prophylaxis for heterosexual HIV transmission in Botswana. N Engl J Med. 2012;367(5):423–34.
9. McCormack S, Dunn DT, Desai M, Dolling DI, Gafos M, Gilson R, Sullivan AK, Clarke A, Reeves I, Schembri G, et al. Pre-exposure prophylaxis to prevent the acquisition of HIV-1 infection (PROUD): effectiveness results from the pilot phase of a pragmatic open-label randomised trial. Lancet. 2016; 387(10013):53–60.
10. Molina JM, Capitant C, Spire B, Pialoux G, Cotte L, Charreau I, Tremblay C, Le Gall JM, Cua E, Pasquet A, et al. On-demand Preexposure prophylaxis in men at high risk for HIV-1 infection. N Engl J Med. 2015;373(23):2237–46.
11. Consolidated guidelines on the use of antiretroviral drugs for treating and preventing HIV infection. Recommendations for a public health approach. 2nd ed. France: World Health Organization; 2016.
12. Centers for Disease Control and Prevention. Preexposure Prophylaxis for the Prevention of HIV Infection in the United States - 2014 Clinical Practice Guideline. Atlanta: Centers for Disease Control and Prevention; 2014.

13. Van Damme L, Corneli A, Ahmed K, Agot K, Lombaard J, Kapiga S, Malahleha M, Owino F, Manongi R, Onyango J, et al. Preexposure prophylaxis for HIV infection among African women. N Engl J Med. 2012; 367(5):411–22.

14. Marrazzo JM, Ramjee G, Richardson BA, Gomez K, Mgodi N, Nair G, Palanee T, Nakabiito C, van der Straten A, Noguchi L, et al. Tenofovir-based preexposure prophylaxis for HIV infection among African women. N Engl J Med. 2015;372(6):509–18.

15. Grant RM, Anderson PL, McMahan V, Liu A, Amico KR, Mehrotra M, Hosek S, Mosquera C, Casapia M, Montoya O, et al. Uptake of pre-exposure prophylaxis, sexual practices, and HIV incidence in men and transgender women who have sex with men: a cohort study. Lancet Infect Dis. 2014; 14(9):820–9.

16. Nunn AS, Brinkley-Rubinstein L, Oldenburg CE, Mayer KH, Mimiaga M, Patel R, Chan PA. Defining the HIV pre-exposure prophylaxis care continuum. AIDS. 2017;31(5):731–4.

17. Haberer JE, Baeten JM, Campbell J, Wangisi J, Katabira E, Ronald A, Tumwesigye E, Psaros C, Safren SA, Ware NC, et al. Adherence to antiretroviral prophylaxis for HIV prevention: a substudy cohort within a clinical trial of serodiscordant couples in East Africa. PLoS Med. 2013;10(9):e1001511.

18. Baeten JM, Donnell D, Mugo NR, Ndase P, Thomas KK, Campbell JD, Wangisi J, Tappero JW, Bukusi EA, Cohen CR, et al. Single-agent tenofovir versus combination emtricitabine plus tenofovir for pre-exposure prophylaxis for HIV-1 acquisition: an update of data from a randomised, double-blind, phase 3 trial. *Lancet Infect Dis*. 2014;14(11):1055–64.

19. (CASP) CASP. Randomised Controlled Trials Checklist. Oxford: Critical Appraisal Skills Programme; 2013.

20. Patterson KB, Prince HA, Kraft E, Jenkins AJ, Shaheen NJ, Rooney JF, Cohen MS, Kashuba AD. Penetration of tenofovir and emtricitabine in mucosal tissues: implications for prevention of HIV-1 transmission. Sci Transl Med. 2011;3(112):112re114.

21. Anderson PL, Liu AY, Castillo-Mancilla JR, Gardner EM, Seifert SM, McHugh C, Wagner T, Campbell K, Morrow M, Ibrahim M, et al. Intracellular Tenofovir-diphosphate and Emtricitabine-triphosphate in dried blood spots following directly observed therapy. Antimicrob Agents Chemother. 2018;62(1):e01710–17.

22. Molina JM, Charreau I, Spire B, Cotte L, Chas J, Capitant C, Tremblay C, Rojas-Castro D, Cua E, Pasquet A, et al. Efficacy, safety, and effect on sexual behaviour of on-demand pre-exposure prophylaxis for HIV in men who have sex with men: an observational cohort study. Lancet HIV. 2017;4(9):e402–10.

23. Liu AY, Cohen SE, Vittinghoff E, Anderson PL, Doblecki-Lewis S, Bacon O, Chege W, Postle BS, Matheson T, Amico KR, et al. Preexposure prophylaxis for HIV infection integrated with municipal- and community-based sexual health services. JAMA Intern Med. 2016;176(1):75–84.

24. Marcus JL, Hurley LB, Hare CB, Nguyen DP, Phengrasamy T, Silverberg MJ, Stoltey JE, Volk JE. Preexposure prophylaxis for HIV prevention in a large integrated health care system: adherence, renal safety, and Discontinuation. J Acquir Immune Defic Syndr. 2016;73(5):540–6.

25. Lahuerta M, Zerbe A, Baggaley R, Falcao J, Ahoua L, DiMattei P, Morales F, Ramiro I, El-Sadr WM. Feasibility, acceptability and adherence with short term HIV pre-exposure prophylaxis in female sexual partners of migrant miners in Mozambique. J Acquir Immune Defic Syndr. 2017;76:343–7.

26. Balavoine S, Noret M, Loze B, Pintado C, Leplatois A, Charbonneau P, Moudachirou K, Djessima-Taba A, Niedbalski L, Siguier M, Aslan A, Ponscarme D, Penot P, Gatey C, Clavel F, Crémieux A-C, Lorho F, Dalle E, Parlier S, Delgado J, Veron R, Fonsart J, Delauerre C, Rozenbaum W, Molina JM. PrEP uptake, safety and efficacy in a hospital-based clinic in Paris. Paris: 9th AIS conference on HIV science. p. 2017.

27. Zablotska IV, S Bloch M, Carr A, Foster R, Grulich A, Guy R, McAllister JO, C Poynten M, Templton D. No HIV infections despite high-risk behaviour and STI incidence among gay/bisexual men taking daily pre-exposure prophylaxis (PrEP): the PRELUDE demonstration project. Paris: 9th AIS conference on HIV science. p. 2017.

28. Vaccher SM, M Grulich AE, Ooi C, Carr A, Haire BG, Sctdhmclz I. Very high adherence to HIV PrEP over one year confirmed by four measures in an open-label demonstration project (PRELUDE) in NSW, Australia. Paris: 9th IAS conference on HIV science. p. 2017.

29. Gafos MW, E White D, Clarke A, Apea V, Brodnicki E, Mackie NS, A Schembri G, Lacey C, Horne R, Dunn D, McCormack S. Adherence intentions, long-term adherence and HIV acquisition among PrEP users in the PROUD open-label randomised control trial of PrEP in England. Paris: 9th AIS conference on HIV science. p. 2017.

30. Gill KD, J Gray G, Pidwell T, Kayamba F, Bennie T, Myer L, Johnson LS, H Slack C, Elharrar V, Strode A, Rooney J, Bekker L. Pluspills: an open label, safety and feasibility study of oral pre-exposureprophylaxis (PrEP) in 15-19 year old adolescents in two sites in South Africa. Paris: 9th AIS conference on HIV science. p. 2017.

31. Choopanya K, Martin M, Suntharasamai P, Sangkum U, Mock P, Leethochawalit M, Chiamwongpaet S, Kitisin P, Natrujirote P, Kittimunkong S, et al. Antiretroviral prophylaxis for HIV infection in injecting drug users in Bangkok, Thailand (the Bangkok Tenofovir study): a randomised, double-blind, placebo-controlled phase 3 trial. Lancet. 2013;381(9883):2083–90.

32. King HL, Keller SB, Giancola MA, Rodriguez DA, Chau JJ, Young JA, Little SJ, Smith DM. Pre-exposure prophylaxis accessibility research and evaluation (PrEPARE study). AIDS Behav. 2014;18(9):1722–5.

33. Kesler MA, Kaul R, Myers T, Liu J, Loutfy M, Remis RS, Gesink D. Perceived HIV risk, actual sexual HIV risk and willingness to take pre-exposure prophylaxis among men who have sex with men in Toronto, Canada. AIDS Care. 2016;28(11):1–8.

34. Merchant RC, Corner D, Garza E, Guan W, Mayer KH, Brown L, Chan PA. Preferences for HIV pre-exposure prophylaxis (PrEP) information among men-who-have-sex-with-men (MSM) at community outreach settings. J Gay Lesbian Ment Health. 2016;20(1):21–33.

35. Kibengo FM, Ruzagira E, Katende D, Bwanika AN, Bahemuka U, Haberer JE, Bangsberg DR, Barin B, Rooney JF, Mark D, et al. Safety, adherence and acceptability of intermittent tenofovir/emtricitabine as HIV pre-exposure prophylaxis (PrEP) among HIV-uninfected Ugandan volunteers living in HIV-serodiscordant relationships: a randomized, clinical trial. PLoS One. 2013;8(9):e74314.

36. Bekker L-G, Hughes J, Amico R, Roux S, Hendrix C, Anderson PL, Dye B, Elharrar V, Sirratt MJ, Grant R. HPTN 067/ADAPT Cape Town: a comparison of daily and nondaily PrEP dosing in African women: Conference on retroviruses and opportunistic infections, Seattle. p. 2015.

37. Frankis J, Young I, Flowers P, McDaid L. Who will use pre-exposure prophylaxis (PrEP) and why?: understanding PrEP awareness and acceptability amongst men who have sex with men in the UK - a mixed methods study. PLoS One. 2016;11(4):e0151385.

38. Mutua G, Sanders E, Mugo P, Anzala O, Haberer JE, Bangsberg D, Barin B, Rooney JF, Mark D, Chetty P, et al. Safety and adherence to intermittent pre-exposure prophylaxis (PrEP) for HIV-1 in African men who have sex with men and female sex workers. PLoS One. 2012;7(4):e33103.

39. van de Wijgert J, McCormack S. Vaginal dysbiosis and pre-exposure prophylaxis efficacy. Lancet HIV. 2017;4(10):e427–9.

40. Heffron R, McClelland RS, Balkus JE, Celum C, Cohen CR, Mugo N, Bukusi E, Donnell D, Lingappa J, Kiarie J, et al. Efficacy of oral pre-exposure prophylaxis (PrEP) for HIV among women with abnormal vaginal microbiota: a post-hoc analysis of the randomised, placebo-controlled partners PrEP study. Lancet HIV. 2017;4(10):e449–56.

41. Selinger C, Kirtane A, Abouzid O, Langer R, Traverso CG, Bershteyn A. Anticipated adherence, efficacy, and impact of weekly oral preexposure prophylaxis: Conference on retroviruses and opportunistic infections, Seattle. p. 2017.

42. The Stigma Factor [http://www.washingtontimes.com/news/2008/aug/6/the-stigma-factor/].

43. Att leva med hiv i sverige. In. Järfälla: Folkhälsomyndigheten; 2016.

44. van der Straten A, Stadler J, Montgomery E, Hartmann M, Magazi B, Mathebula F, Schwartz K, Laborde N, Soto-Torres L. Women's experiences with oral and vaginal pre-exposure prophylaxis: the VOICE-C qualitative study in Johannesburg, South Africa. PLoS One. 2014;9(2):e89118.

45. Van der Elst EM, Mbogua J, Operario D, Mutua G, Kuo C, Mugo P, Kanungi J, Singh S, Haberer J, Priddy F, et al. High acceptability of HIV pre-exposure prophylaxis but challenges in adherence and use: qualitative insights from a phase I trial of intermittent and daily PrEP in at-risk populations in Kenya. AIDS Behav. 2013;17(6):2162–72.

46. Trust TH. Shh... No talking: LGBT-inclusive Sex and Relationships Education in the UK. London: Terrence Higgins Trust; 2016.

47. Scotland H. HIV and Education: Guaranteeing lessons for all. Edinburgh, Scotland: HIV Scotland; 2017.

48. Sex and HIV Education [https://www.guttmacher.org/state-policy/explore/sex-and-hiv-education].

49. UNAIDS. AIDS by the Numbers. Geneva: UNAIDS; 2016.

50. Daughtridge GW, Conyngham SC, Ramirez N, Koenig HC. I am men's health: generating adherence to HIV pre-exposure prophylaxis (PrEP) in young men of color who have sex with men. J Int Assoc Provid AIDS Care. 2015;14(2):103–7.

51. Hunter M. The materiality of everyday sex: thinking beyond 'prostitution'. Afr Stud. 2002;61(1):99–120.

52. Hoenigl M, Graff-Zivin J, Little SJ. Costs per diagnosis of acute HIV infection in community-based screening strategies: a comparative analysis of four screening algorithms. Clin Infect Dis. 2016;62(4):501–11.

53. Knox D, Tan D, Harrigan P, Anderson P. HIV-1 infection with multiclass resistance despite preexposure prophylaxis (PrEP). Boston: Conference on retroviruses and opportunistic infections. p. 2016.

54. Hosek SG, Siberry G, Bell M, Lally M, Kapogiannis B, Green K, Fernandez MI, Rutledge B, Martinez J, Garofalo R, et al. The acceptability and feasibility of an HIV preexposure prophylaxis (PrEP) trial with young men who have sex with men. J Acquir Immune Defic Syndr. 2013;62(4):447–56.

55. Anand T, Kerr SJ, Apornpong T, Nitpolpraset C, Ananworanich J, Phanuphak P, Phanuphak N. Self-perceived' pre-exposure prophylaxis adherence and its relationship to self-reported 'actual adherence' among Thai men who have sex with men and transgender women. Glasgow: HIV Drug Therapy Glasgow; 2016.

56. Macdonald V, Verster A, Baggaley R. A call for differentiated approaches to delivering HIV services to key populations. J Int AIDS Soc. 2017; 20(Suppl 4):21658.

57. Golub SA, Pena S, Hilley A, Pachankis J, Radix A. Brief behavioural intervention increases PrEP drug levels in a real-world setting: Conference on retroviruses and opportunistic infections, Seattle. p. 2017.

58. Marcus JL, Buisker T, Horvath T, Amico KR, Fuchs JD, Buchbinder SP, Grant RM, Liu AY. Helping our patients take HIV pre-exposure prophylaxis (PrEP): a systematic review of adherence interventions. HIV Med. 2014;15(7):385–95.

59. Khosropour CM, Lester RT, Golden MR, Dombrowski JC. Text messaging is associated with improved retention in a clinic-based PrEP program: Conference on retroviruses and opportunistic infections, Seattle. p. 2017.

60. Poushter J. Smartphone ownership and internet usage continues to climb in emerging economies. Pew Research Center: Washington; 2016.

61. The Mobile Economy. Africa 2016. London: GSM Association; 2016.

62. Evidence brief. Pre-exposure prophylaxis for the prevention of HIV in Europe. In: ECDC evidence brief. Stockholm: European Centre for Disease Prevention and Control. p. 2016.

63. Cambiano V, Miners A, Dunn D, McCormack S, Ong KJ, Gill ON, Nardone A, Desai M, Field N, Hart G, et al. Cost-effectiveness of pre-exposure prophylaxis for HIV prevention in men who have sex with men in the UK: a modelling study and health economic evaluation. Lancet Infect Dis. 2017;18:85–94.

64. Moher D, Liberati A, Tetzlaff J, Altman DG, Group P. Preferred reporting items for systematic reviews and meta-analyses: the PRISMA statement. BMJ. 2009;339:b2535.

65. Grinsztejn BH, B Moreira R, Kallas E, Madruga J, Leite I, de Boni R, Anderson P, Liu A, Luz P, Veloso V. High level of retention and adherence at week 48 for MSM and TGW enrolled in the PrEP Brasil demonstration study. Paris: 9th IAS conference on HIV science. p. 2017.

13

Rapid detection of respiratory organisms with the FilmArray respiratory panel in a large children's hospital in China

Jin Li[1†], Yue Tao[2†], Mingyu Tang[1†], Bailu Du[1], Yijun Xia[3], Xi Mo[2*] and Qing Cao[1*]

Abstract

Background: Respiratory tract infections (RTIs) are the most common illness in children, and rapid diagnosis is required for the optimal management of RTIs, especially severe infections.

Methods: Nasopharyngeal swab or sputum specimens were collected from children aged 19 days to 15 years who were admitted to a hospital in Shanghai and diagnosed with RTIs. The specimens were tested with the FilmArray Respiratory Panel, a multiplex PCR assay that detects 16 viruses, *Mycoplasma pneumoniae* (*M. pneumoniae*), *Bordetella pertussis* (*B. pertussis*) and *Chlamydophila pneumoniae* (*C. pneumoniae*).

Results: Among the 775 children studied, 626 (80.8%, 626/775) tested positive for at least one organism, and multiple organisms were detected in 198 (25.5%). Rhinoviruses/enteroviruses (25.5%, 198/775) were detected most often, followed by respiratory syncytial virus (19.5%, 151/775), parainfluenza virus 3 (14.8%, 115/775), influenza A or B (10.9%), adenovirus (10.8%), *M. pneumoniae* (10.6%) and *B. pertussis* (6.3%). The prevalence of organisms differed by age, and most of the viruses were more common in winter. Of the 140 children suspected of having pertussis, 35.0% (49/140) tested positive for *B. pertussis*.

Conclusions: FilmArray RP allows the rapid simultaneous detection of a wide number of respiratory organisms, with limited hands-on time, in Chinese pediatric patients with RTIs.

Keywords: Respiratory tract infections, FilmArray respiratory panel, Respiratory organisms, Children

Background

Acute respiratory tract infections (RTIs) are the leading causes of outpatient visits and hospitalizations in all age groups, especially during winter and spring. For children under 5 years of age, RTIs are the second leading cause of death [1]. Most acute RTIs in children are caused by respiratory viruses, such as respiratory syncytial virus (RSV), adenovirus (ADV), rhinovirus (RV) and influenza viruses. In addition to viruses, atypical pathogens are major causes of pediatric RTIs. One of the most common atypical pathogens is *Mycoplasma pneumoniae* (*M.*

pneumoniae), accounting for 10–40% of hospitalized children with community-acquired pneumonia [2, 3]. In addition to *M. pneumoniae*, the incidence of pertussis in China has significantly increased since 2010. Nevertheless, multiple epidemiological studies have suggested that the incidence of pertussis in China has been significantly underestimated [4, 5]. The early diagnosis of the pathogen is beneficial for the precise selection of medication, which can largely avoid the overuse or even abuse of the antibiotics and improve the clinical care of patients. More importantly, the early diagnosis of contagious pathogens, such as *Bordetella pertussis* (*B. pertussis*) and influenza viruses, can enable early isolation of patients, thus reducing the spread of pathogens.

At present, the routine detection methods for respiratory pathogens in China are mostly based on immunological methods, which include the detection of *M. pneumoniae* and several major viruses, such as RSV,

* Correspondence: moxi@scmc.com.cn; caoqing@scmc.com.cn
†Jin Li, Yue Tao and Mingyu Tang contributed equally to this work.
²The Laboratory of Pediatric Infectious Diseases, Pediatric Translational Medicine Institute, Shanghai Children's Medical Center, Shanghai Jiaotong University School of Medicine, Shanghai, China
¹Department of Infectious Diseases, Shanghai Children's Medical Center, Shanghai Jiaotong University School of Medicine, Shanghai, China
Full list of author information is available at the end of the article

ADV, RV, parainfluenza virus (Para), influenza A virus (FluA) and influenza B virus (FluB). Other respiratory viruses and atypical bacteria, such as *Chlamydophila pneumoniae* (*C. pneumoniae*) and *B. pertussis*, are typically not routinely detected. Given their poor sensitivity and long turn-around time (TAT), immunological methods usually lead to broad-spectrum therapy and have been gradually replaced by molecular-based methods, such as conventional and real-time polymerase chain reaction (PCR), in developed countries [6, 7]. However, most of these molecular tests are technically challenging and require independent spaces, such as pre-PCR and post-PCR rooms, to eliminate the potential risk of cross-contamination, and such requirement limits their applications in China. Therefore, faster, more sensitive and easy-to-use assays for multiplex respiratory pathogen detection are urgently needed.

FilmArray (BioFire Diagnostics, Utah, USA, owned by bioMérieux) is a small, desktop, fully automated multiplex PCR device. The molecular system includes automated nucleic acid extraction, an initial reverse transcription step and multiplex nested PCR, followed by a melting curve analysis [8]. The FilmArray Respiratory Panel (FilmArray RP) is both FDA-approved and CE IVD-marked. The current version of FilmArray RP (v1.7) is able to detect 16 viral and 3 atypical respiratory organisms. The test is performed in a closed system that requires 5 min of hands-on time and 65 min of instrumentation time. Several comparison studies between FilmArray and other tests for respiratory organisms showed comparable results [9–11].

The aim of this study was to evaluate the application of FilmArray RP for the detection of respiratory organisms, and to provide information about the seasonality and prevalence of these organisms in pediatric patients with RTIs in a large children's hospital in China.

Methods
Subjects and specimens
The study population was enrolled according to protocol definitions and inclusion criteria. Patients with respiratory infections, with or without fever (defined as body temperature ≥ 37.5 °C), were included if they had at least one of the following symptoms: (1) cough; (2) nasal obstruction; (3) tachypnoea; (4) nasal flaring; or (5) hypoxia. Patients admitted to the hospital had at least one of the following conditions: (1) unabating high fever; (2) dyspnea, tachypnea or hypoxemia; (3) anorexia or dehydration; (4) radiological confirmation of lung infection; or (5) respiratory infection with underlying diseases, such as congenital heart disease, bronchopulmonary dysplasia, airway malformations, severe malnutrition.

According to the Chinese Center for Disease Control and Prevention (CDC), patients suspected of having pertussis should have a cough for more than 2 weeks and have at least one of the following symptoms: (1) paroxysmal cough; (2) inspiratory whoop; or (3) post-tussive vomiting. In the present study, patients suspected of having pertussis were diagnosed with pertussis when *B. pertussis* was positive by FilmArray RP detection and were otherwise diagnosed with pertussis-like syndrome.

Nasopharyngeal swab (NPS) or sputum specimens were obtained from patients with symptoms of RTIs on the day of hospitalization at Shanghai Children's Medical Center (SCMC) from December 1, 2016 to November 30, 2017. Demographic data and clinical features, as well as laboratory test and imaging results, were obtained for each enrolled patient. The study was approved by the Institutional Review Board and the Ethics Committee of Shanghai Children's Medical Center (SCMCIRB-K2017044), and written informed consent was obtained from the parents of each patient.

FilmArray RP v1.7 testing
The FilmArray RP v1.7 targets 19 organisms, including ADV, influenza A viruses H1, 2009H1, H3 (FluA-H1, FluA-2009H1, FluA-H3) and FluB, parainfluenza virus types 1 to 4 (Para 1–4), coronaviruses 229E, HKU1, OC43, and NL63 (Cov-HKU1, NL63, 229E, OC43), human metapneumovirus (hMPV), RSV, human rhinovirus/enterovirus (Rhino/Entero), *C. pneumoniae*, *M. pneumoniae* and *B. pertussis*. The FilmArray RP assay was performed according to the manufacturer's instructions. The principle of the assay has been previously described [8, 12]. Each pouch included internal run controls for every step, and results for the assay were only provided by the software if the quality control reactions showed appropriate results.

Statistical analysis
SPSS software package v21.0 was used for all statistical analyses. Categorical variables were expressed as frequencies and percentages. The chi-square and Fisher's exact tests were used to compare groups. Continuous variables are expressed as the mean and standard deviation. Student's *t*-test was used to assess the statistical significance between groups. $p < 0.05$ was considered to be statistically significant.

Results
Clinical characteristics of patients
A total of 775 patients diagnosed with upper or lower respiratory tract infections, aged 19 days to 15 years, were enrolled in the present study between December 1, 2016, and November 30, 2017. Congenital heart disease, congenital biliary atresia, malignancy and congenital immunodeficiency were the most frequently observed underlying

diseases in these patients and contributed to 50% of the deaths observed in this study. The general characteristics of the patients enrolled are presented in Table 1.

Overall detection rate of FilmArray RP v1.7

Among the 775 specimens, 428 (55.2%, 428/775) had a single organism, 198 (25.5%, 198/775) had multiple organisms, and 149 (19.2%, 149/775) had no organism. The overall positive rate of the specimens was 80.8% (626/775). Rhino/Entero was the most prevalent organism (25.5%, 198/775), followed by RSV (19.5%, 151/775) and Para 3 (14.8%, 115/775). The positivity rates of other organisms were as follows: ADV, 10.8% (84/775); *M. pneumoniae*, 10.6% (82/775); *B. pertussis*, 6.3% (49/775); FluA, 6.1% (47/775); FluB, 4.8% (37/775); hMPV, 4.8% (37/775); CoV, 4.3% (33/775); Para 1, 3.2% (25/775); Para

4, 1.3% (10/775); Para 2, 0.4% (3/775); and *C. pneumoniae*, 0.1% (1/775).

Analysis of the positive rates and prevalence in different age groups

All the patients were grouped by age as follows: infants (age: < 1 year), toddlers (age: 1–2 years), preschoolers (age: 3–5 years) and school-aged children (age: 6–15 years) (Table 2). The highest specimen positivity rate, at 82.2% (278/338), was in the < 1-year age group, followed by 80.5% (149/185), 80.1% (117/146) and 77.4% (82/106) in the 1–2-year, 3–5-year and 6–15-year groups, respectively. There were no significant differences in the positivity rate of the different age groups. In contrast, the prevalence of organisms were different between the different age groups (Table 2). Rhino/Entero, Para 3, RSV and *B. pertussis* showed the highest prevalence in the < 1-year age group, while ADV, hMPV and FluA showed the highest prevalence in the 3–5-year age group. The most prevalent organism in the 6–15-year age group was *M. pneumoniae*. No organism showed a notably high prevalence in the 1–2-year age group. There was only one *C. pneumoniae*-positive patient during the study period, and this patient was in the 3–5-year age group.

Analysis of specimens detected with multiple organisms

Among the 775 specimens, 198 (25.5%, 198/775) were positive for more than one organism. The largest proportion (49.0%, 97/198) of multi-organism-positive specimens had combinations with Rhino/Entero. Rhino/Entero plus Para 3 was the most common combination, making up 10.6% (21/198) of all multi-organism-positive specimens, while the combination of Rhino/Entero plus ADV was the second most common type (6.1%, 12/198), followed by Rhino/Entero plus RSV (5.6%, 11/198). The multi-organism combinations are listed in Additional file 1: Table S1.

Seasonal prevalence of respiratory organisms from December 1, 2016 to November 30, 2017

The number of positive specimens was determined during different months of the year to demonstrate the epidemiology of the respiratory organisms. Regarding the atypical bacteria, *M. pneumoniae* was detected throughout the year, with the highest incidence occurring in September and three minor peaks in December, January and June (Fig. 1a). The highest incidences of *B. pertussis* were observed in March and May. Only one case of *C. pneumoniae* was detected in July.

The seasonal prevalence of viruses with high detection rates were as follows. Both FluA and hMPV had two peaks that occurred in January and March, and ADV showed a peak in January (Fig. 1b). The prevalence of Para 3 remained high from February–August. The peaks

Table 1 General characteristics of the patients

Characteristic	Value for patients
Total	775
Age, No. (%)	
< 1 year	338 (43.6)
1–2 years	185 (23.9)
3–5 years	146 (18.9)
6–15 years	106 (13.7)
Sex, No. (%)	
Male	430 (55.5)
Female	345 (44.5)
Clinical diagnosis, No. (%)	
URI	50 (6.5)
LRI	725 (93.5)
Underlying diseases, No. (%)	
None	538 (69.4)
CHD	148 (19.1)
Congenital biliary atresia	25 (3.2)
Malignancy	19 (2.5)
Congenital immunodeficiency	6 (0.8)
Other diseases	39 (5.0)
Prognosis after treat, No. (%)	
Alive	731 (94.3)
Death[b]	12 (1.5)
Unknown[c]	32 (4.1)

[a]Abbreviations: *URI* Upper respiratory tract infection; *LRI* Lower respiratory tract infection; *CHD* Congenital heart disease
[b]Most of the children died from underlying diseases, including malignancy, congenital heart disease, Niemann-Pick Disease, etc.
[c]Including the patients who transfer to other hospitals for treatment or abandon treatment. Upon follow-up by phone, 7 patients showed clinical improvement after transfer to other hospitals, 11 patients died after giving up treatment and discharged from our hospital, and 14 patients cannot be contacted and their prognosis were finally unknown

Table 2 Prevalence of respiratory organisms tested in different age groups

Analyte	< 1 year		1-2 years		3-5 years		6-15 years		χ^2	p
	No. Pos	Prevalence (n = 338)	No. Pos	Prevalence (n = 185)	No. Pos	Prevalence (n = 146)	No. Pos	Prevalence (n = 106)		
ADV	17	5.0%	29	15.7%	27	18.5%	11	10.4%	25.157	0.000
CoV total	21	6.2%	7	3.8%	2	1.4%	3	2.8%	6.788	0.079
229E	4	1.2%	1	0.5%	0	0%	2	1.9%	2.750	0.339
HKU1	6	1.8%	1	0.5%	1	0.7%	1	0.9%	1.542	0.696
OC43	11	3.3%	5	2.7%	1	0.7%	0	0%	5.548	0.117
hMPV	9	2.7%	12	6.5%	14	9.6%	1	0.9%	15.751	0.001
Rhino/Entero	101	29.9%	48	25.9%	27	18.5%	22	20.8%	8.453	0.038
FluA total	12	3.6%	13	7.0%	15	10.3%	7	6.6%	8.647	0.034
H3	10	3.0%	11	5.9%	11	7.5%	7	6.6%	5.825	0.120
2009 H1	2	0.6%	2	1.1%	4	2.7%	0	0%	4.550	0.134
FluB	2	0.6%	8	4.3%	15	10.3%	12	11.3%	32.794	0.000
Para total	94	27.8%	36	19.5%	20	13.7%	4	3.8%	34.146	0.000
1	9	2.7%	8	4.3%	8	5.5%	1	0.9%	4.842	0.176
2	0	0%	1	0.5%	1	0.7%	1	0.9%	3.714	0.203
3	81	24.0%	24	13.0%	8	5.5%	2	1.9%	46.976	0.000
4	4	1.2%	3	1.6%	3	2.1%	0	0%	2.095	0.559
RSV	105	31.1%	32	17.3%	11	7.5%	3	2.8%	61.491	0.000
B. pertussis	45	13.3%	2	1.1%	1	0.7%	1	0.9%	49.486	0.000
C. pneumoniae	0	0%	0	0%	1	0.7%	0	0%	3.750	0.325
M. pneumoniae	16	4.7%	16	8.6%	17	11.6%	33	31.1%	60.438	0.000
Total	278	82.2%	149	80.5%	117	80.1%	82	77.4%	1.314	0.726

in RSV cases occurred in both the fall and the winter months. The number of Rhino/Entero cases was relatively high throughout the year regardless of season.

The detection rates for the NPS and sputum samples

Among the 775 patients in our study, NPS samples were collected from 662 (85.4%). Among the other 113 (14.6%) patients, 88 used ventilators, 13 were hypoxic, and 12 were cyanotic after spasmodic coughing or crying, preventing NPS samples from being obtained from these patients; instead, sputum samples were collected and sent for FilmArray RP detection. The positivity rates of the NPS and sputum samples were 83.5% (553/662) and 64.6% (73/113), respectively. Detailed organism information on the two sample types collected from the different age groups is provided in Additional file 2: Tables S2 and S3.

Respiratory organisms detected in patients with suspected pertussis

According to the government policy, all cases of positive pertussis have to be reported to CDC. Because no routine examination could distinguish the patients with pertussis from those with pertussis-like syndrome, we paid special attention to the 140 patients who were clinically diagnosed with suspected pertussis in the present study. Among these patients, 95.0% (133/140) were positive for at least one organism by FilmArray RP, with 50.0% (70/140) and 45.0% (63/140) having single and multiple organisms detected, respectively. Detailed information on the organisms detected is presented in Fig. 2. 49 in the 140 patients (35%) were detected pertussis positive, among whom 42 (85.7%) were under 6 months, and 25 (71.4%) were co-detected with at least one virus.

Discussion

In our study, 775 specimens were collected from pediatric patients with RTIs over a period of one year and analyzed with FilmArray RP v1.7. The overall results yielded a positivity rate of 80.8%, with multiple organisms detected in 25.5% of specimens, which is in accordance with Litwin and Piralla's reports [13, 14]. As in other studies, a notable variation in the pathogen prevalence with season and age was observed. Most viruses had their highest positivity rates in winter, except that Para 3 positivity rate was well distributed through the spring and summer, and the epidemiologic peaks for hMPV occurred 1 to 2 months later than those for RSV

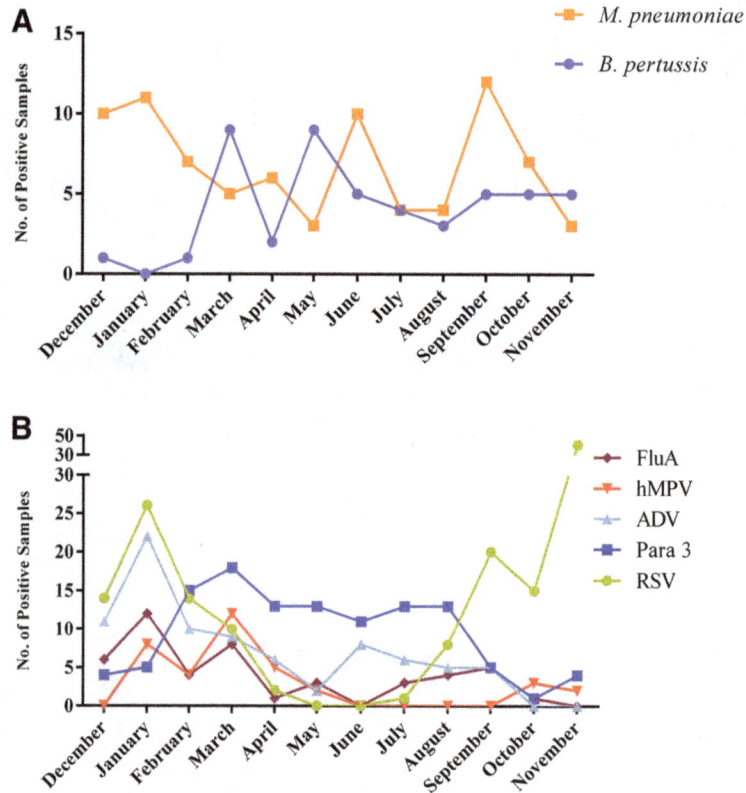

Fig. 1 Seasonal distribution of respiratory organisms detected by FilmArray RP. **a** Monthly prevalence of *B. pertussis* and *M. pneumoniae*. **b** Monthly prevalence of FluA, hMPV, ADV, Para 3 and RSV

[15, 16]. The majority of respiratory viruses were observed in children younger than 5 years old. Notably, RSV was the most prevalent virus in the < 1-year age group, and the prevalence decreased with age; while the incidence of *M. pneumoniae* increased with age [17].

Multiple respiratory organisms were detected in 25.5% of the specimens in our study, the largest proportion of which included Rhino/Entero. Other studies in adults reported lower multi-pathogen detection rates of approximately 8.7–

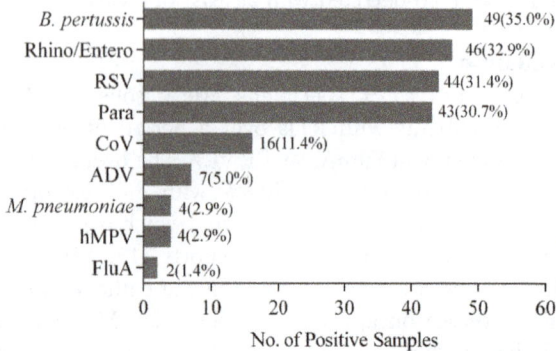

Fig. 2 Detection of respiratory organisms in 140 children suspected with pertussis. 35% (49/140) of the children were tested positive for *B. pertussis* with FilmArray RP

15.9% [14, 18–20], suggesting that pediatric patients with RTIs are more likely to be infected by multiple pathogens than adults. However, the clinical significance, including disease severity and hospitalization time, of multi-pathogen infection, especially Rhino/Entero combination infections, is not clear. A previous report indicated that dual-positive results with RSV and Rhino/Entero specimens might be due to viral shedding from a previous Rhino/Entero infection [21]. Nokso-Koivisto et al. also found that rhinovirus was the most prevalent virus in asymptomatic carriers [22].

The most unexpected result in our study is the high detection rate of *B. pertussis*, with an overall detection rate of 6.32% in the group of 775 patients, further demonstrating the value of FilmArray RP in clinical application. At present, the diagnosis of pertussis in China is based on culture and serology results. However, both the CDC and World Health Organization (WHO) use positive PCR results as the criteria for diagnosis, suggesting that FilmArray RP testing, in addition to culture, can be considered for patients with suspected pertussis in order to better monitor disease outbreaks. Additionally, the early diagnosis of patients with *B. pertussis*, which is typically difficult to distinguish from pertussis-like syndrome, can also help to reduce unnecessary macrolide treatment. The limitation of the panel is the lack of *B.*

parapertussis, which contributes to more than 5% of pertussis cases [23]. However, it has been added to the second-generation panel, FilmArray RP2 v1.1 [24], and the prevalence of *B. parapertussis* in our patients is currently under investigation.

As stated in the manufacturer's instructions, "FilmArray Respiratory Panel (RP) is a multiplexed nucleic acid test intended for use with FilmArray systems for the simultaneous qualitative detection and identification of multiple respiratory viral and bacterial nucleic acids in nasopharyngeal swabs (NPS) obtained from individuals suspected of respiratory tract infections". Therefore, NPS samples are recommended for FilmArray RP, but there are also studies demonstrating a comparable or even higher detection rate in sputum [25, 26]. However, the detection rate in sputum in our study was lower than that in NPS samples. This might partially be attributed to the fact that most of the sputum samples (86.7%, 98/113) were from ICU patients, and the sputum-providing patients showed a higher positivity rate in their sputum culture than the NPS-providing patients (33.6% vs 20.5%). In addition to sputum, bronchoalveolar lavage fluid (BALF) is a common type of respiratory sample, and Azadah et al. showed that detection in BALF by FilmArray RP can provide new and useful microbiological information within 7 days after a negative NPS result is obtained [27]. Therefore, the choice of the most appropriate sample type and time-point for each patient, particularly in specific clinical contexts, such as undergoing fiberoptic bronchoscopy or ventilator use, may require further investigation.

As with other molecular methods, distinguishing whether the microbes detected in the FilmArray analysis, especially those that are also detected in asymptomatic children, such as human rhinovirus, are causative pathogens or colonizers is not feasible [28–30]. Therefore, the clinicians should take caution when judging pathogens because the results are sometimes "false positive". On the other hand, despite the high detection rate of FilmArray RP, a negative result does not mean the patient is not infected; moreover, a positive result does not mean there is no other co-infecting agent, especially in critically ill patients, in whom a bacterial co-infection often occurs. For this "false-negative" limitation, BioFire has a new pneumonia panel that also targets BALF/sputum and covers 9 common viruses, as well as 15 bacteria, including *Klebsiella pneumonia*, *Haemophilus influenza*, *Streptococcus pneumonia* and *Staphylococcus aureus*. Nevertheless, the FilmArray panel only aims to rapidly provide results for potential pathogens as a reference. A more appropriate method is to comprehensively consider the results from other examinations, such as routine blood testing, C-reactive protein (CRP), procalcitonin (PCT), the erythrocyte sedimentation rate (ESR), culture and radiography, as well as the patients' symptoms, including body temperature, breathing, blood oxygen, heart rate, and mental condition.

Our study also has several limitations. First, our study was performed in a single center and may not be representative of the entire Chinese pediatric population. Second, we did not have data from a more appropriate assay to evaluate the specificity of FilmArray RP. Additionally, we do not provide detailed information on the effects of FilmArray RP on the use of antibiotics, clinical outcomes and health economics, which require further investigation.

Conclusion

In conclusion, the FilmArray RP assay significantly expands our ability to diagnose multiple respiratory infections caused by viruses and atypical bacteria. The array can detect 19 respiratory organisms simultaneously, with a high detection rate, in 65 min. Our study provided the age groups and seasonal distributions of different organisms for pediatric RTI patients. This study also provides new insights into the current status of pertussis infection in China. Whether FilmArray RP can enhance clinical decision-making and limit the unnecessary use of antibiotics in China as in other countries still requires further investigation.

Abbreviations
ADV: Adenovirus; *B. pertussis*: *Bordetella pertussis*; *C. pneumoniae*: *Chlamydophila pneumoniae*; CAP: Community-acquired pneumonia; CoV: Coronaviruses; FilmArray RP: FilmArray Respiratory Panel; FluA: Influenza A viruses; FluB: Influenza B viruses; hMPV: Human metapneumovirus; *M. pneumoniae*: *Mycoplasma pneumoniae*; NPS: Nasopharyngeal swab; Para: Parainfluenza virus; PCR: Polymerase chain reaction; Rhino/Entero: Human rhinovirus/enterovirus; RITs: Respiratory tract infections; RSV: Respiratory syncytial virus; SCMC: Shanghai Children's Medical Center

Acknowledgements
We would like to thank the patients and their parents for the support and cooperation in publishing this work.

Funding
This work was financially supported by the Key Developing Disciplines Project from Shanghai Municipal Commission of Health and Family Planning (2016ZB0104), the Collaborative Innovation Center for Translational Medicine at Shanghai Jiaotong University School of Medicine (TM201616), and the Love Charity Foundation Research Project in Shanghai Children's Medical Center (2017SCMC-AY004).

Authors' contributions
QC and XM initiated the study. JL, YT, MYT and BLD performed the detection of respiratory organisms. JL, YT, MYT, QC and XM wrote the manuscript and analyzed the data. YJX provided technical support and assisted in the data analysis. All authors read and approved the final manuscript.

Competing interests
Yijun Xia is an employee of bioMérieux. He was involved in the technical support and data analysis. All the other authors declare they have no conflict of interests to disclose. All the other authors declare that they have no competing interests.

Author details
[1]Department of Infectious Diseases, Shanghai Children's Medical Center, Shanghai Jiaotong University School of Medicine, Shanghai, China. [2]The Laboratory of Pediatric Infectious Diseases, Pediatric Translational Medicine Institute, Shanghai Children's Medical Center, Shanghai Jiaotong University School of Medicine, Shanghai, China. [3]Medical Affairs, Great China | bioMérieux (Shanghai) Company, Limited, Shanghai, China.

References

1. Monto AS. Epidemiology of viral respiratory infections. Am J Med. 2002; 112(Suppl 6A):4S–12S.

2. Jain S, Williams DJ, Arnold SR, Ampofo K, Bramley AM, Reed C, Stockmann C, Anderson EJ, Grijalva CG, Self WH, et al. Community-acquired pneumonia requiring hospitalization among U.S. children. N Engl J Med. 2015;372(9): 835–45.

3. Liu WK, Liu Q, Chen DH, Liang HX, Chen XK, Chen MX, Qiu SY, Yang ZY, Zhou R. Epidemiology of acute respiratory infections in children in Guangzhou: a three-year study. PLoS One. 2014;9(5):e96674.

4. Xu Y, Wang L, Xu J, Wang X, Wei C, Luo P, Ma X, Hou Q, Wang J. Seroprevalence of pertussis in China: need to improve vaccination strategies. Hum Vaccin Immunother. 2014;10(1):192–8.

5. Zhang Q, Zheng H, Liu M, Han K, Shu J, Wu C, Xu N, He Q, Luo H. The seroepidemiology of immunoglobulin G antibodies against pertussis toxin in China: a cross sectional study. BMC Infect Dis. 2012;12:138.

6. Brendish NJ, Malachira AK, Armstrong L, Houghton R, Aitken S, Nyimbili E, Ewings S, Lillie PJ, Clark TW. Routine molecular point-of-care testing for respiratory viruses in adults presenting to hospital with acute respiratory illness (ResPOC): a pragmatic, open-label, randomised controlled trial. Lancet Respir Med. 2017;5(5):401–11.

7. Caliendo AM. Multiplex PCR and emerging technologies for the detection of respiratory pathogens. Clin Infect Dis. 2011;52(Suppl 4):S326–30.

8. Poritz MA, Blaschke AJ, Byington CL, Meyers L, Nilsson K, Jones DE, Thatcher SA, Robbins T, Lingenfelter B, Amiott E, et al. FilmArray, an automated nested multiplex PCR system for multi-pathogen detection: development and application to respiratory tract infection. PLoS One. 2011;6(10):e26047.

9. Wahrenbrock MG, Matushek S, Boonlayangoor S, Tesic V, Beavis KG, Charnot-Katsikas A. Comparison of Cepheid Xpert flu/RSV XC and BioFire FilmArray for detection of influenza a, influenza B, and respiratory syncytial virus. J Clin Microbiol. 2016;54(7):1902–3.

10. Andersson ME, Olofsson S, Lindh M. Comparison of the FilmArray assay and in-house real-time PCR for detection of respiratory infection. Scand J Infect Dis. 2014;46(12):897–901.

11. Renaud C, Crowley J, Jerome KR, Kuypers J. Comparison of FilmArray respiratory panel and laboratory-developed real-time reverse transcription-polymerase chain reaction assays for respiratory virus detection. Diagn Microbiol Infect Dis. 2012;74(4):379–83.

12. Loeffelholz MJ, Pong DL, Pyles RB, Xiong Y, Miller AL, Bufton KK, Chonmaitree T. Comparison of the FilmArray respiratory panel and Prodesse real-time PCR assays for detection of respiratory pathogens. J Clin Microbiol. 2011;49(12):4083–8.

13. Piralla A, Lunghi G, Percivalle E, Vigano C, Nasta T, Pugni L, Mosca F, Stronati M, Torresani E, Baldanti F. FilmArray(R) respiratory panel performance in respiratory samples from neonatal care units. Diagn Microbiol Infect Dis. 2014;79(2):183–6.

14. Litwin CM, Bosley JG. Seasonality and prevalence of respiratory pathogens detected by multiplex PCR at a tertiary care medical center. Arch Virol. 2014; 159(1):65–72.

15. Aberle JH, Aberle SW, Redlberger-Fritz M, Sandhofer MJ, Popow-Kraupp T. Human metapneumovirus subgroup changes and seasonality during epidemics. Pediatr Infect Dis J. 2010;29(11):1016–8.

16. Madhi SA, Ludewick H, Kuwanda L, van Niekerk N, Cutland C, Klugman KP. Seasonality, incidence, and repeat human metapneumovirus lower respiratory tract infections in an area with a high prevalence of human immunodeficiency virus type-1 infection. Pediatr Infect Dis J. 2007;26(8):693–9.

17. Jiang W, Wu M, Zhou J, Wang Y, Hao C, Ji W, Zhang X, Gu W, Shao X. Etiologic spectrum and occurrence of coinfections in children hospitalized with community-acquired pneumonia. BMC Infect Dis. 2017;17(1):787.

18. Bierbaum S, Konigsfeld N, Besazza N, Blessing K, Rucker G, Kontny U, Berner R, Schumacher M, Forster J, Falcone V, et al. Performance of a novel microarray multiplex PCR for the detection of 23 respiratory pathogens (SYMP-ARI study). Eur J Clin Microbiol Infect Dis. 2012;31(10):2851–61.

19. Olofsson S, Brittain-Long R, Andersson LM, Westin J, Lindh M. PCR for detection of respiratory viruses: seasonal variations of virus infections. Expert Rev Anti-Infect Ther. 2011;9(8):615–26.

20. Mahony JB. Detection of respiratory viruses by molecular methods. Clin Microbiol Rev. 2008;21(4):716–47.

21. Brittain-Long R, Westin J, Olofsson S, Lindh M, Andersson LM. Prospective evaluation of a novel multiplex real-time PCR assay for detection of fifteen respiratory pathogens-duration of symptoms significantly affects detection rate. J Clin Virol. 2010;47(3):263–7.

22. Nokso-Koivisto J, Kinnari TJ, Lindahl P, Hovi T, Pitkaranta A. Human picornavirus and coronavirus RNA in nasopharynx of children without concurrent respiratory symptoms. J Med Virol. 2002;66(3):417–20.

23. Hong JY. Update on pertussis and pertussis immunization. Korean J Pediatr. 2010;53(5):629–33.

24. Leber AL, Everhart K, Daly JA, Hopper A, Harrington A, Schreckenberger P, McKinley K, Jones M, Holmberg K, Kensinger B. Multicenter evaluation of BioFire FilmArray respiratory panel 2 for detection of viruses and Bacteria in nasopharyngeal swab samples. J Clin Microbiol. 2018;56(6):e01945–17.

25. Branche AR, Walsh EE, Formica MA, Falsey AR. Detection of respiratory viruses in sputum from adults by use of automated multiplex PCR. J Clin Microbiol. 2014;52(10):3590–6.

26. Doern CD, Lacey D, Huang R, Haag C. Evaluation and implementation of FilmArray version 1.7 for improved detection of adenovirus respiratory tract infection. J Clin Microbiol. 2013;51(12):4036–9.

27. Azadeh N, Sakata KK, Brighton AM, Vikram HR, Grys TE. FilmArray respiratory panel assay: comparison of nasopharyngeal swabs and Bronchoalveolar lavage samples. J Clin Microbiol. 2015;53(12):3784–7.

28. Self WH, Williams DJ, Zhu Y, Ampofo K, Pavia AT, Chappell JD, Hymas WC, Stockmann C, Bramley AM, Schneider E, et al. Respiratory viral detection in children and adults: comparing asymptomatic controls and patients with community-acquired pneumonia. J Infect Dis. 2016;213(4):584–91.

29. Korten I, Mika M, Klenja S, Kieninger E, Mack I, Barbani MT, Gorgievski M, Frey U, Hilty M, Latzin P. Interactions of respiratory viruses and the nasal microbiota during the first year of life in healthy infants. mSphere. 2016;1(6): e00312-16.

30. Shann F. Etiology of severe pneumonia in children in developing countries. Pediatr Infect Dis. 1986;5(2):247–52.

14

Genetic characterization of norovirus GII.4 variants circulating in Canada using a metagenomic technique

Nicholas Petronella[1], Jennifer Ronholm[2,3], Menka Suresh[4], Jennifer Harlow[4], Oksana Mykytczuk[4], Nathalie Corneau[4], Sabah Bidawid[4] and Neda Nasheri[4]* (iD)

Abstract

Background: Human norovirus is the leading cause of viral gastroenteritis globally, and the GII.4 has been the most predominant genotype for decades. This genotype has numerous variants that have caused repeated epidemics worldwide. However, the molecular evolutionary signatures among the GII.4 variants have not been elucidated throughout the viral genome.

Method: A metagenomic, next-generation sequencing method, based on Illumina RNA-Seq, was applied to determine norovirus sequences from clinical samples.

Results: Herein, the obtained deep-sequencing data was employed to analyze full-genomic sequences from GII.4 variants prevailing in Canada from 2012 to 2016. Phylogenetic analysis demonstrated that the majority of these sequences belong to New Orleans 2009 and Sydney 2012 strains, and a recombinant sequence was also identified. Genome-wide similarity analyses implied that while the capsid gene is highly diverse among the isolates, the viral protease and polymerase genes remain relatively conserved. Numerous amino acid substitutions were observed at each putative antigenic epitope of the VP1 protein, whereas few amino acid changes were identified in the polymerase protein. Co-infection with other enteric RNA viruses was investigated and the astrovirus genome was identified in one of the samples.

Conclusions: Overall this study demonstrated the application of whole genome sequencing as an important tool in molecular characterization of noroviruses.

Keywords: Norovirus, Next-generation sequencing, Metagenomics, Recombination, Antigenic drift, Co-infection

Introduction

Norovirus (NoV) is a major cause of acute gastroenteritis worldwide, being responsible for sporadic and outbreak cases in various epidemiological settings [1, 2]. To date, there is no licensed antiviral therapy or vaccine available for the treatment or prevention of NoV infections [3, 4]. In the absence of a robust and readily available cell culture system, most of our understanding regarding NoV transmission, evolution, and molecular characteristics has been inferred from the analyses of epidemiological and clinical data [5].

Based on genetic diversity NoVs are classified into 7 genogroups (I–VII). Only genogroups I, II and IV have been found to infect humans. NoV genogroups are further categorized into 38 genotypes [6]. Genogroup II genotype 4 (GII.4) is the most prevalent, comprising many variants which have caused 62% to 80% of all NoV outbreaks globally since the mid-1990s [7, 8]. NoV GII.4 has evolved rapidly during the past 4 decades [9] resulting in new genetic clusters every 2–5 years [10, 11]. While some GII.4 variants such as Cairo 2007, Asia 2003 and Japan 2008 caused local epidemics, variants such as US95/96 1995, Farmington Hills 2002, Hunter

* Correspondence: neda.nasheri@canada.ca
[4]National Food Virology Reference Centre, Bureau of Microbial Hazards, Food Directorate, Health Canada 251 Sir Frederick Banting Driveway, Ottawa, ON K1A 0K9, Canada
Full list of author information is available at the end of the article

2004, Den Haag 2006b, New Orleans 2009 and Sydney 2012 led to global NoV pandemics [11–14].

Noroviruses are single-stranded, positive sense RNA viruses that belong to the family *Caliciviridae*. The genome is approximately 7.6 kb and contains 3 open reading frames (ORFs). ORF1 encodes a ~ 1700 amino acid polyprotein that is cleaved into 6 non-structural proteins: the p48 protein, an N-terminal protein of unknown function; the 2C-like helicase protein; a 3A-like protein; the VPg protein, a viral genome-linked protein; a 3C-like protease; and the RNA-dependent RNA polymerase (RdRp) [15]. ORF2 encodes the VP1 major capsid protein, which contains two domains: the shell (S) domain and the protruding (P) domain. The P domain of VP1 is further divided into two subdomains: P1 and P2. P2 is the most variable and exposed region of the VP1 protein, which contains antigenic epitopes (A-E) and sites for histo-blood group antigens (HBGAs) binding [16–18]. ORF3 encodes VP2, which is a small basic structural protein [19].

Prior to the advent of next generation sequencing (NGS) technologies, Sanger sequencing was the method of choice for analyzing viral samples, and Sanger sequencing still remains the gold standard for many clinical, environmental, and food-related applications. For characterization of infections associated with NoV, certain regions of the capsid or the polymerase genes are amplified and subjected to Sanger sequencing. While Sanger sequencing is suitable for routine laboratory testing and genotyping, this approach requires the use of standard primers for both amplification and sequencing. The use of standardized primers introduces amplification biases in favor of dominant variants. In addition, less abundant mutations are not detected since base calling methods currently have a 20% detection threshold [20]. Despite not being detected through standard methods, low-frequency mutations in viral populations are associated with drug resistance and strain emergence [21–25]. Also low frequency variants have been employed to elucidate transmission directions in viral infections [21, 22]. Therefore, dependant on the application, studying the genetic diversity of the viral quasispecies can be more informative than focusing on the dominant variants that appear in consensus sequences [20]. Full-length genomic sequences are also required for proper epidemiological analysis and efficient source attribution during sporadic or outbreak infections.

In the present study, we employed next-generation sequencing to expand our knowledge regarding the genetic diversity of GII.4 strains circulating in Canada during a 5-year period, between 2012 and 2016, with a particular focus on GII.4 Sydney 2012 variants. We also analyzed amino acid variations in the major capsid protein and the polymerase protein. Finally, we used the metagenomics data generated by our whole genome sequencing (WGS) approach to identify co-infections with other enteric viruses in the studied samples, and identified that one patient may have had an astrovirus co-infection.

Methods

Sample collection and preparation

Fifty-two NoV GII.4 positive fecal samples that were submitted to the National Food Virology Reference Centre at Health Canada and Viral Diseases Division at Public Health Agency of Canada, between 2012 and 2016, were chosen for this study. Samples were collected from five Canadian provinces (Ontario, Newfoundland and Labrador, Nova Scotia, Saskatchewan, and Alberta). Sample preparation, RNA extraction, and amplification were performed as described previously [22]. Sanger sequencing was performed to verify the presence of NoV GII.4. Viral loads were determined by droplet digital PCR (Bio-Rad, Hercules, California, USA) using the conditions that were described previously [22, 26]. A total of 44 samples had viral loads higher than 250 genome copies/μl, and were selected for deep-sequencing using the Illumina MiSeq platform.

Library preparation and Illumina sequencing

The quality and quantity of extracted RNA was examined using Agilent RNA 6000 Pico Assay Kit and Protocol (Agilent Technologies, Santa Clara, California, USA). Ethanol precipitation of RNA was performed prior to proceeding to TruSeq Stranded mRNA (Illumina, San Diego, California, USA) sample preparation. Library preparation was performed as described previously [22]. The prepared cDNA library was subjected to paired end sequencing on a MiSeq Reagent Kit v3 (150-cycle).

De novo assembly and analysis

Reads were assembled de novo using SPAdes version 3.9.0. Contigs containing NoV sequence data were identified using BLASTn against a continually updated in-house database, as described previously [22], comprised of all NoV sequences available from NCBI. Once NoV contigs were identified and extracted, PROKKA v1.11 was used to identify all the ORFs.

In order to identify the total number of NoV reads per sample in addition to coverage, all reads were subject to a reference guided assembly using SMALT v0.7.4 (https://sourceforge.net/projects/smalt/).

The sequencing reads (SRA) for each sample were deposited in GenBank under the accession numbers SRR6743837 to SRR6743880.

Construction of phylogenetic trees

Phylogenetic trees consisted of either aligned ORFs found in Fig. 1 or whole NoV genomes found in Fig. 2. Nucleotide sequences were aligned using MUSCLE [27] and phylogenetic trees were constructed from resulting alignments with RAxML v8.1.1 implementing a GTR Gamma nucleotide substitution model [28] for 1000 bootstrap replicates.

Recombination analysis

Potential recombination within the complete genome sequences was screened using seven methods (RDP, GENECONV, MaxChi, Bootscan, Chimera, SiScan, and 3Seq) implemented in the Recombination Detection Program version 4.46 (RDP4) [29]. The breakpoints were also defined by RDP4. Similarity between the recombinants and their possible major and minor parents was estimated using BootScan, embedded in RDP4 [28]. SimPlot [30] was used to visualize the relationships between the recombinant and its possible parents. The annotation of the nucleotide is based upon NCBI nucleotide accession number JX445164.

Similarity analysis

Similarities between the aligned Sydney 2012 nucleotide sequences were visualized using the SimPlot program [30]. The similarity was examined using a window size of 200 nucleotides in length (nt) and a step size of 20 nt in the full-length NoV genomes.

Results

Overall sequencing outcome

A total of 24 Giga base-pairs (Gb) raw sequencing data from 4 paired end Illumina MiSeq runs (6 Gb on average)

was generated. The sequencing reads were assembled into contigs via de novo genome assembly. From the 44 samples that were subjected to Illumina MiSeq sequencing, near full-genome sequences (coverage > 90%) were obtained from 19 samples and partial sequences were acquired from the rest of the samples, with a median read depth of 376-fold for the full genome sequences (Additional file 1: Table S1). Despite a large sequencing depth allocated to each sample (on average: 2.75 million reads), only a relatively small proportion of the obtained reads were mapped to NoV genomes in the samples that generated full-genome sequences (on average 2.5% mapped to NoV genome). Genome-wide depth of coverage for each genome was examined by measuring the number of reads per position, and as shown in Additional file 1: Figure S1, the depth of coverage was not uniform across the genomes; the 5′ and 3′ ends of the genomes consistently showed lower coverage. This observation has already been reported by others, as well as our group [22, 31, 32], and it has been explained by the inherent difficulty in recovering readable sequences at the ends of DNA fragments from the short sequences produced by Illumina. Consistent with our previous observations and other reports, samples with higher load had better coverage [22, 33].

Phylogenetic analysis

Nineteen near-full length genomes generated in this study were chosen for further analyses. Four GII.4

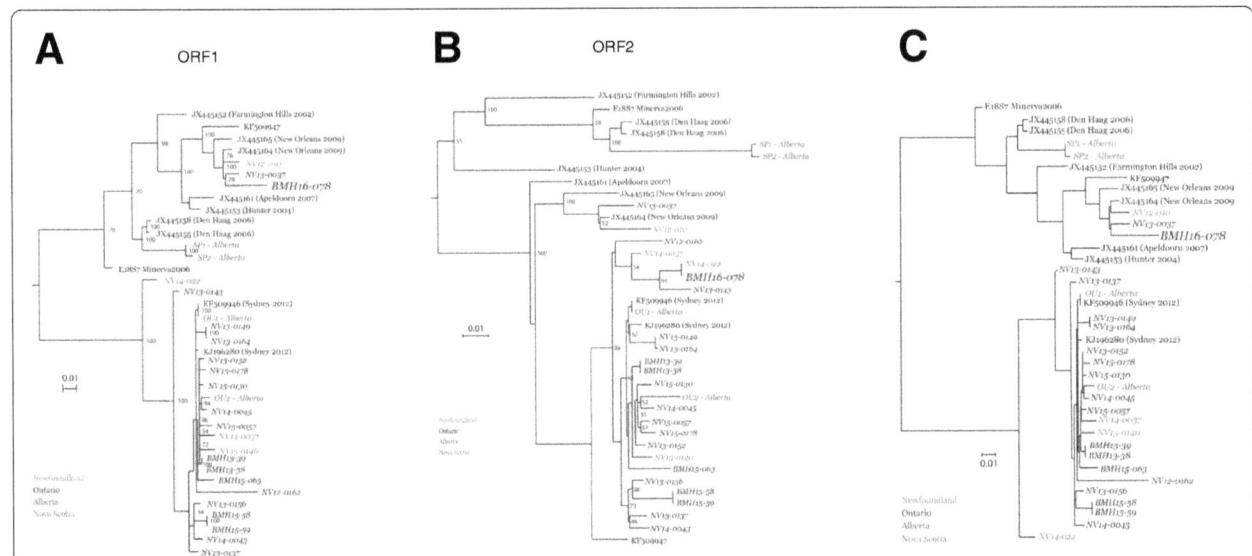

Fig. 1 Phylogenetic analysis of individual ORFs. Consensus sequences obtained in this study along with certain full-length Canadian sequences and reference sequences were aligned and phylogenetic trees were constructed for ORF1 (**a**), ORF2 (**b**) and ORF3 (**c**) using the Maximum Likelihood method. The robustness of the phylogeny was assessed through bootstrap analysis of 1000 pseudo-replicates. Sequences in brown are isolated from Ontario, orange from Alberta, blue for Nova Scotia, green from Newfoundland and Labrador. The recombinant sequence is shown in bold. The sequences generated in this study are italicized

Sydney 2012 near full-genome sequences were obtained from our previous work (BMH15–58, BMH15–59, BMH13–38, and BMH13–39) [22], and 4 Canadian GII.4 full genome sequences have already been deposited in GenBank (SP1-Alberta, SP2-Alberta, OU1-Alberta, and OU2-Alberta) [34]. Phylogenetic analysis was performed on these sequences along with a collection of reference sequences representing a variety of NoV GII.4 strains. Three phylogenetic trees were constructed, one for each ORF (Fig. 1a-c). The majority of sequences are most closely related to Sydney 2012 strains (GenBank accession No KF509946 and KJ196280) (Fig. 1), whereas SP1-Alberta and SP2-Alberta cluster with Den Haag 2006 strains (GenBank accession No JX445155 and JX445158), and NV12–010 and NV13–0037 cluster with New Orleans 2009 strains (GenBank accession No JX445164 and JX445165). Evidence indicates that BMH15–58 and BMH15–59, BMH13–38 and BMH13–39, SP1-Alberta and SP2-Alberta, which have high sequence homology, are epidemiologically linked [22, 34]. The NV13–0149 and NV13–0164

sequences also demonstrate significant homology to one another at each ORF (Fig. 1a-c). These samples were collected from the same province within the same calendar year. However, further epidemiological data are needed to confirm whether these cases were linked as well.

The ORF2 of BMH16–078 resembles GII.4 Sydney 2012 (Fig. 1b), while the ORF1 and ORF3 show a higher similarity to New Orleans 2009 sequences (Fig. 1a and c, respectively). This observation is indicative of a recombination event, and therefore, further analysis was performed.

In order to analyze the sequence homology between the sequenced Canadian GII.4 isolates and the variants circulating globally, selected full-length GII.4 sequences from different geographical regions were acquired from GenBank and aligned with some of the sequences obtained in this study. As depicted in Fig. 2, except for NV14–0045, which clusters with the sequences from South East Asia, the rest of the sequences demonstrate homology to the sequences from the United States, South Africa, United Kingdom and Australia.

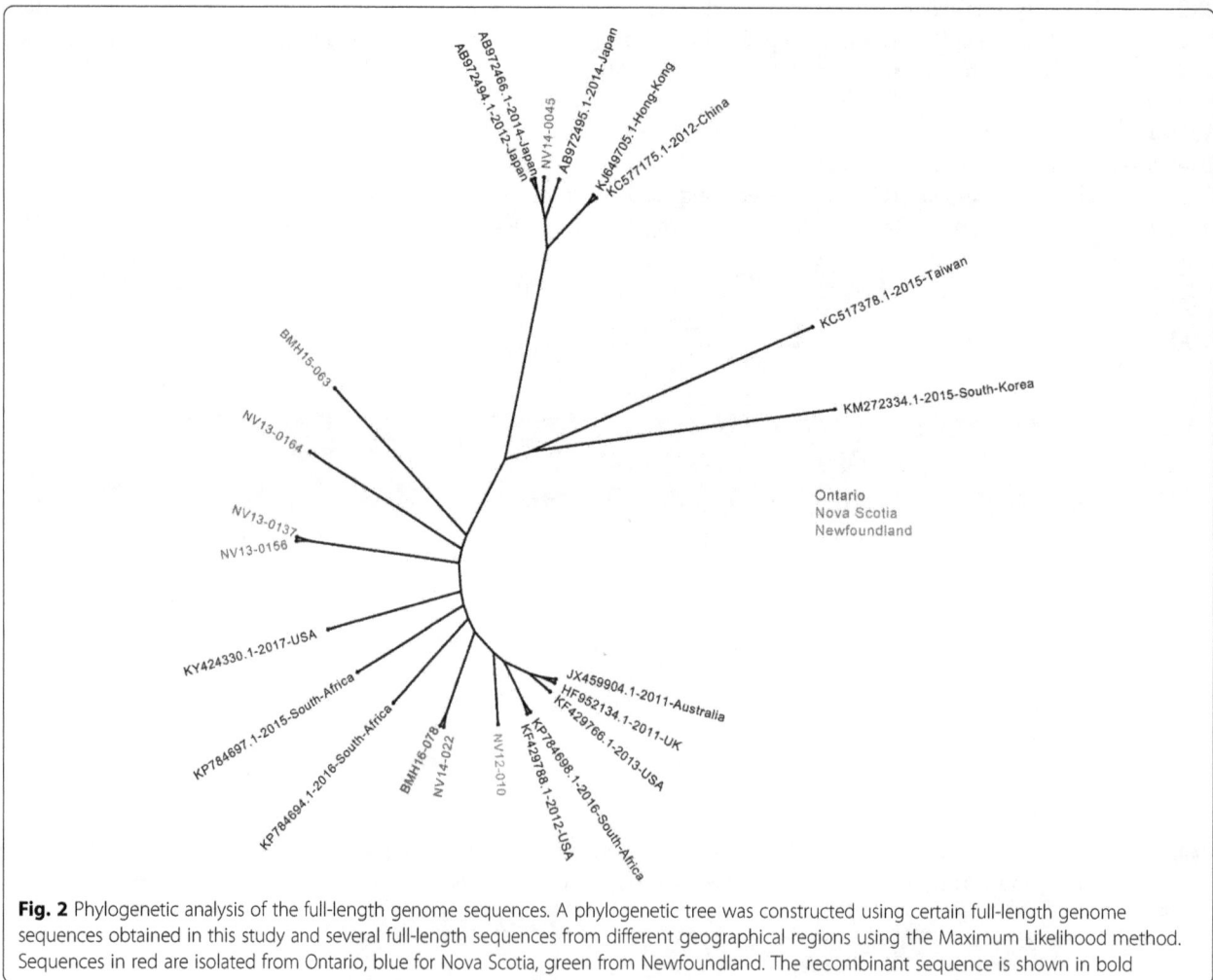

Fig. 2 Phylogenetic analysis of the full-length genome sequences. A phylogenetic tree was constructed using certain full-length genome sequences obtained in this study and several full-length sequences from different geographical regions using the Maximum Likelihood method. Sequences in red are isolated from Ontario, blue for Nova Scotia, green from Newfoundland. The recombinant sequence is shown in bold

Genetic recombination analysis

Genetic recombination is a major driving force in the evolution and emergence of novel GII.4 variants [11, 12, 33, 35]. Genetic recombination occurs when a single cell is co-infected with two NoV variants and, therefore, indicates co-infection of an individual with both variants. Consequently, the detection of a recombination event is important for understanding local and global epidemiology. Since most recombination events between norovirus genomes take place at or near the ORF1/ORF2 or ORF2/ORF3 overlap regions, it is necessary to analyze all three ORFs to identify recombinant viruses [2, 36].

The complete genome sequences obtained in this study were analyzed by RDP4 to determine the presence of NoV genomic recombination. As depicted in Fig. 3, BMH16–078 shared a high level of identity in nucleotide sequences in ORF1 and ORF3 with the New Orleans 2009 (JX445164) strains, but in ORF2 with the Sydney 2012 (KF509946) strains. The breakpoints of recombination were located near the ORF1/2 and ORF2/3 overlap regions, hence, creating a recombinant New Orleans 2009 virus with a Sydney 2012 capsid.

Similarity analysis

In order to investigate sequence heterogeneity and identify potential mutation "hot-spots", full sequences from the Sydney 2012 variants were aligned and nucleotide differences were visualized using SimPlot software. The diversity plot reveals a homogenous distribution of sequence variability in the genome (Fig. 4). The diversity between the genomes increases at the major and minor capsid genes (5085 nt to 6705 nt and 6707 nt to 7513nt, respectively), while the regions corresponding to the viral protease and RNA dependent RNA polymerase (RdRP) genes (3029 nt to 3571 nt and 3572 nt to

5101 nt) seem to be more conserved. The average distance score in the hypervariable region of the VP1 gene (5841 nt to 6031 nt) is 3.9% ± 0.45% and for the VP2 gene (7101 nt to 7321 nt) is 4.7% ± 0.75%. While the average distance score for the protease genes and conserved regions of RdRP (3572 nt to 4351 nt are 1.8% ± 0.54% and 1.6% ± 0.37%, respectively (Fig. 4). Furthermore, relatively higher sequence heterogeneity was observed in parts of the p48, NTPase and VPg genes (5–994, 995–2092, 2093–2629, respectively). Altogether, these results suggest that while the capsid proteins are under selective pressure for rapid evolution and diversification, little genetic diversity can be tolerated in the viral protease and RdRP proteins.

Amino acid variations in the VP1 protein

We performed comprehensive analyses of amino acid changes in the entire VP1 protein for each of the sequences present in our GII.4 alignment, and mapped amino acid substitutions to functional domains plus putative epitopes. Sixty variable sites were detected, representing over 11% of the total VP1 protein of 540 residues. Sixty percent of the variable sites (36 positions) were located in the P2 region of the capsid, with substitutions falling in all 5 recognized blockade epitopes (epitopes A (aa294–298, aa362, aa368), B (aa333, aa382), C (aa340, aa376), D (aa393–395), and E (aa407, aa412–413) [16, 17]. Amino acid variations were identified in 4 out of 5 conformational epitopes (regions 1–5) [9]. However, no substitution was observed in HGBA binding pocket sites I, II, and III (i.e., aa343–347, 374, and 442–443), respectively [37], further validating the conservation of human histo-blood group antigens (HBGAs) binding site among GII.4 variants.

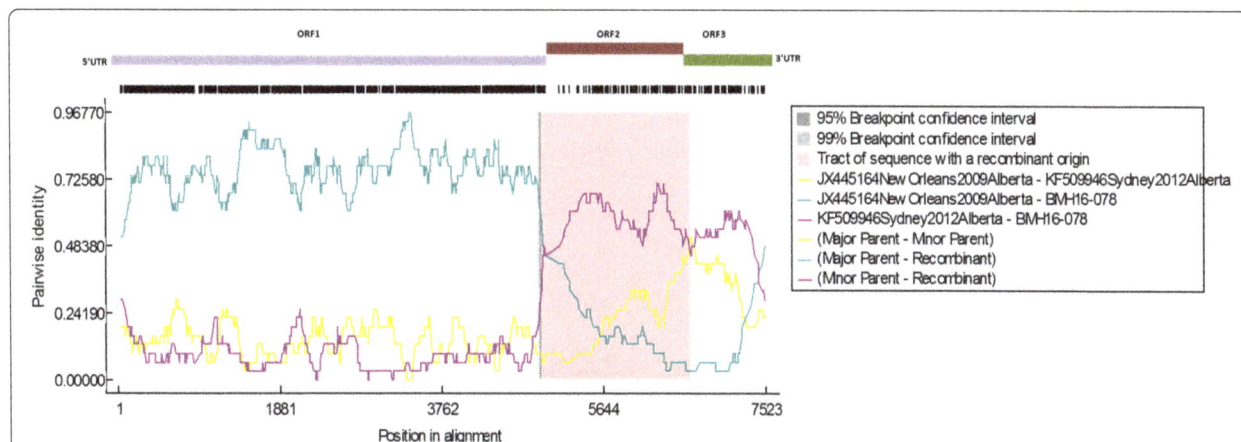

Fig. 3 SimPlot analysis of the complete genomic sequence of BMH16–078 recombination. SimPlot was constructed using the RDP4 Software version 4.72 with a slide window width of 200 bp and a step size of 20 bp. At each position of the window, the query sequence was compared to each of the reference strains. The X-axis indicates the nucleotide positions in the multiple alignments of the NoV sequences; and the Y-axis indicates nucleotide identities between the query sequence and the NoV reference strains

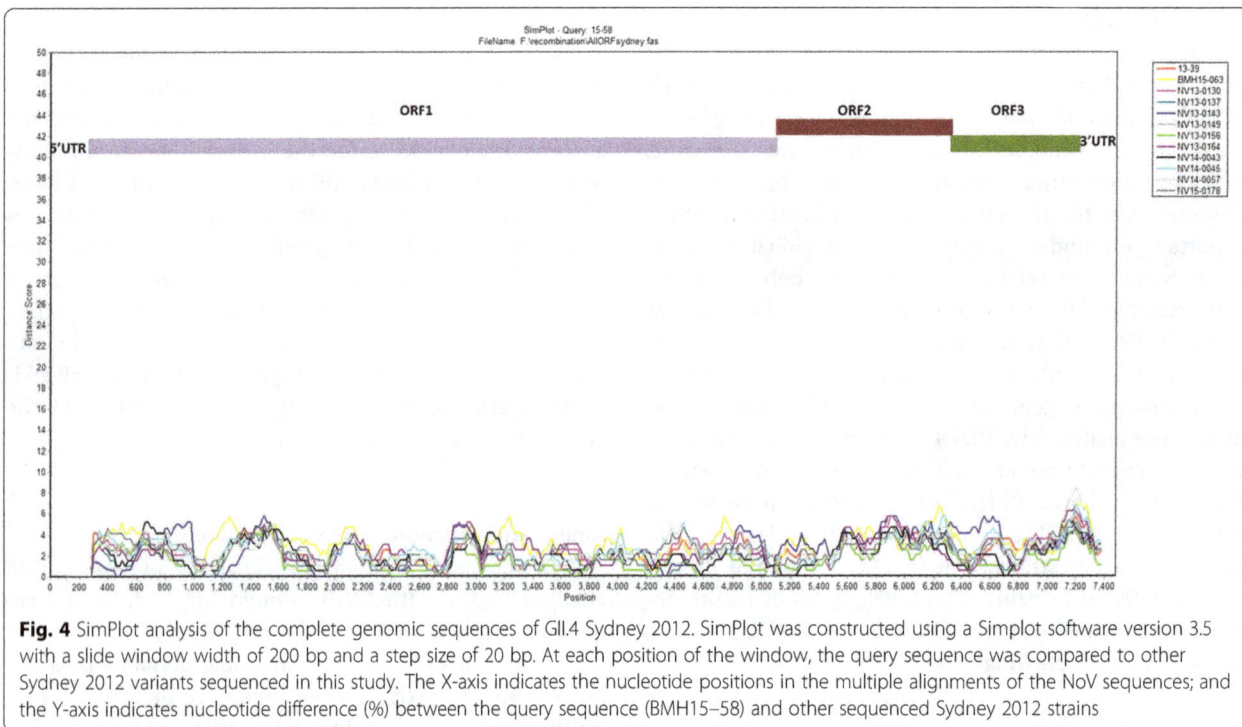

Fig. 4 SimPlot analysis of the complete genomic sequences of GII.4 Sydney 2012. SimPlot was constructed using a Simplot software version 3.5 with a slide window width of 200 bp and a step size of 20 bp. At each position of the window, the query sequence was compared to other Sydney 2012 variants sequenced in this study. The X-axis indicates the nucleotide positions in the multiple alignments of the NoV sequences; and the Y-axis indicates nucleotide difference (%) between the query sequence (BMH15–58) and other sequenced Sydney 2012 strains

Overall, 17 amino acid residues (indicated by an asterisk in the sequence alignment) were present only in one isolate (unique variants). Also, amino acid heterogeneity was observed for 9 sites where two variants for the same location were observed at ratios higher than 30% (Fig. 5).

Amino acid variations in the polymerase protein

The amino acid variations within the polymerase protein of the aligned Sydney 2012 variants were also examined. Overall 33 amino acid changes were identified, which represent 6.4% of the total residues in this protein. The degree of physico-chemical (polarity, hydrophobicity, charge, molecular weight, etc.) conservation was analyzed using Jalview 2.1 software [38] (Fig. 6). No amino acid change was observed within the active site cleft [39–41], and only 5 residues had medium to low conserved physico-chemical properties $(5 \geq \text{Score})$ [42]. However, in vivo studies would be required to determine whether these amino acid variations have any effect on the polymerase activity.

Analysis of co-infection

Due to the metagenomics approach that was employed, we were able to explore the possibility of the presence of other pathogenic RNA viruses that may have co-infected each patient. We were especially interested in investigating whether other enteric viruses such as astrovirus, aichi virus, sapovirus, and coxsackievirus B2 would be present in any of the studied samples. For this reason, assembled contigs for each patient were searched against the complete BLAST nucleotide database for the presence of the nearest homologues to these enteric viruses. The BLAST results identified several short contigs for astrovirus in patient NV13–0152 (Additional file 1: Figure S2), which may indicate a co-infection with this virus. This finding is not surprising as human astrovirus is a common cause of pediatric diarrhea worldwide [43], and co-infection with NoV is likely in childcare facilities.

Discussion

In the field of food safety, quick and accurate detection and characterization of foodborne pathogens is crucial for effective source attribution and risk mitigation. NGS technologies allow for comprehensive investigation of viral genomes without prior knowledge of the target sequences and can sequence full genomes without introducing amplification biases [44]. The sequenced genomes can then be used for epidemiological studies and source tracking. In this study, we employed a metagenomics approach to sequencing NoV genomes directly from clinical samples. The sequence reads generated by this technique can also be mined to investigate the presence of other RNA viruses, pathogenic (co-infections) or non-pathogenic (viral indicators).

Although multiple NoV genotypes co-circulate every season, GII.4 has been the dominant variant worldwide since the early 1990s, and has been responsible for the majority of NoV outbreaks during the last 20 years [2, 14, 42]. In Canada, GII.4 continued to be the most predominant genotype, responsible for 47.6% to 80.2% of all

Antigenic Epitopes
- A
- B
- C
- D
- E

Fig. 5 Non-synonymous differences within the structural domains of the capsid protein (VP1, ORF2), which are the N-terminal (N), shell (S), P1, and P2 domains. Individual epitope sites are highlighted in different colors and putative conformational epitopes are shown as regions 2–4. Unique variants are shown by *. Accession numbers for Farmington Hills 2002, Hunter 2004, Den Haag 2006 1, Den Haag 2006 2, Apeldoorn 2007, New Orleans 2009 1, New Orleans 2009 2, Sydney 2012 1, Sydney 2012 2, and Sydney 2012 3 are JX445152, JX445153, JX445158, JX445155, JX445161, JX445164, JX445145, KF509946, KF509947, KJ96280, respectively

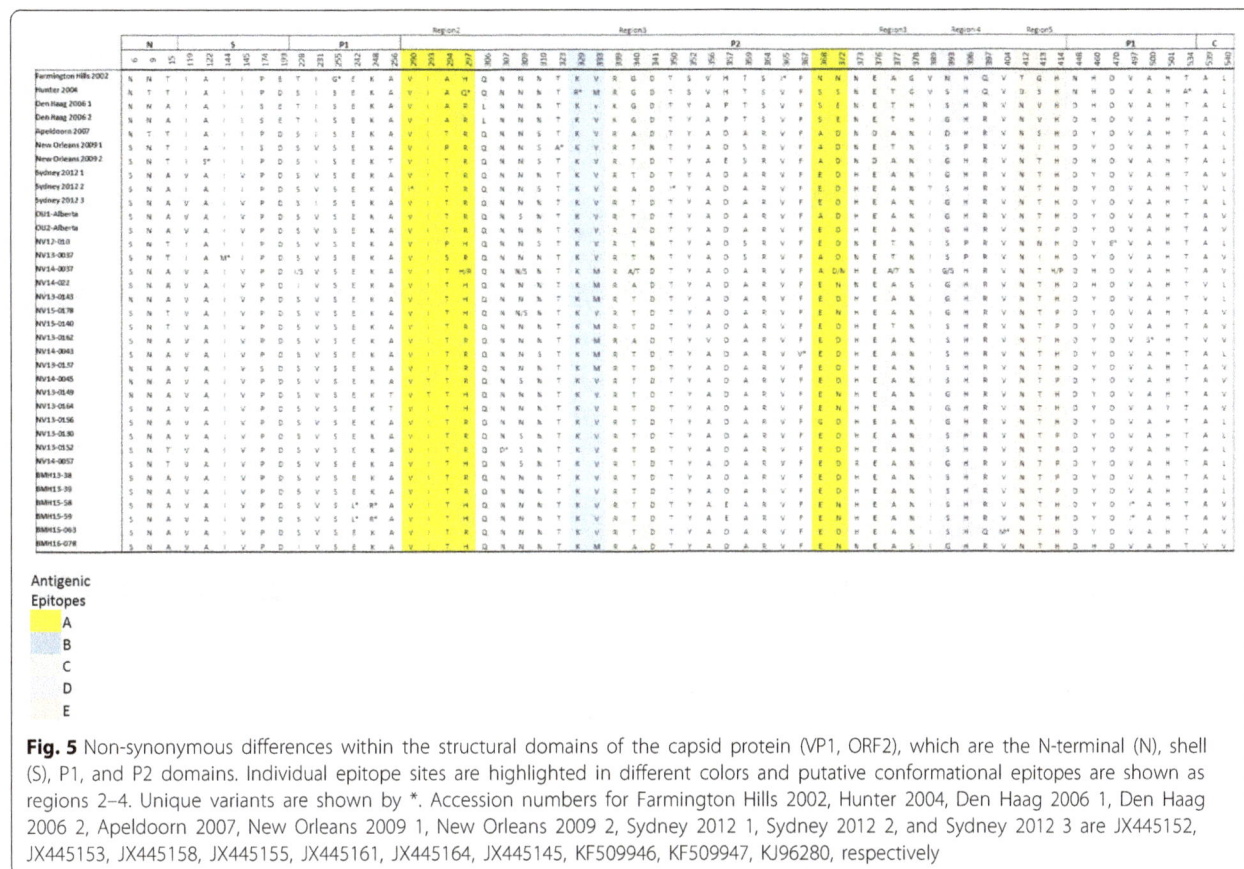

NoV outbreaks [14]. Due to high prevalence and evolution rate of GII.4, we set out to perform genomic characterization of this virus to identify factors that could be associated with its increased epidemic activity.

We have previously demonstrated that the viral titre, and therefore the quantity of viral RNA present in the sample, has a strong effect on the proportion of sequence reads that can be mapped to the NoV genome, and, therefore, on the coverage of the viral genome [22]. Consequently, Illumina sequencing was only performed on 44 samples with viral titres higher than 250 genome copies/µl. Full-genome sequences were obtained from 19 samples, and partial sequences with varying degrees of coverage were retrieved form the remaining 25 samples. For comprehensive analysis of the NoV genome, in this study we only focused on the full-genome sequences whereas the partial sequences will be included in future studies.

The phylogenetic analysis of the obtained genome sequences, along with reference sequences from GenBank for individual ORFs, revealed that most sequences from this study were homologous to Sydney 2012 strains, while the rest showed homology to New Orleans 2009 strains. The timing of sampling also supports our observation; due to its high transmissibility, Sydney 2012

became the predominant strain in Canada in years subsequent to 2012 [14]. We also performed phylogenetic analysis on full-genome sequences and selected sequences that belong to different geographical regions. NV14–0045 that clustered with several sequences from this study showed homology to isolates from South East Asia, while the remaining sequences were homologous with isolates from South Africa and the United States. Due to the lack of epidemiological data, travel cannot be ruled out for NV14–0045 patient. Unfortunately, small numbers of publicly available full-genomic sequences for GII.4 New Orleans 2009 and Sydney 2012 limited our phylogenetic analysis, and we were unable to include sequences from many geographical regions.

Another common source of variability in RNA viruses is recombination. In this study, we obtained near-full genomic NoV sequences from our samples, which enabled us to perform genome-wide recombination analysis. An intra-genotypic recombination event was observed for BMH16–078, which contains Sydney 2012 ORF2, and New Orleans 2009 ORF1 and ORF3 including the GII.P4 New Orleans 2009 pol gene. This strain circulated in Ontario in 2016. ORF1/2 recombinants of New Orleans 2009 and Sydney 2012 have been previously reported [14, 35, 45]. Additionally, it has been

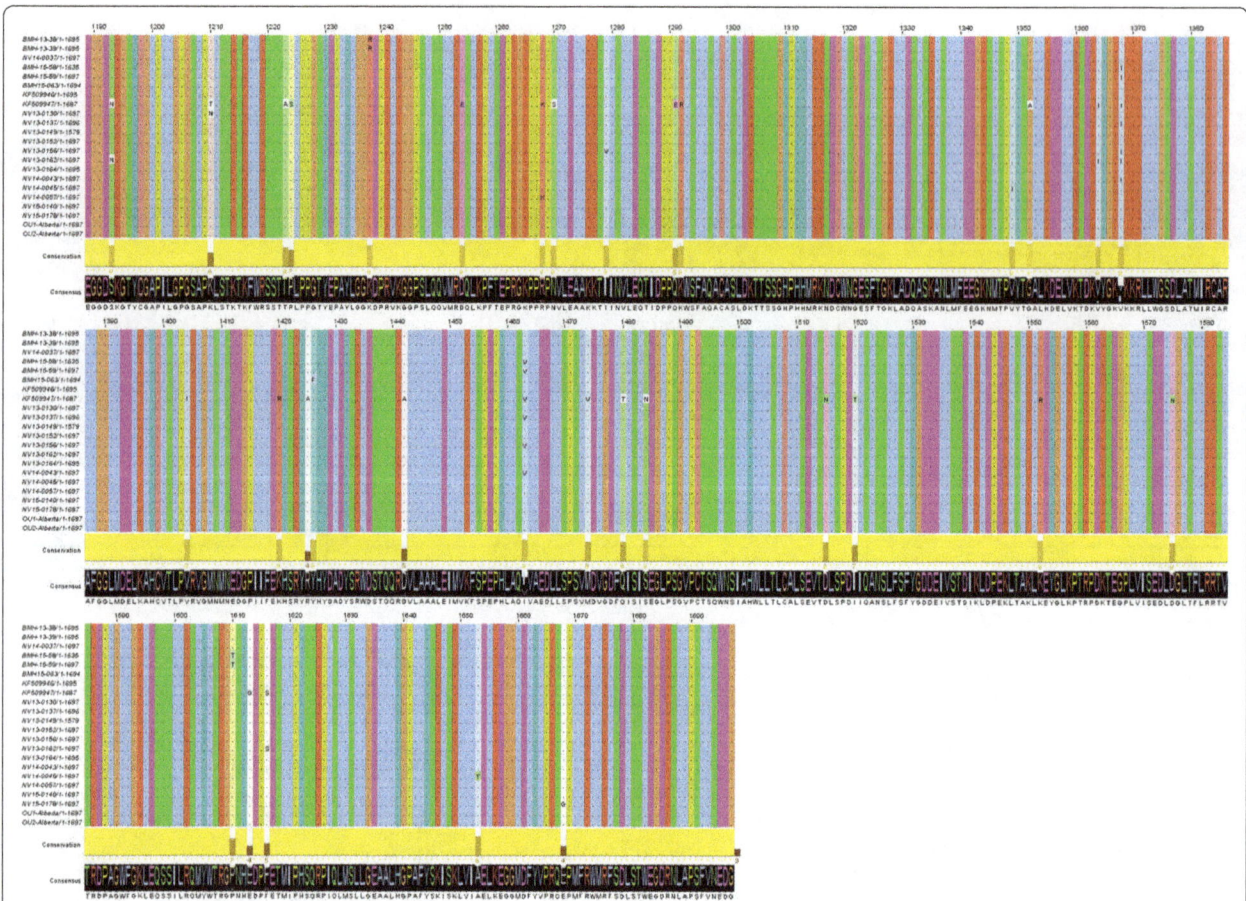

Fig. 6 Amino acid variations within the RNA-dependent RNA polymerase (RdRP) protein of the Sydney 2012 sequences. The Jalview histogram below the alignment indicates the conservation of the physico-chemical properties for each column (lower bars with lower numbers, lower conservation; completely conserved columns are in yellow)

demonstrated that the New Orleans 2009 ORF2 variant has almost disappeared because of recombination with the GII.4 Sydney 2012 ORF2 variant [46]. However, unlike previously reported New Orleans 2009/Sydney 2012 recombinants, the recombination breakpoints of BMH16–078 flank the ORF2, creating a mosaic New Orleans 2009 virus with Sydney 2012 capsid. Due to limited number of full-length GII.4 sequences available, such a sequence has not been reported previously; however, its existence has been inferred from phylogenetic analysis [47]. Comprehensive molecular epidemiological studies are required in order to determine the source and mechanisms facilitating the emergence of this GII.4 variant.

Amino acid substitutions were observed throughout the VP1 protein, but the majority of the changes were located on the outer surface of the P domain, near or at blockade epitopes and conformational epitopes. Further in vivo and in vitro investigations are required in order to validate whether these substitutions alter the antigenic profile of these viruses. None of the studied

samples from patients contained a virus that showed changes in the receptor-binding pocket sites, indicating that the receptor specificity was unchanged among these strains. These results further validate that the P domain of the VP1 protein in GII.4 variants is subject to strong selective pressure that may produce immune escape variants while the receptor binding sites remain relatively conserved.

While genomic similarity analysis verifies that the capsid region is quite heterogeneous between members of the same strain, it indicates that the protease and the polymerase genes are relatively conserved. Another study has also reported that these genes can tolerate few nucleotide changes [48]. This observation is not unexpected due to their critical functions in viral replication, viral protease and RdRP genes are highly conserved [40, 49] and have been attractive targets for the design and development of antiviral strategies. Nucleotide diversity was also observed in regions of the p48, NTPase and VPg genes. Certain regions of these genes have been shown to be able to tolerate drastic nucleotide changes [48], and are evolutionarily less conserved [50].

The presence of other pathogens can have a significant effect on the severity and outcome of NoV infection. For proper metagenomics analysis of a microbial community such as intestinal microbiota, shotgun sequencing of DNA and RNA as well as 16S rRNA sequencing should be conducted [51]. As a-proof-of-concept, by performing 16S rRNA gene sequencing, and metagenomic shotgun sequencing, a wide variety of enteric pathogens were identified in diarrhea stool samples [52]. Since stool filtrates were used in this study, the presence of pathogenic enteric bacteria in the samples was not explored. However, shotgun RNA sequencing of stool filtrates enabled us to examine the presence of other enteric RNA viruses. Herein, we identified a number of sequencing reads that mapped to human astrovirus in sample NV-13-0152. Human astrovirus is a major cause of gastroenteritis in children under the age of 5 [53] and this patient was 15 months old at the time of sample collection. It seems that norovirus-astrovirus co-infection is likely to occur in childcare facilities, however due to the lack of epidemiological and metagenomics data, they may have been under reported.

Overall, in this study, limited numbers of prevailing GII.4 strains were characterized and an accumulation of data from molecular epidemiological studies with continuous surveillance are required for developing prediction systems for NoV outbreaks or an efficient vaccine strategy.

The use of NGS for molecular epidemiology advances our understanding regarding the transmission dynamics of NoV and allows for timely interventions and outbreak control practices, thus reducing transmission and decreasing the burden of norovirus infection. In summary, our study provides detailed analyses of the genetic diversity of NoV GII.4 in Canada. Nevertheless, it is important to continue to monitor and characterize circulating NoV strains in real-time to identify emerging variants that can escape from previously acquired immunity and cause epidemics.

Conclusion

In conclusion, 19 near-full GII.4 genome sequences were retrieved by RNA-Seq method from stool filtrates. The majority of genomes belong to Sydney 2012 strains, while two isolates showed homology to New Orleans 2009 strains. Also, one recombinant sequence was identified. The genomic data were further analyzed for genetic similarity between the isolates as well as identification of non-synonymous changes in the major capsid protein and the viral polymerase protein. Co-infection with other enteric RNA viruses was also investigated.

Abbreviations
NGS: Next-generation Sequencing; NoV: Norovirus; ORF: Open reading frame; RdRp: RNA dependent RNA polymerase; WGS: Whole genome sequencing

Acknowledgements
We would like to thank Dr. Timothy Booth and Elsie Grudeski from the National Microbiology Laboratory for providing the stool filtrates. We also thank Dr. Erling Rud and Dr. Sandeep Tamber from the Research Division of the Bureau of Microbial Hazards Health Canada for reviewing the manuscript and offering helpful comments. This work was financially supported by the Research Division of the Bureau of Microbial Hazards, Health Canada. NN acknowledges support from the Visiting Fellow in a Government Laboratory Program.

Funding
Research Division, Bureau of Microbial Hazards, Food Branch, Health Canada.

Authors' contributions
NN and JR designed and initiated the project. NN, JH, OM, and MS carried out all the wet laboratory works including RNA extraction, quantification and RNA-Seq library preparation and data analysis. NP performed all the bioinformatics analysis, sequence assembly. NN, NP, JR prepared the manuscript. SB, and NC supervised the project and critically reviewed the manuscript. All authors agreed with the final draft of the manuscript. All authors have read and approved the final manuscript.

Competing interests
The authors declare that they have no competing interests.

Author details
[1]Biostatistics and Modeling Division, Bureau of Food Surveillance and Science Integration, Food Directorate, Health Canada Ottawa, Ottawa, ON, Canada. [2]Department of Food Science and Agricultural Chemistry, Faculty of Agricultural and Environmental Sciences, Macdonald Campus, McGill University, Montreal, QC, Canada. [3]Department of Animal Sciences, Faculty of Agricultural and Environmental Sciences, Macdonald Campus, McGill University, Montreal, QC, Canada. [4]National Food Virology Reference Centre, Bureau of Microbial Hazards, Food Directorate, Health Canada 251 Sir Frederick Banting Driveway, Ottawa, ON K1A 0K9, Canada.

References
1. Havelaar AH, Kirk MD, Torgerson PR, Gibb HJ, Hald T, Lake RJ, Praet N, Bellinger DC, de Silva NR, Gargouri N, Speybroeck N, Cawthorne A, Mathers C, Stein C, Angulo FJ, Devleesschauwer B, World Health Organization foodborne disease burden epidemiology reference group: World Health Organization global estimates and regional comparisons of the burden of foodborne disease in 2010. PLoS Med 2015; 12(12):e1001923.
2. de Graaf M, van Beek J, Koopmans MP. Human norovirus transmission and evolution in a changing world. Nat Rev Microbiol. 2016.
3. Rocha-Pereira J, Van Dycke J, Neyts J. Norovirus genetic diversity and evolution: implications for antiviral therapy. Curr Opin Virol. 2016;20:92–8.
4. Lopman BA, Steele D, Kirkwood CD, Parashar UD. The vast and varied global burden of norovirus: prospects for prevention and control. PLoS Med. 2016; 13(4):e1001999.
5. Moore MD, Goulter RM, Jaykus LA. Human norovirus as a foodborne pathogen: challenges and developments. Annu Rev Food Sci Technol. 2015;6:411–33.
6. Vinje J. Advances in laboratory methods for detection and typing of norovirus. J Clin Microbiol. 2015;53(2):373–81.
7. Botha JC, Taylor MB, Mans J. Comparative analysis of south African norovirus GII.4 strains identifies minor recombinant variants. Infect Genet Evol. 2017; 47:26–34.
8. Boon D, Mahar JE, Abente EJ, Kirkwood CD, Purcell RH, Kapikian AZ, Green KY, Bok K. Comparative evolution of GII.3 and GII.4 norovirus over a 31-year period. J Virol. 2011;85(17):8656–66.
9. Motoya T, Nagasawa K, Matsushima Y, Nagata N, Ryo A, Sekizuka T, Yamashita A, Kuroda M, Morita Y, Suzuki Y, Sasaki N, Katayama K, Kimura H. Molecular evolution of the VP1 gene in human norovirus GII.4 variants in 1974-2015. Front Microbiol. 2017;8(2399).
10. Mori K, Chu PY, Motomura K, Somura Y, Nagano M, Kimoto K, Akiba T, Kai A, Sadamasu K. Genomic analysis of the evolutionary lineage of norovirus GII.4 from archival specimens during 1975-1987 in Tokyo. J Med Virol. 2017;89(2): 363–7.

11. Bull RA, Eden JS, Rawlinson WD, White PA. Rapid evolution of pandemic noroviruses of the GII.4 lineage. PLoS Pathog. 2010;6(3):e1000831.

12. Bull RA, White PA. Mechanisms of GII.4 norovirus evolution. Trends Microbiol. 2011;19(5):233–40.

13. van Beek J, Ambert-Balay K, Botteldoorn N, Eden JS, Fonager J, Hewitt J, Iritani N, Kroneman A, Vennema H, Vinje J, White PA, Koopmans M. NoroNet: indications for worldwide increased norovirus activity associated with emergence of a new variant of genotype II.4, late 2012. Euro Surveill. 2013;18(1):8–9.

14. Hasing ME, Hazes B, Lee BE, Preiksaitis JK, Pang XL. Detection and analysis of recombination in GII.4 norovirus strains causing gastroenteritis outbreaks in Alberta. Infect Genet Evol. 2014;27:181–92.

15. Green KY. Caliciviridae: The Noroviruses. In: Knipe DM, Howley PM, editors. Fields Virology. 6th ed. United States: Lippincott Williams & Wilkins; 2013. p. 948.

16. Debbink K, Donaldson EF, Lindesmith LC, Baric RS. Genetic mapping of a highly variable norovirus GII.4 blockade epitope: potential role in escape from human herd immunity. J Virol. 2012;86(2):1214–26.

17. Lindesmith LC, Costantini V, Swanstrom J, Debbink K, Donaldson EF, Vinje J, Baric RS. Emergence of a norovirus GII.4 strain correlates with changes in evolving blockade epitopes. J Virol. 2013;87(5):2803–13.

18. Shanker S, Choi JM, Sankaran B, Atmar RL, Estes MK, Prasad BV. Structural analysis of histo-blood group antigen binding specificity in a norovirus GII.4 epidemic variant: implications for epochal evolution. J Virol. 2011;85(17):8635–45.

19. Vongpunsawad S, Venkataram Prasad BV, Estes MK. Norwalk virus minor capsid protein VP2 associates within the VP1 Shell domain. J Virol. 2013; 87(9):4818–25.

20. Posada-Cespedes S, Seifert D, Beerenwinkel N. Recent advances in inferring viral diversity from high-throughput sequencing data. Virus Res. 2016.

21. Kundu S, Lockwood J, Depledge DP, Chaudhry Y, Aston A, Rao K, Hartley JC, Goodfellow I, Breuer J. Next-generation whole genome sequencing identifies the direction of norovirus transmission in linked patients. Clin Infect Dis. 2013;57(3):407–14.

22. Nasheri N, Petronella N, Ronholm J, Bidawid S, Corneau N. Characterization of the genomic diversity of norovirus in linked patients using a metagenomic deep sequencing approach. Front Microbiol. 2017;8(73).

23. Fernandez-Caballero JA, Chueca N, Poveda E, Garcia F. Minimizing next-generation sequencing errors for HIV drug resistance testing. AIDS Rev. 2017;19(4):231–8.

24. Quer J, Rodriguez-Frias F, Gregori J, Tabernero D, Soria ME, Garcia-Cehic D, Homs M, Bosch A, Pinto RM, Esteban JI, Domingo E, Perales C. Deep sequencing in the management of hepatitis virus infections. Virus Res. 2017;239:115–25.

25. Trebbien R, Christiansen CB, Fischer TK. Antiviral resistance due to deletion in the neuraminidase gene and defective interfering-like viral polymerase basic 2 RNA of influenza a virus subtype H3N2. J Clin Virol. 2018;102:1–6.

26. Kageyama T, Kojima S, Shinohara M, Uchida K, Fukushi S, Hoshino FB, Takeda N, Katayama K. Broadly reactive and highly sensitive assay for Norwalk-like viruses based on real-time quantitative reverse transcription-PCR. J Clin Microbiol. 2003;41(4):1548–57.

27. Edgar RC. MUSCLE: a multiple sequence alignment method with reduced time and space complexity. BMC Bioinformatics. 2004;5:113-2105-5.113.

28. Stamatakis A. RAxML version 8: a tool for phylogenetic analysis and post-analysis of large phylogenies. Bioinformatics. 2014;30(9):1312–3.

29. Martin DP, Murrell B, Golden M, Khoosal A, Muhire B. RDP4: detection and analysis of recombination patterns in virus genomes. Virus evolution. 2015.

30. Lole KS, Bollinger RC, Paranjape RS, Gadkari D, Kulkarni SS, Novak NG, Ingersoll R, Sheppard HW, Ray SC. Full-length human immunodeficiency virus type 1 genomes from subtype C-infected seroconverters in India, with evidence of intersubtype recombination. J Virol. 1999;73(1):152–60.

31. Batty EM, Wong TH, Trebes A, Argoud K, Attar M, Buck D, Ip CL, Golubchik T, Cule M, Bowden R, Manganis C, Klenerman P, Barnes E, Walker AS, Wyllie DH, Wilson DJ, Dingle KE, Peto TE, Crook DW, Piazza P. A modified RNA-Seq approach for whole genome sequencing of RNA viruses from faecal and blood samples. PLoS One. 2013;8(6):e66129.

32. Mortazavi A, Williams BA, McCue K, Schaeffer L, Wold B. Mapping and quantifying mammalian transcriptomes by RNA-Seq. Nat Methods. 2008; 5(7):621–8.

33. Yang Z, Mammel M, Papafragkou E, Hida K, Elkins CA, Kulka M. Application of next generation sequencing toward sensitive detection of enteric viruses isolated from celery samples as an example of produce. Int J Food Microbiol. 2017;261:73–81.

34. Hasing ME, Hazes B, Lee BE, Preiksaitis JK, Pang XL: A next generation sequencing-based method to study the intra-host genetic diversity of norovirus in patients with acute and chronic infection. BMC Genomics 2016, 17;480– doi: 10.1186/s12864 016-2831-y.

35. Fonager J, Stegger M, Rasmussen LD, Poulsen MW, Ronn J, Andersen PS, Fischer TK: A universal primer-independent next-generation sequencing approach for investigations of norovirus outbreaks and novel variants. Sci Rep 2017, 7(1);813– doi: 10.1038/s41598-017-00926-x.

36. Ludwig-Begall LF, Mauroy A, Thiry E. Norovirus recombinants: recurrent in the field, recalcitrant in the lab - a scoping review of recombination and recombinant types of noroviruses. J Gen Virol. 2018.

37. Tan M, Xia M, Chen Y, Bu W, Hegde RS, Meller J, Li X, Jiang X. Conservation of carbohydrate binding interfaces: evidence of human HBGA selection in norovirus evolution. PLoS One. 2009;4(4):e5058.

38. Waterhouse AM, Procter JB, Martin DM, Clamp M, Barton GJ. Jalview version 2--a multiple sequence alignment editor and analysis workbench. Bioinformatics. 2009;25(9):1189–91.

39. Ng KK, Pendas-Franco N, Rojo J, Boga JA, Machin A, Alonso JM, Parra F. Crystal structure of Norwalk virus polymerase reveals the carboxyl terminus in the active site cleft. J Biol Chem. 2004;279(16):16638–45.

40. Shu B, Gong P. Structural basis of viral RNA-dependent RNA polymerase catalysis and translocation. Proc Natl Acad Sci U S A. 2016;113(28):E4005–14.

41. Shaik MM, Bhattacharjee N, Feliks M, Ng KK, Field MJ. Norovirus RNA-dependent RNA polymerase: a computational study of metal-binding preferences. Proteins. 2017;85(8):1435–45.

42. Livingstone CD, Barton GJ. Protein sequence alignments: a strategy for the hierarchical analysis of residue conservation. Comput Appl Biosci. 1993;9(6):745–56.

43. Cortez V, Meliopoulos VA, Karlsson EA, Hargest V, Johnson C, Schultz-Cherry S. Astrovirus biology and pathogenesis. Annu Rev Virol. 2017; 4(1):327–48.

44. Iles JC, Njouom R, Foupouapouognigni Y, Bonsall D, Bowden R, Trebes A, Piazza P, Barnes E, Pepin J, Klenerman P, Pybus OG. Characterization of hepatitis C virus recombination in Cameroon by use of nonspecific next-generation sequencing. J Clin Microbiol. 2015;53(10):3155–64.

45. Martella V, Medici MC, De Grazia S, Tummolo F, Calderaro A, Bonura F, Saporito L, Terio V, Catella C, Lanave G, Buonavoglia C, Giammanco GM: Evidence for recombination between pandemic GII.4 norovirus strains New Orleans 2009 and Sydney 2012. J Clin Microbiol 2013, 51(11);3855–3857.

46. van Beek J, de Graaf M, Al-Hello H, Allen DJ, Ambert-Balay K, Botteldoorn N, Brytting M, Buesa J, Cabrerizo M, Chan M, Cloak F, Di Bartolo I, Guix S, Hewitt J, Iritani N, Jin M, Johne R, Lederer I, Mans J, Martella V, Maunula L, McAllister G, Niendorf S, Niesters HG, Podkolzin AT, Poljsak-Prijatelj M, Rasmussen LD, Reuter G, Tuite G, Kroneman A, Vennema H, Koopmans MPG. NoroNet: molecular surveillance of norovirus, 2005-16: an epidemiological analysis of data collected from the NoroNet network. In: Lancet infect dis; 2018.

47. Eden JS, Tanaka MM, Boni MF, Rawlinson WD, White PA. Recombination within the pandemic norovirus GII.4 lineage. J Virol. 2013;87(11):6270–82.

48. Thorne L, Bailey D, Goodfellow I. High-resolution functional profiling of the norovirus genome. J Virol. 2012;86(21):11441–56.

49. Prasad BV, Shanker S, Muhaxhiri Z, Deng L, Choi JM, Estes MK, Song Y, Palzkill T, Atmar RL. Antiviral targets of human noroviruses. Curr Opin Virol. 2016;18:117–25.

50. Cotten M, Petrova V, Phan MV, Rabaa MA, Watson SJ, Ong SH, Kellam P, Baker S. Deep sequencing of norovirus genomes defines evolutionary patterns in an urban tropical setting. J Virol. 2014;88(19):11056–69.

51. Knight R, Callewaert C, Marotz C, Hyde ER, Debelius JW, McDonald D, Sogin ML. The microbiome and human biology. Annu Rev Genomics Hum Genet. 2017;18:65–86.

52. Zhou Y, Wylie KM, El Feghaly RE, Mihindukulasuriya KA, Elward A, Haslam DB, Storch GA, Weinstock GM. Metagenomic approach for identification of the pathogens associated with diarrhea in stool specimens. J Clin Microbiol. 2016;54(2):368–75.

53. Siqueira JAM, Oliveira DS, Carvalho TCN, Portal TM, Justino MCA, da Silva LD, Resque HR, Gabbay YB. Astrovirus infection in hospitalized children: molecular, clinical and epidemiological features. J Clin Virol. 2017;94:79–85.

54. Okonechnikov K, Conesa A, Garcia-Alcalde F. Qualimap 2: advanced multi-sample quality control for high-throughput sequencing data. Bioinformatics. 2016;32(2):292–4.

15

Blood-borne and sexually transmitted infections: a cross-sectional study in a Swiss prison

Komal Chacowry Pala[1], Stéphanie Baggio[1*], Nguyen Toan Tran[1,4], François Girardin[2], Hans Wolff[1] and Laurent Gétaz[1,3]

Abstract

Background: Incarcerated people carry a high burden of infection, including blood-borne diseases (BBDs). It is also known that one million people contract a sexually transmitted infection (STI) every day worldwide, which represents a global public health challenge. However, data regarding the prevalence of STIs and the risk factors among incarcerated populations are lacking. The objective of this study was to determine the prevalence and associated factors of BBDs and STIs among detainees in the largest pre-trial prison in Switzerland.

Methods: In a cross-sectional study conducted at the Champ-Dollon pre-trial prison, 273 male detainees answered a standardized questionnaire and were screened for syphilis, herpes simplex virus 2 (HSV-2), HIV, and hepatitis C (HCV). Prevalence rates and associations of BBDs and STIs with risk factors were computed.

Results: Most participants (90.9%) were migrants from outside Western Europe, and 5.9% were injecting drug users. HCV was diagnosed among 6.2% of participants (antibody prevalence). The prevalence of HCV was higher among injecting drug users (81.2%) than non-injectors (1.6%). The prevalence of HIV, syphilis, and HSV-2 was 0.4%, 1.1%, and 22.4%, respectively. HCV was associated with a history of injecting drug use and HSV-2 with a lower education level and being older than 26 years.

Conclusions: This study showed the infection prevalence of 2–9 times higher among detainees than in the Swiss community. It also illustrated that these infections are associated with sociodemographic and risk factors. Therefore, the prison environment offers an opportunity to strengthen infectious disease control programs targeting specific subgroups of at-risk people. Such programs would benefit both the prison population and broader society.

Keywords: HIV, Syphilis, Herpesvirus 2, human, Hepatitis C, Prison, Epidemiology

Background

Blood-borne and sexually transmitted infections in prison

Incarcerated people are members of a vulnerable group and carry a high burden of medical conditions, including infectious diseases [1, 2]. Furthermore, precarious living conditions in jails, such as a sedentary lifestyle, a poor diet, inadequate hygiene habits, and drug use, contribute to the transmission of infectious diseases [3]. In prisons, high prevalence rates of blood-borne diseases (BBDs) and sexually transmitted infections (STIs) may be related

to the accumulation of negative health risks. Due to the long asymptomatic periods, the prevalence rate of STIs could also be related to the epidemiology reported in detainees' countries of origin, where they spent part of their lives and where they acquired most of their infections prior to the migration process [4]. Approximately one million people contract an STI every day worldwide. Despite progress in diagnosis, treatment, and prevention, STIs continue to represent a global public health challenge with substantial socio-economic burden [5].

Syphilis and herpes simplex virus 2 (HSV-2) are known to be major global causes of acute illness and long-term disability and cause significant complications [5]. Both can also increase the risk of acquiring and

* Correspondence: stephanie.baggio@hcuge.ch
[1]Division of Prison Health, Geneva University Hospitals, University of Geneva, Chemin de Champ-Dollon 22, 1241 Puplinge, Geneva, Switzerland
Full list of author information is available at the end of the article

transmitting other infections [6], particularly HSV-2, which is associated with an increased risk of HIV acquisition by two- to threefold [7, 8]. Since 2010, many countries, particularly in Western Europe, saw a sharp upsurge in the number of reported syphilis infections [9], which is a public health concern, as 15% of people infected with latent syphilis will present with severe complications if left untreated [9]. Data regarding the prevalence of STIs and risk factors among incarcerated populations are missing [10]. HIV and HCV affect millions of people around the globe and cause profound morbidity and mortality [11]. Of the estimated 10.2 million people incarcerated worldwide, it is reported that 3.8% are infected with HIV (389,000 living with HIV) and 15.1% with HCV (1,546,500) [12]. This prevalence is much higher than in the general population, primarily because of high-risk behaviors, in particular, sharing needles to inject drugs [12, 13].

Correctional facilities are known to provide a valuable and unique opportunity to offer accessible and acceptable health interventions [12]. Therefore, identifying and treating incarcerated people carrying BBDs and STIs may not only limit the disease burden and increased costs by means of early treatment, but also contribute to decrease the overall transmission of STIs, HCV, and HIV in the general population upon their release from prison [14].

The case of Switzerland

Our study took place in Switzerland, which has a prison population of 6,869 people, among whom approximately 71% are foreigners [15]. These foreign detainees come mostly from poor and vulnerable communities [16] and may suffer from a higher burden of disease compared to Swiss prisoners. Undocumented detainees do not have any health insurance coverage and therefore have limited access to health care when living in Switzerland. This lack of health care access includes the access to vaccination, diagnosis and treatment of HIV, HCV, syphilis, and HSV-2.

In Switzerland, Champ-Dollon prison is the largest and most overcrowded (177%) pre-trial prison [17]. It accommodated, on average, 540 prisoners between 2009 and 2011. This prison is also characterized by a high turnover rate of detainees (73%) [17]; approximately half of the prisoners are released within one month of initial incarceration. The medical unit of this prison is attached to Geneva University Hospitals and is completely independent of the prison's administration. It offers a low-threshold primary care approach to health care. All detainees admitted to the facility undergo a health assessment by primary health care nurses. This evaluation acts as triage to identify any health problems that require medical attention, such as allergies; injuries;

breathing problems; mental health problems, including suicidal ideas; addiction; regular medical treatment; suspicion of tuberculosis; or allegations of violence during arrest. When necessary, nurses immediately refer detainees to a primary care physician. A proposal for screening for infectious diseases (hepatitis, HIV, syphilis) is discussed at this time, but these problems are often not considered a priority by inmates at the time of entry into prison. In case of initial refusal, as these screenings are not systematically proposed again later during incarceration, a large proportion of prisoners does not benefit from these diagnoses before being released. In Geneva's prisons, when detainees are diagnosed as positive, they are treated in accordance with good medical practices, respecting the principle of equivalence of care and corresponding to the care provided to people who are free [18]. Regarding the prevention of infectious disease transmission in this prison, specific harm-reduction measures, such as needle and syringe exchange programs, condom distribution, and opioid substitution treatment are provided [19, 20].

Study's objectives

This study aims to determine the prevalence of syphilis, HSV-2, HIV, and HCV serological markers and their associated factors among detainees in the Champ-Dollon prison in Geneva, the largest pre-trial detention center in Switzerland.

Methods

A cross-sectional study was conducted at the Champ-Dollon prison during two varicella outbreaks, which occurred in the male detention units at two distinct times (2009 and 2011).

Study population and setting

Capitalizing on the blood samples taken to test for varicella immunity in all varicella-exposed detainees, we offered these same consenting participants the opportunity to test for HIV, HCV, and syphilis (HSV-2 was only offered to the 2011 cohort) and to take a structured socio-demographic survey. We offered consenting participants of entire affected prison units the opportunity to participate. Women, representing 5% of the prison population in Champ-Dollon, are detained in a separate unit. Since the varicella outbreaks did not affect this unit, all participants were men. We made sure that detainees were not included twice in the study (i.e., in case of re-arrest). There were no exclusion criteria. Of the 281 detainees, 273 agreed to participate in the study ($n = 116$ in 2009, and $n = 157$ in 2011; participation rate = 97.2%).

Ethics statement

The Ethics Research Committee of the Geneva University Hospitals approved the study (EC: 09–137).

Data collection

Each participant underwent serological testing for HIV, HCV, and syphilis. One participant refused the HIV serology. Serum was insufficient to process HSV-2 in one participant and syphilis and HIV in two participants. HSV-2 was tested for only among participants recruited in 2011 (n = 157). Serum samples were tested by commercial immunoenzymatic assays for HIV (HIV, Ag/Ab Combo, Architect, Abbott) and HCV (anti-HCV, Architect, Abbott). Anti-HIV and anti-HCV reactivity were always confirmed via INNO-LIA™ HIV I/II Score and INNO-LIA™ HCV score line immune assays (Innogenetics, Belgium), respectively. HSV-2 serostatus was determined using an HSV-2 IgG enzyme-linked immunosorbent assay (ELISA) (Immunowell, HSV type 2, IgG test, GenBio). A positive HSV-2 serology indicates present or past infection. Syphilis was screened using a two-step Chemiluminescent Microparticle ImmunoAssay (CMIA) (Syphilis TP, Architect, Abbot). Positive cases were confirmed via Treponema Pallidum Particle Agglutination (TPPA) (Serodia®) and the serum Rapid Plasma Reagin (RPR) test (Human). Those CMIA+/RPR+/TPHA+ and without a history of syphilis treatment were assumed to have syphilis. Participants answered a standardized questionnaire administered by a physician. Questions (provided in six different languages: English, French, German, Italian, Spanish, and Russian) explored socio-demographic characteristics (age, sex, country of birth, self-reported socioeconomic status, and education level) and exposure to factors potentially related to STIs and/or BBDs (sexual behavior and past and current injecting drug use). The recall period for sexual behaviors and history of injecting drug use was lifetime.

Clinical management of participants

All participants with confirmed HIV, HCV, HSV-2, and syphilis underwent a clinical evaluation. In cases presenting with HIV and HCV, patients were referred to the Geneva University Hospitals for specialized care. HCV-positive patients whose length of incarceration allowed doctors to consider possible treatment (interferon at the time of the study) benefited from a viremia and a liver biopsy. In accordance with the principle of equivalence of care, the indications for treatment were the same as those used in the general Swiss population. Participants with latent syphilis were treated with intramuscular penicillin (three times once a week). Participants with HSV-2 and recurrent genital ulcers received a prescription for antiviral medication to reduce symptoms during the next recurrent infection or antiviral prophylactic treatment (according to the frequency of relapses). All positive participants were also educated to limit the risk of transmission.

Statistical analysis

Associations between infections (HCV, HSV-2) and other categorical variables (age, gender, region of origin, being an injecting drug user [IDU], and sexual health characteristics) were tested using Chi-square tests. We also computed Cramer's V to provide an overview of the importance of the relationships for significant associations. The Cramer's V ranges from 0 (no association) to 1 (perfect association), with .10 being a small association, .30 a medium association, and .50 a high association. Two multivariate logistic regressions that used HVC and HSV-2 as dependent variables and categorical factors as independent variables were performed. Stepwise regressions including variables (i.e., age, gender, region of origin, being an IDU, and sexual health characteristics) used in the bivariate analyses were performed. Odd ratios are reported. For HIV and syphilis, only descriptive statistics were computed because of the low prevalence rate of infected participants ($n = 1$ and $n = 4$ respectively). Descriptive and bivariate analyses were performed for the whole sample and then separately for 2009 and 2011 to test whether there were significant differences between the two time points. All analyses were performed using SPSS (version 24).

Results

Table 1 summarizes the socio-demographic characteristics of the all-male participants. The mean age was 29.8 ± 9.0 years. The age range was 18–64 years, with 25% of the participants being younger than 23, 50% younger than 28, and 75% younger than 34. A total of 90.9% were migrants originating from outside Western Europe, and 63.7% were undocumented (no Swiss or European Union passport or residence permit in Switzerland). Overall, 72.1% attended secondary school (among all participants, 50.6% completed secondary school).

In terms of sexual health, 2.3% of participants reported homosexual or bisexual behavior. More than half (52.8%) reported having had sexual activities with sex workers. Two-thirds (67.0%) reported occasional or no condom use. Almost three-quarters (73.0%) reported having had more than five sexual partners in their lifetime, and 5.9% of the participants declared a history of injecting drug use.

There were some differences between the two years of data collection: participants were more likely to come from North Africa in 2009 and Latin America in 2011, and the participants' socio-economic level was lower in 2011. There were no differences for other risk factors included in the analyses presented below (history of sexual intercourse with sex workers, being an IDU, and history of genital ulcers).

Table 1 Socio-demographic characteristics

Variable		N (%)	2009	2011	p-value[a]
Sex (male)		273 (100)	116 (100)	157 (100)	–
Region of origin[b]					
	Central and Eastern Europe	104 (38.1)	41 (35.3)	63 (40.1)	**.001**
	Sub-Saharan Africa	77 (28.2)	37 (31.9)	40 (25.5)	
	North Africa	39 (14.3)	26 (22.4)	13 (8.3)	
	Latin America	26 (9.5)	3 (2.6)	23 (14.6)	
	Western Europe	25 (9.2)	8 (6.9)	17 (10.8)	
	Asia	2 (0.7)	1 (0.9)	1 (0.6)	
Age					
	< 28 years	131 (48.0)	63 (54.3)	68 (43.3)	.072
	≥ 28 years	142 (52.0)	53 (45.7)	89 (56.7)	
Education level (8 missing values)					
	Secondary school not completed	74 (27.9)	78 (69.0)	113 (74.3)	.340
	Secondary school completed	191 (72.1)	35 (31.0)	39 (25.7)	
Self-reported socioeconomic status (8 missing values)					
	Low	43 (16.2)	101 (87.1)	121 (79.6)	**.033**
	Intermediate or high	222 (81.3)	12 (10.3)	31 (20.4)	

[a]Chi-square tests or Fisher exact tests. Significant p-values are highlighted in bold
[b]Countries of origin: Central and Eastern Europe: Albania ($n = 44$), Byelorussia ($n = 3$), Bosnia ($n = 2$), Georgia ($n = 9$), Israel ($n = 1$), Kosovo ($n = 24$), Lithuania ($n = 1$), Macedonia ($n = 5$), Romania ($n = 6$), Russia ($n = 3$), Serbia ($n = 5$), Slovakia ($n = 1$); Sub Saharan Africa: Angola ($n = 4$), Benin ($n = 1$), Cameroun ($n = 2$), Cap Verde ($n = 1$), Congo ($n = 1$), Eritrea ($n = 2$), Gambia ($n = 1$), Ghana ($n = 3$), Guinea ($n = 7$), Guinea Bissau ($n = 2$), Guinea Conakry ($n = 20$), Ivory Coast ($n = 6$), Liberia ($n = 1$), Mali ($n = 3$), Nigeria ($n = 12$), Senegal ($n = 1$), Sierra Leone ($n = 5$), Soudan ($n = 1$), Tanzania ($n = 1$), Togo ($n = 2$), Zimbabwe ($n = 1$); North Africa: Algeria ($n = 15$), Egypt ($n = 1$), Iraq ($n = 2$), Libya ($n = 3$), Morocco ($n = 10$), Palestine ($n = 5$), Tunisia ($n = 3$); Latin America: Brazil ($n = 4$), Bolivia ($n = 1$), Chili ($n = 1$), Colombia ($n = 6$), Dominican Republic ($n = 12$), Equateur ($n = 1$), Paraguay ($n = 1$); Western Europe: Belgium ($n = 1$), Germany ($n = 1$), Greece ($n = 1$), Italia ($n = 2$), France ($n = 8$), Portugal ($n = 1$), Spain ($n = 1$), Switzerland ($n = 9$), UK ($n = 1$); Asia: China ($n = 1$), India ($n = 1$)

Table 2 shows the prevalence of infections among participants. Antibody prevalence of HIV, HCV, syphilis, and HSV-2 were 0.4%, 6.2%, 1.1%, and 22.4%, respectively. There were no significant differences between 2009 and 2011. Only HSV-2 was comorbid with other infectious diseases: one participant also had HIV, two had syphilis, and one had HCV. There was no case of co-infection between HIV, syphilis, and HCV.

A total of 76.5% of participants with HCV were aware of their infection before screening. Among HCV-positive participants who were aware of their status before screening, 92.5% reported being IDUs, whereas 25% of participants who were HCV-positive and unaware of their status before screening reported being IDUs, representing a statistically significant difference ($p = 0.04$).

The HIV positive participant was aware of his infection before screening.

According to bivariate analysis, associations of HCV positivity with a history of being an IDU, originating from European countries, having sexual intercourse with sex workers, and having a low education level were statistically significant. We found an important association between HCV and injecting drug use. The other associations were small (max. = .181) (Table 3). Results showed no association between HCV-positivity and age, self-reported socioeconomic level, non-use of condoms, same-sex sexual activities, and the number of sexual partners in a participant's lifetime. In the multivariate model, only IDUs were significantly associated with HCV. Participants who were IDUs were 227 times more

Table 2 Serological prevalence of HIV, HCV, syphilis and HSV-2

	n	% (95% CI)	2009	2011	p-value[a]
HIV (Ag/Ab Combo+ & Inno-Lia+)	1/270	**0.4%** (0.1–2.1)	0/115 (0%)	1/155 (0.7%)	1
Syphilis (ELISA+ & TPHA+ & RPR+)	3/271	**1.1%** (0.4–3.2)	2/114 (1.8%)	2/157 (1.3%)	1
HSV-2 (ELISA HSV-2+)	35/156	**22.4%** (16.6–29.6)	–	35/156 (22.4%)	–
HCV (EIA+ & Inno-Lia+)	17/273	**6.2%** (3.9–9.7)	8/116 (6.9%)	9/157 (5.7%)	.694

95% CI: 95% confidence interval
[a]Chi-square tests or Fisher exact tests. Significant p-values are highlighted in bold

Table 3 Bivariate and multivariate analyses of HCV and HSV-2 according to sociodemographic and sexual health factors

Variable [c]	HCV			HSV-2		
	$n = 17$	p-value bivariate model	p-value multivariate model[d]	$n = 35$	p-value bivariate model	p-value multivariate model[d]
		V-Cramer	OR		V-Cramer	OR[d]
Region of origin						
European countries	14/129 (**10.9%**)	**.003**[a]		12/79 (**15.2%**)	**.028**[a]	
Other regions	3/144 (**2.0%**)	0.181		23/77 (**29.8%**)	0.176	
Age						
< 28 years	5/131 (3.8%)	.113[a]		10/67 (14.9%)	.051[a]	**.019**
≥ 28 years	12/142 (8.5%)	–		25/89 (28.1%)	0.156	2.63
Education level						
Secondary school not completed	1/74 (**1.4%**)	**.047**[b]		15/39 (**38.5%**)	**.009**[a]	**.034**
Secondary school completed	16/191 (**8.4%**)	0.129		20,112 (**17.9%**)	0.214	3.21
Condom use for sexual protection						
Always	3/87 (3.5%)	.165[a]		16/63 (25.4%)	.585[a]	
Sometimes or never	14/177 (7.9%)	–		19/88 (21.6%)	–	
Sexual intercourse with sex workers						
Never	4/125 (**3.2%**)	**.044**[a]		13/65 (20%)	.421[a]	
At least once	13/140 (**9.3%**)	0.124		22/86 (25.6%)	–	
Sexual orientation						
Homosexual/bisexual	1/6 (16.7%)	.662[b]		0/3 (0%)	.999[b]	
Heterosexual	16/259 (6.2%)	–		35/148 (23.6%)	–	
Number of sexual partners						
0 to 5	3/71 (4.2%)	.369[a]		8/44 (18.2%)	.450[a]	
6 or more	14/192 (7.3%)	–		25/105 (23.8%)	–	
Injection drug use						
Yes	13/16 (**81.2%**)	**<.001**[b]	**<.001**	0/7 (0%)	.138[a]	
No	4/253 (**1.6%**)	0.774	227.00	35/145 (24.1%)	–	
History of genital ulcers						
Yes	2/28 (7.1%)	.695[b]		7/15 (**46.7%**)	**.045**[b]	
No	15/239 (6.3%)	–		28/138 (**20.3%**)	0.187	

95% CI: 95% confidence interval, OR: odd-ratio
[a] Chi square tests and [b] Fisher exact tests were performed with Cramers' V as effect size
[c] No statistically significant association between HCV or HSV-2 and socio-economic status, condom use, same-sex sexual activities, and number of sexual partners lifetime ($p > .05$). No inferential statistics were performed on HIV and syphilis because of the low prevalence rate of infected people living in detention
Significant p-values and associated prevalence rates are highlighted in bold
[d] Multiple logistic stepwise regressions with HCV and HSV-2 as dependent variables were performed. p-values of Wald chi-square and odd-ratio with the second category of each variable being the reference category are reported

likely to have HCV compared with participants who were not IDUs ($p < .001$).

Bivariate analyses showed that HSV-2 was significantly associated with education level, region of origin, history of genital ulcers, and marginally associated with age. As for region of origin, 29.8% of participants from Africa and Latin America were seropositive against 15.2% of those originating from European countries. All effect sizes were small (max. = .214), with the highest being

between HSV-2 and education level (Table 3). Results showed no association between HSV-2 infection and self-reported socioeconomic level, non-use of condoms, same-sex sexual activities, number of sexual partners in a participant's lifetime, and sexual intercourse with sex workers. In the multivariate model, level of education and age were significantly associated with HSV-2. Participants with a low educational level (respectively, younger) were 3.21 (respectively 2.63) times more likely to have HSV-2 compared to participants with a higher level of education (respectively, older).

Discussion

This study aimed to estimate the prevalence rate of HIV, syphilis, HCV, and HSV-2 in a sample of male detainees and to investigate associated risk factors. Overall, we found a high prevalence of HIV, HCV, syphilis, and HSV-2. Findings on hepatitis B are reported in a previous study (prevalence rate = 5.9%) [21].

Prevalence rates of infectious diseases

The prevalence of HIV (0.4%) was two times higher in comparison with the general Swiss population (0.2%) [22]. However, this prevalence of 0.4% may be seen as low when considering the profile of the detainees (large proportion of migrants and multiple drug use) and in comparison with the prevalence found in other European prisons. For example, a previous study [23] established that the HIV prevalence in detainees in developed countries ranges from 0.2% in Australia to more than 10% in some European nations. The countries with the highest prevalence rates were in sub-Saharan Africa and Eastern Europe [12].

The prevalence of HCV (6.2%) was nine times higher in comparison withthe general Swiss population (0.71%) [24], but 2.5-fold lower than the average (15.5%) reported in prisons in Western European countries [12].

HSV-2 prevalence (22.4%) was more than two times higher in comparison with the Swiss general population of men of similar age (10.6% among 25–34-year-old participants) [25]. Studies investigating HSV-2 seroprevalence in prison are scarce. Among male detainees in Italy and Portugal, two studies reported an HSV-2 seroprevalence (21.0% and 19.9%) close to that reported in our study population [26]. In one prison in New South Wales, Australia, the prevalence of HSV-2 was estimated to be 21% among males [27].

Finally, the prevalence of syphilis among participants (1.1%) was sevenfold higher in comparison with the general population in European countries (0.16%) [28]. This high prevalence rate suggested that future studies should explore the cost-effectiveness of systematic screening. Indeed, it is estimated that a third of people infected with latent syphilis will present with significant complications if left untreated [29]. Syphilis remains a frequent infectious disease in low- and middle-income countries, and its prevalence rate has recently increased in Western countries [30]. Therefore, screening and treatment of such high-risk populations as detainees would help to reduce this burden of disease.

Risk factors for HCV and HSV-2

We investigated risk factors for the two infectious diseases with a sufficient sample size for analysis. The factor most strongly associated with HCV was the history of drug injection (Cramer's V = .774). This was also the only factor associated with HCV in the multivariate analysis. This observation was consistent with earlier findings [31], which showed that the HCV prevalence among detainees was higher compared to the general population due to the high proportion of IDU. The prevalence of HCV was lower among detainees originating from Africa, Latin America, and Asia than among those from Europe, a higher proportion of whom are IDUs. The proportion of migrants from Africa and Latin America, who are rarely IDUs (only 1.2%), is higher among detainees in Switzerland than in other Western European countries; this fact may explain the lower prevalence of HCV in Swiss prisons than in other Western European countries.

HCV-positive IDUs were more aware of their status (92.5%) than HCV-positive participants who did not inject drugs (25%). Therefore, the subgroup of detainees who did not inject drugs should not be neglected. Complementary studies targeting this subgroup are necessary to investigate HCV epidemiology, particularly among participants from countries with high HCV prevalence and where transmission is not predominantly due to injection drug use. Prisons should be a place that offers screenings and treatment for HCV to this vulnerable population, as members of this population are often hard to reach outside the prison. A study has shown that HCV treatment of detainees is cost-effective [32].

A low education level and increased age were the main risk factors associated with HSV-2 (as well as in the multivariate analysis). These factors corresponded to those identified in the literature [33]. Region of origin and a history of genital ulcers were significant only in the bivariate analyses. Participants from Africa and Latin America with HSV-2 positivity were twice as prevalent as European participants. According to Looker et al., the global burden of HSV-2 varies by region. The HSV-2 prevalence among 15–49-year-old men is the highest in Africa (25%), followed by the Americas (10%), Southeast Asia (7%), and European countries (4%) [34]. However, the region of origin was no longer significant in the multivariate analysis. This was probably due to a multicollinearity with socio-economic level, because migrants originating from low-income countries were likely to have a low educational level.

Factors related to sexual risk history did not efficiently discriminate HSV-2-infected detainees, but history of genital ulcers was associated with HSV-2 in bivariate analyses. Nevertheless, 79% of HSV-2-positive participants did not report a history of genital ulcers. This proportion is consistent with data reported in the literature, where only 9–25% of people who are HSV-2 positive report a history of symptoms suggestive of genital herpes [35]. Among our HSV-2-positive participants, 15% reported recurrent genital ulcers. Four out of five participants with recurrent genital ulcers did not seek medical care because they thought that no treatment was available. These people could be treated with antiviral medication to help reduce symptoms during recurrent infections, while antiviral prophylactic treatment could be prescribed to limit contagiousness and the frequency of relapses [8]. Moreover, these patients need to be educated regarding their contagiousness during and outside symptomatic episodes [36].

HSV-2 was also the only sexual infection associated with other diseases. The participant infected with HIV also had HSV-2, as did the two participants who had syphilis. The number of cases of HIV and syphilis was too small to conclude regarding the comorbidity between sexual infections, and future studies should focus on this important research question.

Strengths and limitations

The strengths of our study included the high participation rate and the use of reliable indicators necessary for planning preventive measures. However, this study had some limitations. First, it included a relatively low number of participants and a limited number of positive cases; thus, it is difficult to make a definite statement about the risk factors, particularly for HIV and syphilis. Nevertheless, the sample size was sufficient to identify the burden of BBDs and STIs in the study population, as well as factors associated with HCV and HSV-2. Second, this study focused on men, so data among women are needed, even if women represent only 5% of the total prison population in Switzerland. Third, because participants were asked to answer sensitive questions (e.g., sexual practices), this information may be less reliable due to reporting bias, social desirability [37], and because the questionnaire was completed face-to-face with a physician. Fourth, for HCV and HSV-2, only serological markers were tested, indicating previous contact with the virus, but not necessarily current infection. Fifth, we used a self-reported measure of socioeconomic status. Future studies should use more reliable ways to assess this important factor. Finally, our findings may not necessarily be generalizable to detention centers in other countries. We hypothesize, however, that the profiles of infections described here would be comparable to other detention centers, where the sociodemographic profiles correspond to those described here. The study population was similar to other pre-trial prisons in Switzerland, which are also characterized by high proportions of migrants and males [15].

Recommendations

This study highlighted some gaps in the policies designed to fight infectious diseases in Swiss prisons. As the burden of HIV, HCV, and STIs was high in this Swiss prison and because risk factors contributed to a higher risk of BBD transmission among prisoners [38], effective measures should be improved to mitigate BBD and STI transmission. Effective and internationally recommended strategies, such as opioid substitution treatment, condom distribution, and needle and syringe exchange programs [39], must be continued in the population study and introduced in other Swiss prisons where they are not yet enforced. Safer tattooing strategies should also be implemented, as tattooing is currently done in a clandestine and unsafe way by using inappropriate handcrafted equipment. Moreover, inmates share these tattoo devices, enhancing the risk of BBD transmission [37, 40]. Identification of BBDs and STIs must be strengthened in detention facilities in a way that makes it possible to ethically screen as many people as manageable, ensuring individual autonomy and access to treatment [39, 41].

Overall, we recommend strengthening preventive strategies in correctional settings, especially for detainees with a low education level and from countries with high HSV-2 endemicity [34]. Region of origin, even if non-significant in the multivariate model, is an important factor when screening for disease at entry to a prison. The socio-economic level is not assessed, whereas the region of origin is. Therefore, this factor might be used as an indicator of the likelihood for the presence of HSV-2. For this subgroup, we also recommend integrating genital ulcers into the participants' medical history and strengthening preventive measures, such as encouraging people to use condoms.

Conclusions

The prevalence of BBDs and STIs found in our incarcerated population was worryingly high. Screening, educational, and preventive programs to promote low-risk and health-seeking behaviors, as well as access to quality treatment and care should be guaranteed to detainees [42]. Infection control should be an important health care focus in prison to prevent possible health complications and further transmission of infectious diseases. Reducing BBD- and STI-related morbidity and breaking the existing transmission chain in prison settings would eventually benefit the larger communities into which detainees will be reintegrated [43].

Acknowledgements
The authors would like to thank the medical and nurses' team of the prison Champ-Dollon, as well as Agnès Lehmann and Giuseppe Togni (Laboratory Unilabs, Geneva) for their active collaboration.

Funding
This work was supported by the Federal Office of Public Health (grant number 09.003678), Bern, Switzerland, and by the Medical Direction of the Geneva University Hospitals.

Authors' contributions

LG conceived and designed the study, KCP drafted the manuscript, KCP and SB analysed data, LG, SB, NTT, FG and HW helped to interpret the data and revised the manuscript critically for important intellectual content. All authors approved the final version of the manuscript to be submitted.

Competing interests

The authors declare that they have no competing interests.

Author details

[1]Division of Prison Health, Geneva University Hospitals, University of Geneva, Chemin de Champ-Dollon 22, 1241 Puplinge, Geneva, Switzerland. [2]Medical Direction and Division of Clinical Pharmacology, Toxicology Geneva University Hospitals, University of Geneva, Geneva, Switzerland. [3]Division of Tropical and Humanitarian Medicine, Geneva University Hospitals, University of Geneva, Geneva, Switzerland. [4]Australian Centre for Public and Population Health Research, Faculty of Health, University of Technology, Sydney, Australia.

References

1. Hammett TM. HIV/AIDS and other infectious diseases among correctional inmates: transmission, burden, and an appropriate response. Am J Public Health. 2006;96(6):974–8.
2. Negro F. Epidemiology of hepatitis C in Europe. Dig Liver Dis. 2014; 46(Supplement 5):S158–64.
3. Felisberto M, Saretto AA, Wopereis S, Treitinger A, Machado MJ, Spada C. Prevalence of human immunodeficiency virus infection and associated risk factors among prison inmates in the City of Florianópolis. Rev Soc Bras Med Trop. 2016;49(5):620–3.
4. Fakoya I, Álvarez-del Arco D, Woode-Owusu M, Monge S, Rivero-Montesdeoca Y, Delpech V, Rice B, Noori T, Pharris A, Amato-Gauci AJ, et al. A systematic review of post-migration acquisition of HIV among migrants from countries with generalised HIV epidemics living in Europe: mplications for effectively managing HIV prevention programmes and policy. BMC Public Health. 2015;15:561.
5. Carmona-Gutierrez D, Kainz K, Madeo F. Sexually transmitted infections: old foes on the rise. Microb Cell. 2016;3(9):361–2.
6. Stamm LV. Syphilis: Re-emergence of an old foe. Microb Cell. 2016;3(9):363–70.
7. Looker KJ, Elmes JAR, Gottlieb SL, Schiffer JT, Vickerman P, Turner KME, Boily M-C. Effect of HSV-2 infection on subsequent HIV acquisition: an updated systematic review and meta-analysis. Lancet Infect Dis. 2017;17(12):1303–16.
8. Schiffer JT, Corey L. New concepts in understanding genital herpes. Curr Infect Dis Rep. 2009;11(6):457–64.
9. CDC: STD Facts - Syphilis (Detailed). In. Atlanta, USA: Centers for Disease Control and Prevention; 2017.
10. Marques NMS, Margalho R, Melo MJ, da Cunha JGS, Meliço-Silvestre AA. Seroepidemiological survey of transmissible infectious diseases in a Portuguese prison establishment. Braz J Infect Dis. 2011;15(3):272–5.
11. Scott JA, Chew KW. Treatment optimization for HIV/HCV co-infected patients. Ther Adv Infect Dis. 2017;4(1):18–36.
12. Dolan K, Wirtz AL, Moazen B, Ndeffo-Mbah M, Galvani A, Kinner SA, Courtney R, McKee M, Amon JJ, Maher L, et al. Global burden of HIV, viral hepatitis, and tuberculosis in prisoners and detainees. Lancet (London, England). 2016;388(10049):1089–102.
13. UNAIDS: The gap report 2014. In. Geneva, Switzerland: The gap report 2014; 2014.
14. Kouyoumdjian FG, Leto D, John S, Henein H, Bondy S. A systematic review and meta-analysis of the prevalence of chlamydia, gonorrhoea and syphilis in incarcerated persons. Int J STD AIDS. 2012;23(4):248–54.
15. Office SFS: Swiss statistics - prisons, detention - key figures. In.: Swiss federal statistical Office; 2011.
16. Rieder JP, Bertrand D, Wolff H, Gravier B, Pasche C, Bodenmann P. Santé en milieu pénitentiaire : vulnérabilité partagée entre détenus et professionnels de la santé. Rev Méd Suisse. 2010;6:1462–5.
17. Baggio S, Gétaz L, Tran NT, Peigné N, Chacowry Pala K, Golay D, Heller P, Bodenmann P, Wolff H. Association of overcrowding and turnover with self-harm in a Swiss pre-trial prison. Int J Environ Res Public Health. 2018;15(4):1-6.
18. Wolff H, Sebo P, Haller DM, Eytan A, Niveau G, Bertrand D, Gétaz L, Cerutti B. Health problems among detainees in Switzerland: a study using the ICPC-2 classification. BMC Public Health. 2011;11:245.
19. Barro J, Casillas A, Gétaz L, Rieder J-P, Baroudi M, François A, Broers B, Wolff H. Retractable syringes in a Swiss prison needle and syringe exchange program: experiences of drug-using inmates and prison staff perceptions. Int J Ment Health Addiction. 2014;12(5):648–59.
20. Favrod-Coune T, Baroudi M, Casillas A, Rieder J-P, Gétaz L, Barro J, Gaspoz J-M, Broers B, Wolff H. Opioid substitution treatment in pretrial prison detention: a case study from Geneva, Switzerland. Swiss Med Wkly. 2013;143:w13898.
21. Gétaz L, Casillas A, Siegrist C-A, Chappuis F, Togni G, Tran NT, Baggio S, Negro F, Gaspoz J-M, Wolff H. Hepatitis B prevalence, risk factors, infection awareness and disease knowledge among inmates: a cross-sectional study in Switzerland's largest pre-trial prison. J Glob Health. 2018;8(2):020407 Accepted.
22. Kohler P, Schmidt AJ, Cavassini M, Furrer H, Calmy A, Battegay M, Bernasconi E, Ledergerber B, Vernazza P, Swiss HIVCS. The HIV care cascade in Switzerland: reaching the UNAIDS/WHO targets for patients diagnosed with HIV. AIDS. 2015;29(18):2509–15.
23. Hellard ME, Aitken CK. HIV in prison: what are the risks and what can be done? Sex Health. 2004;1(2):107–13.
24. Sakem B, Madaliński K, Nydegger U, Stępień M, Godzik P, Kołakowska A, Risch L, Risch M, Zakrzewska K, Rosińska M. Hepatitis C virus epidemiology and prevention in polish and Swiss population - similar and contrasting experiences. Ann Agric Environ Med. 2016;23(3):425–31.
25. Bünzli D, Wietlisbach V, Barazzoni F, Sahli R, Meylan PRA. Seroepidemiology of herpes simplex virus type 1 and 2 in Western and southern Switzerland in adults aged 25-74 in 1992-93: a population-based study. BMC Infect Dis. 2004;4:10.
26. Sarmati L, Babudieri S, Longo B, Starnini G, Carbonara S, Monarca R, Buonomini AR, Dori L, Rezza G, Andreoni M, et al. Human herpesvirus 8 and human herpesvirus 2 infections in prison population. J Med Virol. 2007;79(2):167–73.
27. Butler T, Donovan B, Taylor J, Cunningham AL, Mindel A, Levy M, Kaldor J. Herpes simplex virus type 2 in prisoners, New South Wales, Australia. Int J STD AIDS. 2000;11(11):743–7.
28. Newman L, Rowley J, Hoorn SV, Wijesooriya NS, Unemo M, Low N, Stevens G, Gottlieb S, Kiarie J, Temmerman M. Global estimates of the prevalence and incidence of four curable sexually transmitted infections in 2012 based on systematic review and global reporting. PLoS One. 2015;10(12):e0143304.
29. Ficarra G, Carlos R. Syphilis: the renaissance of an old disease with oral implications. Head Neck Pathol. 2009;3(3):195–206.
30. Barnett R. Syphilis. Lancet. 2018;391(10129):1471.
31. Vescio MF, Longo B, Babudieri S, Starnini G, Carbonara S, Rezza G, Monarca R. Correlates of hepatitis C virus seropositivity in prison inmates: a meta-analysis. J Epidemiol Community Health. 2008;62(4):305–13.
32. Tan JA, Joseph TA, Saab S. Treating hepatitis C in the prison population is cost-saving. Hepatology. 2008;48(5):1387–95.
33. Wald A. Herpes simplex virus type 2 transmission: risk factors and virus shedding. Herpes. 2004;11(Suppl 3):130A–7A.
34. Looker KJ, Magaret AS, May MT, Turner KME, Vickerman P, Gottlieb SL, Newman LM. Global and regional estimates of prevalent and incident herpes simplex virus type 1 infections in 2012. PLoS One. 2015;10(10):e0140765.
35. Jolivet R, Sahli R, Meylan PRA. Herpès génital : l'épidémie silencieuse ? Rev Méd Suisse. 2001;3:21258.
36. Koelle DM, Wald A. Herpes simplex virus: the importance of asymptomatic shedding. J Antimicrob Chemother. 2000;45(Suppl T3):1–8.
37. Moazen B, Saeedi Moghaddam S, Silbernagl MA, Lotfizadeh M, Bosworth RJ, Alammehrjerdi Z, Kinner SA, Wirtz AL, Bärnighausen TW, Stöver HJ, et al. Prevalence of drug injection, sexual activity, tattooing, and piercing among prison inmates. Epidemiol Rev. 2018;40(1):58–69.
38. Ndeffo-Mbah ML, Vigliotti VS, Skrip LA, Dolan K, Galvani AP. Dynamic models of infectious disease transmission in prisons and the general population. Epidemiol Rev. 2018;40(1):40–57.
39. Rich JD, Beckwith CG, Macmadu A, Marshall BDL, Brinkley-Rubinstein L, Amon JJ, Milloy MJ, King MRF, Sanchez J, Atwoli L, et al. Clinical care of incarcerated people with HIV, viral hepatitis, or tuberculosis. Lancet (London, England). 2016;388(10049):1103–14.

40. Tran NT, Dubost C, Baggio S, Gétaz L, Wolff H. Safer tattooing interventions in prisons: a systematic review and call to action. BMC Public Health. 2018;18(1):1015.

41. Tavoschi L, Vroling H, Madeddu G, Babudieri S, Monarca R, Vonk Noordegraaf-Schouten M, Beer N, Gomes Dias J, O'Moore É, Hedrich D, et al. Active case finding for communicable diseases in prison settings: increasing testing coverage and uptake among the prison population in the European Union/European economic area. Epidemiol Rev. 2018;40(1):105–20.

42. Nokhodian Z, Yazdani MR, Yaran M, Shoaei P, Mirian M, Ataei B, Babak A, Ataie M. Prevalence and risk factors of HIV, syphilis, hepatitis B and C among female prisoners in Isfahan, Iran. Hepat Mon. 2012;12(7):442–7.

43. Kazi AM, Shah SA, Jenkins CA, Shepherd BE, Vermund SH. Risk factors and prevalence of tuberculosis, human immunodeficiency virus, syphilis, hepatitis B virus, and hepatitis C virus among prisoners in Pakistan. Int J Infect Dis. 2010;14(Suppl 3):e60–6.

16

Oseltamivir in pregnancy and birth outcomes

Vera Ehrenstein[1]* ⓘ, Nickolaj Risbo Kristensen[1], Brigitta Ursula Monz[2], Barry Clinch[3], Andy Kenwright[3] and Henrik Toft Sørensen[1]

Abstract

Background: Prenatal exposure to influenza or fever is associated with risk of congenital malformations. Oseltamivir is used to treat influenza and to provide post-exposure prophylaxis. We examined the association between oseltamivir use during pregnancy and birth outcomes.

Methods: This was a nationwide registry-based prevalence study with individual level data linkage, in a setting of universal health care access. We included all recorded pregnancies in Denmark in 2002–2013, and used data from population registries to examine associations between dispensings for oseltamivir during pregnancy (first trimester, second/third trimester, none) and congenital malformations, foetal death, preterm birth, foetal growth, and low 5-min Apgar score. Adjusted odds ratios (ORs) and 95% confidence intervals (CIs) were computed using propensity score matching.

Results: The study included 946,176 pregnancies. Of these, 449 had first-trimester exposure and 1449 had second/third-trimester exposure to oseltamivir. Adjusted ORs following first-trimester exposure were 0.94 (95% CI 0.49 to 1.83) for any major congenital malformation and 1.75 (95% CI 0.51 to 5.98) for congenital heart defects, based on 7 exposed cases. The association with congenital heart defects was present for etiologically implausible exposure periods and for known safe exposures. There was no evidence of an association between prenatal exposure to oseltamivir and any of the other birth outcomes assessed.

Conclusions: The study does not provide evidence of risk associated with oseltamivir treatment additional to that associated with influenza infection.

Keywords: Congenital abnormalities, Epidemiology, H1N1 influenza, Oseltamivir

Background

Influenza infection during first trimester of gestation is associated with a 2.0-fold increased risk of any major malformation; a 3.3-fold increased risk of neural tube defects; a 1.6-fold increased risk of congenital heart defects; and with increased risks of several other types of malformations [1, 2]. Congenital heart defects are common, affecting 5–11 of 1000 live births [3], underscoring the importance of treatment and prevention of first-trimester viral infections and their sequelae. During the 2009–2010 pandemic, H1N1 influenza A infection was associated with adverse pregnancy outcomes [4, 5],

while treatment with a neuraminidase inhibitor (NAI) was associated with reduced risks of admission to intensive care units and lower mortality among pregnant women [4, 6]. Oseltamivir is a NAI used in treatment and post-exposure prophylaxis of influenza [7]. Evidence about pregnancy outcomes following oseltamivir exposure is reassuring [8–16], including a recent study based on routine health records from four European countries reporting no evidence of an increased risk of several birth outcomes following a NAI dispensing any time during gestation [16]. Nevertheless, previous studies had limitations, which include, potential selection bias from lack of data on abortuses, and potential misclassification of the outcome, which could dilute associations.

We examined safety of prenatal exposure to oseltamivir as measured by major congenital malformations,

* Correspondence: ve@clin.au.dk
[1]Department of Clinical Epidemiology, Aarhus University Hospital, Olof Palmes Allé 43-45, 8200 Aarhus N, Denmark
Full list of author information is available at the end of the article

preterm birth, reduced foetal growth, low 5-min Apgar score, or foetal death. We addressed several limitations of previous studies by including pregnancies ending in abortive outcomes and ascertaining malformations through the first birthday; using a validated algorithm for congenital heart defects; and applying advanced methods of confounding control.

Methods

Data sources

We linked data from four population-based nationwide registries in Denmark: Danish Civil Registration System [17], Danish Medical Birth Registry [18], Danish National Patient Registry [19], and Danish National Prescription Registry [20]. Additional file 1: Table S1 provides a detailed description of all data sources, including specific types of data originating from each.

Study design, population, and period

We included all pregnancies in Denmark that started and ended between 01 January 2002 and 31 December 2013. Pregnancies ending in a live birth or a stillbirth (≥22 gestational weeks) were identified in the Danish Medical Birth Registry. Pregnancies ending earlier than 22 gestational weeks in abortive outcomes were identified from hospital diagnoses recorded in the Danish National Patient Registry. Starting in 2007, the Danish National Patient Registry had information on congenital malformations identified during second-trimester therapeutic pregnancy terminations.

Exposure

The Danish National Prescription Registry provided information on dispensings for oseltamivir at outpatient (community) pharmacies. The following mutually exclusive categories of oseltamivir exposure during pregnancy were defined: exposure during the first trimester regardless of exposure in the second or third trimester; exposure during the second or the third trimester but not in the first trimester; and no exposure at any time during pregnancy (the reference category). Because organogenesis is complete in the first trimester, we examined association of first-trimester oseltamivir exposure with congenital malformations. For the remaining birth outcomes, oseltamivir exposure at any trimester was considered.

Outcomes

Congenital malformations, identified from diagnoses recorded at therapeutic second trimester abortions (2007–2013), at stillbirth, and up to 1 year postnatally in liveborn infants, were classified according to the major EUROCAT categories [3]. The Danish National Patient Registry is nearly 99% complete for diagnoses of

congenital malformations [21]. For congenital heart defects, we used an algorithm developed specifically for the Danish National Patient Registry, based on the EUROCAT-specified diagnostic codes combined with therapeutic cardiac procedures [22]. The positive predictive value of this algorithm, estimated on a random sample of cases observed in this study, was 94.6% (95% confidence interval 89.2% to 97.7%). The other pregnancy outcomes were stillbirth at ≥22 weeks of gestation; foetal death (spontaneous or induced abortion before 22 weeks of gestation); preterm birth (gestational age 22- < 37 weeks) among live and stillbirths; small for gestational age (SGA) (birth weight below 10th percentile of the sex- and gestational-week-specific weight distribution) among live and stillbirths; and low 5-min Apgar score (< 7) among live births. For non-singleton pregnancies, a given outcome was considered present if recorded in at least one foetus/newborn.

Covariates

We assessed the following covariates based on their known associations with the birth outcomes: maternal age at conception, calendar year of conception, smoking as reported at the first prenatal visit (for live and stillbirths); pre-pregnancy body mass index (BMI) for live and stillbirths; mode of delivery; parity; marital status; birth of a previous child with a malformation (since 1994); indicators of maternal health care utilization (hospitalizations, visits to hospital outpatient specialist clinics, emergency room visits, dispensings for specific drug classes); maternal inpatient or outpatient morbidity (respiratory disease, cardiovascular disease, haematological disease, diabetes, neurological disease, liver or kidney disease, rheumatic disease, inflammatory bowel disease, obesity, immunodeficiency, disorders of female pelvic organs/genital tract, hospital contact for injury or poisoning); maternal outpatient dispensings for antidepressants, antiepileptics, antidiabetics, antihypertensives, drugs for ulcer/gastroesophageal reflux, oral contraceptives, drugs for in-vitro fertilization, thyroid hormones, systemic corticosteroids, non-steroidal anti-inflammatory drugs, opiates, and systemic anti-infective agents other than oseltamivir. Data on all diagnoses originated from inpatient or outpatient hospital diagnoses (secondary care), while data on medication dispensings originated from primary care and outpatient prescribing. The covariates were ascertained during 12 months preconception. Information on influenza status was not available from any data source. Definitions of the study variables appear in Additional file 1: Table S2 and Table S3.

Statistical analyses

We described the distributions of the pregnancy characteristics according to exposure to oseltamivir using appropriate descriptive statistics. For all outcomes except spontaneous or induced abortions, prevalence was used as the measure of occurrence. Crude and adjusted odds ratios (ORs) were computed using logistic regression. Pregnancies that ended before the second trimester were excluded from the analyses of second/third trimester exposure. For abortions, incidence rate was used, with hazard ratios estimated via Cox's proportional-hazards regression, with oseltamivir exposure treated as a time-varying variable [23]. All estimates were reported with 95% confidence intervals (CIs).

Confounding was addressed using two approaches: propensity score matching and conventional adjustment using multivariate regression with generalised estimating equations to account for within-woman correlation. Propensity score matching was considered superior in control of measured confounding, while conventional adjustment allowed use of all available observations and provided the context to evaluate the direction of estimates' change in response to tighter confounding control [24].

A propensity score for each pregnancy was computed, using logistic regression, as the probability of an oseltamivir dispensing given the covariates. Separate propensity scores were computed for the first-trimester and for the second/third-trimester exposure. Unexposed pregnancies were matched to exposed pregnancies on propensity score using nearest-neighbour matching with a caliper width of 0.2 standard deviations of the logit of the propensity score [25]. The balance of baseline characteristics was assessed post-matching, using standardised mean differences, whereby a value of ≤0.1 was considered indicative of balance. Per protocol, up to 100 oseltamivir-unexposed pregnancies were planned to be matched to each oseltamivir-exposed pregnancy. Post-matching assessment of the resulting balance indicated that only 1:1 matching achieved the target covariate balance. This 1:1 matched sample was used in propensity-score analysis, as it was deemed to remove most of the measured confounding. The covariates included in the propensity scores and the balancing statistics before and after matching are described in Additional file 1: Tables S4–S5, and Figure S1.

In conventionally adjusted analyses, we included all covariates with prevalence ≥5% or those inducing a >10% change in the crude OR. The final model included binary variables for parity (0 vs. > 0); marital status; smoking; obesity (BMI ≥30 kg/m^2 or a hospital-based diagnosis of obesity); any chronic illness (cardiovascular disease, haematological disease, diabetes, neurological disease, liver or kidney disease, rheumatic disease or inflammatory bowel disease); and respiratory disease. In addition, all models included variables for mother's age at conception (as a cubic spline) and for prior delivery of a child with a malformation. Smoking is not recorded for pregnancies ending in abortive outcomes; therefore the sensitivity analyses that contained such pregnancies were not adjusted for smoking.

The main analyses were conducted based on pregnancies ending in a live or stillbirth using propensity score to control for confounding. Since confounding by indication was expected to persist in this setting, several prespecified and post hoc sensitivity analyses were conducted for the malformation outcomes to obtain indirect evidence on confounding extent. First, we repeated the main analyses while including malformation diagnoses from terminated pregnancies (for pregnancies in 2007–2013). Second, we excluded mothers with a prior delivery of a child with a malformation. Third, we assessed risks of malformations associated with dispensing for oseltamivir during the main organogenesis period (gestational weeks 4–10 [26]). Fourth, we conducted several 'negative control' analyses [27]: examining effects of oseltamivir dispensing during periods etiologically implausible with respect to inducing major malformations (12 to 3 months preconception; second/third trimester of pregnancy). Fifth, we repeated the analysis replacing first-trimester exposure to oseltamivir with first-trimester exposure to penicillin, which is an anti-infective agent without evidence of teratogenicity [28] but presumed to correlate with presence of an infectious process, including fever. Finally, we examined the distribution of specific types of congenital heart defects for potential clustering, as clustering would support a causal association.

The analyses were conducted using SAS®, version 9.4 (Cary, NC, USA). Results were presented only when the individual cell counts in tables exceeded 5 observations, as specified by the Danish Data Protection Law (www.datatilsynet.dk) and/or regulations of Statistics Denmark (www.dst.dk).

Results

Between 01 January 2002 and 31 December 2013, 948,819 pregnancies started and ended in Denmark. After excluding 2643 (0.3%) pregnancies with invalid personal identifiers, 946,176 pregnancies remained in the analysis. Among these, 1898 (0.2%) pregnancies were exposed to oseltamivir: 449 during the first trimester and 1449 during the second or third trimester (Fig. 1). Of the oseltamivir-exposed pregnancies, 92% were exposed during 2009–2010. Table 1 presents characteristics of pregnancies included in the main analysis according to oseltamivir exposure, before and after propensity score matching.

Table 2 shows crude and adjusted odds ratios for the association of first-trimester exposure to oseltamivir with congenital malformations. Of the 19 first-trimester-exposed pregnancies with major congenital malformations, 8 were congenital heart defects. Among the 670,602

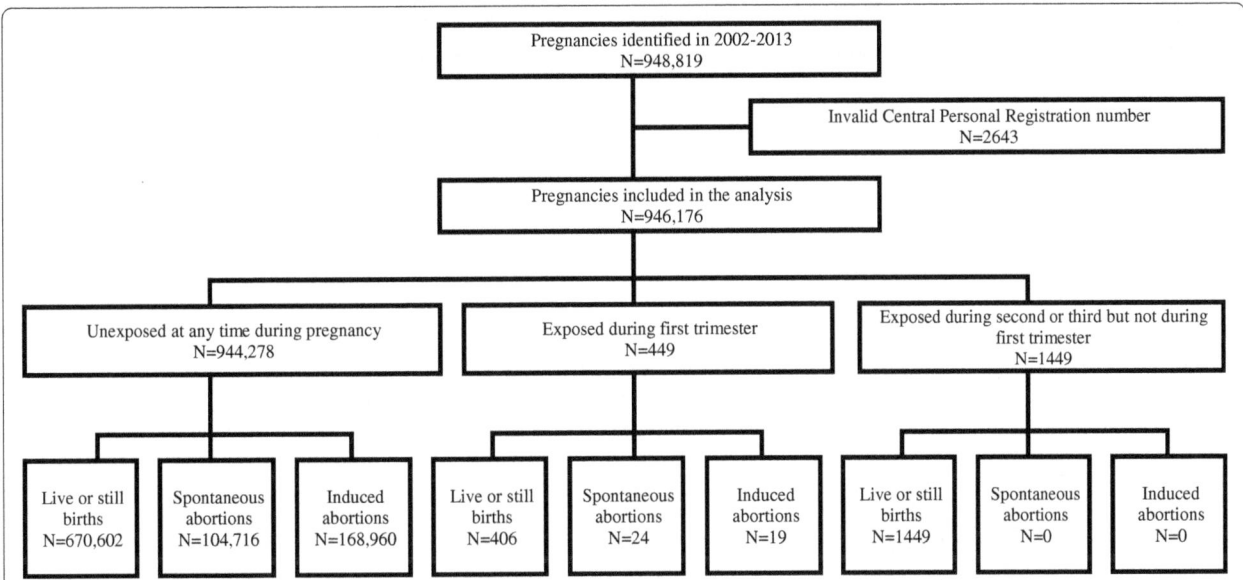

Fig. 1 Identification of pregnancies beginning and ending in 2002–2013, Denmark

oseltamivir-unexposed pregnancies, prevalence of any major malformation was 3.7% and prevalence of congenital heart defects was 0.7%. Among the 406 pregnancies with first-trimester oseltamivir exposure, the prevalence of any malformation was 4.7% and the prevalence of congenital heart defects was 2.0%. The odds ratios from propensity-score matched regression analysis were 0.94 (95% CI 0.49 to 1.83) for any malformation and 1.75 (95% CI 0.51 to 5.98) for congenital heart defects. Associations for congenital heart defects were also observed in the negative control sensitivity analyses of dispensing during second or third trimester (Table 3).

Table 4 presents results for the outcomes SGA, preterm birth, low 5-min Apgar score, and stillbirth. Based on propensity-score adjusted analyses, most odds ratios were close to 1.0. Some propensity-score-matched estimates were imprecise and therefore should be interpreted with caution. Table 5 shows the association between pregnancy exposure to oseltamivir and spontaneous or induced abortions, with oseltamivir as a time-varying exposure, based on 861 pregnancies exposed to oseltamivir. Adjusted incidence rate ratios associated with oseltamivir exposure were 0.99 (95% CI 0.66 to 1.48) for spontaneous abortion and 0.64 (95% CI 0.41 to 1.00) for induced abortion. No clustering of specific congenital heart defects was observed (data not shown).

Discussion
Main findings
In this population-based study, prenatal exposure to oseltamivir was not associated with increased risks of any major congenital malformation, foetal death,

preterm birth, SGA or low 5-min Apgar score. For congenital heart defects, defined using a validated algorithm with high positive predictive value and completeness, exposure to oseltamivir during the first trimester was associated with an adjusted odds ratio of 1.75 (95% CI 0.51 to 5.98) based on live and stillbirths, and with an adjusted odds ratio of 2.00 (95% CI 0.60 to 6.64) after inclusion of malformations from terminated pregnancies. The association persisted for oseltamivir exposure in the second or third trimester, i.e., after completion of the organogenesis. There was no clustering of specific congenital heart defects among foetuses with first-trimester oseltamivir exposure. Because of low prevalence of oseltamivir exposure, associations with other major congenital malformations could not be evaluated.

Limitations
Important limitations of the present analysis are the low number of exposed cases and the lack of systematic data on influenza status. It is plausible to assume that during the 2009–2010 H1N1 influenza A pandemic, most oseltamivir use in pregnancy was therapeutic rather than prophylactic. This essentially guaranteed confounding by indication, especially since the unexposed pregnancies, the overwhelming majority of which were not affected by influenza, were used as the comparator in the analysis. An ideal comparator population would be composed of pregnancies affected by influenza but not treated with oseltamivir to provide the background risk of outcomes in influenza affected population. Instead, the comparator population of unexposed pregnancies

Table 1 Characteristics of pregnancies resulting in a live or still birth, by exposure to oseltamivir

Characteristic	Before propensity score matching			After propensity score matching			
	Unexposed to oseltamivir during pregnancy	Exposed during first trimester	Exposed during second or third trimester	Unexposed to oseltamivir during pregnancy	Exposed during first trimester	Unexposed to oseltamivir during pregnancy	Exposed during second or third trimester
Number	670,602	406	1449	397	397	1420	1420
Age at conception (years)							
< 20	14,636 (2.2)	11 (2.7)	32 (2.2)	6 (1.5)	11 (2.8)	23 (1.6)	31 (2.2)
20-35	549,563 (82.0)	310 (76.4)	1114 (76.9)	301 (75.8)	303 (76.3)	1109 (78.1)	1088 (76.6)
≥ 35	106,403 (15.9)	85 (20.9)	303 (20.9)	90 (22.7)	83 (20.9)	288 (20.3)	301 (21.2)
Age at conception (years)							
Median (IQR)	30 (26–33)	30 (27–34)	30 (27–34)	31 (27–34)	30 (27–34)	31 (27–34)	30 (27–34)
Mean (SD)	30.0 (4.9)	30.7 (5.0)	30.8 (4.9)	31.1 (4.9)	30.8 (5.0)	31.0 (4.8)	30.8 (4.9)
Calendar year of conception							
2002-2008	426,697 (63.6)	18 (4.4)	60 (4.1)	241 (60.7)	18 (4.5)	845 (59.5)	60 (4.2)
2009-2010	118,496 (17.7)	376 (92.6)	1335 (92.1)	78 (19.6)	367 (92.4)	265 (18.7)	1310 (92.3)
2011-2013	125,409 (18.7)	12 (3.0)	54 (3.7)	78 (19.6)	12 (3.0)	310 (21.8)	50 (3.5)
Unmarried	357,106 (53.3)	191 (47.0)	663 (45.8)	184 (46.3)	185 (46.6)	623 (43.9)	645 (45.4)
Pre-pregnancy body mass index (kg/m²)							
< 18.5	24,336 (3.6)	20 (4.9)	46 (3.2)	6 (1.5)	20 (5.0)	55 (3.9)	46 (3.2)
18.5- < 25.0	355,498 (53.0)	238 (58.6)	835 (57.6)	204 (51.4)	233 (58.7)	766 (53.9)	822 (57.9)
25.0- < 30.0	118,521 (17.7)	84 (20.7)	305 (21.0)	75 (18.9)	83 (20.9)	269 (18.9)	300 (21.1)
≥ 30	70,259 (10.5)	54 (13.3)	212 (14.6)	48 (12.1)	52 (13.1)	166 (11.7)	206 (14.5)
Missing	101,988 (15.2)	10 (2.5)	51 (3.5)	64 (16.1)	9 (2.3)	164 (11.5)	46 (3.2)
Smoking							
No	561,830 (83.8)	351 (86.5)	1258 (86.8)	358 (90.2)	351 (88.4)	1275 (89.8)	1258 (88.6)
Yes	95,528 (14.2)	46 (11.3)	162 (11.2)	39 (9.8)	46 (11.6)	145 (10.2)	162 (11.4)
Missing[a]	13,244 (2.0)	9 (2.2)	29 (2.0)	–	–	–	–
Parity							
0	314,229 (46.9)	136 (33.5)	441 (30.4)	122 (30.7)	132 (33.2)	415 (29.2)	427 (30.1)
1	242,531 (36.2)	183 (45.1)	637 (44.0)	187 (47.1)	179 (45.1)	654 (46.1)	627 (44.2)
2	86,863 (13.0)	64 (15.8)	296 (20.4)	67 (16.9)	63 (15.9)	270 (19.0)	292 (20.6)
> 2	26,979 (4.0)	23 (5.7)	75 (5.2)	21 (5.3)	23 (5.8)	81 (5.7)	74 (5.2)
Prior delivery of a child with a malformation (since 1994)	20,171 (3.0)	16 (3.9)	67 (4.6)	19 (4.8)	16 (4.0)	72 (5.1)	64 (4.5)
Hospital history during 12 months before conception[b]							
At least one inpatient hospitalization	124,627 (18.6)	83 (20.4)	334 (23.1)	75 (18.9)	79 (19.9)	270 (19.0)	327 (23.0)
At least one visit to outpatient specialist clinic	232,129 (34.6)	169 (41.6)	609 (42.0)	155 (39.0)	165 (41.6)	570 (40.1)	597 (42.0)
At least one emergency room visit	85,760 (12.8)	80 (19.7)	215 (14.8)	69 (17.4)	77 (19.4)	180 (12.7)	211 (14.9)
Respiratory diseases	33,405 (5.0)	39 (9.6)	90 (6.2)	38 (9.6)	39 (9.8)	89 (6.3)	89 (6.3)
Cardiovascular disease	7760 (1.2)	7 (1.7)	30 (2.1)	5 (1.3)	6 (1.5)	15 (1.1)	29 (2.0)
Haematological disease	2364 (0.4)	5 (1.2)	15 (1.0)	0 (0.0)	5 (1.3)	8 (0.6)	15 (1.1)
Diabetes	10,590 (1.6)	5 (1.2)	38 (2.6)	7 (1.8)	5 (1.3)	29 (2.0)	37 (2.6)
Neurological disease[b]	5654 (0.8)	5 (1.2)	20 (1.4)	–	–	–	–
Obesity[c]	73,216 (10.9)	56 (13.8)	222 (15.3)	49 (12.3)	54 (13.6)	174 (12.3)	216 (15.2)

Table 1 Characteristics of pregnancies resulting in a live or still birth, by exposure to oseltamivir *(Continued)*

Characteristic	Before propensity score matching			After propensity score matching			
	Unexposed to oseltamivir during pregnancy	Exposed during first trimester	Exposed during second or third trimester	Unexposed to oseltamivir during pregnancy	Exposed during first trimester	Unexposed to oseltamivir during pregnancy	Exposed during second or third trimester
Disorders of female pelvic organs/genital tract	44,730 (6.7)	32 (7.9)	86 (5.9)	25 (6.3)	32 (8.1)	70 (4.9)	84 (5.9)
Hospital contact for injury or poisoning	60,037 (9.0)	51 (12.6)	148 (10.2)	51 (12.8)	50 (12.6)	130 (9.2)	144 (10.1)
Use of prescription medication in the 12 months before conception							
Antidepressants	34,293 (5.1)	30 (7.4)	115 (7.9)	29 (7.3)	29 (7.3)	105 (7.4)	109 (7.7)
Drugs for ulcer/ gastroesophageal reflux	26,456 (3.9)	27 (6.7)	84 (5.8)	18 (4.5)	26 (6.5)	80 (5.6)	83 (5.8)
Oral contraceptives	243,936 (36.4)	156 (38.4)	534 (36.9)	173 (43.6)	153 (38.5)	517 (36.4)	523 (36.8)
Drugs for in-vitro fertilization	54,563 (8.1)	43 (10.6)	116 (8.0)	35 (8.8)	43 (10.8)	103 (7.3)	114 (8.0)
Thyroid hormones	7284 (1.1)	8 (2.0)	25 (1.7)	8 (2.0)	8 (2.0)	31 (2.2)	24 (1.7)
Systemic corticosteroids	13,005 (1.9)	17 (4.2)	49 (3.4)	17 (4.3)	16 (4.0)	41 (2.9)	49 (3.5)
Non-steroidal anti-inflammatory drugs	98,907 (14.7)	78 (19.2)	268 (18.5)	66 (16.6)	77 (19.4)	252 (17.7)	261 (18.4)
Opiates	21,777 (3.2)	18 (4.4)	58 (4.0)	17 (4.3)	17 (4.3)	76 (5.4)	57 (4.0)
Systemic anti-infective agents other than oseltamivir	278,680 (41.6)	195 (48.0)	734 (50.7)	189 (47.6)	190 (47.9)	740 (52.1)	719 (50.6)
Number of different drugs classes dispensed, median (IQR)	1 (1–2)	2 (1–3)	2 (1-3)	2 (1–3)	2 (1–3)	2 (1–3)	2 (1–3)

IQR interquartile range, *SD* standard deviation

[a]Matching of the unexposed pregnancies was done separately for those exposed in the first trimester and those exposed in the second or third trimester. No matching of pregnancies with missing data on smoking

[b]Not reported for the following protocol-specified characteristics because of low (< 5) group counts: liver and kidney disease; rheumatic disease; inflammatory bowel disease; immunodeficiency, and use of antiepileptics. In the propensity-score matched dataset neurologic diseases also not reported. [c]Defined by pre-pregnancy body mass index or a hospital diagnosis of obesity. Data are n (%) unless otherwise specified

represented the prevalence of congenital malformations in the general Danish population, i.e., an overall prevalence of malformations close to that reported for Denmark by the EUROCAT, based on a representative sample (2002–2012 total prevalence per 1000 births: 30 [95% CI 28 to 31] for any malformation; 9.1 [95% CI 8.4 to 10.0] for congenital heart defects [3]). The most recent analysis involving Scandinavian data [16] excluded pregnancies with a hospital-based diagnosis of influenza. This was done to reduce confounding by

indication, but may have potentially introduced selection bias by excluding the most severely affected pregnancies from the study population. In our study, excluding women with a hospital diagnosis of influenza did not materially affect the findings (conventionally adjusted OR for any major congenital malformation 1.20 [95% CI: 0.74 to 1.95]).

Several considerations point to residual confounding These include increasing attenuation of odds ratios in response to closer confounding control; persisting

Table 2 First-trimester exposure to oseltamivir and congenital malformations among live or stillbirths

Outcome	Unexposed N = 670,602	Exposed N = 406	Crude odds ratio (95% CI)	Adjusted odds ratio (95% CI)	
				Conventional regression analysis[a]	Propensity-score matched regression analysis[b]
Any major congenital malformation	24,773 (3.7%)	19 (4.7%)	1.28 (0.81 to 2.03)	1.25 (0.78 to 2.01)	0.94 (0.49 to 1.83)
Congenital heart defects	4795 (0.7%)	8 (2.0%)	2.79 (1.39 to 5.62)	2.51 (1.19 to 5.31)	1.75 (0.51 to 5.98)

CI confidence interval

[a]Adjusted for age at conception, parity, smoking, marital status, obesity, prior delivery of a child with a malformation, respiratory diseases, any other chronic illness (cardiovascular disease, haematological disease, diabetes, neurological disease [including antidepressants or antiepileptics use], liver or kidney disease, rheumatic disease or inflammatory bowel disease) during the 12 months before conception

[b]Sample size: exposed = 397; unexposed = 397; prevalence of any major malformation, exposed/unexposed: 4.5%/4.8%; prevalence of congenital heart defects, exposed/unexposed: 1.8%/1.0%

Table 3 Sensitivity analyses of the outcome of congenital malformations following exposure to oseltamivir in pregnancy

	Conventional regression analysis			Propensity-score matched regression analysis		
	Unexposed	Exposed	Odds ratio (95% CI) [a]	Unexposed	Exposed	Odds ratio (95% CI) [b]
Analysis including pregnancies terminated due to congenital malformations (2007-2013), prespecified						
Number	521,037	432		432	432	
Any major congenital malformation	16,692 (3.2%)	22 (5.1%)	1.58 (1.03 to 2.44)	20 (4.6%)	22 (5.1%)	1.10 (0.60 to 2.02)
Congenital heart defects	3005 (0.6%)	8 (1.9%)	3.17 (1.57 to 6.40)	4 (0.9%)	8 (1.9%)	2.00 (0.60 to 6.64)
Pregnancies among women without an earlier pregnancy resulting in a malformed child, post hoc						
Number	650,431	390		381	381	
Any major malformation	23,712 (3.7%)	18 (4.6%)	1.26 (0.77 to 2.04)	20 (5.3%)	17 (4.5%)	0.84 (0.43 to 1.64)
Congenital heart defects	4598 (0.7%)	8 (2.1%)	2.68 (1.27 to 5.68)	5 (1.3%)	7 (1.8%)	1.50 (0.42 to 5.32)
First trimester exposure to oseltamivir, defined as oseltamivir dispensing during 4-10 weeks of gestation, post hoc						
Number	670,602	212		205	205	
Any major malformation	24,773 (3.7%)	8 (3.8%)	0.91 (0.43 to 1.95)	8 (3.9%)	7 (3.4%)	0.88 (0.32 to 2.41)
Congenital heart defects	4795 (0.7%)	5 (2.4%)	2.70 (1.00 to 7.29)	N/A		
Oseltamivir dispensing in second or third trimester (post-organogenesis), prespecified						
Number	670,602	1449		1420	1420	
Any major malformation	24,773 (3.7%)	64 (4.4%)	1.18 (0.91 to 1.53)	51 (3.6%)	61 (4.3%)	1.21 (0.82 to 1.77)
Congenital heart defects	4795 (0.7%)	21 (1.5%)	2.10 (1.36 to 3.24)	6 (0.4%)	21 (1.5%)	3.50 (1.41 to 8.67)
Exposure to oseltamivir between 12 and 3 months preconception, post hoc						
Number	669,934	538		530	530	
Any major malformation	24,745 (3.7%)	24 (4.5%)	1.20 (0.80 to 1.80)	19 (3.6%)	24 (4.5%)	1.28 (0.69 to 2.37)
Congenital heart defects	N/A					
First-trimester exposure to penicillin, post hoc [c]						
Number	471,117	70,309		Analysis not conducted		
Any major malformation	17,148 (3.6%)	2798 (4.0%)	1.09 (1.04 to 1.13)			
Congenital heart defects	3296 (0.7%)	599 (0.9%)	1.17 (1.07 to 1.29)			

CI confidence interval, N/A not applicable (counts too low to report)
[a]Adjusted for age at conception, parity, smoking, marital status, obesity, prior delivery of a child with a malformation, respiratory diseases, any other chronic illness (cardiovascular disease, haematological disease, diabetes, neurological disease [including use of antidepressants or antiepileptics], liver or kidney disease, rheumatic disease, or inflammatory bowel disease) during 12 months before conception
[b]Variables included in estimation of propensity scores are listed in the Additional file 1
[c]Exposure to penicillin for malformations (any, congenital heart defects) among live born and stillborn infants conceived and delivered in 2002-2013 in Denmark

associations for the negative control exposures, for which no association was expected unless caused by confounding – i.e., in periods after the organogenesis is expected to be complete. At the same time, the ORs for congenital heart defects were similar to those reported in other studies for first-trimester fever (1.54 [95% CI 1.37 to 1.74]) [29] or first-trimester influenza infection (1.56 [95% CI 1.13 to 2.14]) [1]. The lower precision of the odds ratios obtained in the propensity score matched analysis was the trade-off taken for maximising validity via 1:1 matching. Other limitations of this analysis are potential misclassification of exposure status by relying on dispensing records, by lack of information on oseltamivir dispensed during hospital stays, and by potential errors in recorded gestational age.

Other evidence
Taken together, the available evidence is not consistent with harmful pregnancy effects of oseltamivir or other NAIs [8, 10–16]. A Canadian study of more than 55,000 pregnant women, including 1237 exposed to oseltamivir during the H1N1 pandemic, reported no evidence of an association between prenatal exposure to oseltamivir and preterm birth, low Apgar scores, or poor foetal growth [12]. Similarly, a study in Texas based on 135 oseltamivir-exposed pregnancies did not suggest harmful pregnancy effects [13]. The most recent study, conducted by Graner et al. [16], used linked databases from four European countries, including the same source data for Denmark as used in the current study and investigated similar outcomes.

Table 4 Prenatal exposure to oseltamivir and SGA, preterm birth, low 5-min Apgar score, and stillbirth

	Unexposed	Exposed	Crude odds ratio (95% CI)	Conventional regression analysis, odds ratio (95% CI)	Propensity score-matched regression analysis, odds ratio (95% CI)[c]
First trimester					
Number	670,602	406			
Small for gestational age	64,944 (9.7%)	32 (7.9%)	0.80 (0.56 to 1.14)	0.88 (0.61 to 1.26)	0.75 (0.46 to 1.24)
Preterm birth	42,399 (6.3%)	28 (6.9%)	1.10 (0.75 to 1.61)	1.21 (0.83 to 1.79)	0.87 (0.52 to 1.46)
Low 5-min Apgar score[a]	5429 (0.8%)	5 (1.2%)	1.52 (0.63 to 3.68)	1.64 (0.68 to 3.97)	1.00 (0.29 to 3.45)
Second/third trimester					
Number	670,602	1449			
Small for gestational age	64,944 (9.7%)	121 (8.3%)	0.85 (0.71 to 1.02)	0.94 (0.77 to 1.13)	0.84 (0.64 to 1.10)
Preterm birth	42,399 (6.3%)	79 (5.4%)	0.85 (0.68 to 1.07)	0.89 (0.70 to 1.12)	0.85 (0.62 to 1.16)
Low 5-min Apgar score[a]	5429 (0.8%)	10 (0.7%)	0.85 (0.46 to 1.59)	0.92 (0.49 to 1.71)	1.25 (0.49 to 3.17)
Stillbirth[b]	3047 (0.4%)	7 (0.5%)	1.06 (0.51 to 2.24)	1.13 (0.50 to 2.52)	1.20 (0.37 to 3.93)

Data are n (%) or odds ratio (95% CI) unless otherwise specified
SGA small for gestational age, CI confidence interval
[a]Live born only
[b]Live or stillborn at ≥22 weeks of gestation; data not shown for first-trimester exposure because of low counts
[c]Variables included in estimation of propensity scores are listed in the Additional file 1

Graner et al. identified seven cases of congenital heart malformations in 814 first trimester oseltamivir-exposed pregnancies, resulting in a (conventionally) adjusted odds ratio of 0.96 (95% CI 0.43 to 2.15). Our study detected eight congenital heart defects in less than half as many exposed pregnancies ($N = 406$). This may be explained by the extension of the case detection period to up to 1 year postnatally. The differences in the conventionally adjusted odds ratios in our study compared with the study by Graner et al. (2.51 versus 0.96) may have resulted from our decision not to exclude pregnancies with hospital influenza diagnoses, combined with the higher prevalence of congenital heart defects among offspring of exposed women in our study population.

Interpretation
The OR for congenital heart defects associated with the first-trimester exposure to oseltamivir was of comparable size to that reported for influenza infection or fever, indicating that despite close control of confounding, in

the setting of pregnancy, a nearly full confounding by influenza status is likely. The association was also observed during etiologically implausible periods, such as periods after completion of organogenesis; furthermore, the ORs weakened in response to successive control of measured confounding, from crude ORs (fully confounded) to conventionally adjusted ORs (some residual confounding) to propensity-score adjusted ORs (least residual confounding). Lack of clustering of specific congenital heart defects among foetuses with first-trimester oseltamivir exposure although does not disprove it, argues against the causality underlying the observed association [30]. Thus, this study in the context of the available evidence is consistent with adverse pregnancy outcomes being associated with influenza infection itself.

Conclusions
The study does not provide evidence of risk associated with oseltamivir treatment additional to that previously known to be associated with influenza infection.

Table 5 Exposure to oseltamivir in pregnancy and spontaneous or induced abortions

Type of abortion	Exposed[a]		Unexposed		Crude hazard ratio (95% CI)	Adjusted[b] hazard ratio (95% CI)
Spontaneous or induced	43	122	273,676	293,663	0.77 (0.57 to 1.04)	0.79 (0.59 to 1.07)
Spontaneous	24	122	104,716	293,663	1.00 (0.67 to 1.50)	0.99 (0.66 to 1.48)
Induced	19	122	168,960	293,663	0.59 (0.38 to 0.93)	0.64 (0.41 to 1.00)

CI confidence interval
[a]Based on 861 gestations exposed to oseltamivir
[b]Adjusted for age at conception, parity, smoking, marital status, obesity, prior delivery of a child with a malformation, respiratory diseases, any other chronic illness [cardiovascular disease, haematological disease, diabetes, neurological disease (including use of antidepressants or antiepileptics), liver or kidney disease, rheumatic disease or inflammatory bowel disease] during 12 months before conception
[c]Exposure to oseltamivir is analysed as time-varying variable

Abbreviations

BMI: Body mass index; CI: Confidence interval; ICD-10: International Classification of Diseases, Tenth Revision; IQR: Interquartile range; N/A: Not applicable; NAI: Neuraminidase inhibitor; OR: Odds ratio; SD: Standard deviation; SGA: Small for gestational age

Acknowledgements

We are grateful to Dr. Morten Olsen for expert advice on cardiac malformations and for conducting the case adjudication; and to the research nurses Henriette Kristoffersen and Hanne Moeslund Madsen for medical chart abstraction.

Funding

This study was funded by F. Hoffmann-La Roche Ltd. through an institutional research agreement with Aarhus University. It was designed as a Post-Authorization Safety Study in consultation with the European Medicines Agency). Employees of the funding source (BM, BC, and AK) were involved in the study design, the interpretation of data, writing of the manuscript, and the decision to submit the paper for publication. The funding source was not involved in collection or analysis of data. All authors had full access to all analysis outputs and results. The corresponding author had final responsibility for the decision to submit for publication.

Authors' contributions

VE contributed to the study design, oversaw the analyses, drafted the manuscript, and revised it critically for important intellectual content. NRK contributed to the study design, conducted the data analyses, and revised the manuscript critically for important intellectual content. BUM contributed to study design, oversaw the analyses and contributed to interpretation of results. BC provided clinical expertise, and contributed to study design. AK provided statistical expertise and contributed to the analytic strategy. HTS contributed to the study design, acquired the data, and provided clinical and epidemiologic expertise. All authors critically revised the manuscript for intellectual contents. The authors listed above approved the version to be submitted and agree to be accountable for all aspects of the work in ensuring that questions related to the accuracy or integrity of any part of the work are appropriately investigated and resolved. All authors read and approved the final manuscript.

Competing interests

BM, BC and AK are full-time employees and hold stock and/or stock options in Roche, the manufacturer of oseltamivir. VE, NRK, and HTS are salaried employees of Aarhus University/Aarhus University Hospital. HTS is supported by the Program for Clinical Research Infrastructure (PROCRIN), established by the Lundbeck Foundation and the Novo Nordisk Foundation and administered by the Danish Regions. This study was funded by F. Hoffmann-La Roche Ltd. through a research agreement to and administered by Aarhus University.

Author details

[1]Department of Clinical Epidemiology, Aarhus University Hospital, Olof Palmes Allé 43-45, 8200 Aarhus N, Denmark. [2]F. Hoffmann-La Roche Ltd., Basel, Switzerland. [3]Roche Products Ltd., Welwyn Garden City, UK.

References

1. Luteijn JM, Brown MJ, Dolk H. Influenza and congenital anomalies: a systematic review and meta-analysis. Hum Reprod. 2014;29:809–23.
2. Acs N, Banhidy F, Puho E, Czeizel AE. Maternal influenza during pregnancy and risk of congenital abnormalities in offspring. Birth Defects Res A Clin Mol Teratol. 2005;73:989–96.
3. European Surveillance of Congenital Anomalies EUROCAT Guide 1.4, Section 3.3 EUROCAT Subgroups of Congenital Anomalies (Version 2014). 2014. http://www.eurocat-network.eu/content/EUROCAT-Guide-1.4-Section-3.3.pdf. Accessed 16 July 2017.
4. Mosby LG, Rasmussen SA, Jamieson DJ. 2009 pandemic influenza A (H1N1) in pregnancy: a systematic review of the literature. Am J Obstet Gynecol. 2011;205:10–8.
5. Pierce M, Kurinczuk JJ, Spark P, Brocklehurst P, Knight M. Perinatal outcomes after maternal 2009/H1N1 infection: national cohort study. BMJ. 2011;342: d3214.
6. Muthuri SG, Venkatesan S, Myles PR, Leonardi-Bee J, Al Khuwaitir TS, Al Mamun A, Anovadiya AP, Azziz-Baumgartner E, Baez C, Bassetti M, et al.
7. McKimm-Breschkin JL. Influenza neuraminidase inhibitors: antiviral action and mechanisms of resistance. Influenza Other Respir Viruses. 2013;7(Suppl 1):25–36.
8. Beau AB, Hurault-Delarue C, Vial T, Montastruc JL, Damase-Michel C, Lacroix I. Safety of oseltamivir during pregnancy: a comparative study using the EFEMERIS database. BJOG. 2014;121:895–900.
9. Berveiller P, Mir O, Vinot C, Bonati C, Duchene P, Giraud C, Gil S, Treluyer JM. Transplacental transfer of oseltamivir and its metabolite using the human perfused placental cotyledon model. Am J Obstet Gynecol. 2012;206:92 e1–6.
10. Dunstan HJ, Mill AC, Stephens S, Yates LM, Thomas SH. Pregnancy outcome following maternal use of zanamivir or oseltamivir during the 2009 influenza a/H1N1 pandemic: a national prospective surveillance study. BJOG. 2014;121:901–6.
11. Wollenhaupt M, Chandrasekaran A, Tomianovic D. The safety of oseltamivir in pregnancy: an updated review of post-marketing data. Pharmacoepidemiol Drug Saf. 2014;23:1035–42.
12. Xie HY, Yasseen AS 3rd, Xie RH, Fell DB, Sprague AE, Liu N, Smith GN, Walker MC, Wen SW. Infant outcomes among pregnant women who used oseltamivir for treatment of influenza during the H1N1 epidemic. Am J Obstet Gynecol. 2013;208:293 e1–7.
13. Greer LG, Sheffield JS, Rogers VL, Roberts SW, McIntire DD, Wendel GD Jr. Maternal and neonatal outcomes after antepartum treatment of influenza with antiviral medications. Obstet Gynecol. 2010;115:711–6.
14. Donner B, Niranjan V, Hoffmann G. Safety of oseltamivir in pregnancy: a review of preclinical and clinical data. Drug Saf. 2010;33:631–42.
15. Saito S, Minakami H, Nakai A, Unno N, Kubo T, Yoshimura Y. Outcomes of infants exposed to oseltamivir or zanamivir in utero during pandemic (H1N1) 2009. Am J Obstet Gynecol. 2013;209:130.e1–9.
16. Graner S, Svensson T, Beau AB, Damase-Michel C, Engeland A, Furu K, Hviid A, Haberg SE, Molgaard-Nielsen D, Pasternak B, et al. Neuraminidase inhibitors during pregnancy and risk of adverse neonatal outcomes and congenital malformations: population based European register study. BMJ. 2017;356:j629.
17. Schmidt M, Pedersen L, Sorensen HT. The Danish civil registration system as a tool in epidemiology. Eur J Epidemiol. 2014;29:541–9.
18. Knudsen LB, Olsen J. The Danish medical birth registry. Dan Med Bull. 1998; 45:320–3.
19. Schmidt M, Schmidt SA, Sandegaard JL, Ehrenstein V, Pedersen L, Sorensen HT. The Danish National Patient Registry: a review of content, data quality, and research potential. Clin Epidemiol. 2015;7:449–90.
20. Kildemoes HW, Sorensen HT, Hallas J. The Danish National Prescription Registry. Scand J Public Health. 2011;39:38–41.
21. Larsen H, Nielsen GL, Bendsen J, Flint C, Olsen J, Sorensen HT. Predictive value and completeness of the registration of congenital abnormalities in three Danish population-based registries. Scand J Public Health. 2003;31:12–6.
22. Olsen M, Garne E, Svaerke C, Sondergaard L, Nissen H, Andersen HO, Hjortdal VE, Johnsen SP, Videbaek J. Cancer risk among patients with congenital heart defects: a nationwide follow-up study. Cardiol Young. 2014;24:40–6.
23. Savitz DA, Hertz-Picciotto I, Poole C, Olshan AF. Epidemiologic measures of the course and outcome of pregnancy. Epidemiol Rev. 2002;24:91–101.
24. Lawlor DA, Tilling K, Davey Smith G. Triangulation in aetiological epidemiology. Int J Epidemiol. 2016;45:1866–86.
25. Austin PC. A tutorial and case study in propensity score analysis: an application to estimating the effect of in-hospital smoking cessation counseling on mortality. Multivariate Behav Res. 2011;46:119–51.
26. Buhimschi CS, Weiner CP. Medications in pregnancy and lactation: part 1. Teratology. Obstet Gynecol. 2009;113:166–88.
27. Dusetzina SB, Brookhart MA, Maciejewski ML. Control outcomes and exposures for improving internal validity of nonrandomized studies. Health Serv Res. 2015;50:1432–51.
28. Jepsen P, Skriver MV, Floyd A, Lipworth L, Schonheyder HC, Sorensen HT. A population-based study of maternal use of amoxicillin and pregnancy outcome in Denmark. Br J Clin Pharmacol. 2003;55:216–21.
29. Dreier JW, Andersen AM, Berg-Beckhoff G. Systematic review and meta-analyses: fever in pregnancy and health impacts in the offspring. Pediatrics. 2014;133:e674–88.
30. Weiss NS. Can the "specificity" of an association be rehabilitated as a basis for supporting a causal hypothesis? Epidemiology. 2002;13:6–8.

Effectiveness of neuraminidase inhibitors in reducing mortality in patients admitted to hospital with influenza A H1N1pdm09 virus infection: a meta-analysis of individual participant data. Lancet Respir Med. 2014;2:395–404.

17

Treatment completion for latent tuberculosis infection in Norway: a prospective cohort study

Yvette Louise Schein[1], Tesfaye Madebo[2], Hilde Elise Andersen[3], Trude Margrete Arnesen[4], Anne Ma Dyrhol-Riise[5,6,7], Hallgeir Tveiten[8], Richard A. White[9] and Brita Askeland Winje[10]* (iD)

Abstract

Background: Successful treatment of latent tuberculosis infection (LTBI) is essential to reduce tuberculosis (TB) incidence rates in low-burden countries. This study measures treatment completion and determinants of non-completion of LTBI treatment in Norway in 2016.

Methods: This prospective cohort study included all individuals notified with LTBI treatment to the Norwegian Surveillance System for Infectious Diseases (MSIS) in 2016. We obtained data from MSIS and from a standardized form that was sent to health care providers at the time of patient notification to MSIS. We determined completion rates. Pearson's chi squared test was used to study associations between pairs of categorical variables and separate crude and multivariable logistic regression models were used to identify factors associated with treatment completion and adverse drug effects.

Results: We obtained information on treatment completion from 719 of the 726 individuals notified for LTBI treatment in 2016. Overall, 91% completed treatment. Treatment completion was highest in the foreign-born group [foreign-born, $n = 562$ (92%) vs Norwegian-born, $n = 115$ (85%), $p = 0.007$]. Treatment completion did not differ significantly between prescribed regimens ($p = 0.124$). Adverse events were the most common reason for incomplete treatment. We found no significant differences in adverse events when comparing weekly rifapentine (3RPH) with three months daily isoniazid and rifampicin (3RH). However, there were significantly fewer adverse events with 3RPH compared to other regimens ($p = 0.037$). Age over 35 years was significantly associated with adverse events irrespective of regimen ($p = 0.024$), whereas immunosuppression was not significantly associated with adverse events after adjusting for other variables ($p = 0.306$). Treatment under direct observation had a significant effect on treatment completion for foreign-born (multivariate Wald p-value = 0.017), but not for Norwegian-born (multivariate Wald p-value = 0.408) individuals.

Conclusions: We report a very high treatment completion rate, especially among individuals from countries with high TB incidence. The follow-up from tuberculosis-coordinators and the frequent use of directly observed treatment probably contributes to this. Few severe adverse events were reported, even with increased age and in individuals that are more susceptible. While these results are promising, issues of cost-effectiveness and targeting treatment to individuals at highest risk of TB are important components of public health impact.

Keywords: Latent tuberculosis infection, Preventive treatment, Rifapentine, Isoniazid, Rifampicin, Chemoprophylaxis, Compliance, Screening, Surveillance

* Correspondence: brita.winje@fhi.no
[10]Department of Vaccine Preventable Diseases, Norwegian Institute of Public Health, Oslo, Norway
Full list of author information is available at the end of the article

Background

Treatment of latent tuberculosis infection (LTBI) in groups at high risk for tuberculosis (TB) disease is a cornerstone in the global strategy to eliminate TB [1]. Norway has a mandatory screening program for TB and LTBI, which includes immigrants from high TB incidence countries, pre-employment screening, and outbreak management [2]. In addition, LTBI management is recommended prior to iatrogenic immunosuppression. In 2016, immigrants under the age of 35 from countries with TB incidence rates (IR) > 40 per 100,000 population (as estimated by WHO) were eligible for screening with IGRA (or equivalent) upon arrival in Norway. In addition, immigrants $\geq$ 15 years of age were screened for TB with a chest X-ray. In Norway's national guidelines, LTBI treatment is strongly recommended for children under the age of 5, contacts, those with fibrotic lesions on chest X-ray, or those with select immunosuppressive conditions (HIV-infection, haemodialysis, solid organ transplants, malignancies, or prior to iatrogenic immunosuppression). LTBI treatment is conditionally recommended for children aged 5–14 years, those with calcifications on chest X-ray, those who are underweight, and individuals with long-term steroid treatment, diabetes mellitus, or drug addiction. Being foreign-born was not considered a single criterion for priority for treatment at the time of the study [3].

The use of LTBI treatment has rapidly increased in Norway in recent years, stabilizing at around 750 cases per year [4, 5]. Individuals prescribed LTBI treatment are reported to the Norwegian Surveillance System for Infectious Diseases (MSIS) [6]. However, treatment completion, an important indicator of the impact, safety, and cost effectiveness of the screening program, is not routinely reported.

LTBI treatment completion rates vary considerably across risk-groups and settings [7], and long duration and adverse events are well-known barriers to treatment completion [7–12]. A Norwegian study from 2009 found overall high LTBI treatment completion, and no adverse events requiring hospital admission [13]. Since then, Norwegian guidelines have increasingly targeted groups at high risk for TB reactivation, including older individuals with more comorbidities and recent immigrants to Norway [3]. Recent immigrants are often difficult to follow-up due to their mobility and a lack of government-issued identification numbers [14, 15]. Additionally, the increasing use of immunosuppressants may pose new challenges to LTBI treatment strategy.

The most common LTBI regimen is a daily combination of rifampicin and isoniazid for three months (3RH). The increasing use of weekly-administered rifapentine (3RPH) [8], a newer and less-studied regimen, highlights the need for strengthened LTBI treatment surveillance. National guidelines currently recommend directly observed treatment (DOT) for this new 3RPH regimen.

Severe adverse events due to preventive treatment are primarily related to isoniazid induced peripheral neuropathy and hepatotoxicity, with higher rates found in those aged $\geq$ 35 years [12, 16], and hepatotoxicity, gastrointestinal intolerance, and hypersensitivity from rifamycins [12]. We question whether tolerance to adverse effects may be context specific, with lower tolerance in a country where TB is rare. If significant scale-up of LTBI treatment is indicated, information about adverse events and treatment completion by regimen will be highly relevant.

In Norway, prescription of TB drugs, including LTBI treatment, is the responsibility of pulmonologists, infectious disease specialists, or paediatricians who work primarily in hospital settings. The role of "TB coordinator" was introduced in the national TB control programme in 2003 to strengthen patient support and coordinate TB control between all healthcare levels [2]. One key responsibility of the coordinator is to establish a treatment plan for every individual starting TB treatment. The plan clearly states the responsibilities of all partners involved and seeks to maximize patient-involvement.

The objective of this study is to measure LTBI treatment completion and determinants of non-completion in all individuals notified to MSIS in 2016. We also assess the risk of severe adverse events related to treatment, and their consequences for the LTBI treatment strategy, and explore the use of associated healthcare resources.

Methods

Study participants

This is a nationwide prospective cohort study, including all individuals reported with LTBI treatment to MSIS between January 1, 2016 and December 31, 2016. The protocol is available as supplementary material (Additional file 1:). Data included demographic and clinical information available through MSIS, and additional data on treatment completion, adverse events, patient support, and use of healthcare resources collected through a standardized treatment completion form that was sent to prescribing clinicians and TB coordinators at the time the individual was reported to MSIS (form with translation, see Additional file 2: a, b). If the form was not returned, we sent one reminder by mail before calling the prescribing clinician or responsible TB coordinator. If multiple forms were returned for the same individual, we verified conflicting data with a call to the responsible physician or TB coordinator. If we were unable to verify conflicting data, such as the number of visits with a physician or TB coordinator, we calculated the mean value of the reported data before inclusion in the analyses.

Definitions

LTBI treatment completion was measured as reported by the responsible clinician, and verified by the duration of treatment (measured in days) for the different regimens. Information on adverse events was only reported if it led to interruption (treatment was stopped temporarily, but later continued) or termination (stopped completely) of treatment. Severity of hepatotoxicity was based on reported increase in the liver enzymes alanine aminotransferase (ALAT) and aspartate transaminase (ASAT) and bilirubin in blood samples. Severity was classified by upper limits of normal values (ULN) for serum levels of ALAT or ASAT, consistent with the Common Terminology Criteria for Adverse Events (CTCAE4) [17]: grade 1 (>ULN -3.0 x ULN), grade 2 (> 3.0–5.0 x ULN), grade 3 (> 5.0–20.0 x ULN), and grade 4 (> 20.0 x ULN). Other blood test results were not routinely collected. Remaining adverse events were classified by their clinical symptoms.

Statistical analysis

We used STATA 2015 for statistical analysis. We present descriptive statistics for continuous variables as means and standard deviations for symmetrical data, and medians and interquartile range (IQR) for skewed data. Pearson's chi squared or Fisher's exact test, as appropriate, assessed associations between pairs of variables.

Additionally, we ran two separate logistic regression models. The first model analysed the association between treatment non-completion and origin (Norwegian-born/foreign-born), age ($\geq$/< 35 years), gender, and type of treatment support (self-administered treatment/ daily DOT/weekly DOT). Treatment regimen could not be included in the model because of its association with DOT. Similarly, we could not include both establishment of treatment plan and use of DOT in the model because the two are related. The final model did not include either the establishment of a treatment plan or immunosuppression because these were not found to be significantly associated with treatment completion in crude analyses.

To investigate if the association between treatment non-completion and treatment support was modified by age, sex, or origin we ran separate models. We ran the baseline model (treatment non-completion = treatment support + origin + age + sex) and then subsequently tested for interaction between treatment support and age, sex, or origin, i.e. (treatment support*age)/ (treatment support*sex)/ (treatment support*origin). We then performed likelihood ratio tests comparing the separate models to the baseline model. We found no statistically significant effect of age or sex on treatment support. We found a significant effect of origin on treatment support and therefore stratified the effect of treatment support

on treatment non-completion by origin in the model. We also tested for an interaction between origin and age and origin and sex. No such interactions were identified.

Information on age and origin was complete. Information on treatment completion was missing for six individuals, and treatment support was missing for 13. Since missing information is unlikely random, we used multiple imputations to investigate the effect of missing data on the model. We imputed five datasets using chained equations ("mi impute chained" command) and recreated the complete-case analyses using the imputed data.

The second model analysed the association between interruption or termination of treatment because of adverse events (yes/no), and treatment regimens (3HR/3RPH/Other), age ($\geq$/< 35 years), and immunosuppression (yes/no). One individual had missing information for treatment regimen, and for this person we coded treatment regimen as "other".

To investigate if the association between adverse events and treatment regimen was modified by age or immunosuppression, we ran two models. We ran the baseline model (adverse effect = treatment regimens + age + immunosuppression) and subsequently tested for interaction between treatment regimens and age or immunosuppression, i.e. (treatment regimens*age)/ (treatment regimens*immunosuppression). We also ran a model investigating whether there was an interaction between age and immunosuppression, i.e. (age*immunosuppression). We then performed likelihood ratio tests comparing the separate models to the baseline model. We found no statistically significant effect of age or immunosuppression on treatment regimens. We could not test the interaction between age and immunosuppression due to the small number of cases.

Results

Study population

In 2016, MSIS received 747 notifications of the prescription of LTBI treatment. We later excluded 21 cases because the treatment was completed in 2015 (delay in reporting), which left 726 individuals for follow-up in the prospective cohort. Table 1 presents baseline characteristics of the study population by origin.

Eighteen percent of the individuals ($n = 131$) were Norwegian-born and 82% ($n = 595$) were foreign-born. Information on country of birth was missing for four individuals. Among foreign-born, 197 (33%) were born in a country with a WHO estimated [18] TB incidence rate (IR) of $\geq$ 200 per 100,000 population, Table 1. Forty-three percent of immigrants ($n = 253$) had no additional risk factors for TB progression other than being foreign-born. Of these, 94 (35%) arrived from countries with TB IR < 150, 66 (52%) with IR 150–200, and 91 (46%) with IR > 200 per 100,000 population (2

Table 1 Baseline characteristics of the study population by origin, n = 726

Baseline Characteristics	Norwegian-born	Foreign-born	Total	p-value
Number of individuals	131 (100)	595 (100)	726 (100)	
Gender				0.115
Male	69 (53)	358 (60)	427 (59)	
Age at notification				> 0.001
< 5 years	37 (28)	25 (4)	62 (9)	
5–14 years	10 (8)	132 (22)	142 (20)	
15–34 years	33 (25)	315 (53)	348 (48)	
35–64 years	36 (27)	115 (19)	151 (21)	
≥ 65 years	15 (11)	8 (1)	23 (3)	
Risk groups[a]				
Any risk factor[a]	121 (92)	342 (58)	463 (64)	
Recent exposure, contacts	68 (52)	95 (16)	163 (22)	> 0.001
Contacts < 5 years	35 (27)	3 (0.5)	38 (5)	
Positive chest X-ray, any	7 (5)	60 (10)	67 (9)	0.090
Fibrotic lesions	2 (2)	17 (3)	19 (3)	0.388
Immunosuppressive condition	51 (39)	72 (12)	123 (17)	> 0.001
HIV infection	–	12 (2)	12 (2)	
Chronic renal disease	1 (1)	4 (1)	5 (1)	
Diabetes, any	1 (1)	4 (1)	5 (1)	
Underlying disease relevant for Immunosuppressive treatment[b]	13 (10)	10 (2)	23 (3)	
Other medical conditions[c]	36 (7)	42 (7)	78 (15)	
Interferon Gamma Release Assay (IGRA)				> 0.001
Positive	94 (72)	577 (97)	671 (92)	
Negative	15 (11)	5 (1)	20 (3)	
Inconclusive	2 (2)	–	2 (0)	
Missing or unknown	20 (15)	13 (2)	33 (5)	
Regimen				> 0.001
3RH daily[I]	97 (74)	302 (51)	399 (55)	
3RPH weekly[II]	30 (23)	276 (46)	306 (42)	
4R or 6H monotherapy daily[III]	3 (2)	15 (3)	18 (2)	
Other[IV]	–	2 (0)	2 (0)	
Missing	1 (1)	–	1 (0)	
TB IR (per 100,000) in country of birth[#]				
< 150	na	267 (45)	267 (45)	
150–200	na	127 (21)	127 (21)	

Table 1 Baseline characteristics of the study population by origin, n = 726 (Continued)

Baseline Characteristics	Norwegian-born	Foreign-born	Total	p-value
> 200	na	197 (33)	197 (33)	
Missing	na	4 (1)	4 (1)	

Data are presented as n (%) or median [interquartile range]. % refers to columns and not rows
[a]According to Norwegian guidelines for the management and control of tuberculosis: with strong or conditional recommendation for LTBI treatment (age < 15 years, known exposure, positive chest X-ray or immunosuppressive condition)
[b]Includes rheumatologic-, dermatologic-, neurologic- and gastroenterological medical conditions
[c]Other medical conditions include unspecified immunosuppressive conditions reported by the clinician
[I]3RH: rifampicin (R) and isoniazid (H) daily for three months
[II]3RPH: rifapentine (RP) and isoniazid (H) in 12 weekly doses
[III]Rifampicin (R) monotherapy daily for four months or isoniazid (H) monotherapy daily for six months
[IV]Others include full-course TB treatments for two individuals for two and four months respectively
Four immigrants had missing information on country of birth

missing). In total, 314 (53%) of the immigrants had lived in Norway for less than one year at the time of notification, and were therefore classified as recent immigrants.

The Norwegian-born group was more likely to be part of contact tracing, have at least one medical risk factor, and have a negative interferon-gamma release assay result (IGRA; QuantiFERON TB-Gold (QFT®)) prior to treatment onset, Table 1. Age distribution differed between Norwegian and foreign-born, with a higher proportion of either young or old patients in the Norwegian-born group. 3RH (55%) was the most common regimen, although the use of the newest regimen, 3RPH (42%), was frequent, and its use increased over the study period. The 3RPH regimen was more commonly prescribed among foreign-born (46%) compared to Norwegian-born (23%).

Treatment completion

Information on treatment completion was obtained for 719 (99%) of the individuals who started LTBI treatment. Table 2 presents treatment completion and the reasons for not completing treatment. Overall, 91% completed their treatment course as reported by the prescribing physician.

Treatment completion did not differ significantly for different regimens ($p = 0.124$). Foreign-born individuals were more likely to complete treatment compared to Norwegian-born [foreign-born, $n = 562$ (92%) vs Norwegian-born, $n = 115$ (85%), $p = 0.007$]. They were also more likely to be prescribed with 3RPH [foreign-born, $n = 276$ (46%) vs Norwegian-born $n = 30$ (23%) p-value 0.001], a regimen for which DOT is recommended. Foreign-born individuals were also more likely to be treated under DOT, even for regimens for which DOT is not routinely recommended [foreign-born, $n = 151$ (47%) vs Norwegian-born $n = 28$ (28%) $p = 0.002$]. Among recent immigrants, 294 (94%) completed their treatment, 48%

Table 2 Treatment completion and reasons for non-completion by treatment regimen, Norway 2016

Treatment completion	3RH[I] daily	3RPH[II] weekly	Other[III]	Total
Number of individuals	399	306	21	726
Duration of treatment (days), median [IQR]*	90 [73–156]	77 [70–98]	–	–
Treatment completion				
Completed according to physician[a]	357 (89.5)	284 (92.8)	17 (80.9)	658 (90.6)
Missing information	3 (0.8)	4 (1.3)	–	7 (1.0)
Incomplete treatment	39 (10)	18 (5.9)	4 (19.0)	61 (8.4)
Reasons for incomplete treatment				
LTBI excluded	4 (1.0)	–	–	4 (0.6)
Diagnosed with TB disease	1 (0.3)	–		1 (0.1)
Patient choice	4 (1.0)	2 (0.7)	–	6 (0.8)
Lost to follow-up	1 (0.3)	3 (1.0)	–	4 (0.6)
Other or unknown	3 (0.8)	2 (0.7)		5 (0.7)
Termination due to adverse effects[b]	26 (6.5)	11 (3.4)	4 (19.0)	41 (5.6)
Hepatotoxicity (grade 1–2)[c]	8 (2.0)	–	–	8 (1.1)
Hepatotoxicity (grade 3–4)[c]	5 (1.6)	2 (0.7)	1 (4.8)	8 (1.1)
Gastrointestinal symptoms	10 (2.5)	8 (2.6)	2 (9.5)	20 (2.8)
Fatigue	6 (1.5)	8 (2.6)	1 (4.8)	15 (2.1)
Flu-like symptoms	2 (0.5)	4 (1.3)	1 (4.8)	7 (1.0)
Skin rash	2 (0.5)	1 (0.3)	1 (4.8)	4 (0.6)
Peripheral neuropathy	1 (0.3)			1 (0.1)
Joint pain	–	2 (0.6)	–	2 (0.3)
Other symptoms[d]	2 (0.5)	3 (1.0)	2 (9.5)	7 (1.0)

Data are presented as n (%) or median [interquartile range]
[I]3RH: rifampicin (R) and isoniazid (H) daily for three months
[II]3RPH: rifapentine (RP) and isoniazid (H) in 12 weekly doses
[III]Other: rifampicin (R) monotherapy daily for four months ($n = 5$), Isoniazid (H) monotherapy for six months ($n = 13$) or combination therapy for TB disease ($n = 2$) and missing information about drug regimen (n = 1)
*Duration of treatment for those where the clinician reported the treatment as completed
[a]The responsible clinician reported that the planned treatment was completed
[b]Many reported more than one adverse effect
[c]Severity of hepatotoxicity was classified according to Common Terminology Criteria for Adverse Events (CTCAE), ULN = upper limits of normal value for serum levels of liver function, grade 1 (>ULN -3.0 × ULN), grade 2 (> 3.0–5.0 × ULN), grade 3 (> 5.0–20.0 × ULN), and grade 4 (> 20.0 × ULN)
[d]Includes headache, sleep disorder, and unstable international normalized ratio (INR) for prothrombin time

were prescribed with 3RPH, and 65% were treated under DOT while on regimens other than 3RPH.

In crude logistic regression models, origin, age, sex, and treatment support were significantly associated with treatment non-completion. In a multivariable logistic regression model, we found that neither origin, age over 35 years, or sex were significantly associated with treatment non-completion. However, the effect of treatment support was modified by origin, with significantly lower risk of non-completion with daily and weekly DOT compared to self-administration in the foreign-born group. Treatment support had no significant effect on treatment completion in the Norwegian-born group, Table 3.

We ran a sensitivity analysis by rerunning the analyses in Table 3 with a multiple imputed dataset (using chained equations). The sensitivity analysis showed no impact on the overall results, and the results are available as supplementary material (Additional file 3).

Adverse events

Adverse events was the most common reason reported for incomplete treatment in all groups. The total number of adverse events according to the study definitions was 47 (6.5%). In total, 41 (5.6%) individuals terminated treatment, Table 2, and an additional six (0.8%) individuals interrupted treatment to control adverse events but later continued and completed treatment. These six individuals are recorded as complete treatment in Table 2. Three of these temporary interruptions (3RH) were due to hepatotoxicity (one grade 2 and two grade 3), two were due to gastrointestinal symptoms, (3RPH and H)

Table 3 Associations between the outcome of treatment non-completion and the variables treatment support, origin, age and sex (*n* = 726)

Covariates	Univariable			Multivariable			
	n	c OR	p	a OR	SE	p	95% CI
Origin							
Foreign-born	595	1 (ref)		1(ref)			
Norwegian-born	131	2.1	0.016	0.8	0.342	0.602	0.34–1.84
Age group							
≤ 35	561	1 (ref)		1 (ref)			
> 35 years	165	1.9	0.026	1.7	0.521	0.093	0.92–3.09
Sex							
Female	299	1 (ref)		1 (ref)			
Male	427	0.5	0.017	0.6	0.093	0.106	0.36–1.10

Treatment support. Model with interaction term for origin: LRT p-value of interaction term = 0.049

Effect of treatment support on treatment completion in foreign-born (multivariate wald p-value 0.017)

Self-administered[a]	174	1 (ref)		1 (ref)			
DOT daily[b]	151	0.2	0.005	0.3	0.150	0.017	0.10–0.80
DOT weekly[c]	261	0.4	0.009	0.4	0.162	0.027	0.22–0.91

Effect of treatment support on treatment completion in Norwegian-born (multivariate wald p-value 0.468)

Self-administered[a]	80	1 (ref)		1 (ref)			
DOT daily[b]	28	1.7	0.374	2.1	1.332	0.229	0.62–7.26
DOT weekly[c]	19	0.9	0.928	1.0	0.868	0.961	0.20–5.34

OR Odds ratio, *SE* standard error, *DOT* Direct Observed Treatment for part of or the full treatment period
[a]Self-administered include those who managed their treatment themselves or were given weekly pill boxes
[b]daily DOT: those who were administered daily treatment under direct observation
[c]weekly DOT: those who were administered weekly rifapentine and isoniazid under direct observation

and one to fatigue (3RPH). The duration of the interruption was 2, 4, 7, 22, 28 and 113 days respectively.

In a multivariable logistic regression model, we found that regimen was borderline associated with adverse events (*p*-value = 0.065). There were no significant differences when comparing 3RH vs 3RPH, nor 3RH vs Other (R or H monotherapy or full course TB treatment). However, there were significantly fewer adverse events with 3RPH compared to "other" regimens (*p* = 0.037). Age over 35 years was significantly associated with having more adverse events, even after adjusting for regimen, whereas immunosuppression was not significantly associated with having adverse events after adjusting for other variables, Table 4. No deaths were reported.

Duration of treatment prior to termination ranged from 2 to 122 days, with a median of 25 days (IQR 6–84). For the two 3-month regimens combined (3RH +3RPH), 61% of those who terminated treatment completed less than half of the prescribed regimen.

Among those who met the study-definition for adverse effects, 22 (47%) had one symptom, 16 (34%) had two, and nine (19%) had three. There was no significant difference in number of symptoms reported between those who interrupted and those who terminated treatment (*p* = 0677). Gastrointestinal symptoms was the most common complaint in both age groups, followed by hepatotoxicity and fatigue, Table 2. Two individuals were classified with grade 4 hepatotoxicity. One was a child who was diagnosed with toxic hepatitis after two weeks of LTBI treatment. Treatment was immediately stopped, allowing transaminase values to normalize, and the patient fully recovered. The other was a middle-aged individual who developed hepatotoxicity with high transaminase values after eight weeks of LTBI treatment.

Table 4 Associations between adverse events[a], regimen, age, and immunosuppression, n = 726

Covariates		Univariable		Multivariable			
	n	c OR	p	a OR	SE	p	95% CI
Regimen (Wald test for overall variable in adjustment model, *p* = 0.065)							
3RH[b]	399	1 (ref)		1 (ref)			
3RPH[c]	306	0.57	0.097	0.60	0.209	0.141	0.30–1.18
Other[d]	21	3.99	0.012	2.37	1.360	0.131	0.78–7.30
Age							
≤ 35 yrs	561	1 (ref)		1 (ref)			
> 35 yrs	165	3.62	< 0.001	2.51	2.25	0.024	1.13–5.60
Immunosuppression							
No immunosuppression	603	1 (ref)		1 (ref)			
Immunosuppression, any	123	3.39	< 0.001	1.55	0.66	0.306	0.67–3.57

OR Odds ratio, *SE* standard error
[a]Adverse effects leading to termination or interruption of treatment, *n* = 47
[b]3HR, 3 months daily rifampicin and isoniazid
[c]3RPH, 12 weekly doses of rifapentine and isoniazid
[d]Other; rifampicin monotherapy (*n* = 5), isoniazid monotherapy (*n* = 13), combination therapy for TB disease (*n* = 2) and 1 missing information

The treatment was immediately stopped, and transaminase values normalized after six weeks. Both individuals received 3RH regimen and were managed as outpatients. Additionally, eight individuals were classified as having hepatotoxicity grade 3. Two of these were hospitalized due to complex comorbidities. The remaining were treated as outpatients, and transaminase values normalized after treatment was stopped. The 3RH regimen was prescribed in 16 out of 19 (84%) patients who interrupted or terminated treatment due to hepatotoxicity.

Patient support, drug administration, and use of healthcare resources

A treatment plan was established prior to treatment for 655 (90%) individuals. Foreign-born individuals were more likely to have a treatment plan compared with Norwegian-born individuals ($n = 544$, 91% vs $n = 111$, 85%, p 0.017).

DOT, either for part of or the whole treatment period, was reported in 173 (43%) of individuals prescribed with 3RH, in 280 (92%) with 3RPH, and in six (29%) with "other", Table 5. Home-visiting nurses provided DOT in 324 (71%) cases, the family in 11 (2%), and outpatient hospital clinics, assisted living facilities, refugee centres, work places, or general practitioners in 57 (12%). Information about the DOT provider was missing for 65 (15%) individuals.

The median number of consultations with a medical doctor was 1.5 (IQR 1–8, range 1–11), and 1.5 (IQR 0–7, range 0–14) with nurse. Almost half (48%) had only one consultation with a doctor. We found no significant difference in the mean number of consultations with a doctor or nurse between foreign-born and Norwegian-born individuals. Among the 658 individuals who completed treatment, 397 (60%) had their last consultation in the hospital before ($n = 334$, 51%), or at the time of treatment initiation ($n = 63$, 9%). Only 193 (29%) had a consultation in the hospital more than six weeks after the treatment start date.

Table 5 Drug-administration by regimen, n = 726

Drug administration	3RH[a] daily	3RPH[b] weekly	Other[c]	Total
Number of individuals	399 (100)	306 (100)	21 (100)	726 (100)
Self-administered	220 (55)	20 (7)	14 (67)	254 (35)
Direct observed treatment				
Whole period	132 (33)	269 (88)	3 (14)	404 (56)
Part of period	41 (10)	11 (4)	3 (14)	55 (8)
Missing information	6 (2)	6 (2)	1 (5)	13 (2)

Data are presented as n (%)
[a]rifampicin (R) and isoniazid (H) daily for three months
[b]rifapentine (RP) and isoniazid (H) in 12 weekly doses
[c]rifampicin (R) monotherapy daily for four months (n = 5), Isoniazid (H) monotherapy for six months (n = 13) or combination therapy for TB disease (n = 2) and missing information (n = 1)
[d]Other included: hospital outpatient clinic, assisted living facilities, refugee centres, work-places or with general practitioners.

Discussion

This one-year prospective study found a 91% LTBI treatment completion rate in Norway. Treatment completion did not differ significantly by regimen. Completion was higher among foreign-born than Norwegian-born individuals. Treatment under DOT had a significant effect on treatment completion for foreign-born individuals, but not in the Norwegian-born group. The primary reason for not completing treatment was adverse events. The majority of these were mild to moderate in severity, although medically significant (grade 3) and severe (grade 4) hepatotoxicity led to termination of treatment in 1.1% of participants. Few individuals were lost to follow-up. Individual treatment plans were established for the majority, and DOT was common, even with regimens where this is not routinely recommended.

Treatment completion

The treatment completion rate of 91% is consistent with the 89% previously reported in Norway [13]. Direct comparison with previous studies is difficult due to differences in study designs, regimens, and the populations under study. Completion rates are commonly reported as inversely related to treatment length [7]. Unsupervised six to nine months of isoniazid treatments in the US have shown around 50% completion rates [10, 11, 19, 20], 3–4 months RH regimens are reported at 85–90% [13, 21–23] and recent studies report similarly high completion rates with weekly (supervised) 3RPH administration [24–28]. Our results are consistent with a 2017 review [29] reporting no important differences in efficacy and completion rates for the 3RPH regimen when compared to other regimens. The review, however, did support a higher likelihood of completion with a shorter regimen. Additionally, lower loss to follow up has been associated with immunocompromised patients, being part of a contact investigation, and the shorter, rifamycin-based regimens [30].

Our high completion rate is surprising given that the majority of patients were recent arrivals to Norway and were born in countries with a high TB prevalence, factors often associated with poor access and adherence to health services. A Swedish study reported 76% LTBI treatment completion over a six year period (2002–2007) overall, but only 68% completion among recent immigrants, (< 1 years residence) with immigrants of Somali origin having the lowest completion rates [23]. Similarly in Japan, a study reported significantly higher completion rates in Japanese versus foreign-born individuals [31]. In our setting, the most recent immigrants completed treatment at a higher rate than other immigrants, and immigrants as a whole completed treatment to a higher extent than Norwegian-born individuals. This finding is unexpected because immigrants in Norway tend to under-utilize other preventive health services, such as mammography [32]. Foreign-born individuals in this study were more likely to have a treatment plan established prior to LTBI treatment, be treated under direct observation, and were more commonly prescribed the 3RPH weekly regimen compared to Norwegian-born individuals. These findings may explain such high rates of completion among recent immigrants. Treatment support, which was coded separately for daily or weekly DOT to reflect treatment regimens, was significantly associated with treatment completion among foreign-born individuals when controlling for other co-variates. However, we were unable to control for adverse effects as a co-variate in the analyses, since this information was only recorded when not completing treatment.

Another explanation may be the role of TB coordinators, mostly specialized nurses, which is unique in a northern European setting. The TB coordinators are actively involved in implementation of TB control activities, both on individual and system levels. They know their patients well, and this may mitigate loss to follow-up. Previous studies have shown that social interventions such as adherence coaching, contingency contracting, enhanced outreach, and home visits improve treatment completion and may benefit patients who are at risk of progressing to active TB [33, 34]. In Norway, such activities are initiated by TB coordinators.

Adverse events

Adverse events was the most common reason for not completing treatment in both the Norwegian and foreign-born groups. This is consistent with other studies [35]. The proportion of individuals who discontinued LTBI treatment due to side-effects (5.6%) in this study is similar to the 7.6% reported in the Netherlands [21], 6.4 and 5.9% reported in the USA [35], and 7% reported in Norway in 2009 [13], but lower than the 12% reported from Australia [36]. Similarly, a recent study in Taiwan that compared treatment completion and cost effectiveness for 3RPH versus H reported higher completion in the 3RPH regimen due to the shorter treatment period and reduced likelihood of severe side effects [37]. This is also consistent with our results.

The severity of reported adverse events varied. Since the treatment is preventive rather than curative, mild to moderate side effects may influence both the patient's and the doctor's motivation to continue treatment. The rate of clinically significant and severe hepatotoxicity (grade 3 and 4) reported in this study (1.1%) is lower than a median rate of 1.8% (range 0.1–11.9%) reported in a study on age-related hepatotoxicity following 6-9 months of isoniazid [16]. In accordance with other studies, we found a higher rate of grade 3 and 4 hepatotoxicity with increasing age [7, 16, 36], lower rates with 3RPH compared with

other regimens [20, 26, 35, 38], rare need for hospitalization, and no deaths [13, 16, 27, 36, 39, 40].

Patient support and use of health care resources

Norway's high completion rate must also be seen in relation to the resources used to achieve it. Two elements that make preventive treatment in Norway relatively costlier than elsewhere are the frequent use of DOT and the highly specialized care levels. Almost two thirds of the patients involved in the study received treatment under DOT. Norwegian guidelines do not routinely recommend DOT for treatment regimens other than 3RPH. The increasing use of this 12-dose regimen (3RPH), with weekly administration rather than a prolonged daily regimen, will reduce DOT associated costs. Further, a recent randomized clinical trial found that there was not a significant difference in completion rates for directly observed 3RPH versus self-administered 3RPH treatment, which may change current recommendations for supervised 3RPH treatment [41].

Providing preventive treatment through subspecialist physicians rather than primary care is costly. However, training a larger group of primary care doctors about the details of TB and its prevention and treatment in low incidence settings such as Norway would require substantial effort. The greatest cost, as well as the greatest benefit, may be attributable to having dedicated TB coordinators. In the current study, 90% of patients had treatment plans established by TB coordinators.

Strengths and limitations

The strengths of the study include the population-wide approach, the comprehensive information available for every individual, the standardized classification of severity of hepatotoxicity, and our very low rate of loss to follow-up. The sensitivity of our reporting system for LTBI treatment is assumed to be high since information on TB-related prescriptions is collected independently, and missing data is routinely monitored to ensure complete information.

Limitations include that completion rates and adverse events for the various regimens may reflect systematic differences in treatment assignment and clinician assessment rather than differences in the regimens themselves. We have, when possible, adjusted for this in our analyses. Judgment of treatment completion was made by the treating physician, often based on only one consultation at the beginning of the treatment course, in addition to information received from the TB coordinator and the DOT-provider. The question about completion was, however, followed up with a statement of the number of days on treatment and overseen by the TB coordinator. Adverse drug events that did not lead to interruption or termination of treatment were not recorded. Therefore, we could not control for this as a co-variate. We may have also missed some adverse effects and mild degrees of toxicity.

Conclusions

This study indicates that with well-organized health services, high LTBI treatment completion is possible, even in high-risk immigrant groups. We report high treatment completion across all subgroups. Treatment completion is the end-point of Norway's LTBI screening strategy. Knowledge of the treatment completion rate and adverse events are crucial in the assessment of the screening program's impact and cost effectiveness. Although adverse events were the primary determinants of treatment non-completion, our results seem reassuring, even for more elderly and immunocompromised individuals, given adequate monitoring and follow-up during treatment. While this study has shown that DOT is very effective in ensuring treatment completion among hard to reach populations, further research is necessary to evaluate best practices from a cost-effectiveness standpoint.

Abbreviations

3RH: Daily Rifampicin and Isoniazid for 3 Months; 3RPH: Weekly Rifapentine and Isoniazid for 3 months; ALAT: Alanine aminotransferase; ASAT: Aspartate aminotransferase; CTCAE: Common Terminology Criteria for Adverse Events; DOT: Directly Observed Treatment; H: Daily Isoniazid for 6 months; IGRA: Interferon-gamma release assay; IR: Incidence Rate; LTBI: Latent Tuberculosis Infection; MSIS: Norwegian Surveillance System for Infectious Diseases; NIPH: Norwegian Institute of Public Health; R: Daily Rifampicin for 4 months; TB: Tuberculosis; ULN: Upper Limits of Normal values; WHO: World Health Organization

Acknowledgements

We thank clinicians and tuberculosis coordinators throughout Norway for their strong efforts in submitting treatment completion forms for the study. We also thank Kirsten Konsmo and Annette Tyvand at the Norwegian Institute of Public Health for their support in data-collection and data-cleaning. Finally, we thank the U.S.-Norway Fulbright Foundation for their support of YS's efforts on this project.

Funding

The Norwegian Health association funded the project leader (BAW) and a Fulbright Grant funded the first author (YS) throughout the study period. The Norwegian Institute of Public Health allocated administrative resources to the project.

Authors' contributions

BAW initiated the study, wrote the protocol, obtained necessary approvals and set up the data-collection. All authors were involved in the final version of the protocol. YS was responsible for the major part of data-collection and data-entry, data-analyses, and for drafting the manuscript. TM evaluated and classified adverse drug events, RW was responsible for the statistical analyses, BAW and YS drafted the manuscript and YS, HEA, TMA, AMDR, HT, RW and BAW critically revised and approved the final version of the manuscript.

Competing interests

The authors declare that they have no competing interests.

Author details

[1]Perelman School of Medicine at the University of Pennsylvania, Philadelphia, PA, USA. [2]Department of Pulmonary Medicine, Stavanger University Hospital, Stavanger, Norway. [3]Department of Pulmonary Medicine, TB unit, Stavanger University Hospital, Stavanger, Norway. [4]Department of Tuberculosis, Blood Borne and Sexually Transmitted Infections, Norwegian Institute of Public Health, Oslo, Norway. [5]Department of Infectious Diseases, Oslo University Hospital, Oslo, Norway. [6]Institute of Clinical Medicine, University of Oslo, Oslo, Norway. [7]Dep. of Clinical Science, University of Bergen, Oslo, Norway. [8]Department of Pulmonary Medicine, Oslo University Hospital, Oslo, Norway. [9]Department of Infectious Disease Epidemiology and Modelling, Norwegian Institute of Public Health, Oslo, Norway. [10]Department of Vaccine Preventable Diseases, Norwegian Institute of Public Health, Oslo, Norway.

References

1. WHO. Global strategy and targets for tuberculosis prevention, care and control after 2015 [http://apps.who.int/gb/ebwha/pdf_files/EB134/B134_12-en.pdf?ua=1].
2. Helse- og omsorgsdepartementet: Forskrift om tuberkulosekontroll FOR-2009-02-13-205; 2009.
3. Norwegian Institute of Public Health Guidelines for Prev Control of tuberculosis [https://www.fhi.no/nettpub/tuberkuloseveilederen/].
4. Arnesen TM, Heldal E, Mengshoel AT, Nordstrand K, Rønning K. In: Folkehelseinstituttet, editor. Tuberkulose i Norge i 2016 med behandlingsresultater for 2015. Oslo: Norwegian Institute of Public Health; 2017. isbn:ISSN 1894–4868.
5. Arnesen TM, Eide KA, Norheim G, Mengshoel AT, Sandbu S, Winje BA. In: Folkehelseinstituttet, editor. Tuberkulose i Norge i 2013 med behandlingsresultater for 2012; 2014.
6. Helse- og omsorgsdepartementet: Forskrift om Meldingssystem for smittsomme sykdommer (MSIS-forskriften) FOR-2003-06-20-740. 2003.
7. WHO. Guidelines for the management of latent tuberculosis infection [http://www.who.int/tb/publications/ltbi_document_page/en/].
8. Sharma SK, Sharma A, Kadhiravan T, Tharyan P. Rifamycins (rifampicin, rifabutin and rifapentine) compared to isoniazid for preventing tuberculosis in HIV-negative people at risk of active TB. Cochrane Database Syst Rev. 2013;7:CD007545.
9. Aspler A, Long R, Trajman A, Dion MJ, Khan K, Schwartzman K, Menzies D. Impact of treatment completion, intolerance and adverse events on health system costs in a randomised trial of 4 months rifampin or 9 months isoniazid for latent TB. Thorax. 2010;65(7):582–7.
10. Horsburgh CR Jr, Goldberg S, Bethel J, Chen S, Colson PW, Hirsch-Moverman Y, Hughes S, Shrestha-Kuwahara R, Sterling TR, Wall K, et al. Latent TB infection treatment acceptance and completion in the United States and Canada. Chest. 2010;137(2):401–9.
11. Page KR, Sifakis F, Montes de Oca R, Cronin WA, Doherty MC, Federline L, Bur S, Walsh T, Karney W, Milman J, et al. Improved adherence and less toxicity with rifampin vs isoniazid for treatment of latent tuberculosis: a retrospective study. Arch Intern Med. 2006;166(17):1863–70.
12. Getahun H, Matteelli A, Abubakar I, Aziz MA, Baddeley A, Barreira D, Den Boon S, Borroto Gutierrez SM, Bruchfeld J, Burhan E, et al. Management of latent Mycobacterium tuberculosis infection: WHO guidelines for low tuberculosis burden countries. Eur Respir J. 2015;46(6):1563–76.
13. Olsen AIM, Andersen HE, Amus J, Djupvik JA, Gran G, Skaug K, Mørkve O. Management of latent tuberculosis infection in Norway in 2009: a descriptive cross-sectional study. Public Health Action. 2013;3(2):166–71.
14. Harstad I, Heldal E, Steinshamn SL, Garasen H, Jacobsen GW. Tuberculosis screening and follow-up of asylum seekers in Norway: a cohort study. BMCPublic Health. 2009;9:141.
15. Harstad I, Heldal E, Steinshamn SL, Garasen H, Winje BA, Jacobsen GW. Screening and treatment of latent tuberculosis in a cohort of asylum seekers in Norway. ScandJ Public Health. 2010;38(3):275 82.

16. Kunst H, Khan KS. Age-related risk of hepatotoxicity in the treatment of latent tuberculosis infection: a systematic review. International Journal of Tuberculosis & Lung Disease. 2010;14(11):1374–81.

17. Common Terminology Criteria for Adverse Events (CTCAE) Version 4. https://www.eortc.be/services/doc/ctc/CTCAE_4.03_2010-06-14_QuickReference_5x7.pdf.

18. WHO. Global Tuberculosis Report. Geneva: World Health Organization; 2016.

19. Lardizabal A, Passannante M, Kojakali F, Hayden C, Reichman LB. Enhancement of treatment completion for latent tuberculosis infection with 4 months of rifampin. Chest. 2006;130(6):1712–7.

20. Perez AP, Seo SK, Schneider WJ, Eisenstein C, Brown AE. Management of Latent Tuberculosis Infection among Health Care workers: 10-year experience at a single center. Clin Infect Dis. 2017;65(12):2105–11.

21. Erkens CG, Slump E, Verhagen M, Schimmel H, de Vries G, Cobelens F, van den Hof S. Monitoring latent tuberculosis infection diagnosis and management in the Netherlands. Eur Respir J. 2016;47(5):1492–501.

22. Geijo MP, Herranz CR, Vano D, Garcia AJ, Garcia M, Dimas JF. Short-course isoniazid and rifampin compared with isoniazid for latent tuberculosis infection: a randomized clinical trial. Enferm Infecc Microbiol Clin. 2007;25(5):300–4.

23. Kan B, Kalin M, Bruchfeld J. Completing treatment for latent tuberculosis: patient background matters. Int J Tuberc Lung Dis. 2013;17(5):597–602.

24. Lines G, Hunter P, Bleything S. Improving treatment completion rates for latent tuberculosis infection: a review of two treatment regimens at a community health center. J Health Care Poor Underserved. 2015;26(4):1428–39.

25. Martinson NA, Barnes GL, Moulton LH, Msandiwa R, Hausler H, Ram M, McIntyre JA, Gray GE, Chaisson RE. New regimens to prevent tuberculosis in adults with HIV infection. N Engl J Med. 2011;365(1):11–20.

26. Sterling TR, Villarino ME, Borisov AS, Shang N, Gordin F, Bliven-Sizemore E, Hackman J, Hamilton CD, Menzies D, Kerrigan A, et al. Three months of rifapentine and isoniazid for latent tuberculosis infection. N Engl J Med. 2011;365(23):2155–66.

27. Sandul AL, Nwana N, Holcombe JM, Lobato MN, Marks S, Webb R, Wang SH, Stewart B, Griffin P, Hunt G, et al. High rate of treatment completion in program settings with 12-dose weekly isoniazid and Rifapentine (3HP) for latent Mycobacterium tuberculosis infection. Clin Infect Dis. 2017. https://doi.org/10.1093/cid/cix505.

28. McClintock AH, Eastment M, McKinney CM, Pitney CL, Narita M, Park DR, Dhanireddy S, Molnar A. Treatment completion for latent tuberculosis infection: a retrospective cohort study comparing 9 months of isoniazid, 4 months of rifampin and 3 months of isoniazid and rifapentine. BMC Infect Dis. 2017;17(1):146.

29. Pease C, Hutton B, Yazdi F, Wolfe D, Hamel C, Quach P, Skidmore B, Moher D, Alvarez GG. Efficacy and completion rates of rifapentine and isoniazid (3HP) compared to other treatment regimens for latent tuberculosis infection: a systematic review with network meta-analyses. BMC Infect Dis. 2017;17(1):265.

30. Alsdurf H, Hill PC, Matteelli A, Getahun H, Menzies D. The cascade of care in diagnosis and treatment of latent tuberculosis infection: a systematic review and meta-analysis. Lancet Infect Dis. 2016;16(11):1269–78.

31. Kawatsu L, Uchimura K, Ohkado A. Trend and treatment status of latent tuberculosis infection patients in Japan - analysis of Japan TB surveillance data. PLoS One. 2017;12(11):e0186588.

32. Bhargava S, Tsuruda K, Moen K, Bukholm I, Hofvind S. Lower attendance rates in immigrant versus non-immigrant women in the Norwegian breast Cancer screening Programme. J Med Screen. 2017;1:969141317733771.

33. Stuurman AL, Vonk Noordegraaf-Schouten M, van Kessel F, Oordt-Speets AM, Sandgren A, van der Werf MJ. Interventions for improving adherence to treatment for latent tuberculosis infection: a systematic review. BMC Infect Dis. 2016;16:257.

34. Eastment MC, McClintock AH, McKinney CM, Narita M, Molnar A. Factors that influence treatment completion for latent tuberculosis infection. J Am Board Fam Med. 2017;30(4):520–7.

35. Moro RN, Borisov AS, Saukkonen J, Khan A, Sterling TR, Villarino ME, Scott NA, Shang N, Kerrigan A, Goldberg SV. Factors associated with noncompletion of latent tuberculosis infection treatment: experience from the PREVENT TB trial in the United States and Canada. Clin Infect Dis. 2016; 62(11):1390–400.

36. Denholm JT, McBryde ES, Eisen DP, Pennington JS, Chen C, Street AC. Adverse effects of isoniazid preventative therapy for latent tuberculosis infection: a prospective cohort study. Drug Healthc Patient Saf. 2014;6:145–9.

37. Huang YW, Yang SF, Yeh YP, Tsao TC, Tsao SM. Impacts of 12-dose regimen for latent tuberculosis infection: treatment completion rate and cost-effectiveness in Taiwan. Medicine (Baltimore). 2016;95(34):e4126.

38. Zenner D, Beer N, Harris RJ, Lipman MC, Stagg HR, van der Werf MJ. Treatment of latent tuberculosis infection: an updated network meta-analysis. Ann Intern Med. 2017;167(4):248–55.

39. McElroy PD, Ijaz K, Lambert LA, Jereb JA, Iademarco MF, Castro KG, Navin TR. National survey to measure rates of liver injury, hospitalization, and death associated with rifampin and pyrazinamide for latent tuberculosis infection. Clin Infect Dis. 2005;41(8):1125–33.

40. Menzies D, Long R, Trajman A, Dion MJ, Yang J, Al Jahdali H, Memish Z, Khan K, Gardam M, Hoeppner V, et al. Adverse events with 4 months of rifampin therapy or 9 months of isoniazid therapy for latent tuberculosis infection: a randomized trial. Ann Intern Med. 2008;149(10):689–97.

41. Belknap R, Holland D, Feng PJ, Millet JP, Cayla JA, Martinson NA, Wright A, Chen MP, Moro RN, Scott NA, et al. Self-administered versus directly observed once-weekly isoniazid and Rifapentine treatment of latent tuberculosis infection: a randomized trial. Ann Intern Med. 2017;167(10):689–97.

Associations between perceived barriers and benefits of using HIV pre-exposure prophylaxis and medication adherence among men who have sex with men in Western China

Ying Hu[1], Xiao-ni Zhong[1*], Bin Peng[1], Yan Zhang[1], Hao Liang[2], Jiang-hong Dai[3], Ju-ying Zhang[4] and Ai-long Huang[5]

Abstract

Background: To investigate the associations between the perceived barriers and benefits of using HIV pre-exposure prophylaxis medication, including worries about the side effects, disliking taking drugs, perceived burden of taking medication, positive expectations as to the efficacy of the drugs, favourable doctor-patient relationships, and medication adherence among men who have sex with men (MSM) to provide a target for improving medication adherence and reducing HIV infection among MSM.

Methods: MSM were recruited in western China from April 2013 to October 2014, administered oral tenofovir (TDF) daily and followed up every 12 weeks for 2 years. At each follow-up, the medication rate was calculated based on the self-reported number of missed doses over 2 weeks, and then, the medication adherence was evaluated. The barriers and benefits perceived during medication were obtained by a self-administered questionnaire, and their effects on medication adherence were analysed by linear mixed models.

Results: A total of 411 participants were enrolled in this study, and 1561 follow-up observation points were obtained. The average medication rate was 0.62 ± 0.37, and the medication rate increased with longer follow-up ($P < 0.05$). The medication rate was higher among MSM who were divorced (compared to those who were unmarried, $P < 0.0001$). MSM with more positive expectations as to the efficacy of the drugs showed higher rates of medication (P < 0.0001), while those who were more worried about side effects had a lower medication rate ($P = 0.0208$). In contrast, the dislike of taking the drugs and the burden perceived during medication had no effects on the actual medication rate of taking TDF ($P > 0.05$).

Conclusion: How to obtain and maintain high medication adherence among MSM is the key to the PrEP intervention strategy for effective reduction of HIV infection. For MSM in China, we should deepen their understanding of the effectiveness and safety of PrEP and increase their confidence in PrEP, thereby improving their medication adherence.

Keywords: Pre-exposure prophylaxis, PrEP, MSM, Adherence, Barriers and benefits

* Correspondence: zxn133cq@sina.com
[1]Department of Health Statistics and Information Management, School of Public Health and Management, Chongqing Medical University, Chongqing, China
Full list of author information is available at the end of the article

Background

The report of the Joint United Nations Program on HIV/ AIDS [1] points out that the number of HIV infections reached 1.8 million in 2016 and men who have sex with men (MSM) have a higher risk of infection. The Progress Report on AIDS Prevention and Treatment in China [2] shows that the HIV epidemic currently maintains a low-prevalence trend, with a higher-prevalence among MSM, especially in the western part of China [3]. In 2006, MSM accounted for 2.5% of new HIV infections in China, and the rate increased dramatically to 25.5% in 2017 [4, 5].

Pre-exposure prophylaxis (PrEP) has been considered the most promising biomedical HIV prevention strategy so far. The antiviral drug tenofovir (TDF) used in PrEP and combined therapy with TDF and emtricitabine (TDF-FTC) have been approved by the USFDA as preventive drugs for the MSM population [6], and in 2014, comprehensive PrEP guidelines were released [7]. Many international clinical studies have shown the effectiveness of PrEP in different groups, including MSM [8–10], women [11] and injection drug users [12, 13].

In addition, studies have also suggested that adherence to medication is crucial for the efficacy of PrEP [9, 11, 14–16]. The iPrEP study demonstrated that the once-daily oral PrEP drug resulted a 44% reduction in the incidence of HIV among MSM and transgender women, while pill use on 90% or more of days showed greater protection (73%), and it increased to 92% efficacy for participants with detectable drug levels [10]. However, a study conducted among African women unable to show the efficacy of oral PrEP due to their low adherence levels [17]. Therefore, an investigation into barriers and facilities associated with adherence to PrEP is required.

Factors from the perspectives of social, behavioural and psychological areas associated with PrEP adherence have been identified in clinical trials [9, 18–20]. However, in China, only one open-label clinical trial has been conducted among HIV-uninfected MSM in western China to assess the efficacy and safety of oral TDF in preventing HIV infection [21], but little is known about the barriers and facilities of PrEP adherence in China. Based on the fact that PrEP clinical trials have not been widely conducted in China, assessing participants' feelings and attitudes during medication among the very first group of people involved in taking PrEP drugs is important and necessary. For instance, participants who perceive that there are side effects of drugs tend to show low adherence to medication, while sound doctor-patient relationships are a facilitator of adherence [22, 23].

Therefore, in this study, we aimed to investigate the changes in barriers and benefits that HIV-uninfected MSM perceive during the course of medication and examine the associations between perceived barriers and benefits of oral PrEP and actual medication adherence

to provide a basis and some guidance for application and promotion of PrEP strategies among MSM in China.

Methods

Participants and study design

Participants were recruited from Chongqing, Sichuan, Xinjiang and Guangxi by non-probability sampling from April 2013 to October 2014, including via publishing information on gay websites and cooperating with non-governmental organizations. Inclusion criteria: (1) MSM aged 18–65 years; (2) self-reported negative or unknown HIV status; (3) had engaged in sex with male partners at least every two weeks; (4) had at least one or more same-sex partners one month before the trial; and (5) willing to take medicine under guidance and comply with follow-up arrangements. Exclusion criteria: (1) HBsAg- or anti-HBc-positive, (2) having a serious illness that investigators considered could possibly interfere with the interventions, follow-ups or assessments of the participants; (3) advanced cancer; (4) alcohol abuse within one year before entering the study; (5) receiving other drugs 3 months prior to screening; and (6) having a history of severe allergies.

A total of 575 MSM eligible were enrolled in the daily TDF group after the screening, and they were informed about the purpose and content of the study as well as the possible benefits and risks. All participants signed the informed consent and were given standard HIV prevention interventions, including HIV testing, counselling to reduce the risk of HIV infection, free condom distribution, and STI management.

Procedures

Participants were asked to fill in the self-administered quantitative questionnaire for the baseline survey and at each follow-up conducted every 12 weeks, inquiring about their feelings or attitudes during medication, the number of missed pills, as well as the occurrence of adverse events within the last two weeks during the follow-up. In addition, HIV-1 serological detection, blood biochemical examination and haematological examination were performed. At each follow-up, a new round of drugs was supplied. In addition, every two weeks, our trained investigators contacted participants though QQ or telephone to learn about their medication use and provide counselling on adherence.

Participants stopped using the medication if one of the following occurred: confirmed HIV infection; serious adverse reactions; failure to participate in follow-up, planning to leave the research study, or other reasons; or medicine withdrawal for personal reasons.

This study follows the *Declaration of Helsinki* and *Good Clinical Practice* and has been approved and supervised by the Ethics Committee.

Measures

Demographic characteristics

Participants reported their age, household registration, educational level, marital status and average monthly income in the baseline survey.

HIV-related characteristics

HIV-related characteristics included HIV counselling or testing previously, threat perception of HIV, and HIV knowledge, which was addressed by 13 questions concerning HIV infection and transmission (1 point for correct answer, 0 for incorrect answer; the total scores≥11 points was regarded as a high level of HIV knowledge). Additionally, the number of male sexual partners, the frequency of looking for sexual partners through the Internet and whether they had been diagnosed with sexually transmitted diseases (STDs) by doctors in the past six months were assessed in the baseline survey.

Perceived barriers during medication

The barriers included a dislike of taking the drugs, worries about the drug's side effects, and the sense of burden perceived during medication. Participants were asked about the barriers perceived when taking TDF in the face-to-face follow-up surveys every 12 weeks. The barriers were rated as 1 point (not at all) to 5 points (always), and participants rated them according to their feelings during medication.

The dislike of taking drugs was made up of 3 items, including "I don't like the taste", "I don't like the formulation" and "I think the drugs are hard to swallow". Then, the average score of the three was taken. Standard Cronbach's α coefficient varied between 0.72 and 0.79 over eight time points.

In addition, the sense of burden perceived during medication was evaluated by "I'm worried about that sexual partners know that I'm taking medicine", and the worries about the drug side effects were accessed by "I'm worried about drug side effects" directly both at baseline and during follow-up.

Perceived benefits during medication

The benefits included positive expectations to medication and favourable doctor-patient relationships at baseline and during the follow-up surveys.

Participants were asked to provide an answer in response to "I think the drugs kept me safe from AIDS" to evaluate the positive expectations to medication, with the answer scored with 1 point (not at all) to 5 points (always).

The doctor-patient relationship consists of two items: "Doctors here are friendly to me, and they care about my health," and "I trust the doctors here." The Cronbach's α coefficient was 0.71 at baseline and varied between 0.74 and 0.91 over the eight time points.

Definition of adherence

We used the medication rate in the last two weeks to assess the adherence of the participants. At each follow-up, the participants were asked to answer whether they missed some doses or not and to fill in the number of missed doses if they did. Medication rate = (14 – number of missed doses)/14, between 0 and 1.

Statistics analysis

The enumeration data including demographic characteristics were expressed as frequency and rate, while measurement data were expressed as $\overline{X} \pm S$, median and range. Longitudinal data were analysed using a linear mixed model (LMM), reporting the β coefficient and 95% confidence intervals (95% CI). LMM was used to assess the change in medication rate over the follow-up and to evaluate which variables were associated with the trend of change. The medication rate in each follow-up was used as the outcome variable to fit the null model and the random intercept-slope model. After the addition of the level 1 explanatory variable (scores of the barriers and benefits perceived during medication) and the level 2 explanatory variable (demographic characteristics), the final model was fitted. The modelling of the linear mixed models was conducted using the Proc Mixed of SAS software. All statistical analyses were performed using SAS 9.4 software and SPSS 22.0 software. $P < 0.05$ was considered to have statistical significance.

Results

Of 575 participants who completed the baseline survey in the TDF group, 141 who did not participate in at least one follow-up and 23 who did not report the number of missed doses at least once were excluded. Thus, a total of 411 MSM involved in at least one follow-up with a maximum of 8 and an average of 3.54 were included in the final analysis. A total of 1561 follow-up observation points were provided.

The demographical and HIV-related characteristics are shown in Table 1. The average age of the 411 MSM was 29.34 ± 7.85 years, and their age ranged from 18 to 61 years. Among the participants, 73.90% were urban residents, and 26.10% were rural residents; 90% graduated from high school and above, and 78.83% were unmarried. Nearly half (48.27%) had an average monthly income above 3000 yuan. The scores of HIV knowledge ranged from 0 to 13 with a median of 9, and only 26.76% had scores above 11. While 64.63 and 81.91% of participants declared that they had ever engaged in HIV counselling and testing, respectively, only 56.97% believed that AIDS is a great threat to themselves and their families. Only 40.63% had only one male sexual partner in the past six months, but only 9.34% had been diagnosed with an STD in the past six months.

Table 1 Demographic and HIV-related characteristic

Variables	Group	N	%
Age	18–25 years old	163	39.66
	26–35 years old	158	38.44
	older than 35 years old	90	21.90
Household registration[a]	Urban	303	73.90
	Rural	107	26.10
Education level[a]	Junior high or below	39	9.56
	Senior high	116	28.43
	Junior college	93	22.79
	College or above	160	39.22
Marital status	Unmarried	324	78.83
	Married	62	15.09
	Divorced/widowed	25	6.08
Monthly income(RMB)[a]	≤1000	63	15.59
	1001–3000	146	36.14
	3001–5000	138	34.16
	5001–10,000	47	11.63
	≥10,001	10	2.48
HIV knowlegde score	< 11	301	73.24
	≥11	110	26.76
HIV counseling[a]	Yes	265	64.63
	No	145	35.37
HIV testing[a]	Yes	335	81.91
	No	74	18.09
Perceived AIDS severity[a]	Moderate and low	135	32.93
	High	275	67.07
Perceived AIDS threat to themselves and family[a]	Moderate and low	176	43.03
	High	233	56.97
Number of male sexual partners in the past six months[a]	1	154	40.63
	2	89	23.48
	≥3	136	35.88
Looking for sexual partners though the Internet in the past six months[a]	Never	148	37.95
	Occasionally	153	39.23
	Always/Sometimes	89	22.82
Diagnosed with STD by doctors in the past six months[a]	Yes	38	9.34
	No	369	90.66

[a]Partially missing data (numbers might not add up to the total because of missing data)

The scores of the barriers and benefits participants perceived at baseline and during the follow-up are shown in Table 2. The changes in the scores of "worries about drug side effects" and "positive expectation about the efficacy of the drugs" over the follow-up are shown in Fig. 1. At baseline, when participants had not yet started to take PrEP, the score for "worries about drug side effects" was 2.97 ± 1.15, but it showed a decreasing trend during the follow-up. Participants had a relatively high expectation

about the efficacy of the drugs at baseline (3.17 ± 1.36), and even though the score was 2.89 ± 1.41 at first follow-up, there was an increasing trend throughout the follow-up, which reached 3.72 ± 1.37 at the end. The scores of "disliked taking drugs" and "burden perceived during medication" fluctuated at a low and moderate level throughout the follow-ups, respectively. The score of "relationships between doctor and participants" was high both at baseline (4.20 ± 1.13) and throughout the entire follow-up.

Table 2 Overall medication rate and scores of the barriers and benefits perceived during medication (mean ± sd)

	Baseline	12 week	24 week	36 week	48 week	60 week	72 week	84 week	96 week
medication rate	Not applicable	0.57 ± 0.39	0.58 ± 0.37	0.59 ± 0.37	0.61 ± 0.36	0.70 ± 0.34	0.70 ± 0.33	0.69 ± 0.32	0.67 ± 0.39
dislike of taking drugs	Not applicable	1.69 ± 0.77	1.70 ± 0.84	1.65 ± 0.76	1.81 ± 0.87	1.75 ± 0.79	1.64 ± 0.75	1.70 ± 0.87	1.55 ± 0.77
worries about drugside effects	2.97 ± 1.15	2.90 ± 1.33	2.84 ± 1.42	2.74 ± 1.40	2.86 ± 1.45	2.76 ± 1.36	2.63 ± 1.37	2.45 ± 1.23	2.23 ± 1.07
burden perceived during medication	2.07 ± 1.23	2.23 ± 1.42	2.34 ± 1.50	2.32 ± 1.47	2.32 ± 1.53	2.54 ± 1.59	2.78 ± 1.66	2.21 ± 1.57	2.09 ± 1.41
positive expectations to medication	3.17 ± 1.36	2.89 ± 1.41	2.94 ± 1.42	2.98 ± 1.51	3.01 ± 1.54	3.17 ± 1.50	3.50 ± 1.51	3.70 ± 1.54	3.72 ± 1.37
favorable doctor patient relationship	4.20 ± 1.13	4.12 ± 1.16	3.92 ± 1.28	4.06 ± 1.24	4.02 ± 1.26	4.15 ± 1.17	4.30 ± 1.13	4.46 ± 1.03	4.52 ± 1.01

The average medication rate for the entire cohort was 0.62 ± 0.37, and its changes during the follow-ups are shown in Table 2. The results of the linear mixed model used to analyse the factors associated with medication adherence are shown in Table 3. The changes of predictive medication rate over the follow-up are shown in Fig. 1. The β coefficient for "time" (meaning follow-up times and coded as 1 to 8) was significant (β = 0.014; 95% CI = 0.005–0.024), indicating that the medication rate increased slightly during the follow-up. After adjusting for potential confounding variables, participants who were divorced showed a higher medication rate (compared with those who were unmarried, β = 0.179; 95% CI = 0.047–0.311). "Positive expectations towards medication", as a time-varying value, was positively associated with the medication rate over time (β = 0.033; 95% CI = 0.020–0.047), indicating that those with higher scores on positive expectations as to the efficacy of the medicine over time reported better adherence to medication over time. In

addition, the more worried the participant was about drug side effects during the follow-up, the lower the medication rate (β = – 0.019; 95% CI = – 0.035–– 0.003). However, the dislike of taking drugs, burden perceived during medication, and the relationship between the doctor and participant showed no correlation with the medication rate (P > 0.05).

Discussion

This study is among the first to examine the potential factors related to PrEP adherence among MSM in a clinical trial in China, and its findings suggest that MSM's positive expectations towards medication was a facilitator, while their worries about drug side effects was a barrier to PrEP adherence during the whole course of medication.

In the present study, a positive expectation towards medication refers to their trust in the efficacy of the drugs, which was evaluated only at a moderate level during the first follow-up but increased as the follow-up

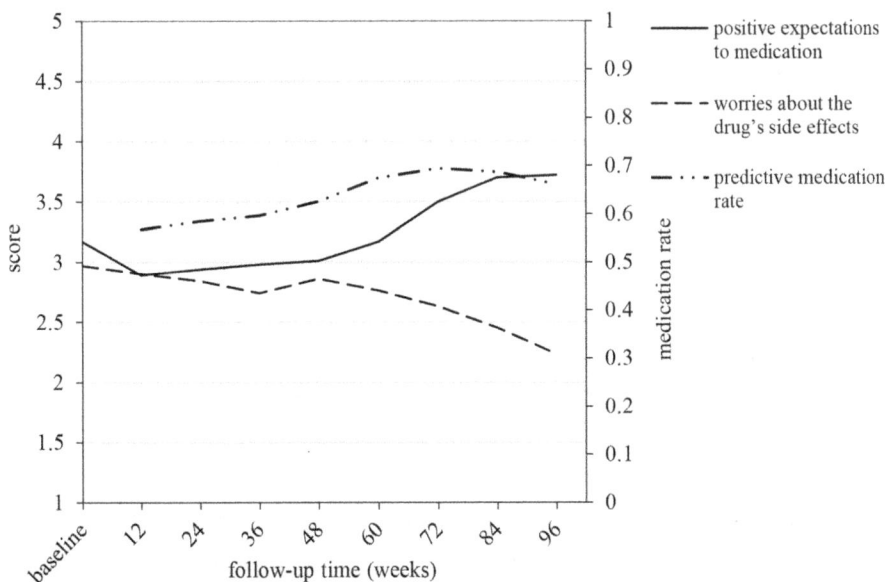

Fig. 1 Graph of the changes in the scores of positive expevtations to medication and worries about the drug's side effects and of predictive medication rate over the follow-up

Table 3 Linear mixed model for medication rate over time

	β	t value	P	95% CI
Variables				
Intercept	0.542	7.49	< 0.0001	0.400~ 0.683
Time	0.014	2.87	0.0046	0.005~ 0.024
Age	0.011	0.42	0.6717	−0.039~ 0.060
Household registration				
Rural	ref			
Urban	− 0.047	−1.20	0.2321	−0.123~ 0.030
Education level	0.018	1.07	0.2837	−0.015~ 0.052
Marital status				
Unmarried	ref			
Married	−0.017	−0.33	0.7429	−0.116~ 0.083
Divorced/widowed	0.179	2.65	0.0085	0.047~ 0.311
Monthly income(RMB)	−0.010	− 0.61	0.5440	− 0.044~ 0.023
Dislike of taking drugs	0.004	0.35	0.7267	−0.019 ~ 0.028
Positive expectations to medication	0.033	4.81	<.0001	0.020~ 0.047
Favorable doctor-patient relationship	−0.017	−1.94	0.0527	−0.033~ 0.001
Worries about drug side effects	−0.019	−2.31	0.0208	−0.035~ − 0.003
Burden perceived during medication	0.014	1.87	0.0621	−0.001~ 0.029

β: longitudinal linear regression coefficient for medication rate

continued. The medication rate became higher along with an increase in their expectations during the follow-up, suggesting that it is still urgent to make efforts to publicize the effectiveness of PrEP drugs. Although many clinical trials of PrEP have been conducted worldwide and TDF was first approved by the FDA as a preventive drug for the MSM population in 2012, this is the first clinical research on PrEP conducted in China and according to the previous surveys on the willingness to use PrEP among MSM in China, only 22% of MSM (308/1402) reported that they had heard of PrEP [24], and a similar rate was observed among female sex workers (16.5%, 264/1611) [25] indicating that MSM in China only have a relatively low awareness of PrEP and that the majority of them have very little understanding of this new biomedical HIV prevention strategy. Therefore, providing more clinical evidence to them may contribute to improving their adherence to medication. It has always been said that the efficacy of drugs depends on patient adherence, but efficacy and adherence may complement each other since positive expectations as to their efficacy encourages people to be more likely to take the medicine on their own initiative.

In addition, the more worried patients are about side effects, the lower the medication rate, which is consistent with not only those studies examining factors associated with willingness to use PrEP [26] but also results found in clinical trials [27, 28]. Unlike therapeutic drugs, few people would take a preventative drug if it has

serious side effects, which is in line with the findings of Mustanski et al. [29] that PrEP is more likely to be used as a preventative strategy for HIV if it has a low burden of side effects and satisfactory benefits are perceived. The worries about drug side effects showed a declining trend in the MSM during the follow-ups, which may be related to the low incidence of adverse events during medication. In our entire follow-up, the main adverse events were nausea, vomiting and diarrhoea, all with a low incidence, and there were no serious adverse events reported. Therefore, in addition to positive expectations of drug efficacy affecting the medication rate, their confidence in the safety of the drugs was also an important facilitator of their medication, which suggested that we should provide them correct information about this drug, inform them of possible side effects, and help them during the follow-ups, thereby reducing their worries about the efficacy and safety of the drugs and improve their adherence to medication.

There was no relationship between disliking taking drugs and the medication rate. In our study, the dislike of taking drugs referred to disliking the drug formulation, taste and pill size. The TDF used in this study were white tablets with 300 mg/tablet. During the follow-ups, the score of the dislike of taking drugs was lowest, which means the drug formulation, taste and size were acceptable by participants to some extent.

No association between the burden perceived during medication and the medication rate was observed. We hypothesized that taking medicine would give their partners a sense that they are in HIV at-risk status, which may impact their adherence. However, we did not find any such relationship and considered that this may be related to the dosing strategy, in which daily oral drugs had more flexibility when compared with dosing 'on demand', another dosing strategy recommended for MSM (a double dose of TDF/FTC 2–24 h before each sexual intercourse, followed by two single doses of TDF/FTC, 24 and 48 h after the first drug intake), and with this dosing strategy (dosed 'on demand'), Mutua et al. [30] found that the burden perceived during medication reduced adherence.

However, the average medication rate during the entire follow-up was not very high. We believed that, other than the factors that we have examined in this study, there were some other barriers that existed and impacted the medication rate. In this study, we mainly focused on some attitudinal factors during medication and examined their relationships with adherence, which could provide some guidelines as to the implementation of clinical trials in China, and thus, it is the very first step in the promotion of PrEP in China. Nevertheless, medication is a long-term process, and long-term adherence to medication may be affected by many factors. For instance, patients may forgot to take their medicine, which has been reported in some studies [28, 31] and in our study; when we asked participants why they missed their doses, some reported that they forgot to take them sometimes. Thus, in the future, interventions should be developed to help remind people to take their medicine. In addition, supplying patients with additional correct information about the benefits and potential risks of the drugs, provided to both MSM and clinicians, their confidence in the drug efficacy could increase, and at the same time, their adherence could be improved.

Limitations

There are some shortcomings in this study. First, we recruited the participants by non-probability sampling, which may lead to some bias and limit the generalizability of this study. In addition, even though we enrolled 575 MSM, 141 did not participate in at least one follow-up. However, when compared with those who were involved in all follow-ups, there were no significant differences in their attitudes (positive expectation about the efficacy of the drugs, worries about the drug side effects, the sense of burden perceived, doctor-participant relationship) in the baseline survey. The average number of follow-ups of the 411 participants was 3.5 times, and there was a certain loss to follow-up. Ensuring a high retention rate should be a priority in future clinical trials. In addition, we used the self-reported number of pills in the past two weeks to evaluate the medication rate. Self-report is the most

widely used method to assess medication adherence; however, it may have some recall bias. [32]. Other approaches used in PrEP clinical trials in other countries such as pill counts, electronic monitoring device data, and blood drug level have their strengths and limitations, and therefore, a combination of two or more methods to evaluate adherence could be used in the next clinical trial [33].

Conclusion

How to obtain and maintain high medication adherence is the key in PrEP to achieve an effective reduction in HIV infection. The results of our study showed that the overall medication rate in the daily medication group is not high. Worries about the efficacy and safety of PrEP were factors influencing the medication rate. For MSM in China, we should work to increase their understanding of the effectiveness and safety of PrEP and increase their confidence in PrEP, thereby improving their medication adherence.

Abbreviations
MSM: Men Who Have Sex With Men Men Who Have Sex With Men; PrEP: Pre-exposure Prophylaxis; TDF: Tenofovir; TDF-FTC: Tenofovir and Emtricitabine; USFDA: US Food and Drug Administration

Acknowledgements
We thank all participants and investigators in Chongqing, Sichuan, Xinjiang and Guangxi for their help.

Funding
This study was supported by the National Key Project for Infectious Diseases of the Ministry of Science and Technology of China (grant number 2012ZX10001007–007) and Chongqing Science & Technology Commission (No. cstc2013jcyjA10009).

Authors' contributions
YH performed the data analyses and wrote the manuscript; XNZ was involved in the design of the study and collecting data in Chongqing, as well as the revision of the manuscript; BP, YZ, HL, JHD, JYZ was involved in the design of the study and collecting data. ALH was in charge of this study. All authors read and approved the final manuscript.

Competing interests
The authors have declared that no competing interests exist.

Author details
[1]Department of Health Statistics and Information Management, School of Public Health and Management, Chongqing Medical University, Chongqing, China. [2]Department of Epidemiology and Medical Statistics, School of Public Health, Guangxi Medical University, Nanning, China. [3]Department of Epidemiology and Health Statistics, School of Public Health, Xinjiang Medical University, Xinjiang, China. [4]Department of Epidemiology and Medical Statistics, School of Public Health, Sichuan University, Sichuan, China. [5]Key Laboratory of Molecular Biology on Infectious Diseases, Ministry of Education, Chongqing Medical University, Chongqing, China.

References

1. UNAIDS, 2017. UNAIDS DATA 2017; Available from: http://www.unaids.org/sites/default/files/media_asset/20170720_Data_book_2017_en.pdf.

2. 2015 China AIDS Response Progress Report. Available from: http://www.unaids.org/sites/default/files/country/documents/CHN_narrative_report_2015.pdf. Accessed 9 Apr 2018.

3. Zhang L, et al. HIV prevalence in China: integration of surveillance data and a systematic review. Lancet Infect Dis. 2013;13(11):955–63.

4. Qin Q, et al. Spatial analysis of the human immunodeficiency virus epidemic among men who have sex with men in China, 2006-2015. Clin Infect Dis. 2017;64(7):956–63.

5. NCAIDS N. Update on the AIDS/STD epidemic in China in December. Chinese J AIDS&STD. 2017;24(2):111.

6. Holmes D. FDA paves the way for pre-exposure HIV prophylaxis. Lancet. 2012;380(9839):325.

7. Smith DK, et al. Preexposure prophylaxis for the prevention of HIV infection in the United States—2014: a clinical practice guideline. Korean J Ophthalmol. 2014;27(4):282–7.

8. Thigpen MC, et al. Antiretroviral preexposure prophylaxis for heterosexual HIV transmission in Botswana. N Engl J Med. 2012;367(5):423–34.

9. Grant RM, et al. Uptake of pre-exposure prophylaxis, sexual practices, and HIV incidence in men and transgender women who have sex with men: a cohort study. Lancet Infect Dis. 2014;14(9):820.

10. Grant RM, et al. Preexposure chemoprophylaxis for HIV prevention in men who have sex with men. N Engl J Med. 2010;363(27):2587–99.

11. Karim QA, et al. Effectiveness and safety of tenofovir gel, an antiretroviral microbicide, for the prevention of HIV infection in women. Science. 2010;329(5996):1168–74.

12. Choopanya K, et al. Antiretroviral prophylaxis for HIV infection in injecting drug users in Bangkok, Thailand (the Bangkok Tenofovir study): a randomised, double-blind, placebo-controlled phase 3 trial. Lancet. 2013;381(9883):2083–90.

13. Alistar SS, Owens DK, Brandeau ML. Effectiveness and cost effectiveness of oral pre-exposure prophylaxis in a portfolio of prevention programs for injection drug users in mixed HIV epidemics. PLoS One. 2014;9(1):e86584.

14. Haberer JE, et al. Adherence to antiretroviral prophylaxis for HIV prevention: a substudy cohort within a clinical trial of Serodiscordant couples in East Africa. PLoS Med. 2013;10(9):e1001511.

15. Marrazzo JM, et al. Tenofovir-based Preexposure prophylaxis for HIV infection among African women. N Engl J Med. 2015;372(6):509–18.

16. Muchomba FM, et al. State of the science of adherence in pre-exposure prophylaxis and microbicide trials. J Acquir Immune Defic Syndr. 2012;61(4):490–8.

17. Van DL, et al. Preexposure prophylaxis for HIV infection among African women. N Engl J Med. 2012;308(9):411–22.

18. Mehrotra ML, et al. The effect of depressive symptoms on adherence to daily Oral PrEP in men who have sex with men and transgender women: a marginal structural model analysis of the iPrEx OLE study. Aids & Behavior. 2016;20(7):1527–34.

19. Defechereux PA, et al. Depression and Oral FTC/TDF pre-exposure prophylaxis (PrEP) among men and transgender women who have sex with men (MSM/TGW). Aids & Behavior. 2016;20(7):1478–88.

20. Minnis AM, et al. Pre-exposure prophylaxis adherence measured by plasma drug level in MTN-001: comparison between vaginal gel and oral tablets in two geographic regions. Aids & Behavior. 2016;20(7):1541–8.

21. Zeng X. Tenofovir-based oral PrEP prevents HIV infection among men who have sex with men in western China:a multicenter, randomized, controlled clinical trial: Chongqing Medical University; 2013 (in Chinese).

22. O'Brien MK, Petrie K, Raeburn J. Adherence to medication regimens: updating a complex medical issue. Med Care Review. 1992;49(4):435.

23. Bakken S, et al. Relationships between perception of engagement with health care provider and demographic. AIDS Patient Care STDs. 2000;14(4):189–97.

24. Zhang Y, et al. Attitudes toward HIV pre-exposure prophylaxis among men who have sex with men in western China. Aids Patient Care & Stds. 2013;27(3):137.

25. Peng B, et al. Willingness to use pre-exposure prophylaxis for HIV prevention among female sex workers: a cross-sectional study in China. Hiv/aids. 2012;4(default):149.

26. Holloway IW, et al. Facilitators and barriers to pre-exposure prophylaxis willingness among young men who have sex with men who use geosocial networking applications in California. Aids Patient Care & Stds. 2017;31(12):517.

27. Gengiah TN, et al. Adherence challenges with drugs for pre-exposure prophylaxis to prevent HIV infection. Int J Clin Pharm. 2014;36(1):70–85.

28. Kebaabetswe PM, et al. Factors associated with adherence and concordance between measurement strategies in an HIV daily Oral Tenofovir/Emtricitibine as pre-exposure prophylaxis (Prep) clinical trial, Botswana, 2007-2010. Aids & Behavior. 2015;19(5):758–69.

29. Mustanski B, et al. Perceived likelihood of using HIV pre-exposure prophylaxis medications among young men who have sex with men. Aids Behavior. 2013;17(6):2173–9.

30. Mutua G, et al. Safety and adherence to intermittent pre-exposure prophylaxis (PrEP) for HIV-1 in African men who have sex with men and female sex workers. PLoS One. 2012;7(4):e33103.

31. Skoler-Karpoff S, et al. Efficacy of Carraguard for prevention of HIV infection in women in South Africa: a randomised, double-blind, placebo-controlled trial. Lancet. 2008;372(9654):1977–87.

32. Williams AB, et al. A proposal for quality standards for measuring medication adherence in research. Aids & Behavior. 2013;17(1):284–97.

33. Abaasa A, et al. Utility of different adherence measures for PrEP: patterns and incremental value. Aids & Behavior. 2017;22(5):1–9.

19

Field suitability and diagnostic accuracy of the Biocentric® open real-time PCR platform for plasma-based HIV viral load quantification in Swaziland

Bernhard Kerschberger[1]*[iD], Qhubekani Mpala[1], Paola Andrea Díaz Uribe[1], Gugu Maphalala[2], Roberto de la Tour[3], Sydney Kalombola[1], Addis Bekele[1], Tiwonge Chawinga[1], Mukelo Mliba[1], Nombuso Ntshalintshali[4], Nomcebo Phugwayo[2], Serge Mathurin Kabore[1], Javier Goiri[3], Sindisiwe Dlamini[2], Iza Ciglenecki[3] and Emmanuel Fajardo[5]

Abstract

Background: Viral load (VL) testing is being scaled up in resource-limited settings. However, not all commercially available VL testing methods have been evaluated under field conditions. This study is one of a few to evaluate the Biocentric platform for VL quantification in routine practice in Sub-Saharan Africa.

Methods: Venous blood specimens were obtained from patients eligible for VL testing at two health facilities in Swaziland from October 2016 to March 2017. Samples were centrifuged at two laboratories (LAB-1, LAB-2) to obtain paired plasma specimens for VL quantification with the national reference method and on the Biocentric platform. Agreement (correlation, Bland–Altman) and accuracy (sensitivity, specificity) indicators were calculated at the VL thresholds of 416 (2.62 $\log_{10}$) and 1000 (3.0 $\log_{10}$) copies/mL. Leftover samples from patients with discordant VL results were re-quantified and accuracy indicators recalculated. Logistic regression was used to compare laboratory performance.

Results: A total of 364 paired plasma samples (LAB-1: $n = 198$; LAB-2: $n = 166$) were successfully tested using both methods. The correlation was high ($R = 0.82$, $p < 0.01$), and the Bland–Altman analysis showed a minimal mean difference (– 0.03 $\log_{10}$ copies/mL; 95% CI: -1.15 to 1.08). At the clinical threshold level of 3.0 $\log_{10}$ copies/mL, the sensitivity was 88.6% (95% CI: 78.7 to 94.9) and the specificity was 98.3% (95% CI: 96.1 to 99.4). Sensitivity was higher in LAB-1 (100%; 95% CI: 71.5 to 100) than in LAB-2 (86.4%; 95% CI: 75.0 to 94.0). Most upward ($n = 8$, 2.2%) and downward ($n = 11$, 3.0%) misclassifications occurred at the 2.62 log threshold, with LAB-2 having a 16 (95% CI: 2.26 to 113.27; $p = 0.006$) times higher odds of downward misclassification. After retesting of discordant leftover samples ($n = 17$), overall sensitivity increased to 93.5% (95% CI: 85.5 to 97.9) and 97.1% (95% CI: 90.1 to 99.7) at the 2.62 and 3.0 thresholds, and specificity increased to 98.6% (95% CI: 96.5 to 99.6) and 99.0% (95% CI: 97.0 to 99.8) respectively.

Conclusions: The test characteristics of the Biocentric platform were overall comparable to the national reference method for VL quantification. One laboratory tended to misclassify VL results downwards, likely owing to unmet training needs and lack of previous hands-on practice.

Keywords: HIV, Biocentric, Open platform, Viral load, Accuracy, Swaziland

* Correspondence: bernhard.kerschberger@gmail.com
[1]Medecins Sans Frontieres (OCG), P.O. Box 18, Eveni, Lot No. 331, Sheffield Road, Industrial Area, Mbabane, Swaziland
Full list of author information is available at the end of the article

Background

The World Health Organization (WHO) recommends routine viral load (VL) testing at 6 and 12 months after initiation of antiretroviral therapy (ART) and annually thereafter [1]. Quantifying the patient's VL allows clinicians to monitor the effectiveness of ART, to trigger adherence counselling interventions when VL is elevated above a clinical threshold (e.g. ≥1000 copies/mL), to diagnose virological failure, and to make timely and correct decisions on treatment switching [1–3]. Because the WHO recommends immediate initiation of ART at the time of HIV diagnosis irrespective of CD4 cell count and WHO staging criteria [1, 4], the number of patients needing routine VL testing will increase in the coming years. Although HIV programmes using routine VL monitoring have shown decreased morbidity and mortality [3], the expansion of VL testing creates clinical and programmatic challenges in resource-limited settings (RLS) [5, 6] and access to HIV monitoring services remains suboptimal [7, 8].

An important bottleneck is the suboptimal capacity of national laboratories in RLS to perform VL testing at scale. The supply weakness is often due to lack of funding to procure VL testing platforms and consumables, inability to recruit and retain qualified staff, lack of adequate training, and suboptimal servicing and maintenance of equipment [7]. Establishment of multiple laboratories in one country and the deployment of various platforms by different stakeholders (e.g. non-governmental organizations) is one strategy to overcome supply chain shortfalls and stimulate market competition [5]. This approach, however, raises concerns about comparability of VL test results between platforms and laboratories as well as about quality assurance and control.

Swaziland is increasing access to routine VL monitoring. The Ministry of Health performs VL testing using the Roche method, and Médecins Sans Frontières (MSF) has been performing VL quantification using the Biocentric method [9]. In 2015, the decision was taken to perform an in-country assessment of the Biocentric method to assess its suitability for contributing to expansion of VL testing in Swaziland. Thus, we compared the performance of the Biocentric platform under field conditions using plasma for VL testing in comparison with the national reference platform. The findings reported here are part of a larger prospective evaluation study comparing the test characteristics of the Biocentric platform, using different sampling and processing procedures (plasma and dried-blood spots [DBS]) for VL testing.

Methods

Setting

Swaziland is the country with the highest HIV prevalence (32% in people aged 18–49 years) in the world

[10]. HIV care and treatment has been expanded, and close to 150,000 people received ART in 2015 [11]. Swaziland is expanding routine VL monitoring, and several VL platforms have been established. Three Roche platforms are operated, one at the National Reference Laboratory at Mbabane and two at decentralized sites (Manzini, Siteki). Since 2012, the Biocentric platform has been used in Nhlagano Laboratory in southern Swaziland, serving 25 rural primary and secondary healthcare facilities, with approximately 25,000 VL tests performed annually. It has been enrolled in the External Quality Assurance Program with the US Centers for Disease Control and Prevention (CDC) for proficiency testing. In addition, a second Biocentric platform was established at the National Reference Laboratory in 2016 but had not been used before this study. This study used the more recent Biocentric platform which was released in 2016. It was upgraded at Nhlangano laboratory (LAB-1) and newly installed at the National Reference Laboratory in Mbabane (LAB-2).

VL platforms

The reference platform was the quantitative COBAS AmpliPrep/COBAS TaqMan (CAP/CTM) HIV-1 Test, Version 2.0 (Roche Molecular Diagnostics, Indiana, USA), operated at LAB-2 (Mbabane). It is a fully automated, closed system testing 63 samples per run with 5–8 h needed to obtain results. The lower limit of detection is 20 copies/mL (corresponding to 1.3 $\log_{10}$ copies/mL). Standardized internal quality control samples are provided and the reference laboratory is enrolled with the CDC laboratory external quality assurance program, monitoring the quality of VL testing and reporting twice per year.

The comparator comprised two Biocentric platforms operated at LAB-1 (Nhlangano) and at LAB-2 (Mbabane). This multi-manufacturer open platform consists of an open automated RNA and DNA extractor (Arrow®) and a real-time PCR system (FluoroCycler® 96) for nucleic acid amplification and detection. It uses the Generic HIV Charge Virale assay and test kits, which were developed by the French Agency for Research on AIDS and viral hepatitis (ANRS) and are manufactured and commercialized by Biocentric (Bandol, France) [12]. Internal quality control is provided by standards in the assay. This somewhat manual system has a time to results of approximately 3 h, with 96 samples per run (82 patient samples, five standards per duplicate, and one positive and one negative control per duplicate). The average limit of detection of HIV RNA at a positivity rate of > 95% with 250 µL plasma input volume is 416 (95% CI: 388 to 450) copies/mL [12]. The Biocentric assay received CE certification by a European Notified Body (British Standards Institution) and has been

Field suitability and diagnostic accuracy of the Biocentric® open real-time PCR platform...

173

submitted for WHO pre-qualification of in vitro diagnostics. Further details on the method are available elsewhere [13].

Study sample and procedures

Experienced laboratory technologists at LAB-1 received short refresher training on the Biocentric platform. Most laboratory technologists at LAB-2 had no experience in the Biocentric method and they received training over 3 days as per recommendation of the manufacturer. Figure 1 shows the study flow chart. From 12 October 2016 to 1 March 2017, HIV-infected adults (≥18 years) were recruited at Nhlangano Health Centre and Lobamba Clinic when they were eligible for VL testing according to the local VL testing algorithm (a baseline VL before ART initiation and during ART). During the recruitment phase, Lobamba Clinic introduced universal ART provision (thus many patients were eligible for ART initiation and received a pre-treatment VL test), while most patients in Nhlangano Health Centre were already established on ART (and thus received a follow-up VL test). The nurse obtained written consent, collected baseline information and referred patients for phlebotomy. A phlebotomist obtained one 4 mL venous blood ethylenediaminetetraacetic acid (EDTA) tube from each participant. In addition, a second EDTA tube and DBS cards were prepared as part of the larger study (details and results not reported here). The blood tubes obtained at Nhlangano Health Centre were sent to LAB-1 and those obtained at Lobamba Clinic to LAB-2.

In both laboratories, technologists centrifuged the EDTA tube to obtain two paired plasma specimens of 1 mL, which were stored in two separate sterile tubes at − 20 °C before testing. As the reference method was located at the National Reference Laboratory (and collocated to Biocentric LAB-2), deep frozen plasma samples were shipped (2 h) from LAB-1 to LAB-2 for testing on the reference platform. All testing runs were performed with a plasma input volume of 250 μL on the Biocentric method and 1 mL on the Roche method. VL results that were discrepant between the two methods at LAB-1 and LAB-2 were repeated on the Biocentric method in the same laboratory when leftover plasma samples were available. The laboratory personnel were blinded to the results of both methods.

Statistical analysis

This study is reported according to the STARD guidelines [14]. Patients without a plasma test result on both platforms were removed from analysis. Baseline characteristics of the study population were described and summarized in frequency statistics and percentages. To compare baseline characteristics of patients by recruitment site, differences in continues (e.g. age) and categorical (e.g. sex) data were assessed with the Wilcoxon rank sum test and the Pearson's chi-squared test. We regarded the VL results from the reference method (CAP/CTM) as the national gold standard. Because the two assays had different lower and upper detection limits, VL test results were equalized at the common lowest ($2.62 \log_{10}$ copies/mL) and highest reliable ($7.0 \log_{10}$ copies/mL) detection limits. We assessed the correlation between the two methods graphically and with the Pearson's correlation coefficient for quantifiable VL values $\geq 2.62 \log_{10}$ copies/mL on the two platforms. Then we used Bland–Altman analysis to describe agreement between the two platforms by calculating the mean difference along with 95% limits of agreement [15]. Sensitivity and specificity were calculated using the threshold of $2.62 \log_{10}$ copies/mL

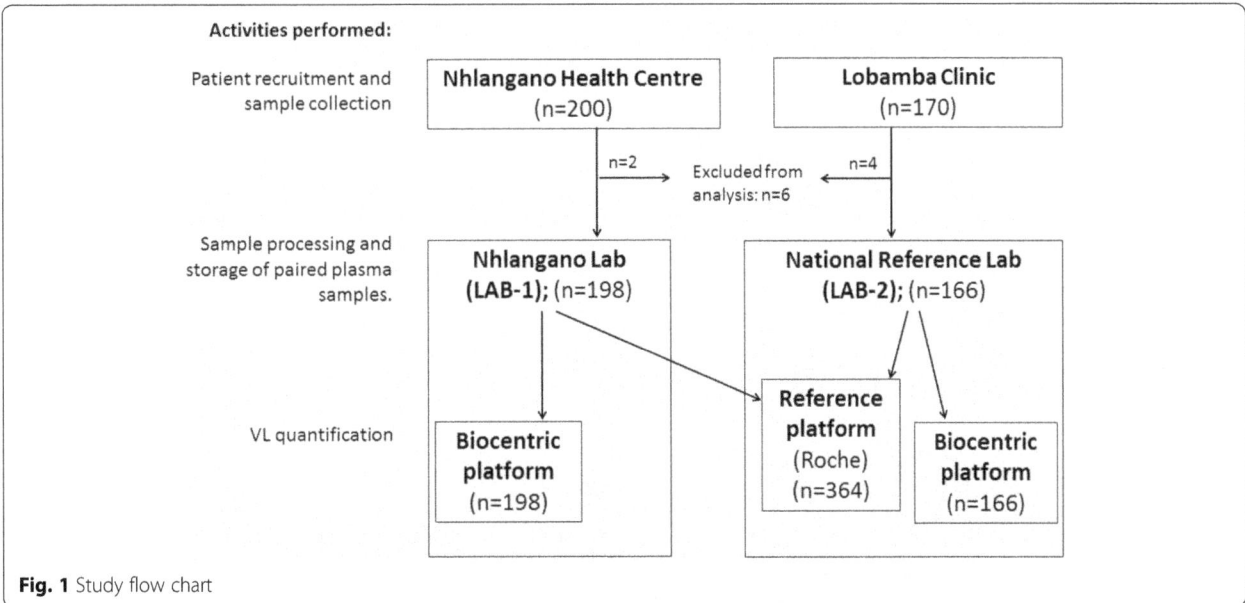

Fig. 1 Study flow chart

(lower limit of detection, corresponding to 416 copies/mL) and 3.0 $\log_{10}$ copies/mL (clinical threshold, corresponding to 1000 copies/mL). The positive and negative predictive values (PPV and NPV) were computed assuming 10 and 20% VL elevations in a hypothetical population undergoing VL testing. All analyses were conducted separately for each laboratory and both laboratories combined.

In sensitivity analyses, to account for prolonged turnaround times from sample collection to freezing of paired plasma samples, diagnostic accuracy estimates (sensitivity, specificity) were recalculated for samples with processing times of ≤4.0 h. In addition, misclassified values were described separately at the patient level and accuracy estimates recalculated after re-quantification of discordant VL results. Discordance was defined as VL results which were categorized differently by the Biocentric platform (above or below) compared with the reference test, using a binary VL cut-off at 2,62 and 3.0 $\log_{10}$ copies/mL. Because LAB-2 appeared to have had higher rates of misclassification, we evaluated a possible association between laboratory (LAB-2 vs LAB-1) and VL result misclassification. Potential confounding factors were identified a priori using directed acyclic graphs (DAGs) [16] and included in multivariable penalized maximum likelihood logistic regression models. All analyses were performed with STATA v14.1 (StataCorp, Texas, USA).

Results

Baseline characteristics

We recruited 370 patients, of whom six (1.6%) were excluded from analysis: three were less than 18 years of age and three had insufficient or sub-optimal quality plasma samples for VL quantification (Fig. 1). Of the remaining 364 patients with paired VL testing results available (Table 1), the median age was 36 (interquartile range [IQR]: 30–44.5) years, 231 (64.7%) and 15 (4.2%) were non-pregnant and pregnant women respectively, and 305 (83.8%) patients received a VL test while on ART (median time on ART 5.0 (IQR 2.0–7.5) years). Nhangano Health Centre recruited 198 (54.4%) patients who, compared with Lobamba Clinic, were more likely to be men (32.5% vs 29.4%) and non-pregnant women (67.0% vs 61.9%), were older (39 vs 32.5 years), were more likely to have received a VL test during ART (98.0% vs 66.9%) and had been on ART for longer (6.2 vs 2.9 years). All samples from Nhlangano Health Centre (n = 198) were sent for processing to LAB-1 and all samples from Lobamba Clinic (n = 166) to LAB-2 (Fig. 1). The median time from EDTA collection to plasma storage at − 20 °C (processing time) was 1.9 (IQR: 1.1–3.3) hours, and it was shorter for LAB-1 (1.2, IQR: 0.9–1.9) than for LAB-2 (3.1, IQR: 2.2–4.1) (p < 0.01). Overall, 54 (14.8%) samples were stored for between 4 and 6 h, and one sample for 6.9 h. The median time from freezing of the plasma sample to testing on the reference and Biocentric platforms was 21.5 (IQR: 13–28) and 89 (IQR: 56–103) days respectively.

Results of VL quantification using the reference method

According to the reference method, 236 (64.8%) specimens had a VL below the detection limit, and 58 (15.9%) had a VL of 1.3–< 3.0, 17 (4.7%) of 3.0–< 4.0 and 53 (14.6%) of ≥4.0 $\log_{10}$ copies/mL. The median

Table 1 Baseline characteristics of the study population by recruitment site/ laboratory and overall

	Both facilities combined	Nhlangano (LAB-1)[a]	Lobamba (LAB-2)[a]	p-value
Total	364	198 (54.4)	166 (45.4)	
Age; median (IQR), years	36 (30–44.5)	39 (33–48)	32.5 (27–39)	< 0.01
Gender and pregnancy status (missing = 7)				< 0.01
Men	111 (31.1)	64 (32.5)	47 (29.4)	
Non-pregnant women	231 (64.7)	132 (67.0)	99 (61.9)	
Pregnant women	15 (4.2)	1 (0.5)	14 (8.8)	
Reason for VL test				< 0.01
Pre-ART	59 (16.2)	4 (2.0)	55 (33.1)	
ART	305 (83.8)	194 (98.0)	111 (66.9)	
Time on ART; median (IQR), years	5.0 (2.0–7.5)	6.2 (3.3–8.3)	2.9 (1.8–5.4)	< 0.01
VL values on the reference method; $\log_{10}$ copies/mL				< 0.01
< 1.3	236 (64.8)	150 (75.8)	86 (51.8)	
1.3–< 3.0	58 (15.9)	37 (18.7)	21 (12.7)	
3.0–< 4.0	17 (4.7)	5 (2.5)	12 (7.2)	
≥ 4.0	53 (14.6)	6 (3.0)	47 (28.3)	

ART Antiretroviral therapy, IQR Interquartile range, VL Viral load
[a]VL samples obtained in Nhlangano Health Centre were tested at LAB-1 (Nhlangano), and VL samples obtained in Lobamba Clinic were tested at LAB-2 (Mbabane)

VL of specimens with detectable VLs ($n = 128$) on the reference method was 3.42 (IQR: 1.66–4.91) $\log_{10}$ copies/mL. LAB-1 received more undetectable (< 1.3 $\log_{10}$ copies/mL) paired specimens ($n = 150$, 75.8%) than LAB-2 ($n = 86$, 51.8%; $p < 0.01$), and the median VL among detectable measurements was also lower (LAB-1: 1.57, IQR: 1.3–2.76; LAB-2: 4.26, IQR: 2.91–5.10; $p < 0.01$) (Table 1).

Correlation and agreement

The Pearson's correlation coefficient for quantifiable VL values above the threshold level of 2.62 $\log_{10}$ copies/mL on both methods ($n = 66$) showed a strong positive correlation between the reference method and Biocentric ($R = 0.82$, $p < 0.01$) and appeared higher in LAB-1 ($R = 0.98$, $p < 0.01$) compared with LAB-2 ($R = 0.75$, $p < 0.01$) (Fig. 2). Figure 3 shows the Bland–Altman difference plots for quantifiable VL results ($n = 66$) on both methods. The overall mean difference was minimal at − 0.03 (95% CI: -1.15 to 1.08) $\log_{10}$ copies/mL. It was 0.24 (95% CI: -0.54 to 1.03) $\log_{10}$ copies/mL for LAB-1 and -0.09 (95% CI: -1.24 to 1.05) $\log_{10}$ copies/mL for LAB-2. All values were within ±1.0 $\log_{10}$ copies/mL from the mean, and 60 (90.9%) were within ±0.5 $\log_{10}$ copies/mL from the mean.

Diagnostic accuracy

Accuracy was calculated at two threshold levels (2.62 and 3.0 $\log_{10}$ copies/mL), and findings are presented in Table 2. The overall accuracy of the Biocentric platform was excellent at the 2.62 log threshold, with

an area under the receiver operating characteristic (ROC) curve of 0.92 (95% CI: 0.87 to 0.96), and was similar for the two laboratories (LAB-1: 0.94, 95%CI: 0.87 to 1.00; LAB-2: 0.92, 0.87 to 0.96).

For the threshold levels of 2.62 and 3.0 $\log_{10}$ copies/mL, the overall (both laboratories combined) sensitivity was 85.7% (95% CI: 75.9 to 92.6) and 88.6% (78.7 to 94.9) respectively, and the specificity was 97.2% (94.6 to 98.8) and 98.3% (96.1 to 99.4). Although the specificity was similar in both laboratories, ranging from 96.2 to 99.1% at both threshold levels, the sensitivity was lower in LAB-2 at both log thresholds (at 2.62 $\log_{10}$ copies/mL: 84.4%, 73.1 to 92.1) compared with LAB-1 (at 2.62 $\log_{10}$ copies/mL: 92.3%, 64.0 to 99.8) (Table 2). While the sensitivity at the 3.0 log threshold was high at 100% (71.5 to 100) in LAB-1, it remained low in LAB-2 (86.4%, 75.0 to 94.0). At the 2.62 log threshold, the combined PPV was 77.4 (63.2 to 87.2) and the NPV was 98.4 (97.3 to 99.1) assuming a prevalence of 10% VL elevation, and 88.5 (79.4 to 93.9) and 96.5 (94.0 to 97.9) respectively assuming a prevalence of 20%. Both the PPV and NPV remained similar when calculated at the 3.0 log threshold.

In sensitivity analyses, the sensitivity and specificity estimates at both VL log thresholds remained similar after removal of samples with > 4.0 h ($n = 55$) or missing ($n = 1$) processing times (2.62 log threshold: sensitivity 85.7% (74.6 to 93.3), specificity 96.7 (93.7 to 98.6); 3.0 log threshold: sensitivity 89.5% (78.5 to 96.0), specificity (98.0% (95.4 to 99.4)).

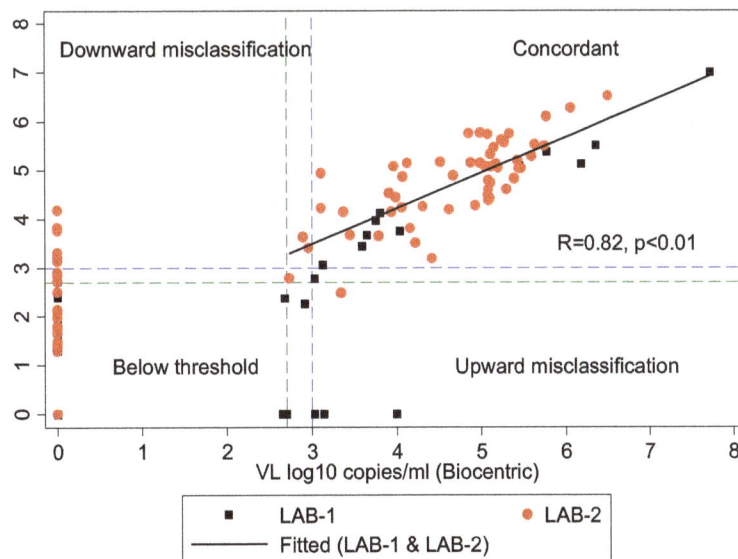

Fig. 2 Assay correlation and concordance between the Biocentric platform and the reference method. VL, viral load; R, Pearson's correlation coefficient; p, p-value; LAB-1, laboratory 1 in Nhlangano; LAB-2, laboratory 2 in Mbabane. The correlation graph shows paired VL values obtained from the reference and Biocentric platforms. The Pearson's correlation coefficient and the fitted linear regression line were calculated for quantifiable VL values above the threshold level of 2.62 log10 copies/mL on both methods ($n = 66$)

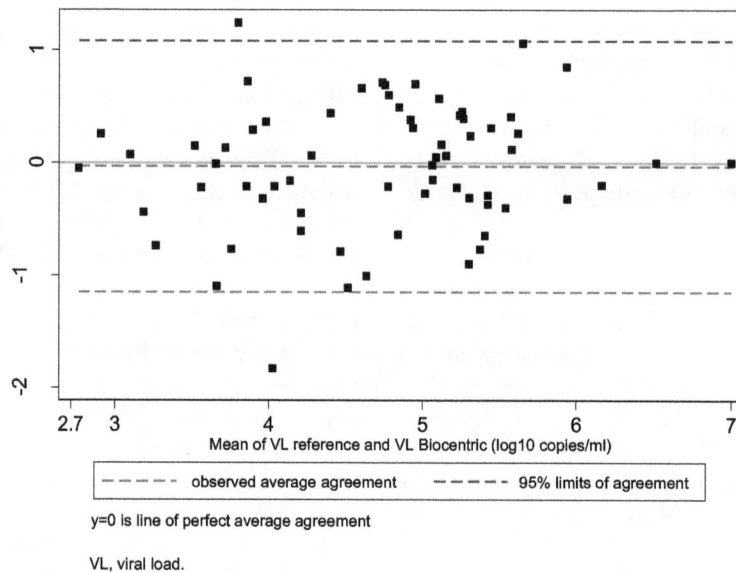

Fig. 3 Bland–Altman mean difference analysis between the Biocentric platform and the reference method (n = 66). The analysis was performed for paired samples with a VL ≥2.62 $\log_{10}$ copies/mL on both the Biocentric and the reference platform

Misclassification

At the threshold of 2.62 $\log_{10}$ copies/mL, 19/364 (5.2%) samples were misclassified: 11/364 (3.0%) samples were misclassified downwards and 8/364 (2.2%) were misclassified upwards (Table 3). Among these, five samples were below the lower detection limit of the reference method but were detected on the Biocentric platform, and 11 samples were quantified on the reference method but not detected on the Biocentric platform. Misclassification occurred across all quantification levels of the reference method: five in the VL range of < 1.3 $\log_{10}$ copies/mL, eight in the range of 1.3–< 3.0 $\log_{10}$ copies/mL, five

in the range of 3.0–< 4.0 $\log_{10}$ copies/mL, and one at ≥4.0 $\log_{10}$ copies/mL. Of note, 57.9% (n = 11) of misclassification occurred in LAB-2, of which 10/11 (90.9%) were downward misclassifications. Overall, 18/19 (94.7%) discordant samples differed more than 0.5 $\log_{10}$ copies/mL at the threshold of 2.62 $\log_{10}$ copies/mL and 11/13 (84.6%) at the threshold of 3.0 $\log_{10}$ copies/mL.

After adjustment for potential factors associated with misclassification (see Additional file 1), multivariate analysis showed that LAB-2 had a 15.99 (95% CI: 2.26 to 113.27; p = 0.002) higher odds of downward

Table 2 Test characteristics of the Biocentric platform at two VL threshold levels

	At 2.62 $\log_{10}$ copies/mL			At 3.0 $\log_{10}$ copies/mL		
	LAB-1 (n = 198)	LAB-2 (n = 166)	Combined (n = 364)	LAB-1 (n = 198)	LAB-2 (n = 166)	Combined (n = 364)
Sensitivity % (95% CI)	92.3 (64.0–99.8)	84.4 (73.1–92.2)	85.7 (75.9–92.6)	100 (71.5–100)	86.4 (75.0–94.0)	88.6 (78.7–94.9)
Specificity % (95% CI)	96.2 (92.4–98.5)	99.0 (94.7–100)	97.2 (94.6–98.8)	97.9 (94.6–99.4)	99.1 (94.9–100.0)	98.3 (96.1–99.4)
ROC area % (95% CI)	0.94 (0.87–1.00)	0.92 (0.87–0.96)	0.92 (0.87–0.96)	0.99 (0.98–1.00)	0.93 (0.88–0.97)	0.93 (0.90–0.97)
PPV (at 10%)[a] % (95% CI)	73.1 (56.3–85.1)	90.5 (57.6–98.5)	77.4 (63.2–87.2)	83.9 (66.3–93.2)	91.1 (59.3–98.6)	85.3 (70.7–93.3)
NPV (at 10%)[a] % (95% CI)	99.1 (94.5–99.9)	98.3 (97.0–99.0)	98.4 (97.3–99.1)	100 (93.3–100)	98.5 (97.2–99.2)	98.7 (97.6–99.3)
PPV (at 20%)[a] % (95% CI)	85.9 (74.4–92.8)	95.6 (75.3–99.3)	88.5 (79.4–93.9)	92.1 (81.6–96.9)	95.9 (76.6–99.4)	92.9 (84.5–96.9)
NPV (at 20%)[a] % (95% CI)	98.0 (88.4–99.7)	96.2 (93.5–97.8)	96.5 (94.0–97.9)	100 (86.1–99.9)	96.7 (93.9–98.2)	97.2 (94.7–98.5)

ROC Receiver operating characteristic, *PPV* Positive predictive value, *NPV* Negative predictive value

[a]For the calculation of predictive values, 10 and 20% prevalence of detectable VLs were assumed in a hypothetical population undergoing routine VL testing

Table 3 Original and reclassified viral load test results between the Biocentric platform and the reference assay

Lab	Reason for VL testing	Time to freezing (hours)[a]	VL results during first round of VL quantification				VL results after re-quantification		
			Reference method (log$_{10}$ copies/mL-l)	Biocentric platform (log$_{10}$ copies/mL-l)	Misclassification		Biocentric platform (log$_{10}$ copies/mL-l)	Misclassification	
					2.62 log$_{10}$ copies/mL	3.0 log$_{10}$ copies/mL		2.62 log$_{10}$ copies/mL	3.0 log$_{10}$ copies/mL
Lab-1	ART	2.7	0	3.14	upward	upward	*	*	*
Lab-1	ART	3.8	0	2.65	upward	CON	0	CON	CON
Lab-1	ART	1.1	0	3.03	upward	upward	0	CON	CON
Lab-1	ART	0.9	0	4.00	upward	upward	0	CON	CON
Lab-1	ART	0.5	0	2.70	upward	CON	*	*	*
Lab-1	ART	0.3	2.25	2.92	upward	CON	*	*	*
Lab-1	ART	1.5	2.37	2.68	upward	CON	0	CON	CON
Lab-2	Pre-ART	2.2	2.48	3.34	upward	upward	2.78	upward	CON
Lab-2	ART	4.4	2.72	0	downward	CON	0	downward	CON
Lab-1	ART	1.6	2.73	0	downward	CON	*	*	*
Lab-1	ART	2.4	2.78	3.03	CON	upward	*	*	*
Lab-2	Pre-ART	2.6	2.84	0	downward	CON	2.84	CON	CON
Lab-2	Pre-ART	1.2	2.90	0	downward	CON	0	downward	CON
Lab-2	Pre-ART	1.4	2.91	0	downward	CON	3.00 (999[b])	CON	upward[b]
Lab-2	Pre-ART	1	3.13	0	downward	downward	0	downward	downward
Lab-2	ART	2.6	3.21	0	downward	downward	3.51	CON	CON
Lab-2	Pre-ART	3	3.31	0	downward	downward	0	downward	downward
Lab-2	Pre-ART	3.2	3.40	2.96	CON	downward	3.84	CON	CON
Lab-2	Pre-ART	4.7	3.63	2.89	CON	downward	3.60	CON	CON
Lab-2	Pre-ART	4.1	3.77	0	downward	downward	3.06	CON	CON
Lab-2	ART	0.3	3.82	0	downward	downward	3.95	CON	CON
Lab-2	Pre-ART	2.5	4.17	0	downward	downward	4.29	CON	CON

*Re-quantification on the Biocentric platform was not possible as no leftover plasma samples were available due to contamination. Reclassification of test results was not performed

Zero values indicate that the VL results were below the detection limit of the VL assays

CON Concordant

[a]Time from sample collection to freezing at − 20 °C before testing

[b]Due to rounding, the 3.00 log$_{10}$ copies/mL values represent a false-positive test result at the 3.0 log$_{10}$ copies/mL threshold but a concordant result according to the non-log$_{10}$ values

misclassification at the 2.62 log threshold compared with LAB-1. No associations were found for the overall probability of discordant VL values (upward and downward misclassification combined), for upward misclassification or at the 3.0 log threshold level. The full regression model is presented in Additional file 2.

Re-quantification of discordant VL values

Discordant VL values at both log thresholds were re-quantified on the Biocentric platform in corresponding LAB-1 and LAB-2 by the more experienced laboratory technologists when leftover samples were available. At the 2.62 log threshold, 15/19 (78.9%) leftover samples were re-quantified, of which 10 samples became concordant, one remained misclassified upwards (2.78 log$_{10}$ copies/mL on the Biocentric platform vs 2.48 log$_{10}$ copies/mL on the reference method) and four remained misclassified

downwards (undetectable on the Biocentric platform vs 2.72, 2.90, 3.13 and 3.31 log$_{10}$ copies/mL on the reference method). Re-quantification at the 3.0 log threshold yielded similar findings. Among the 11/13 (84.6%) successfully re-quantified results, nine VL values became concordant while two remained misclassified downwards (undetectable on the Biocentric platform vs 3.13 and 3.31 log$_{10}$ copies/mL on the reference method). When we considered the re-quantified values and kept the original VL values for non-retested samples, the overall sensitivity estimates increased to 93.5 (95% CI: 85.5 to 97.9) and 97.1% (90.1 to 99.7) at the 2.62 and 3.0 thresholds, and specificity estimates increased to 98.6 (96.5 to 99.6) and 99.0% (97.0 to 99.8) respectively (Table 4). The PPV and NPV increased to 96.0% (88.5–98.7) and 99.3% (97.2–99.8) respectively when a prevalence of 20% VL elevation at the 3.0 log threshold was assumed.

Table 4 Test characteristics of the Biocentric platform (both laboratories combined) after re-quantification of discordant VL samples

	At 2.62 $\log_{10}$ copies/mL ($n = 364$)	At 3.0 $\log_{10}$ copies/mL ($n = 364$)
Sensitivity % (95% CI)	93.5 (85.5–97.9)	97.1 (90.1–99.7)
Specificity % (95% CI)	98.6 (96.5–99.6)	99.0 (97.0–99.8)
ROC area % (95% CI)	0.96 (0.93–0.99)	0.98 (0.96–1.0)
PPV (at 10%)[a] % (95% CI)	88.2 (73.8–95.2)	91.4 (77.4–97.0)
NPV (at 10%)[a] % (95% CI)	99.3 (98.3–99.7)	99.7 (98.8–99.9)
PPV (at 20%)[a] % (95% CI)	94.4 (86.4–97.8)	96.0 (88.5–98.7)
NPV (at 20%)[a] % (95% CI)	98.4 (96.3–99.3)	99.3 (97.2–99.8)

If VL re-quantification was not feasible, the first VL testing result was taken into account

ROC Receiver operating characteristic, *PPV* Positive predictive value, *NPV* Negative predictive value

[a]For the calculation of predictive values, 10 and 20% prevalence of detectable VLs were assumed in a hypothetical population undergoing routine VL testing

Discussion

Improved access to VL monitoring is crucial in RLS to meet the fast growing monitoring needs of large ART cohorts. One strategy is the deployment of multiple platforms by different stakeholders. This study is the first in Swaziland and, to our knowledge, the second internationally [13] to evaluate the utility of the Biocentric platform using plasma for VL quantification under routine conditions in comparison with another method. We showed that the Biocentric platform performs reliably under routine conditions. It had a strong positive correlation with the reference method ($R = 0.81$, $p < 0.01$), and the overall agreement between the two methods was high (mean difference – 0.03) at the 3.0 log threshold. Although 5.2% of samples were misclassified at the threshold of 2.62 $\log_{10}$ copies, most discrepancies were resolved after re-quantification of discordant results, and the sensitivity and specificity increased to 97.1 and 99.0% at the 3.0 $\log_{10}$ VL threshold. These estimates were similar to those reported previously, where the sensitivity and specificity were 100 and 90% respectively compared with the HIV Amplicor Monitor assay (Roche Diagnostics, Basel, Switzerland) [13].

Misclassification of results occurred across all quantification levels and most of them with an absolute difference of more than 0.5 $\log_{10}$ copies/mL. This may indicate that misclassifications were due to factors beyond the technical variation of the platforms (e.g. operator differences). This study also showed inter-laboratory differences. Sensitivity was decreased in LAB-2, and LAB-2 emerged as an

independent risk factor for downward misclassification (false negative) compared with LAB-1. Differences in quality between laboratories were likely due to manual sample preparation and reagent volume pipetting errors by staff who were less trained and experienced in this method. The Biocentric platform was newly established in LAB-2 and the training provided before the evaluation may have been insufficient. Disadvantages of this platform are that it is a manual technique requiring experienced staff, who cannot always be easily found or retained in RLS, and that manual techniques may be more prone to error [5, 6]. Therefore, intra- and inter-laboratory quality assurance mechanisms should be established (in addition to the internal controls provided by the assay) to detect suboptimal performance as soon as possible. As a consequence, the National Reference Laboratory decided to provide further formal and hands-on training before the routine use of this platform in LAB-2. Of note, inter-laboratory differences independent of the VL assay and differences between platforms were also reported in other settings [17, 18]. Because of the inherent variability between VL platforms, it is recommended that patients be monitored using the same technology platform to ensure correct interpretation of VL changes over time [19].

Context specific considerations

When VL testing is introduced into routine settings, viral (e.g. genetic diversity of HIV strains), programmatic, laboratory-specific and clinical (e.g. definitions of viral failure) factors need to be taken into account to establish a contextualized VL testing strategy. Firstly, a positive aspect of this platform is its ability to be implemented in RLS, performing reliably under routine conditions specifically at the clinical threshold level of 3.0 $\log_{10}$ copies/mL. In our experience, maintenance requirements of this open platform are minimal and individual elements are interchangeable, such as RNA extraction techniques [20] and previously validated real-time PCR thermal cyclers [21]. Another positive factor is its high throughput volume. Four of the Biocentric-experienced laboratory technologists were able to perform up to three runs per day (246 tests per day) with four extractors and one thermal cycler under routine conditions.

Secondly, the use of plasma for VL quantification limits its use to settings with strong sample transportation systems in place and/or the capacity to prepare and store samples at clinical sites. According to Biocentric, DBS samples can also be used on the platform, requiring less logistical and cold-chain support. VL quantification on DBS cards on Biocentric is being evaluated in Swaziland and will be reported in future. Thirdly, the Biocentric platform is a polyvalent technology, which allows testing of VL in conditions other than HIV, such as HIV early infant diagnosis (EID) and hepatitis C VL. This is becoming increasingly important for programmes wishing to integrate laboratory services using multi-disease platforms [22].

Fourthly, the Biocentric HIV VL test is priced competitively (ex-works USD14.9 per test) compared with other well-established VL technologies [23]. Finally, the Biocentric VL reagents, as with other VL technologies, contain guanidine thiocyanate (GTC), which is a toxic chemical compound [24] commonly used for the extraction of DNA and RNA in molecular tests [25]. As GTC can release cyanide gases in contact with bleach and due to its toxicity to aquatic life, it has to be managed as hazardous waste, normally through high-temperature incineration [25]. This can pose logistical challenges in RLS and requires proper planning and budgeting.

Limitations and strengths
A limitation of the study is that discrepant test results were not fully investigated. They were also not re-quantified on both methods owing to insufficient leftover plasma samples, with retesting being performed solely on the Biocentric platform. Although retesting of discordant results is not standard of practice in laboratory evaluation studies, retesting was performed to obtain additional information of the nature of discrepant results, assuming that the suboptimal performance of LAB-2 was likely due to less hands-on practice of the laboratory technologists rather than problems with the Biocentric method itself. After retesting, a few samples remained discrepant, for which several explanations exist. Firstly, there is the possibility of false test results on the national reference platforms due to internal quality issues or operator errors. However, internal and external quality control did not indicate quality issues during the study period. Nevertheless, a third VL assay should have been used to resolve discrepant results. Secondly, the two platforms used different plasma input volumes, increasing the likelihood of variations in measurements for values at the detection threshold. Thirdly, transportation and storage conditions may have affected the sample quality, possibly leading to a degradation of RNA. Lastly, we did not test for HIV genotypic diversity. VL assays differ in their ability to quantify genetically diverse HIV strains, largely depending on the design of primers and probes [13, 26–29]. The CAP/CTM HIV-1 v2.0 detects HIV-1 groups M, N and O, and Biocentric detects HIV-1 group M (A–H) [28]. Without a panel of samples with genetic diversity, generalizability is limited, specifically to settings where other strains are endemic. However, according to a recent study in Cameroon, Biocentric performed well in that setting which is characterized by broad HIV genetic variability [30]. Another limitation is that the majority of VL samples were below the detection limit of the Biocentric platform, reducing the sample size for correlation and Bland–Altman

analyses. Finally, we did not assess reproducibility. This study focused on field diagnostic accuracy and is not a pure analytical study. Repeat testing would have been complex to undertake at various conditions (intra and inter-variability) because it would have required more VL samples from patients.

A strength of the study was its conduct under routine real-world conditions; therefore, challenges and constraints are comparable to other RLS in Sub-Saharan Africa. Also, the personnel involved from sample collection (phlebotomist) to VL testing (laboratory technologists) are likely to reflect staff composition of other RLS.

Conclusions
The Biocentric platform using plasma for VL quantification showed results that were comparable overall to the national reference method. This study also revealed inter-laboratory differences in performance, which was likely due to unmet training needs and lack of hands-on practice of technologists in one laboratory, highlighting the need for continuous training of laboratory personnel. In addition to participation in national and international proficiency testing programmes, routine quality control methods should be integrated into laboratories performing at high scale in RLS to detect suboptimal performance as soon as possible. The Biocentric platform is now routinely used in Swaziland to support the expansion of VL testing.

Abbreviations
ART: Antiretroviral therapy; DBS: Dried-blood spots; EDTA: Ethylenediaminetetraacetic acid; LAB-1: Laboratory 1; LAB-2: Laboratory 2; NPV: Negative predictive value; PPV: Positive predictive value; RLS: Resource limited setting; VL: Viral load; WHO: World Health Organization

Acknowledgements
We acknowledge the contribution and support of the following people during the development of the protocol: Sikhathele Mazibuko, Celeste Gracia Edwards, David Etoori, Mpumelelo Ndlangamandla, Mikhael de Souza, Inoussa Zabsonre, Carol Metcalf. We also acknowledge Patience Nxumalo, Aditi Jani, Noziswe Rugongo and Robin Nesbitt for supporting the conduct of the study, and Clare Griffith for editing the manuscript.

Funding
Most of the study was funded by UNITAID, and Biocentric donated some VL testing consumables and devices. The funding sources (UNITAID, Biocentric) did not play any role in design of the study, data collection, analyses, and interpretation of data or in the writing of the manuscript or the decision to publish the findings.

Authors' contributions
Study design and protocol development: BK, QM, GM, EF, RT, SMK, JG, IC. Implementation of the research: BK, PADU, QM, GM, SK, AB, TC, MM, NN, NP, SD, SMK. Statistical analysis: BK. Interpretation of findings: BK, PADU, QM, GM, EF, RT, SK, AB, TC, MM, NN, NP, SMK, JG, SD, IC. Writing of the first draft of the manuscript: BK. All authors read and approved the final manuscript.

Competing interests
The authors declare that they have no competing interests.

Author details

[1]Medecins Sans Frontieres (OCG), P.O. Box 18, Eveni, Lot No. 331, Sheffield Road, Industrial Area, Mbabane, Swaziland. [2]Ministry of Health (National Reference Laboratory), Mbabane, Swaziland. [3]Medecins Sans Frontieres (OCG), Geneva, Switzerland. [4]Clinton Health Access Initiative (CHAI), Mbabane, Swaziland. [5]Medecins Sans Frontieres (Access Campaign), Geneva, Switzerland.

References

1. World Health Organization, Department of HIV/AIDS. Consolidated guidelines on the use of antiretroviral drugs for treating and preventing HIV infection: recommendations for a public health approach. Geneva: World Health Organization; 2016. Available from: http://apps.who.int/iris/bitstream/10665/208825/1/9789241549684_eng.pdf. Cited 31 Jul 2016

2. Sigaloff KCE, Hamers RL, Wallis CL, Kityo C, Siwale M, Ive P, et al. Unnecessary antiretroviral treatment switches and accumulation of HIV resistance mutations; two arguments for viral load monitoring in Africa. JAIDS J Acquir Immune Defic Syndr. 2011;58:23–31.

3. Keiser O, Chi BH, Gsponer T, Boulle A, Orrell C, Phiri S, et al. Outcomes of antiretroviral treatment in programmes with and without routine viral load monitoring in southern Africa. AIDS Lond Engl. 2011;25:1761–9.

4. Progress Report 2016- Prevent HIV, test and treat all. Geneva: World Health Organization; 2016.

5. Making viral load routine- successes and challenges in the implementation of routine HIV viral load monitoring. Part 1: programmatic strategies. Geneva: Médecins Sans Frontières; 2016.

6. Making viral load routine- successes and challenges in the implementation of routine HIV viral load monitoring. Part 2: the viral load laboratory. Geneva: Médecins Sans Frontières; 2016.

7. The availability and use of diagnostics for HIV: a 2012/2013 WHO survey of low- and middle-income countries. Geneva: World Health Organization; 2014.

8. Pham MD, Romero L, Parnell B, Anderson DA, Crowe SM, Luchters S. Feasibility of antiretroviral treatment monitoring in the era of decentralized HIV care: a systematic review. AIDS Res Ther. 2017;14:3.

9. Jobanputra K, Parker LA, Azih C, Okello V, Maphalala G, Jouquet G, et al. Impact and programmatic implications of routine viral load monitoring in Swaziland. J Acquir Immune Defic Syndr 1999. 2014;67:45–51.

10. Bicego GT, Nkambule R, Peterson I, Reed J, Donnell D, Ginindza H, et al. Recent patterns in population-based HIV prevalence in Swaziland. PLoS One. 2013;8:e77101.

11. Annual HIV program report 2015. Mbabane: Swaziland Ministry of Health; 2016.

12. Generic HIV charge virale. Bandol: Biocentric; 2015.

13. Steegen K, Luchters S, De Cabooter N, Reynaerts J, Mandaliya K, Plum J, et al. Evaluation of two commercially available alternatives for HIV-1 viral load testing in resource-limited settings. J Virol Methods. 2007;146:178–87.

14. Cohen JF, Korevaar DA, Altman DG, Bruns DE, Gatsonis CA, Hooft L, et al. STARD 2015 guidelines for reporting diagnostic accuracy studies: explanation and elaboration. BMJ Open. 2016;6 Available from: http://www.ncbi.nlm.nih.gov/pmc/articles/PMC5128957/. Cited 24 May 2017.

15. Bland JM, Altman D. Statistical methods for assessing agreement between two methods of clinical measurement. Lancet. 1986;327:307–10.

16. Shrier I, Platt RW. Reducing bias through directed acyclic graphs. BMC Med Res Methodol. 2008;8:70.

17. Greig J, du Cros P, Klarkowski D, Mills C, Jørgensen S, Harrigan PR, et al. Viral load testing in a resource-limited setting: quality control is critical. J Int AIDS Soc. 2011;14:23.

18. Monleau M, Aghokeng AF, Eymard-Duvernay S, Dagnra A, Kania D, Ngo-Giang-Huong N, et al. Field evaluation of dried blood spots for routine HIV-1 viral load and drug resistance monitoring in patients receiving antiretroviral therapy in Africa and Asia. J Clin Microbiol. 2014;52:578–86.

19. Sollis KA, Smit PW, Fiscus S, Ford N, Vitoria M, Essajee S, et al. Systematic review of the performance of HIV viral load technologies on plasma samples. PLoS ONE. 2014;9 Available from: https://www.ncbi.nlm.nih.gov/pmc/articles/PMC3928047/. Cited 12 Apr 2018.

20. Liégeois F, Boué V, Mouinga-Ondémé A, Lékané DK, Mongo D, Sica J, et al. Suitability of an open automated nucleic acid extractor for high-throughput plasma HIV-1 RNA quantitation in Gabon (Central Africa). J Virol Methods. 2012;179:269–71.

21. Erick KN, Adawaye C, Raphael B, Richard KL, Georges ML, Patrick D, et al. Implementation of an in-house quantitative real-time PCR for determination of HIV viral load in Kinshasa. Open Access Libr J. 2014;1:1.

22. Considerations for adoption and use of multidisease testing devices in integrated laboratory networks (Information note). Geneva: World Health Organization; 2017. Available from: http://www.who.int/tb/publications/2017/considerations_multidisease_testing_devices_2017/en/

23. Putting HIV and HCV to the test | A product guide for point-of-care CD4 tests and laboratory-based and point-of-care HIV and HCV viral load tests. Geneva: Médecins Sans Frontières (MSF); 2017. Available from: https://www.msfaccess.org/PHHT2017

24. Pubchem. National Center for Biotechnology Information | PubChem Compound Database | Guanidinium thiocyanate. Available from: https://pubchem.ncbi.nlm.nih.gov/compound/65046. Cited 1 Nov 2017.

25. Robert E, Farrell J. RNA Isolation Strategies. In: RNA Methodologies. 4th ed. San Diego: Academic Press; 2010. Available from: https://doi.org/10.1016/B978-0-12-374727-3.00002-4.

26. Rouet F, Foulongne V, Viljoen J, Steegen K, Becquart P, Valéa D, et al. Comparison of the generic HIV viral load® assay with the Amplicor™ HIV-1 monitor v1.5 and Nuclisens HIV-1 EasyQ® v1.2 techniques for plasma HIV-1 RNA quantitation of non-B subtypes: the Kesho bora preparatory study. J Virol Methods. 2010;163:253–7.

27. Holguín A, López M, Molinero M, Soriano V. Performance of three commercial viral load assays, versant human immunodeficiency virus type 1 (HIV-1) RNA bDNA v3.0, Cobas AmpliPrep/Cobas TaqMan HIV-1, and NucliSens HIV-1 EasyQ v1.2, testing HIV-1 non-B subtypes and recombinant variants. J Clin Microbiol. 2008;46:2918–23.

28. Peeters M, Aghokeng AF, Delaporte E. Genetic diversity among human immunodeficiency virus-1 non-B subtypes in viral load and drug resistance assays. Clin Microbiol Infect. 2010;16:1525–31.

29. Colson P, Motte A, Tamalet C. Underquantification of plasma HIV-1 RNA levels in a cohort of newly-diagnosed individuals. Int J Infect Dis. 2010;14: e362–3.

30. Ngo-Malabo ET, Ngoupo TPA, Zekeng M, Ngono V, Ngono L, Sadeuh-Mba SA, et al. A cheap and open HIV viral load technique applicable in routine analysis in a resource limited setting with a wide HIV genetic diversity. Virol J. 2017;14 Available from: https://www.ncbi.nlm.nih.gov/pmc/articles/PMC5686852/. Cited 12 Apr 2018.

20

Association of *TLR8* and *TLR9* polymorphisms with tuberculosis in a Chinese Han population: a case-control study

Ming-Gui Wang, Miao-Miao Zhang, Yu Wang, Shou-Quan Wu, Meng Zhang and Jian-Qing He[*]

Abstract

Background: Toll-like receptor (*TLR*) single nucleotide polymorphisms (SNPs) have been associated with regulation of *TLR* expression and development of active tuberculosis (TB). The objectives of this study were to determine whether *TLR8* and *TLR9* SNPs were associated with the development of latent TB infection (LTBI) and the subsequent pulmonary TB (PTB) in a Chinese Han population.

Methods: Two independent samples were enrolled. The first sample contained 584 TB cases and 608 controls; the second sample included 204 healthy controls, 201 LTBI subjects and 209 bacteria-confirmed active PTB patients. Three SNPs (rs3764880, rs187084 and rs5743836) were genotyped. The associations between the SNPs and risk of LTBI or PTB were investigated using unconditional logistic regression analysis.

Results: The A-allele of *TLR8* rs3764880 SNP was protective against the development of TB in males (A vs G, OR = 0.58, 95%CI = 0.37–0.91). The AA genotype of rs3764880 SNP was found to increase the risk of PTB among females with an OR of 4.81 (1.11–20.85). The G allele of *TLR9* SNP rs187084 was found to increase the risk of PTB (G vs A, *P* = 0.01, OR = 1.48, 95% CI = 1.10–2.00), the significance was also observed under dominant genetic models. The GA-genotype of *TLR9* rs187084 SNP was found to increase the risk of PTB with an OR of 1.68 (1.07–2.65), but was found to decrease the risk of MTB infection with an OR = 0.64 (0.41–0.98). *TLR9*_rs5743836 SNP was excluded from the data analyses, because the minimum allele frequency was< 1%.

Conclusions: Our findings in two independent samples indicated that SNPs in *TLR8* and *TLR9* were associated with the development of TB, and highlight that SNPs may have different effects on disease pathogenesis and progression.

Keywords: Toll-like receptors, Single nucleotide polymorphism, Tuberculosis

Background

Tuberculosis (TB), caused by infection with *Mycobacterium tuberculosis* (MTB), remains one of the world's deadliest communicable diseases. According to the World Health Organization, an estimated 10.4 million people developed TB and 1.7 million died of the disease in 2016 [1]. However, most individuals exposed to MTB experience latent MTB infection (LTBI) and do not develop active disease. Considerable evidence suggests that host genetic factors play a key role in determining an individual's susceptibility to TB [2–5].

Toll-like receptors (*TLRs*) are a class of pattern recognition molecules, which are known to play important roles in the innate and adaptive immune system [6], by recognizing pathogen-associated molecular patterns. Most *TLRs* are expressed on the cell surface, whereas other *TLRs* (3, 7, 8, and 9) are expressed intracellularly [7, 8]. *TLR7*, *TLR8*, and *TLR9* have been implicated in immune diseases due to their ability to recognize oligonucleotide-based (RNA-and DNA-based) molecular patterns as agonists [9].

* Correspondence: Jianqhe@gmail.com; jianqing_he@scu.edu.cn
Department of Respiratory and Critical Care Medicine, West China Hospital, Sichuan University, No. 37, Guo Xue Alley, Chengdu 610041, Sichuan Province, People's Republic of China

TLR8 is located in the membranes of the endosomal compartment and recognize single-stranded RNA, regulating in the induction of interferon (IFN) and inflammatory cytokines [10–12]. Previous studies have shown that *TLR8* variants influence the expression of *TLR8* [13–15]. The *TLR8* single nucleotide polymorphism (SNP) rs3764880 (Met1Val) regulates the translation of the two main *TLR8* isoforms, and plays a significant part in the immune response [12, 15]. A study conducted by Davila et al. [14], was the first to demonstrate that SNPs in *TLR8* were associated with TB in adults. Since *TLR8* is located on chromosome X (Xp22.3-p22.2), males carrying a single copy of the defective allele may have higher risk of TB. In addition, several studies have shown that the G allele of *TLR8* rs3764880 was associated with TB susceptibility in males [14, 16–18]. These studies demonstrated that the rs3764880 SNP in *TLR8* play important roles in TB.

The ligands for *TLR9* are DNA-containing CpG motifs [19]. *TLR9* is located in the endosomal compartment of plasmacytoid dendritic cells and monocytes/macrophages [19], and plays a vital role in autoimmune diseases and inflammatory diseases by the regulation of type I IFN and inflammatory cytokines [19–21]. The rs187084 and rs5743836 SNPs located in the promoter are the most important and have been associated with various inflammatory diseases [9, 21–24]. Previous functional analyses have shown that both rs187084 and rs5743836 SNPs influence the transcription of *TLR9* by regulation of promoter activity [22, 25, 26]. Previous studies indicated that *TLR9* is one of the most important receptors in the control of infections with pathogens such as hepatitis C virus [22], Brucella [27], and MTB [23, 28, 29]. Some studies found that the rs187084 in *TLR9* showed no association with TB in Vietnam and Iran [28, 30]. However, no study has explored the association between rs187084 and MTB infection or the process from LTBI to TB. The rs5743836 in *TLR9* showed a strong association with tuberculosis in African-Americans and Caucasians [31], while the association was not found in Vietnam [28] or Mexico population [29]. Wu L et al. [32] also reported that rs5743836 was a risk factor for LTBI.

These findings demonstrated that *TLR8* and *TLR9* play important roles in infectious diseases, and also emphasized the role of the rs3764880 SNP in *TLR8* and rs187084 and rs5743836 SNPs in *TLR9*. To date, the SNPs of *TLR8* and *TLR9* have been studied in association with susceptibility to TB, but such studies addressing host genetic susceptibility to TB was limited, whether an association implies susceptibility for developing active disease or just acquisition of MTB infection is unclear. In this study, we investigated the associations of SNPs of *TLR8* (rs3764880) and *TLR9* (rs187084, rs5743836) with TB in a Chinese Han sample. Then we explored the associations of these SNPs with LTBI or PTB in a second sample of Chinese Han individuals.

Materials and methods
Subjects
First sample
A cohort of 584 new TB patients above 15 years of age were recruited from the West China Hospital of Sichuan University. Diagnosis was based on the following criteria: culture positive and/or smear positive for MTB and/or histopathological findings of TB and clinical and/or radiographic presentation consistent with TB, with positive response to anti-TB therapy. 608 unrelated healthy controls (with unknown status of MTB infection), matched with cases by gender and age, were selected from individuals attending the outpatient department of the West China Hospital for annual physical examination. Healthy controls with a history of prior anti-TB treatment were excluded. All participants diagnosed with diabetes mellitus, human immunodeficiency virus (HIV) co-infection, or in receipt of immunosuppressive therapy, were excluded.

Second sample
A cohort of 614 participants were recruited: patients with pulmonary TB (PTB) ($n = 209$), LTBI subjects ($n = 201$), and healthy controls (HC) without MTB infection ($n = 204$). As with the first sample, the subjects in the second sample were recruited from the West China Hospital in Chengdu. Eligibility criteria for PTB patients included: 1) ≥ 18 years old; 2) diagnosis of PTB based on sputum smear examinations for acid-fast bacilli and/or the culture of MTB. Both LTBI and HC subjects were unrelated and asymptomatic contacts of bacteria-confirmed active TB patients. LTBI was defined as a positive result for the QuantiFERON-TB Gold In-Tube and HC was defined as a negative result for the same assay, and patients belonging to both subgroups had no radiological evidence of active TB, negative sputum smear and culture, and no history of TB. Exclusion criteria included a positive serological test for HIV infection, organ transplantation, primary immunodeficiency, cancer, and treatment with immunosuppressive drugs, endocrine disorders such as diabetes, autoimmune or chronic renal disease, and extrapulmonary TB cases.

All protocols were approved by the ethics committee of the West China Hospital of Sichuan University. Written informed consent was obtained from all participants involved in this study. Demographic characteristics of all participants were collected from a detailed questionnaire.

Genotyping
A volume of 2–5 ml blood samples were collected in EDTA tubes (BD Vacutainers, Franklin Lakes, NJ, USA) from each participant. Genomic DNA was extracted from

whole blood following a protocol described elsewhere [33]. Three SNPs (rs3764880, rs187084, rs5743836) were genotyped using a custom-by-design 2 × 48-Plex SNPscan™ Kit (Cat#: G0104, Genesky Biotechnologies Inc., Shanghai, China) as described previously [34]. This kit was developed according to a patented SNP genotyping technology by Genesky Biotechnologies Inc., which was based on double ligation and multiplex fluorescence PCR. As a quality control measure, 5% of the samples were genotyped in duplicate using the same method to check for concordance. Assessment of genotypes was done by laboratory personnel without any prior knowledge of the diagnosis of the subjects.

Statistical analyses

The clinical and demographic characteristics were compared using the student's test or ANOVA for continuous variables and with the $\chi2$ test or Fisher's exact test for categorical variables. $P < 0.05$ was considered significant.

Hardy-Weinberg Equilibrium (HWE) in healthy controls was tested using asymptotic Pearson's chi-square tests for each SNP, in each study. Because the *TLR8* rs3764880 SNP is located on chromosome X, we tested for HWE in females only. Since we used loose-matching to select cases and controls, associations between polymorphisms and risk of TB, LTBI or PTB were investigated using unconditional logistic regression analysis [35], adjusting for age and gender, and smoking as in the analysis of the first sample. Because this was an exploratory analysis, we did not introduce a correction for multiple comparisons. The results were expressed by odds ratios (ORs) and 95% confidence intervals (95% CIs). All statistical analyses were carried out using SPSS statistical software, release 19.0.

Results

Clinical information of study subjects

Demographic and clinical parameters of the patients are summarized in Table 1. As shown in Table 1, 584 TB cases and 608 controls from the Chinese Han population were enrolled in the first sample, with no significant difference in age and gender ratio. More smokers were found among the TB patients as compared with controls ($P = 0.012$). 614 eligible participants were enrolled in the

second sample, including 209 PTB cases, 201 LTBI, and 204 HC (Table 1). There was no significant difference in gender among the three groups, while the mean age was significantly different among the PTB, LTBI and control groups ($P < 0.001$). No deviations from HWE were detected in all groups ($P > 0.05$). Genotyping data for the three SNPs were successfully obtained for ≥98.8% of the subjects. However, *TLR9*_rs5743836 SNP was excluded from the data analyses, because the minimum allele frequency (MAF) was ≤1%.

TLR8 rs3764880 and TB disease progression

The genotype and allele distributions of this SNP in the first sample are shown in Table 2. Firstly, a decreased frequency of the minor allele A of *TLR8*_rs3764880 was found in the male TB patient group, and found to be protected against TB (OR = 0.58, 95%CI = 0.37–0.91, $P = 0.02$) after adjusting for age and smoking in the first sample. No difference was found in the genotype frequencies among male patients in this sample. There was no difference in both allele and genotype frequencies among female subjects in the first sample. Further analysis was performed in the second sample (Table 3). No significant differences in the allele frequency of *TLR8*_rs3764880 SNP were observed for male or female subjects when comparing PTB disease with LTBI groups or when comparing LTBI group with HC subjects. In contrast, an increased frequency of the AA genotype of rs3764880 was observed in female patients, and found to increase the risk of PTB (OR = 4.81, 95%CI = 1.11–20.85, $P = 0.04$) when comparing PTB disease with LTBI groups. No differences in frequencies of *TLR8*_rs3764880 genotypes were observed for male or female patients when comparing LTBI group with HC subjects.

TLR9 rs187084 and TB disease progression

The genotype and allele distributions of this SNP in the first and second samples are shown in Table 4. Associations between *TLR9* rs187084 and the development of TB, PTB or LTBI were assessed in dominant, and recessive models. Firstly, analysis in the first sample detected no difference in allele and genotype frequencies among TB patients and controls. No significant differences were

Table 1 Clinical characteristics of the study population

	First sample			Second sample			
	TB patients (584)	Control (608)	P value	PTB (209)	LTBI (201)	HC (204)	P value
Age (mean ± SD)	36.68 ± 15.61	37.18 ± 15.68	0.608	38.76 ± 16.97	49.09 ± 15.91	45.71 ± 14.90	< 0.001
Gender							
Males, n	299	302	0.598	107	95	93	0.503
Females, n	285	306		102	106	111	
Smokers, n(%)	173 (29.62%)	141 (23.19%)	0.012	–	–	–	–

Abbreviations: *TB* tuberculosis, *PTB* pulmonary tuberculosis, *LTBI* latent tuberculosis infection, *HC* healthy control

Table 2 The genotype and allele frequencies of rs3764880 in patients with TB and controls

Genotypes and allele frequencies	Cases, n (%)	Controls, n (%)	OR (95%CI)	P value
Males				
TLR8 rs3764880 major allele G	253 (86.6)	236 (79.5)	1	Reference
TLR8 rs3764880 minor allele A	39 (13.4)	61 (20.5)	0.58 (0.37–0.91)	0.02
Females				
TLR8 rs3764880 GG	203 (71.2)	209 (68.8)	1	Reference
TLR8 rs3764880 GA	76 (26.7)	82 (27.0)	0.93 (0.65–1.35)	0.71
TLR8 rs3764880 AA	6 (2.1)	13 (4.3)	0.49 (0.18–1.31)	0.16
TLR8 rs3764880 major allele G	482 (84.6)	500 (82.2)	1	Reference
TLR8 rs3764880 minor allele A	88 (15.4)	108 (17.8)	0.84 (0.61–1.14)	0.26

Abbreviations: TB tuberculosis, OR odds ratio, CI confidence interval. P value adjusted for age and smoking

detected in *TLR9* rs187084 SNP between TB patients and controls under any genetic model in the first sample. To further explore whether this SNP was associated with susceptibility to PTB or MTB infection, the second sample was analyzed. When comparing PTB patients with LTBI group, significant associations with developing disease were observed after adjusting for age and gender (Table 4). The GA-genotype of *TLR9* rs187084 SNP was found more frequent in PTB cases, and was found to increase the risk of PTB with an OR of 1.68 (95% CI: 1.07–2.65). The prevalence of minor allele G of rs187084 was significantly higher in patients with

PTB than that of controls (41.9% vs 32.3%, OR = 1.48, 95% CI = 1.10–2.00, P = 0.01). The significance was also observed under dominant genetic models (Table 4), indicating that the GG and GA genotypes increased risk susceptibility to develop active PTB from LTBI status. When comparing the LTBI group with HC subjects, a significant difference was found in genotype distributions. GA-genotype was found to decrease the risk of MTB infection (GA vs AA, P = 0.04, OR = 0.64, 95% CI = 0.41–0.98). However, no differences in allele distributions or genotype distributions under different genetic models were observed between LTBI group and HC subjects.

Table 3 The genotype and allele frequencies of rs3764880 in the second sample

Genotypes and allele frequencies	Cases, n (%)	Controls, n (%)	OR (95%CI)	P value
PTB and LTBI				
Males				
TLR8 rs3764880 major allele G	84 (79.2)	84 (88.4)	1	Reference
TLR8 rs3764880 minor allele A	22 (20.8)	11 (11.6)	1.92 (0.85–4.32)	0.12
Females				
TLR8 rs3764880 GG	65 (63.7)	71 (67.6)	1	Reference
TLR8 rs3764880 GA	28 (27.5)	31 (29.5)	1.08 (0.56–2.09)	0.83
TLR8 rs3764880 AA	9 (8.8)	3 (2.9)	4.81 (1.11–20.85)	0.04
TLR8 rs3764880 major allele G	158 (77.5)	173 (82.4)	1	Reference
TLR8 rs3764880 minor allele A	46 (22.5)	37 (17.6)	1.56 (0.93–2.62)	0.09
LTBI and HC				
Males				
TLR8 rs3764880 major allele G	84 (88.4)	76 (82.6)	1	Reference
TLR8 rs3764880 minor allele A	11 (11.6)	16 (17.4)	0.53 (0.23–1.25)	0.15
Females				
TLR8 rs3764880 GG	71 (67.6)	70 (63.1)	1	Reference
TLR8 rs3764880 GA	31 (29.5)	36 (32.4)	0.85 (0.47–1.52)	0.58
TLR8 rs3764880 AA	3 (2.9)	5 (4.5)	0.64 (0.15–2.84)	0.56
TLR8 rs3764880 major allele G	173 (82.4)	176 (79.3)	1	Reference
TLR8 rs3764880 minor allele A	37 (17.6)	46 (20.7)	0.83 (0.51–1.34)	0.44

Abbreviations: PTB pulmonary tuberculosis, LTBI latent tuberculosis infection, HC healthy control, OR odds ratio, CI confidence interval. P value adjusted for age

Table 4 Association between rs187084 and TB, LTBI and PTB susceptibility in Chinese Han population

| | First sample | | | | Second sample | | | | | | | |
	TB, n(%)	Controls, n(%)	OR^a (95% CI)	p^a	PTB, n(%)	LTBI, n (%)	OR^b (95% CI)	p^b	LTBI, n(%)	HC, n (%)	OR^b (95% CI)	p^b
Genotype												
GG	75 (12.9)	74 (12.3)	1.07 (0.74–1.55)	0.70	41 (19.6)	29 (14.5)	1.80 (0.99–3.27)	0.06	29 (14.5)	30 (14.8)	0.83 (0.46–1.52)	0.55
GA	267 (46.0)	271 (44.9)	1.06 (0.83–1.36)	0.64	93 (44.5)	71 (35.5)	1.68 (1.07–2.65)	0.03	71 (35.5)	93 (45.8)	0.64 (0.41–0.98)	0.04
AA	238 (41.0)	259 (42.9)	1	Reference	75 (35.9)	100 (50.0)	1	Reference	100 (50.0)	80 (39.4)	1	Reference
Allele												
G	417 (35.9)	419 (34.7)	1.05 (0.88–1.24)	0.6	175 (41.9)	129 (32.3)	1.48(1.10–2.00)	0.01	129 (32.3)	153 (37.7)	0.82 (0.61–1.10)	0.19
A	743 (64.1)	789 (65.3)	1	Reference	243 (58.1)	271 (67.8)	1	Reference	271 (67.8)	253 (62.3)	1	Reference
Dominant												
GG + GA	342 (59.0)	345 (57.1)	1.07 (0.85–1.35)	0.59	134 (64.1)	100 (50.0)	1.70 (1.12–2.57)	0.01	100 (50.0)	123 (60.6)	0.68 (0.46–1.02)	0.06
AA	238 (41.0)	259 (42.9)	1	Reference	75 (35.9)	100 (50.0)	1	Reference	100 (50.0)	80 (39.4)	1	Reference
Recessive												
GG	75 (12.9)	74 (12.3)	1.05 (0.74–1.48)	0.8	41 (19.6)	29 (14.5)	1.40 (0.81–2.42)	0.22	29 (14.5)	30 (14.8)	1.03 (0.59–1.79)	0.93
GA + AA	505 (87.1)	530 (87.7)	1	Reference	168 (80.4)	171 (85.5)	1	Reference	171 (85.5)	173 (85.2)	1	Reference

Abbreviations: TB tuberculosis, *PTB* pulmonary tuberculosis, *LTBI* latent tuberculosis infection, *HC* healthy control, [a], adjusted for age, gender and smoking with logistic regression; [b], adjusted for age and gender with logistic regression; OR, odds ratio; CI, confidence interval

Discussion

Multiple groups have investigated associations between the three SNPs which we examined in the in current study and TB susceptibility in a variety of populations, but the results were inconsistent [14, 17, 18, 28, 30, 32, 36–40]. Few studies have classified LTBI and HC without MTB infection. The current study first analyzed the association between *TLR8/9* SNPs and TB in the first sample, and then further explored the *TLR8/9* variants with LTBI and active PTB in the second sample. Our results suggest that genetic variants might have different roles in the development of active PTB and LTBI.

Davila et al. [14] for the first time found that four SNPs (rs3764879G/C, rs3788935G/A, rs3761624G/A, rs3764880G/A) in *TLR8* showed evidence of association with TB susceptibility with minor alleles showing an increased susceptibility to PTB in males in Russian and Indonesian populations. Furthermore, associations have also been found in Turkish male children [17], Pakistan population [41], and South African population [18]. However, neither Kobayashi et al. [42] nor Chimusa et al. [43] showed any association between rs3764880 and TB susceptibility. Our results showed that the rs3764880 A allele in *TLR8* greatly reduced TB risk in males. This result was consistent with that in a Pakistan population [41], which showed the rs3764880 A allele had a protective role against TB,but different from that in Turkish [17], South African [18], Russian and Indonesian populations [14], which showed the rs3764880 A allele increased susceptibility to TB in males. Subsequently, our data in the second sample provided new evidence for our understanding of the role of rs3764880 in the development of LTBI and PTB. The data suggested that the AA-genotype of rs3764880 increased susceptibility to PTB among females, however, might decrease susceptibility to LTBI. The difference between our results and that of other studies may be due to differences in race, or living environment. Therefore, the detection of this SNP among LTBI subjects may provide important information in the assessment of their risk profiles for susceptibility to development of PTB. Previous studies have found that the SNPs in *TLR8* might have gender effects across the genetic association studies on TB susceptibility [14, 17, 18, 41]. Our results also found a gender difference: male carriers of rs3764880 allele A showed a decreased risk for TB, and females carrying the AA genotype increased the risk of PTB when compared with LTBI. What's more, this gender effect was both demonstrated in the two independent study samples.

Several investigators have studied the roles of *TLR9* SNPs in TB. As reported previously in studies of Vietnam and Iran [28, 30], we found the rs187084 in *TLR9* showed no association with TB in the first sample. In the second sample, the G-allele of *TLR9* rs187084 greatly increased

PTB risk, and this association was also observed under a dominant genetic model, which suggested a risk role of the allele G. However, the GA genotype decreased the risk of MTB infection. A study by Digna Rosa Velez et al. [31] showed a strong association between rs5743836 and tuberculosis in African-Americans and Caucasians population, while the association was not found in Vietnam [28] or Mexico population [29]. Another study conducted by Wu L et al. [32] showed that rs5743836 was a risk factor for LTBI and its MAF was 0.27 in a Chinese population in Shanghai city. The MAF of this SNP is high among African-Americans, Africans and Caucasians [31], while low in the Mexican population [29] and Vietnamese people [28]. These studies, thus indicated that the MAF of rs5743836 may vary between different ethnic groups. In this study, we found the MAF of rs5743836 was less than 1%. Since our sample size may not be large enough for a SNP with low MAF, and may potentially lead to false associations with the phenotype investigated, the rs5743836 was excluded in the data analyses. The MAF of rs5743836 in Beijing Han population from the International HapMap Project (http://www.1000genomes.org/) is less than 0.01, which support our result and indicates a low mutation rate in Chinese Han population. Therefore, the higher rs5743836 MAF in the study of Wu L et al. may suggest that populations other than Chinese Han were included in the study [32].

It has been discussed that some SNPs may actually be associated with MTB infection [36, 37], some may be associated with active TB [38, 39] and other studies suggested some SNPs may have different impacts on the susceptibility to LTBI and PTB [32, 40, 44]. Lu et al. found that an immunity-related GTPase family M SNP was associated with active TB and LTBI, but also plays opposite roles in the development of active TB and LTBI [44]. Our results provide strong evidence that the allele "A" of the polymorphism rs3764880 was associated with decreased risk of tuberculosis in the first sample. The genotype "AA" of rs3764880 was more commonly found in female PTB patients compared with LTBI, indicating this genotype increases the possibility of progression of tuberculosis infection to disease in the second sample. For the polymorphism of rs187084 in *TLR9*, we found the genotype "GA" and allele "G" was more common in PTB patients compared with LTBI, which demonstrated that this allele increased the risk of progression from tuberculosis infection to active disease. However, the GA-genotype was found to reduce the risk of MTB infection, thereby indicating that the results of our two samples were inconsistent and may have been caused by a number of factors. It may be caused by the following reasons. First, we included all TB patients in our first sample without differentiating between the different types of TB, while we only included PTB patients in the second sample. Genetic polymorphisms may have different effects on PTB and extra-pulmonary TB (EPTB), which may be due to the fact that different immune mechanisms are involved in PTB and EPTB [45]. Second, the results in the first sample may be explained, when the distinction between LTBI and HC without the infection of MTB is ignored. In other words, the results may be different because of the differences within the control group. Therefore, it is reasonable that these SNPs showed different results in the two samples.

Our study faced some intrinsic limitations. First, small sample size in the second sample may have limited our ability to detect potential influence of *TLR* SNPs on the susceptibility to both LTBI and PTB. Further studies are therefore necessary to validate these associations in larger sample sizes and other populations. Second, TB case of the first sample included both clinical diagnosed and bacteria confirmed TB patients, regardless of their types, which could potentially reduce the validity of our conclusions. Third, LTBI and HC subjects included in the second sample were asymptomatic contacts of bacteria-confirmed active TB patients, the assessment of exposure to an active TB case relied on self-reported behavior, which may not be accurate among participants and may cause misclassification bias (once exposed, those controls could become cases). Forth, it is likely that linkage disequilibrium patterns differed among other populations and the Han Chinese population in this study, and thus, those associations may not replicate exactly [14, 28, 31]. A plausible explanation is that the SNPs that we identified are in linkage disequilibrium with another mutation that either confers a functional or a regulatory change within those genes. Hence, to interpret results across studies, future experiments should cover all common variation in the associated *TLR8/9* gene region in order to pinpoint the causal polymorphism. Furthermore, one potential limitation in our study was a lack of correction for multiple comparisons. The reported statistically significant results would need to be regarded as nominally significant.

Conclusion

Our study provides another evidence supporting the importance of host genetic variability in TB susceptibility. We identified the allele A of the rs3764880 that appears protective against TB among males of Chinese Han ancestry. Our results also highlight that polymorphisms may have different effects on disease pathogenesis and progression. This study may help to identify those TB-affected individuals most susceptible to disease, and to improve our understanding of the effects of genetic heterogeneity on the development of the different stages of TB.

Abbreviations

CIs: Confidence intervals; EPTB: extra-pulmonary tuberculosis; HC: Healthy controls; HIV: Human immunodeficiency virus; HWE: Hardy-Weinberg Equilibrium; IFN: Interferon; LTBI: Latent Mycobacterium tuberculosis infection; MAF: Minimum allele frequency; MTB: Mycobacterium tuberculosis; ORs: Odds ratios; PTB: Pulmonary Tuberculosis; SNP: Single nucleotide polymorphism; TB: Tuberculosis; TLRs: Toll-like receptors

Acknowledgements

Not applicable.

Funding

This work was supported by the Research Fund for the Doctoral Program of Higher Education of China [grant number 20130181110068], the National Natural Science Foundation of China [grant number 81170042, grant number 81370121], and the National Scientific and Technological Major Project of China [grant number 2012ZX10004-901].

Authors' contributions

MGW performed statistical analysis, wrote the manuscript, and was involved in the interpretation of findings. MMZ developed study protocol, collected data, and supervised this study. Y W developed study protocol and collected data. SQW was involved in data analysis and manuscript revision. MZ developed study protocol and supervised the study. JQH developed study protocol, collected data, revised the manuscript, and interpreted the findings. All authors read and approved the final manuscript.

Competing interests

The authors declare that they have no competing interests.

References

1. World Health Organization. Global Tuberculosis Report 2017. Geneva: World Health Organization; 2017.
2. Bellamy R. Genetic susceptibility to tuberculosis. Clin Chest Med. 2005;26(2): 233–46 vi.
3. Casanova JL, Abel L. Genetic dissection of immunity to mycobacteria: the human model. Annu Rev Immunol. 2002;20:581–620.
4. Baghdadi JE, Orlova M, Alter A, Ranque B, Chentoufi M, Lazrak F, et al. An autosomal dominant major gene confers predisposition to pulmonary tuberculosis in adults. J Exp Med. 2006;203(7):1679–84.
5. Fortin A, Abel L, Casanova JL, Gros P. Host genetics of mycobacterial diseases in mice and men: forward genetic studies of BCG-osis and tuberculosis. Annu Rev Genomics Hum Genet. 2007;8:163–92.
6. Aderem A, Ulevitch RJ. Toll-like receptors in the induction of the innate immune response. Nature. 2000;406(6797):782–7.
7. Pandey S, Agrawal DK. Immunobiology of toll-like receptors: emerging trends. Immunol Cell Biol. 2006;84(4):333–41.
8. Takeda K, Kaisho T, Akira S. Toll-like receptors. Annu Rev Immunol. 2003;21: 335–76.
9. Krieg AM, Vollmer J. Toll-like receptors 7, 8, and 9: linking innate immunity to autoimmunity. Immunol Rev. 2007;220:251–69.
10. Hornung V, Barchet W, Schlee M, Hartmann G. RNA recognition via TLR7 and TLR8. Handb Exp Pharmacol. 2008;183:71–86.
11. Heil F, Hemmi H, Hochrein H, Ampenberger F, Kirschning C, Akira S, et al. Species-specific recognition of single-stranded RNA via toll-like receptor 7 and 8. Science. 2004;303(5663):1526–9.
12. Oh DY, Taube S, Hamouda O, Kucherer C, Poggensee G, Jessen H, et al. A functional toll-like receptor 8 variant is associated with HIV disease restriction. J Infect Dis. 2008;198(5):701–9.
13. Wang CH, Eng HL, Lin KH, Liu HC, Chang CH, Lin TM. Functional polymorphisms of TLR8 are associated with hepatitis C virus infection. Immunology. 2014;141(4):540–8.
14. Davila S, Hibberd ML, Hari Dass R, Wong HE, Sahiratmadja E, Bonnard C, et al. Genetic association and expression studies indicate a role of toll-like receptor 8 in pulmonary tuberculosis. PLoS Genet. 2008;4(10):e1000218.

15. Gantier MP, Irving AT, Kaparakis-Liaskos M, Xu D, Evans VA, Cameron PU, et al. Genetic modulation of TLR8 response following bacterial phagocytosis. Hum Mutat. 2010;31(9):1069–79.

16. Lai YF, Lin TM, Wang CH, Su PY, Wu JT, Lin MC, et al. Functional polymorphisms of the TLR7 and TLR8 genes contribute to Mycobacterium tuberculosis infection. Tuberculosis (Edinb). 2016;98:125–31.

17. Dalgic N, Tekin D, Kayaalti Z, Cakir E, Soylemezoglu T, Sancar M. Relationship between toll-like receptor 8 gene polymorphisms and pediatric pulmonary tuberculosis. Dis Markers. 2011;31(1):33–8.

18. Salie M, Daya M, Lucas LA, Warren RM, van der Spuy GD, van Helden PD, et al. Association of toll-like receptors with susceptibility to tuberculosis suggests sex-specific effects of TLR8 polymorphisms. Infect Genet Evol. 2015;34:221–9.

19. Hemmi H, Takeuchi O, Kawai T, Kaisho T, Sato S, Sanjo H, et al. A toll-like receptor recognizes bacterial DNA. Nature. 2000;408(6813):740–5.

20. Misch EA, Hawn TR. Toll-like receptor polymorphisms and susceptibility to human disease. Clin Sci (Lond). 2008;114(5):347–60.

21. Baccala R, Hoebe K, Kono DH, Beutler B, Theofilopoulos AN. TLR-dependent and TLR-independent pathways of type I interferon induction in systemic autoimmunity. Nat Med. 2007;13(5):543–51.

22. Fischer J, Weber ANR, Bohm S, Dickhofer S, El Maadidi S, Deichsel D, et al. Sex-specific effects of TLR9 promoter variants on spontaneous clearance of HCV infection. Gut. 2017;66(10):1829–37.

23. Bafica A, Scanga CA, Feng CG, Leifer C, Cheever A, Sher A. TLR9 regulates Th1 responses and cooperates with TLR2 in mediating optimal resistance to Mycobacterium tuberculosis. J Exp Med. 2005;202(12):1715–24.

24. Schurz H, Daya M, Moller M, Hoal EG, Salie M. TLR1, 2, 4, 6 and 9 variants associated with tuberculosis susceptibility: a systematic review and meta-analysis. PLoS One. 2015;10(10):e0139711.

25. Ng MT, Van't Hof R, Crockett JC, Hope ME, Berry S, Thomson J, et al. Increase in NF-kappaB binding affinity of the variant C allele of the toll-like receptor 9 -1237T/C polymorphism is associated with helicobacter pylori-induced gastric disease. Infect Immun. 2010;78(3):1345–52.

26. Hamann L, Glaeser C, Hamprecht A, Gross M, Gomma A, Schumann RR. Toll-like receptor (TLR)-9 promotor polymorphisms and atherosclerosis. Clin Chim Acta. 2006;364(1–2):303–7.

27. Copin R, De Baetselier P, Carlier Y, Letesson JJ, Muraille E. MyD88-dependent activation of B220-CD11b+LY-6C+ dendritic cells during Brucella melitensis infection. J Immunol. 2007;178(8):5182–91.

28. Graustein AD, Horne DJ, Arentz M, Bang ND, Chau TT, Thwaites GE, et al. TLR9 gene region polymorphisms and susceptibility to tuberculosis in Vietnam. Tuberculosis (Edinb). 2015;95(2):190–6.

29. Torres-Garcia D, Cruz-Lagunas A, Garcia-Sancho Figueroa MC, Fernandez-Plata R, Baez-Saldana R, Mendoza-Milla C, et al. Variants in toll-like receptor 9 gene influence susceptibility to tuberculosis in a Mexican population. J Transl Med. 2013;11:220.

30. Jahantigh D, Salimi S, Alavi-Naini R, Emamdadi A, Owaysee Osquee H, Farajian Mashhadi F. Association between TLR4 and TLR9 gene polymorphisms with development of pulmonary tuberculosis in Zahedan, southeastern Iran. ScientificWorldJournal. 2013;2013:534053.

31. Velez DR, Wejse C, Stryjewski ME, Abbate E, Hulme WF, Myers JL, et al. Variants in toll-like receptors 2 and 9 influence susceptibility to pulmonary tuberculosis in Caucasians, African-Americans, and west Africans. Hum Genet. 2010;127(1):65–73.

32. Wu L, Hu Y, Li D, Jiang W, Xu B. Screening toll-like receptor markers to predict latent tuberculosis infection and subsequent tuberculosis disease in a Chinese population. BMC Med Genet. 2015;16:19.

33. Liu Q, Wu S, Xue M, Sandford AJ, Wu J, Wang Y, et al. Heterozygote advantage of the rs3794624 polymorphism in CYBA for resistance to tuberculosis in two Chinese populations. Sci Rep. 2016;6:38213.

34. Du W, Cheng J, Ding H, Jiang Z, Guo Y, Yuan H. A rapid method for simultaneous multi-gene mutation screening in children with nonsyndromic hearing loss. Genomics. 2014;104(4):264–70.

35. Kuo CL, Duan Y, Grady J. Unconditional or conditional logistic regression model for age-matched case-control data? Front Public Health. 2018;6:57.

36. Horne DJ, Graustein AD, Shah JA, Peterson G, Savlov M, Steele S, et al. Human ULK1 variation and susceptibility to Mycobacterium tuberculosis infection. J Infect Dis. 2016;214(8):1260–7.

37. Nonghanphithak D, Reechaipichitkul W, Namwat W, Lulitanond V, Naranbhai V, Faksri K. Genetic polymorphisms of CCL2 associated with susceptibility to latent tuberculous infection in Thailand. Int J Tuberc Lung Dis. 2016;20(9):1242–8.

38. Lu Y, Zhu Y, Wang X, Wang F, Peng J, Hou H, et al. FOXO3 rs12212067: T > G association with active tuberculosis in Han Chinese population. Inflammation. 2016;39(1):10–5.

39. Dalgic N, Tekin D, Kayaalti Z, Soylemezoglu T, Cakir E, Kilic B, et al. Arg753Gln polymorphism of the human toll-like receptor 2 gene from infection to disease in pediatric tuberculosis. Hum Immunol. 2011;72(5):440–5.

40. Stein CM, Zalwango S, Chiunda AB, Millard C, Leontiev DV, Horvath AL, et al. Linkage and association analysis of candidate genes for TB and TNFalpha cytokine expression: evidence for association with IFNGR1, IL-10, and TNF receptor 1 genes. Hum Genet. 2007;121(6):663–73.

41. Bukhari M, Aslam MA, Khan A, Iram Q, Akbar A, Naz AG, et al. TLR8 gene polymorphism and association in bacterial load in southern Punjab of Pakistan: an association study with pulmonary tuberculosis. Int J Immunogenet. 2015;42(1):46–51.

42. Kobayashi K, Yuliwulandari R, Yanai H, Naka I, Lien LT, Hang NT, et al. Association of TLR polymorphisms with development of tuberculosis in Indonesian females. Tissue Antigens. 2012;79(3):190–7.

43. Chimusa ER, Zaitlen N, Daya M, Moller M, van Helden PD, Mulder NJ, et al. Genome-wide association study of ancestry-specific TB risk in the south African Coloured population. Hum Mol Genet. 2014;23(3):796–809.

44. Lu Y, Li Q, Peng J, Zhu Y, Wang F, Wang C, et al. Association of autophagy-related IRGM polymorphisms with latent versus active tuberculosis infection in a Chinese population. Tuberculosis (Edinb). 2016;97:47–51.

45. Majorov KB, Lyadova IV, Kondratieva TK, Eruslanov EB, Rubakova EI, Orlova MO, et al. Different innate ability of I/St and a/Sn mice to combat virulent Mycobacterium tuberculosis: phenotypes expressed in lung and Extrapulmonary macrophages. Infect Immun. 2003;71(2):697–707.

Human cytomegalovirus and Epstein-Barr virus infections, risk factors, and their influence on the liver function of patients with acute-on-chronic liver failure

Jianhua Hu[1†], Hong Zhao[1†], Danfeng Lou[2†], Hainv Gao[2], Meifang Yang[1], Xuan Zhang[1], Hongyu Jia[1] and Lanjuan Li[1*] ⓘ

Abstract

Background: Studies on human cytomegalovirus (HCMV) and Epstein-Barr virus (EBV) have focused primarily on the immunosuppressed population. Few studies have considered immunocompetent and not severely immunocompromised patients. We determined the infection rates of HCMV and EBV, their risk factors and their influence on liver function in patients with HBV-related acute-on-chronic liver failure (ACLF).

Methods: Patients infected with ACLF-based hepatitis B virus (HBV) from 1 December 2016 to 31 May 2018 were enrolled in our study and were divided into infected and uninfected groups. The risk factors for HCMV and EBV infection and their influence on liver function were analysed.

Results: A total of 100 hospitalized patients with ACLF due to HBV infection were enrolled in this study. Of these patients, 5% presented HCMV deoxyribonucleic acid (DNA) and 23.0% presented EBV DNA. An HBV DNA count of < 1000 IU/mL increased the occurrence of HCMV infection ($P = 0.003$). Age, especially older than 60 years, was a risk factor for EBV infection ($P = 0.034$, $P = 0.033$). HCMV-infected patients had lower alanine aminotransferase (ALT) levels; albumin levels and Child–Pugh scores in EBV-infected patients were higher than those in uninfected patients.

Conclusions: HCMV and EBV were detected in patients with ACLF caused by HBV infection. Lower replication of HBV (HBV DNA < 1000 IU/mL) may increase the probability of HCMV infection; age, especially older than 60 years of age, was a risk factor for EBV infection. HCMV infection may inhibit HBV proliferation and did not increase liver injury, while co-infection with EBV may influence liver function and may result in a poor prognosis.

Keywords: Acute-on-chronic liver failure, Human cytomegalovirus, Epstein-Barr virus, Hepatitis B virus

Background

Human cytomegalovirus (HCMV) is a β human herpesvirus with positive rates of antibodies of 50–100% [1, 2]. Primary HCMV infection is often acquired during early childhood, and in later development stages, HCMV establishes lifelong latency or persistence within a person through cells of myeloid lineage [1] or granulocyte-monocyte lineage [3]. However, reactivated or exogenous reinfection with HCMV may occur and may become a major viral cause of morbidity and mortality in immunocompromised patients, such as organ or haematopoietic stem cell transplant (HSCT) recipients [4–6] and patients with acquired immune deficiency syndrome (AIDS) [1, 2].

Epstein-Barr virus (EBV) is a γ human herpesvirus with positive rates of antibodies of up to 90% [7, 8]. Primary EBV infection mostly manifests as infectious mononucleosis, with fever, angina, lymphadenopathy,

* Correspondence: ljli@zju.edu.cn

[†]Jianhua Hu, Hong Zhao and Danfeng Lou contributed equally to this work.

[1]State Key Laboratory for Diagnosis and Treatment of Infectious Diseases, Collaborative Innovation Center for Diagnosis and Treatment of Infectious Diseases, The First Affiliated Hospital, College of Medicine, Zhejiang University, 79 QingChun Road, Hangzhou 310003, Zhejiang, China

Full list of author information is available at the end of the article

and liver and spleen enlargement. After a primary infection occurs, EBV also develops a lifelong latency in B cells [9]. Latent EBV may be reactivated under certain conditions, thereby inducing abnormal B cell proliferation and leading to neoplastic disease.

Studies on HCMV have focused mostly on immunosuppressed individuals [2, 4, 5]. Studies on EBV have mostly examined patients with neoplastic disease [10] and post-transplant lymphoproliferative disorder following HSCT [5, 11, 12]. Limited studies have considered immunocompetent and not severely immunocompromised patients.

Acute liver failure (ALF) is a well-established medical emergency defined as a severe liver injury. However, a proportion of patients who present features mimicking ALF suffer from an underlying chronic liver disease or liver cirrhosis. These patients, who have been defined as patients with acute-on-chronic liver failure (ACLF), display various degrees of immune disorders and short-term mortality rates [13]. HCMV may induce fulminant hepatic failure [14, 15], and EBV may trigger acute liver failure [15–17].

HCMV may be reactivated in patients with cirrhosis [18–20]. Rosi, S. et al. [19] recently revealed that HCMV causes or contributes to hepatic decompensation or ACLF in patients with cirrhosis even if they are not severely immunocompromised. However, the patients in the above study [19] had alcohol-related and mixed-aetiology cirrhosis (hepatitis C virus and alcohol-related cirrhosis). To date, studies have yet to describe HCMV or EBV infections in patients with ACLF due to hepatitis B virus (HBV)-related chronic liver disease or liver cirrhosis.

Therefore, this study aims to identify HCMV and EBV infection in patients with ACLF-based HBV in our hospital. The specific objective of this study was to explore the HCMV and EBV infection rate, the risk factors of these infections, and their influence on the liver function of patients with ACLF-based HBV, which will improve the survival of these patients through an effective intervention.

Methods
Patients
The databases of patients with liver disease were reviewed in our hospital, and patients diagnosed with ACLF due to HBV-related chronic liver disease or liver cirrhosis were identified. HCMV/EBV-infected and –uninfected patients were included in this retrospective study. Eligible patients must have been hospitalized at First Affiliated Hospital, College of Medicine, Zhejiang University from 1 January 2016 to 31 May 2018. The demographics, clinical characteristics, and experimental results, such as liver function and HBV DNA level, were reviewed by a trained team of physicians and entered in duplicate into a computerized system.

Enrolment criteria
ACLF was defined in accordance with the following criteria specified by the Asian Pacific Association for the Study of the Liver (2014) [13] and the Guideline for Diagnosis and Treatment of Liver Failure in China [21]: (1) acute deterioration of pre-existing HBV-related chronic liver disease or liver cirrhosis; (2) extreme fatigue with severe digestive symptoms, such as observable anorexia, abdominal distension, or nausea and vomiting; (3) progressively worsening jaundice within a short period (serum total bilirubin of ≥ 10 mg/dL or daily elevation of ≥ 1 mg/dL); (4) a haemorrhagic tendency, with a prothrombin activity of $\leq 40\%$ (or international normalized ratio (INR) ≥ 1.5); (5) decompensation ascites; and (6) with or without hepatic encephalopathy. The absence of any of these six criteria precluded a diagnosis of ACLF.

Exclusion criteria
Patients meeting the following criteria were excluded: (1) ACLF due to HBV-unrelated chronic liver disease or liver cirrhosis, such as alcoholism, autoimmunity, hepatolenticular degeneration, non-alcoholic fatty liver disease, etc.; (2) patients with hepatocellular carcinoma complications; (3) patients aged below 18 years old; (4) women undergoing pregnancy and lactation; (5) patients with AIDS; (6) patients with underlying diseases requiring long-time corticosteroids or immunosuppressive treatments. Patients who met any of these six criteria were excluded from this study.

Quantitative polymerase chain reaction assay for HCMV and EBV deoxyribonucleic acid (DNA)
HCMV and EBV DNA was extracted from whole-blood samples and detected using a commercial DNA extraction kit (Daan Gene Co. Ltd., Zhongshan University, China) following the manufacturer's instructions. Quantitative polymerase chain reaction (PCR) was performed using a TaqMan PCR Kit (Daan Gene Co. Ltd., Zhongshan University, China) following the manufacturer's instructions and run on a real real-time PCR system (Stratagene MX3000P, Agilent Technologies, Santa Clara, CA, USA). Positive and negative controls were included in the quantitative PCR process. The viral loads were denoted in IU/mL. On the basis of the detection limit of the PCR kit, EBV and HCMV DNA loads of <500 copies/mL and ≥ 500 copies/mL were considered negative and positive, respectively. The accuracy was evaluated by an internal quality control, and the coefficient of variation was within an acceptable range.

Human cytomegalovirus and Epstein-Barr virus infections, risk factors, and their influence...

191

Risk factors of HCMV and EBV infection

Previous studies revealed that among organ transplant and HSCT recipients, the risk factors of HCMV and EBV infection were age, male gender, T-cell depletion, immunosuppressive agents, serostatus matching, acute and chronic graft-versus-host disease, rejection and use of human leukocyte antigen (HLA)-mismatched or unrelated donors [3, 5, 6, 11, 12, 22]. However, the potential risk factors of HCMV and EBV infection in immunocompetent and not severely immunocompromised patients, such as those with ACLF due to HBV infection, remain unclear. Previous reports have described the interactions between HBV and HCMV [23, 24], and between HBV and EBV [25]. Thus, we attempted to explore whether in addition to gender and age, HBV-related indexes, including the proliferation state (HBV DNA levels and HBV DNA < 1000 IU/mL), serological status of HBV (HBsAg levels, HBcAb levels, HBeAg positivity (>0.18 PEIU/ml)) and liver cirrhosis are risk factors for HCMV and EBV infection in patients with ACLF due to HBV infection.

Liver function, child-Pugh score, and MELD score

Liver function, including albumin, alanine aminotransferase (ALT), aspartate aminotransferase (AST), albumin/globulin (A/G), total bilirubin (TB); direct bilirubin (DB), and γ-glutamyl transpeptidase (GGT), was reviewed by Student's t tests or Mann-Whitney tests. The indexes above that were significantly different were further analysed by binary logistic regression.

The Child-Pugh [26] and model for end-stage liver disease (MELD) [27] scores can be used to accurately assess the liver function and prognosis of patients with end-stage liver disease and liver failure. In addition to the aforementioned functional indexes, we also calculated the Child-Pugh and MELD scores of the patients. The calculation for the MELD score is as follows: MELD score = $3.8 \times \log_e$ (bilirubin[mg/dL]) + $11.2 \times \log_e$(INR) + $9.6 \times \log_e$ (creatinine [mg/dL]) + 6.4 (aetiology: 0 if cholestatic or alcoholic; otherwise, 1) [27].

Statistical analysis

Statistical analyses were performed using SPSS software. The results were expressed as the means ± standard deviations, median (quartile) and percentages. The means for continuous variables were compared by using independent-group Student's t tests for normally distributed data (age, albumin, TB, DB, MELD score) and Mann-Whitney tests for non-normally distributed data (ALT, AST, GGT, Child-Pugh score). The categorical variables were analysed by performing chi-square or Fisher's exact tests. The risk factors of HCMV and EBV infection as well as the relationship between liver function and HCMV/EBV infection were analysed using binary logistic regression. All p-values were based on a two-tailed test of significance.

Results

HCMV and EBV infection

As described in Fig. 1 and Table 1, a total of 1011 patients hospitalized in our hospital with ACLF were screened between 1 January 2016 and 1 September 2017. A total of 878 subjects were hospitalized due to ACLF due to HBV, and the others were excluded. A total of 100 patients were assessed for HCMV and EBV, of which five (5.0%) patients were HCMV DNA-positive, with a mean of 1.39×10^4 copies/mL, and 23 (23.0%) patients were EBV DNA-positive, with a mean of 2.7×10^3 copies /mL. In addition, one patient was both HCMV DNA- and EBV DNA-positive. The subjects consisted of 81 men and 19 women, with a mean age of 47.7 years old. A total of 19.0% of the patients were at least 60 years old. The demographic and clinical characteristics of the participants are presented in Table 1.

Risk factors for HCMV and EBV infection

Among the aforementioned possible risk factors, we found that HBV DNA < 1000 IU/mL was a risk factor for HCMV infection ($P = 0.003$), with a dramatically increased risk of 34.00-fold (95% CI: 3.453–334.800). The ages of the EBV-infected patients were older than the uninfected patients. A greater number of EBV-infected patients were > 60 years of age. Age, especially older than 60 years ($P = 0.034$, $P = 0.033$) was a risk factors for EBV infection by 1.042-fold and 3.200-fold, respectively (95% CI: 1.003–1.082, 1.098–9.324). (Table 1, Table 2).

Liver function, child-Pugh score, and MELD score

All indexes of liver function, Child-Pugh score, and MELD score were analysed between infected and uninfected patients. Only the ALT and AST levels in HCMV-uninfected patients were significantly lower than in HCMV-infected patients ($P = 0.001$, $P = 0.002$). When the above indexes (ALT and AST) were further analysed using binary logistic regression, we only found that there was relationship between lower ALT levels and HCMV infection ($P = 0.039$, OR 1.067). However, the albumin level was lower in EBV-infected patients (29.72 ± 3.626 g/L) than in uninfected patients (33.19 ± 4.217 g/L). This difference was statistically significant ($P = 0.001$). EBV-infected patients achieved significantly higher Child-Pugh scores (12.0 (11.0, 13.0) VS 10.0 (9.0, 12.0), $P = 0.008$). When we further analysed the relationship between the albumin level, Child-Pugh score and EBV infection using binary logistic regression, we found that EBV-infected patients had lower albumin levels and higher Child-Pugh scores (P = 0.001, OR 1.242; $P = 0.009$, OR 1.493). (Tables 3, 4 and 5).

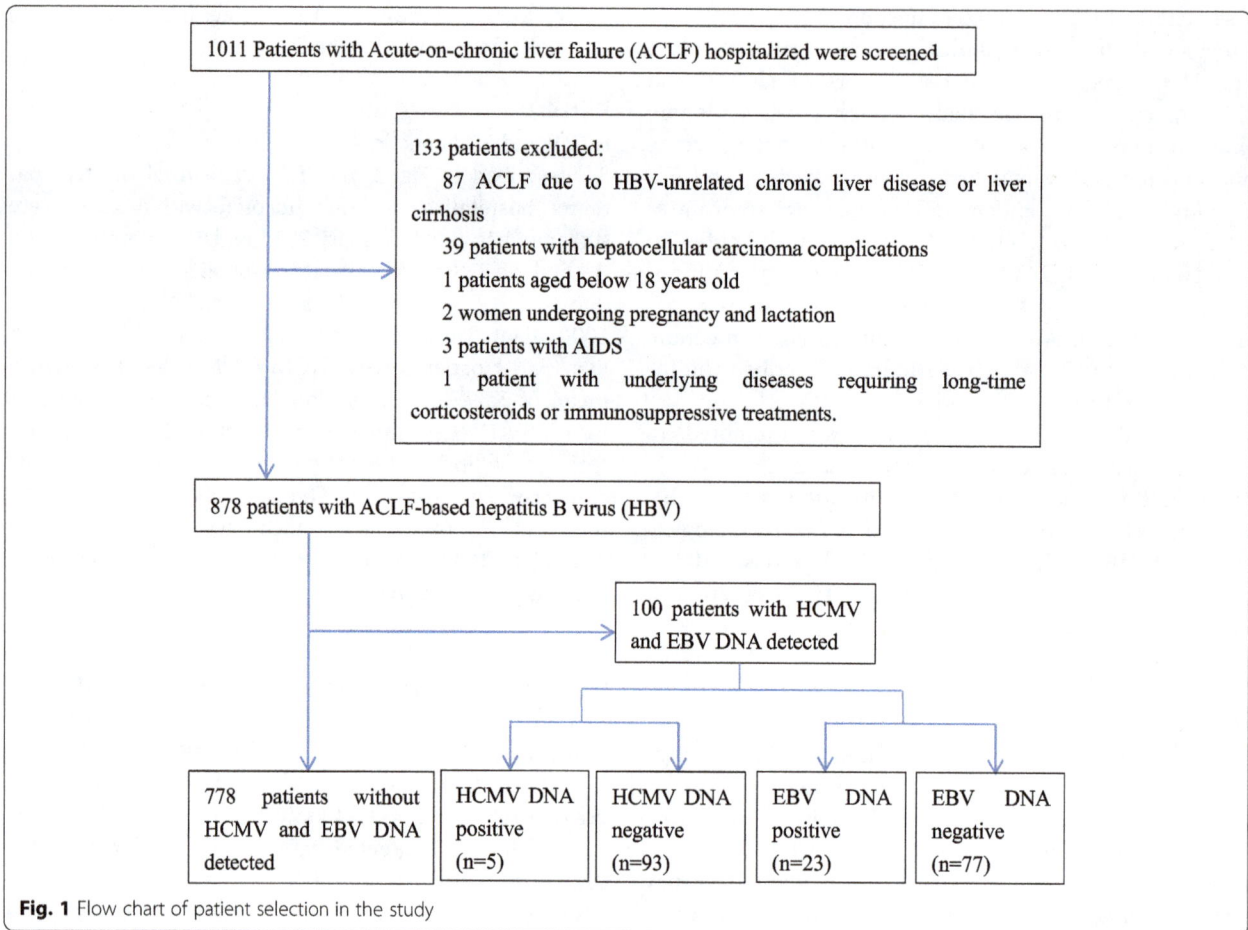

Fig. 1 Flow chart of patient selection in the study

Discussion

Human herpes viruses include herpes simplex virus type 1 (HSV-1), herpes simplex virus type 2 (HSV-2), varicella zoster virus (VZV), HCMV, EBV, human herpesvirus 6 (HHV-6), human herpesvirus 7 (HHV-7), and human herpesvirus 8 (HHV-8). Although HCMV and EBV are more studied in this respect, after initial infections with no or mild symptoms, all human herpes viruses may become latent under certain conditions. However, most studies of latent HCMV and EBV infection have focused on immunosuppressed individuals. In this study, we aimed to focus our investigation on HCMV and EBV in immunocompetent individuals.

Our study evaluates a cohort of 100 hospitalized patients with ACLF due to HBV infection, of which 5.0% patients presented with HCMV DNA, 23.0% patients presented with EBV DNA, and one patient was positive for both HCMV DNA and EBV DNA. HBV DNA < 1000 IU/mL was a risk factor for HCMV infection, and age, especially older than 60 years, were risk factors for EBV infection. HCMV-infected patients had lower ALT levels, indicating that HCMV infection may not increase liver injury. In contrast, EBV infection possibly influenced

liver function, as EBV-infected patients had lower albumin levels and higher Child-Pugh scores.

By reviewing the medical records and laboratory data, we found that of the 69 patients in this study in whom HCMV IgG and EB viral capsid antigen (EB-VCA) IgG were measured, all were HCMV IgG- and EB-VCA IgG-positive. HCMV and EBV primary infection mostly occur in childhood. Thus, in this study, it is likely that the observed HCMV and EBV infections were due to reactivation rather than primary infection.

Previous studies have investigated the association between HCMV infection and HBV infection [23, 28–30]. In the present study, we found that 5.0% of patients were co-infected with HCMV, and this finding was similar to that reported by Lian et al. [30]. Limited studies have explored the association between EBV infection and HBV infection [25]. An et al. [25] reported that compared with HBV infection (9.10%), EBV infection occurred more frequently in patients with HBV-related liver cirrhosis (40.0%) and liver carcinoma patients (25.0%). In the present study, we found that 23.0% of the patients were infected with EBV, which differed from the previously

Table 1 Characteristics of patients with acute-on-chronic liver caused by HBV infection

	Total (n = 100)	HCMV			EBV		
		Infected (n = 5)	Un-infected (n = 95)	P	Infected (n = 23)	Un-infected (n = 77)	P
Sex (M/F)	81/19	5/0	76/19	0.580	17/6	64/13	0.367
Age[a]	47.68 ± 12.520	45.00 ± 13.191	47.82 ± 12.541	0.626	52.65 ± 15.098	46.19 ± 11.335	0.067
≥ 60 yr	19 (19.0%)	1 (20.0%)	18 (18.9%)	1.000	8 (34.8%)	11 (14.3%)	0.037
Liver Cirrhosis	46 (46.0%)	2 (40.0%)	44 (46.3%)	1.000	12 (52.2%)	34 (44.2%)	0.498
Underling Conditions[b]							
Hypertension	13 (13.0%)	1 (20.0%)	12 (12.6%)	0.509	2 (8.7%)	11 (14.3%)	0.727
Diabetes Mellitus	11 (11.0%)	1 (20.0%)	10 (10.5%)	0.449	4 (17.4%)	7 (9.1%)	0.271
Coronary Atherosclerotic Heart Disease	4 (4.0%)	0 (0.0%)	4 (4.2%)	1.000	1 (4.3%)	3 (3.9%)	1.000
Chronic Bronchitis and Pulmonary emphysema	1 (1.0%)	0 (0.0%)	1 (1.1%)	1.000	0 (0.0%)	1 (1.3%)	1.000
Ulcerative Colitis	1 (1.0%)	1 (20.0%)	0 (0.0%)	0.086	0 (0.0%)	1 (1.3%)	1.000
Schizophrenia	2 (2.0%)	0 (0.0%)	2 (2.1%)	1.000	0 (0.0%)	2 (2.6%)	1.000
Chronic kidney disease	1 (1.0%)	0 (0.0%)	1 (1.1%)	1.000	0 (0.0%)	1 (1.3%)	1.000
Neoplasm							
Gastric Carcinoma	1 (1.0%)	0 (0.0%)	1 (1.1%)	1.000	0 (0.0%)	1 (2.2%)	1.000
Renal Carcinoma	1 (1.0%)	0 (0.0%)	1 (1.1%)	1.000	1 (7.7%)	0 (0.0%)	0.224

Note: [a]mean ± standard deviation, years; [b]one patient underling conditions included coronary atherosclerotic heart disease, hypertension, chronic bronchitis and emphysema pulmonum; one patient coexisting conditions included diabetes Mellitus, hypertension; and one patient coexisting conditions included coronary atherosclerotic heart Disease, diabetes mellitus, hypertension

reported infection rate because chronic HBV infection and liver cirrhosis were both included in our study.

Immunosuppressive drugs, high-dose corticosteroids, T-cell depletion, acute and chronic GVHD, rejection, and virus coinfection were identified as the most common risk factors for HCMV or EBV infection [3, 5, 6, 11, 12, 22]. These risk factors were determined mainly based on immunodeficient or immunosuppressed patients, such as organ transplant recipients, HSCT recipients, and patients with AIDS. Few studies have considered immunocompetent and not severely immunocompromised patients. In the present study, we focused on patients with ACLF due to HBV infection.

ACLF is defined as an acute hepatic insult manifesting as jaundice and coagulopathy that is complicated within 4 weeks by ascites and/or encephalopathy in patients with previously diagnosed or undiagnosed chronic liver disease [13, 21] with various degrees of immune disorders. Considering the relationship among HCMV, EBV, and HBV [23, 25, 28–30], we attempted to explore whether HBV-related indexes and liver cirrhosis are potential risk factors in addition to age and gender.

We found that HCMV-infected patients had lower HBV DNA levels than HCMV-uninfected patients (P = 0.001). Eighty percent of the HCMV-infected patients had HBV DNA < 1000 IU/mL, which was greater than

Table 2 Binary logistic analysis for HCMV, EBV risk factors

Variable	HCMV			EBV		
	OR	95% CI	P	OR	95% CI	P
Age	0.981	0.909–1.059	0.623	1.042	1.003–1.082	0.034
Age ≥ 60 yr	1.069	0.113–10.153	0.953	3.200	1.098–9.324	0.033
Male	0.000	0.000–0.000	0.998	1.738	0.575–5.248	0.327
Liver Cirrhosis	0.773	0.123–4.837	0.783	1.380	0.542–3.510	0.499
HBV DNA levels	1.000	0.999–1.000	0.241	1.000	1.000–1.000	0.890
HBV DNA (<1000 IU/ml)	34.000	3.453–334.800	0.003	0.900	0.228–3.546	0.880
HBsAg titer	1.000	1.000–1.000	0.607	1.000	1.000–1.000	0.317
HBcAb titer	1.108	0.859–1.430	0.429	0.956	0.769–1.198	0.687
HBeAg positive (>0.18PEIU/ml)	0.773	0.123–4.837	0.783	2.187	0.844–5.669	0.107

Note: HCMV human cytomegalovirus, EBV Epstein–Barr virus

Table 3 Liver function between HCMV infected and un-infected patients

	HCMV infected (n = 5)	HCMV un-infected (n = 95)	P
ALT (U/L)	34.0 (30.0, 48.0)	166.0 (87.0, 446.0)	0.001
AST (U/L)	45.0 (43.5, 52.0)	134.0 (78.0, 254.0)	0.002
Albumin (g/L)	31.86 ± 3.002	32.42 ± 4.397	0.779
TB (U/L)	358.20 ± 191.525	328.91 ± 119.722	0.606
DB (U/L)	241.80 ± 125.398	228.74 ± 85.521	0.746
GGT (U/L)	46.0 (38.5, 142.5)	75.0 (55.0, 125.0)	0.300
Child-pugh Score	12.0 (9.0, 12.0)	11.0 (10.0, 12.0)	0.994
Meld Score	20.43 ± 2.328	23.54 ± 5.759	0.235

Note: *ALT* alanine aminotransferase, *AST* aspartate aminotransferase, *A/G* Albumin/Globulin, *TB* total bilirubin, *DB* direct bilirubin, *GGT* γ-glutamyl transpeptadase

the number of HCMV-uninfected patients with similar levels (9.5%). In addition, we found that HBV DNA < 1000 IU/mL was a risk factor for HCMV infection. HBV was strongly correlated with HCMV. Our findings were similar to those of previous reports [23, 24]. Cavanaugh, V. J. et al. [24] discovered that cytokines produced by murine cytomegalovirus inhibited HBV replication and gene expression. Bayram, A. et al. [23] revealed that the inflammation caused by HCMV can contribute to viral clearance during chronic HBV infection. Therefore, we suggest that HBV and HCMV replication may mutually inhibit each other. Thus, when HBV replication is inactive, as indicated by a lower titre of HBV DNA, especially HBV DNA < 1000 IU/mL, HCMV replication activity is facilitated. However, the specific mechanism underlying this phenomenon must be further studied.

Our previous study posited that male donors, conditioning regimens including ATG and GVHD prophylaxis, and prednisone increase the risk of EBV infection in patients receiving HSCT [5]. However, EBV infection and its risk factors were rare in patients who are not

Table 4 Liver function between EBV infected and un-infected patients

	EBV infected (n = 23)	EBV un-infected (n = 77)	P
ALT (U/L)	162.0 (76.0, 504.0)	153.0 (74.5.0, 408.0)	0.734
AST (U/L)	133.0 (50.0, 332.0)	130.0 (69.0, 241.0)	0.889
Albumin (g/L)	29.72 ± 3.626	33.19 ± 4.217	0.001
TB (U/L)	291.52 ± 109.996	341.98 ± 124.966	0.084
DB (U/L)	202.10 ± 74.653	237.55 ± 89.320	0.087
GGT (U/L)	70.0 (46.0, 92.0)	78.0 (54.5, 128.0)	0.206
Child-pugh Score	12.0 (11.0, 13.0)	10.0 (9.0, 12.0)	0.008
Meld Score	23.48 ± 4.551	23.35 ± 5.992	0.925

Note: *ALT* alanine aminotransferase, *AST* aspartate aminotransferase, *A/G* Albumin/Globulin, *TB* total bilirubin, *DB* direct bilirubin, *GGT* γ-glutamyl transpeptadase

Table 5 Binary logistic analysis for liver function and HCMV, EBV infection

Virus	variable	OR (95% CI)	P
HCMV	ALT	1.067 (1.003~ 1.135)	0.039
	AST	1.078 (0.994~ 1.169)	0.071
EBV	Albumin	1.242 (1.088~ 1.416)	0.001
	Child-pugh Score	1.493 (1.106~ 2.015)	0.009

Note: *HCMV* human cytomegalovirus, *EBV* Epstein–Barr virus

severely immunocompromised, such as those with ACLF. In the present study, HBV-related indexes, including proliferation state, serological status of HBV and liver cirrhosis, were not risk factors of EBV infection in HBV-related ACLF. However, age was a risk factor for EBV infection, especially in patients > 60 years of age. XM. Zhang [31] previously reported that the rate of EBV-1 infection in this age group was significantly higher than that in the < 40 age group. Age was related to EBV-1 infection in patients with chronic periodontitis. It was suggested that the immune system and the environment of the host change with the age, and thus, latent EBV was released and propagated in the host cell [31].

Bayram, A. et al. [23] indicated that the mean ALT and intrahepatic HBV DNA levels in patients with HCMV co-infected with chronic viral hepatitis B were lower than those in patients without HCMV co-infection. Similarly, we found that the levels of ALT, AST, and HBV DNA were lower in patients with ACLF due to HBV co-infection with HCMV. However, further analysis using binary logistic regression indicated that only the ALT level was related to HCMV infection. Therefore, we suggest that HCMV infection may inhibit HBV proliferation, decrease inflammatory activity, reduce liver cell damage, and reduce ALT levels. However, the specific mechanism underlying this phenomenon must be further studied.

Previous studies have reported that EBV infection causes acute liver failure [15–17]. In the present study, EBV-infected patients had lower albumin levels than uninfected patients. In addition, EBV-infected patients also had higher Child-Pugh scores. Thus, EBV infection may be related to lower albumin and higher Child-Pugh score. EBV infection may increase liver injury and decrease the liver synthesis ability in ACLF patients. Furthermore, Child-Pugh score is a suitable prognostic evaluation indictor for patients with end-stage liver disease; a higher score corresponds to higher mortality in the short term [26]. Thus, the influence of EBV infection on liver function may result in poor prognosis.

This work is limited by a number of factors. First, a slight bias is present in any retrospective study, which will result in a certain statistical bias. Second, we did not conduct follow-up for the included patients and did not analyse the confirmed influence of prognosis on HCMV and EBV infection in the short and long terms. Third, we unfortunately did not include all human herpes viruses in this study. Fourth, we found that HCMV-infected patients had lower HBV DNA levels, and thus HCMV viral replication is likely to be detrimental to HBV replication in these 5 HCMV-infected cases. This may be due to the inflammatory cytokines caused by HCMV contributing to viral clearance during chronic HBV infection. However, we unfortunately did not measure the proinflammatory cytokines released by HCMV that prevent HBV replication. Fifth, we cannot distinguish between primary infection and reactivation of HCMV and EBV infection for all patients, although there all 69 patients in our study who were evaluated were found to be HCMV IgG- and EBV IgG-positive. We will address these drawbacks in our future studies. Finally, although we found that EBV-infected patients had lower albumin levels and higher Child-Pugh scores, as indicated by binary logistic regression, this may be associated with overall physiological decline in these patients. Although this study does have limitations, our evaluation of patients with HBV-related ACLF may begin to fill in gaps of knowledge on HCMV and EBV infection in immunocompetent patients.

Conclusions

This study revealed that HCMV and, more notably, Epstein-Barr virus (EBV) were detected in patients with ACLF due to HBV infection. Lower replication levels of HBV (HBV DNA < 1000 IU/mL) was associated with an increased probability of HCMV infection; age, especially older than 60 years, were associated with EBV infection. HCMV infection may inhibit HBV proliferation and reduce liver injury, while EBV infection possibly influenced liver function, as EBV-infected patients had lower albumin levels and higher Child-Pugh scores. HCMV co-infection did not increase liver injury. However, co-infection with EBV may influence liver function and may induce poor prognosis in HBV-related ACLF. Thus, attention should be paid to the possibility that older patients, especially those older than 60 years with ACLF due to HBV, may be infected with EBV. In this case, effective antiviral therapy may be needed; otherwise, EBV infection may influence the patients'prognosis.

Abbreviations

A/G: Albumin/Globulin; ACLF: Acute-on-chronic liver failure; AIDS: immune deficiency syndrome; ALF: Acute liver failure; ALT: Alanine aminotransferase; AST: Aspartate aminotransferase; DB: Direct bilirubin; DNA: Deoxyribonucleic acid; EBV: Epstein-Barr virus; GGT: γ-glutamyl transpeptadase; HBeAg: Hepatitis B e antigen; HBsAg: Hepatitis B surface antigen; HBV: Hepatitis B virus; HCMV: Human cytomegalovirus; HLA: Human leukocyte antigen; HSCT: Hematopoietic stem cell transplant recipients; INR: International normalized ratio; MELD: Model for end-stage liver disease scores; PCR: Polymerase chain reaction; TB: Total bilirubin

Acknowledgments
Not applicable.

Funding
This study was supported by the national science and technology major project (2017ZX10202202–003-004), which was funded by ministry of science and technology.

Authors' contributions
Study design: LJL, JHH; Data collection: DFL, XZ; Data analysis: HZ, HNG, MFY, HYJ; Paper writing: JHH, HZ, DFL. JHH, HZ, DFL contributed equally to this work. All authors read and approved the final manuscript.

Competing interests
The authors declare that they have no competing interests.

Author details
[1]State Key Laboratory for Diagnosis and Treatment of Infectious Diseases, Collaborative Innovation Center for Diagnosis and Treatment of Infectious Diseases, The First Affiliated Hospital, College of Medicine, Zhejiang University, 79 QingChun Road, Hangzhou 310003, Zhejiang, China. [2]Shulan (Hangzhou) Hospital, 848 Dongxin Road, Hangzhou 310004, Zhejiang, China.

References
1. Gandhi MK, Khanna R. Human cytomegalovirus: clinical aspects, immune regulation, and emerging treatments. Lancet Infect Dis. 2004;4:725–38. https://doi.org/10.1016/S1473-3099(04)01202-2.
2. Jiang XJ, Zhang J, Xiong Y, Jahn G, Xiong HR, Yang ZQ, Liu YY. Human cytomegalovirus glycoprotein polymorphisms and increasing viral load in AIDS patients. PLoS One. 2017;12:e0176160. https://doi.org/10.1371/journal.pone.0176160.
3. Ljungman P, Hakki M, Boeckh M. Cytomegalovirus in hematopoietic stem cell transplant recipients. Infect Dis Clin North Am. 2010;24:319–37. https://doi.org/10.1016/j.idc.2010.01.008.
4. Vietzen H, Gorzer I, Honsig C, Jaksch P, Puchhammer-Stockl E. Association between antibody functions and human cytomegalovirus (HCMV) replication after lung transplantation in HCMV-seropositive patients. J Heart Lung Transplant. 2017. https://doi.org/10.1016/j.healun.2017.07.010.
5. Fan J, Jing M, Yang M, Xu L, Liang H, Huang Y, Yang R, Gui G, Wang H, Gong S, et al. Herpesvirus infections in hematopoietic stem cell transplant recipients seropositive for human cytomegalovirus before transplantation. Int J Infect Dis. 2016;46:89–93. https://doi.org/10.1016/j.ijid.2016.03.025.
6. Preiksaitis JK, Brennan DC, Fishman J, Allen U. Canadian society of transplantation consensus workshop on cytomegalovirus management in solid organ transplantation final report. Am J Transplant. 2005;5:218–27. https://doi.org/10.1111/j.1600-6143.2004.00692.x.
7. Taylor GS, Long HM, Brooks JM, Rickinson AB, Hislop AD. The immunology of Epstein-Barr virus-induced disease. Annu Rev Immunol. 2015;33:787–821. https://doi.org/10.1146/annurev-immunol-032414-112326.
8. Maeda A, Sato T, Wakiguchi H. Epidemiology of Epstein-Barr virus (EBV) infection and EBV-associated diseases. Nihon Rinsho. 2006;64(Suppl 3): 609–12.
9. Vouloumanou EK, Rafailidis PI, Falagas ME. Current diagnosis and management of infectious mononucleosis. Curr Opin Hematol. 2012;19: 14–20. https://doi.org/10.1097/MOH.0b013e32834daa08.
10. Ma J, Li J, Hao Y, Nie Y, Li Z, Qian M, Liang Q, Yu J, Zeng M, Wu K. Differentiated tumor immune microenvironment of Epstein-Barr virus-associated and negative gastric cancer: implication in prognosis and immunotherapy. Oncotarget. 2017;8:67094–103. https://doi.org/10.18632/oncotarget.17945.
11. Peric Z, Cahu X, Chevallier P, Brissot E, Malard F, Guillaume T, Delaunay J, Ayari S, Dubruille V, Le Gouill S, et al. Features of Epstein-Barr Virus (EBV) reactivation after reduced intensity conditioning allogeneic hematopoietic stem cell transplantation. Leukemia. 2011;25:932–8. https://doi.org/10.1038/leu.2011.26.
12. Kullberg-Lindh C, Mellgren K, Friman V, Fasth A, Ascher H, Nilsson S, Lindh M. Opportunistic virus DNA levels after pediatric stem cell transplantation: serostatus matching, anti-thymocyte globulin, and total body irradiation are additive risk factors. Transpl Infect Dis. 2011;13:122–30. https://doi.org/10.1111/j.1399-3062.2010.00564.x

13. Sarin SK, Kedarisetty CK, Abbas Z, Amarapurkar D, Bihari C, Chan AC, Chawla YK, Dokmeci AK, Garg H, Ghazinyan H, et al. Acute-on-chronic liver failure: consensus recommendations of the Asian Pacific Association for the Study of the liver (APASL) 2014. Hepatol Int. 2014;8:453–71. https://doi.org/10.1007/s12072-014-9580-2.

14. Hsu JY, Tsai CC, Tseng KC. Fulminant hepatic failure and acute renal failure as manifestations of concurrent Q fever and cytomegalovirus infection: a case report. BMC Infect Dis. 2014;14:651. https://doi.org/10.1186/s12879-014-0651-8.

15. Gupta E, Ballani N, Kumar M, Sarin SK. Role of non-hepatotropic viruses in acute sporadic viral hepatitis and acute-on-chronic liver failure in adults. Indian J Gastroenterol. 2015;34:448–52. https://doi.org/10.1007/s12664-015-0613-0.

16. Zhang W, Chen B, Chen Y, Chamberland R, Fider-Whyte A, Craig J, Varma C, Befeler AS, Bisceglie AM, Horton P, et al. Epstein-Barr Virus-Associated Acute Liver Failure Present in a 67-Year-Old Immunocompetent Female. Gastroenterology Res. 2016;9:74–8. https://doi.org/10.14740/gr718e.

17. Mellinger JL, Rossaro L, Naugler WE, Nadig SN, Appelman H, Lee WM, Fontana RJ. Epstein-Barr virus (EBV) related acute liver failure: a case series from the US acute liver failure study group. Dig Dis Sci. 2014;59:1630–7. https://doi.org/10.1007/s10620-014-3029-2.

18. Tanaka S, Toh Y, Minagawa H, Mori R, Sugimachi K, Minamishima Y. Reactivation of cytomegalovirus in patients with cirrhosis: analysis of 122 cases. Hepatology. 1992;16:1409–14.

19. Rosi S, Poretto V, Cavallin M, Angeli P, Amodio P, Sattin A, Montagnese S. Hepatic decompensation in the absence of obvious precipitants: the potential role of cytomegalovirus infection/reactivation. BMJ Open Gastroenterol. 2015;2:e000050. https://doi.org/10.1136/bmjgast-2015-000050.

20. Varani S, Lazzarotto T, Margotti M, Masi L, Gramantieri L, Bolondi L, Landini MP. Laboratory signs of acute or recent cytomegalovirus infection are common in cirrhosis of the liver. J Med Virol. 2000;62:25–8.

21. Failure L, Artificial Liver Group CSoID. Chinese Medical Association, severe liver diseases and artificial liver group, Chinese Society of Hepatology, Chinese Medical Association. Guideline for diagnosis and treatment of liver failure. Chin J Clin Infect Dis. 2012;5:321–7.

22. Hanley PJ, Bollard CM. Controlling cytomegalovirus: helping the immune system take the lead. Viruses. 2014;6:2242–58. https://doi.org/10.3390/v6062242.

23. Bayram A, Ozkur A, Erkilic S. Prevalence of human cytomegalovirus co-infection in patients with chronic viral hepatitis B and C: a comparison of clinical and histological aspects. J Clin Virol. 2009;45:212–7. https://doi.org/10.1016/j.jcv.2009.05.009.

24. Cavanaugh VJ, Guidotti LG, Chisari FV. Inhibition of hepatitis B virus replication during adenovirus and cytomegalovirus infections in transgenic mice. J Virol. 1998;72:2630–7.

25. An H, Zhou XJ, Miu CM. Clinical study on the relationship between EBV infection and liver diseases infected by HBV. Zhong Xi Yi Jie He Gan Bing Za Zhi. 2005;15:144–5.

26. Pugh RN, Murray-Lyon IM, Dawson JL, Pietroni MC, Williams R. Transection of the oesophagus for bleeding oesophageal varices. Br J Surg. 1973;60:646–9.

27. Kamath PS, Wiesner RH, Malinchoc M, Kremers W, Therneau TM, Kosberg CL, D'Amico G, Dickson ER, Kim WR. A model to predict survival in patients with end-stage liver disease. Hepatology. 2001;33:464–70. https://doi.org/10.1053/jhep.2001.22172.

28. Aldona K, Jacek W, Maciej Z, Wieslawa B, Joanna SZ. Cellular expression of human cytomegalovirus (HCMV) in children with chronic hepatitis B. Przegl Epidemiol. 2001;55(Suppl 3):146–52.

29. Zuschke CA, Herrera JL, Pettyjohn FS. Cytomegalovirus hepatitis mimicking an acute exacerbation of chronic hepatitis B. South Med J. 1996;89:1213–6.

30. Lian YL, Wu WF, Shi YM, Liu QC, Tang XP. Preliminary study on relationship between different viral pathogenesis and disease prognosis in patients with severe viral hepatitis. Zhonghua Shi Yan He Lin Chuang Bing Du Xue Za Zhi. 1999;13:355–7.

31. Zhang XM, Miu Y, Li L. Analysis of chronic periodontitis EBV -1 (epstein-barr virus −1) and HHV-6 (humanher pesvirus −6) infection and risk factors. J Modern Stomatol. 2011;24:332–6.

22

HIV prevalence, related risk behaviors, and correlates of HIV infection among people who use drugs in Cambodia

Heng Sopheab[1*], Chhorvann Chhea[1], Sovannary Tuot[2] and Jonathan A. Muir[3]

Abstract

Background: Although HIV prevalence in Cambodia has declined to 0.6% among the general population, the prevalence remains high among female sex workers (14.0%) and men who have sex with men (2.3%). Over the past 10 years, the number of people who use drugs (PWUDs) has increased considerably. PWUDs, especially people who inject drugs (PWIDs), who have multiple sex partners or unprotected sex contribute to a higher HIV prevalence. This paper aims to estimate the prevalence of HIV across PWUD groups and to identify factors associated with HIV infection.

Methods: Respondent-driven sampling (RDS) was used to recruit 1626 consenting PWUDs in 9 provinces in 2012. Questionnaires and blood specimens were collected. HIV prevalence estimates were calculated using RDSAT 7.1. Individual weightings for HIV were generated with RDSAT and used for a weighted analysis in STATA 13. Multivariate logistic regression was used to identify the independent factors associated with HIV prevalence.

Results: Most of the PWUDs were men (82.0%), and 7.3% were PWIDs. Non-PWIDs, especially users of amphetamine-type stimulants (ATS), represented the larger proportion of the participants (81.5%). The median age for of the PWUDs was 24.0 years (IQR: 20–29). The HIV prevalence among the PWUDs was 5.1% (95% CI: 4.1–6.2), 24.8%, among PWIDs and 4.0% among non-PWIDs. The HIV prevalence among female PWIDs was 37.5, and 22.5% among male PWIDs. Four factors were independently associated with HIV infection: female sex, with AOR = 7.8 (95% CI: 3.00–20.35); age groups 21–29 and older (AOR = 10.3, 95% CI: 1.2–20.4); and using drugs for ≥12 months (AOR = 4.0, 95% CI: 1.38–11.35). Finally, injecting drugs remained a strong predictor of HIV infection, with an AOR = 4.1 (95% CI: 1.53–10.96).

Conclusion: HIV prevalence remains high among PWIDs. Harm reduction efforts, such as needle and syringe provision programs, must improve their coverage. Innovative strategies are needed to reach sub-groups of PWUDs, especially women who inject drugs. Furthermore, the large proportion of non-PWIDs, especially ATS users, should not be ignored. Therefore, combined HIV prevention and harm reduction programs should integrate ATS users.

Keywords: HIV, People who use drugs, People who inject drugs, PWID, Non-PWID, ATS users, Cambodia

Background

Over the past 25 years, remarkable progress has been made in the fight against HIV in Cambodia. The HIV prevalence has fallen from 2.0% (1999) to 0.6% (2015) among the general population aged 15–49 years [1]. However, a high prevalence is still observed among key populations, such as female sex workers (14.0 to 15.0%) [2, 3] and men who have sex with men (2.3%) [4].

Since 2004, evidence has indicated an increase in the number of people who use drugs (PWUD) and the availability of illicit drugs in Cambodia. The country has changed from a drug trafficking transit location to a site of drug production and use [5, 6]. The country has been affected by illicit drug abuse problems, mainly amphetamine-type stimulant (ATS) use. Notable increases have been observed among youth and sex workers. A study among youth out of school in 2010 showed that approximately 4% of young women and 15% of young men aged 10 to 24 years reported ever having used drugs [7].

---

* Correspondence: hsopheab@niph.org.kh
[1]School of Public Health at the National Institute of Public Health, Lot #80, Samdech Penn Nouth Blvd. Tuol Kork District, Phnom Penh, Cambodia
Full list of author information is available at the end of the article

PWUDs, especially people who inject drugs (PWIDs) who share syringes and needles with multiple partners or have unprotected sex contribute considerably to a higher HIV prevalence. Non-injecting drug users are at a higher risk of experiencing physical and mental health problems [8] and poly-substance abuse disorder. They also may become injecting drug users with an increased risk of HIV infection [9–11]. The 2012 estimate of the size of this key population, conducted by the National Center for HIV/ AIDS, Dermatology and STIs (NCHADS), suggested that there were approximately 28,000 PWUDs in Cambodia; half of them were ATS users, and close to 7% reported injecting heroin [12].

In Asia, the HIV prevalence among PWIDs varies from country to country and within countries. For example, the HIV prevalence among PWIDs was 36.4% in Indonesia (2011), 25.2% in Thailand, 16.6% in Malaysia, 10.5% in Vietnam, and 6.4% in China [13, 14]. Factors that may account for this variability between countries include the intensity of harm reduction programs, overlapping risk behaviors (e.g. interaction with paid sex, and having multiple sex partners) and drug injection and social and sexual networking [15, 16].

In the past, studies have indicated that factors associated with the HIV prevalence among PWIDs include socio-demographic characteristics (e.g., sex, older age, marital status, less education), risky sexual behaviors (e.g., paid sex, sex exchanged for drugs) and risky behaviors during drug use (e.g., needle and syringe sharing, using injected drugs for more than one year) [14, 17, 18].

In Cambodia, there have been a few studies on drug use policy and harm reduction intervention programs, such as needle and syringe distribution programs [19, 20]. For example, Chheng et al indicated that in 2003, the Government of Cambodia acknowledged the importance and necessity of harm reduction approaches to prevent HIV transmission among PWUDs and their sexual partners. However, the harm reduction intervention was never fully implemented due to limited awareness and support from law enforcement at the local level as well as budgeting commitment [19]. The failure of this policy indeed had a negative impact on HIV prevention and harm reduction for the highest-risk groups, such as PWUDs.

Little is known about the characteristics and patterns of drug use in Cambodia. Moreover, the HIV prevalence among this key population has never been estimated nationwide. Therefore, this paper, which used data from a study conducted in late 2012–2013 [12], sought to estimate the prevalence of HIV infection among people who inject drugs (PWIDs) and drug users who do not inject drugs (non-PWIDs), and examine factors associated with HIV infection in these populations.

Methods
Study sites and population
Nine provinces were purposively selected for the study: Phnom Penh, Sihanoukville, Kampong Speu, Battambang, Banteay Meanchey, Siem Reap, Kampong Cham, Prey Veng, and Svay Rieng. These provinces were selected based on a program report indicating that they accounted for 85% of all PWUDs in Cambodia and that drug abuse activity in these provinces was significantly high *(Consultative Technical Working Group on Drug and HIVAIDS, 2012)*. Study participants were individuals at least 15 years old who reported using any illicit drug, including heroin, cocaine, opiates, amphetamines, methamphetamines, yama, ice, crystal and ketamine, in the past 12 months.

In the analysis, the 9 provinces were separated into two groups based on the HIV prevalence among PWUDs: those with an HIV prevalence ≥4% were assigned to the high-risk province group (Sihanoukville, Phnom Penh, Battambang, and Banteay Meanchey), and those with a lower prevalence were assigned to the low-risk province group (Kampong Speu, Kampong Cham, Prey Veng, Svay Rieng and Siem Reap).

Sampling and sample size
We used respondent-driven sampling (RDS), a network referral method, to recruit this hard-to-reach population (PWUDs) to ensure a representative sample [21]. At the beginning, 36 diverse seeds (4 seeds per province) were recruited through local NGOs working with drug users. They were selected based on sex (male/female) and type of drug use (injecting/non-injecting). Each seed was asked to recruit other 2 eligible PWUDs from their personal network using study coupons, with the aim of having 4 or 5 waves of recruitment to reach equilibrium [21]. In total, we approached 1662 participants. However, 36 of the 1662 (2.2%) were not eligible after the initial screening process, resulting in the final sample size of 1626.

Data collection: Risk behaviors and blood specimens
The data collection was conducted from August 2012 to April 2013. Recruitment sites in each province were selected based on the information from provincial HIV/drug programs that worked with the drug users and were aware of places commonly accessible to PWUDs. The main criterion for recruitment sites was that they provide a space to ensure the privacy and confidentiality of the participants. After oral informed consent was received from the participants, the interviews were conducted by gender-matched interviewers (e.g., male interviewers interviewed male participants) and were followed by a request for a blood sample. The interviewers used a questionnaire to collect data on socio-demographic characteristics, drug-taking behaviors, types and frequency of drug use and HIV-related risk

behaviors. The questionnaire was based on a small-scale survey of drug users in Cambodia in 2006 and on pre-testing [22]. The interviews lasted approximately 30 min.

A 5-ml blood sample was drawn and kept in a tube with an anti-coagulant to prevent the blood from clotting. At the end of each day, the blood samples were sent to a laboratory at a Voluntary Counseling and Testing Center (VCT) near the study recruitment site.

Monitoring and HIV testing and quality control
The interviewers and supervisors were selected from among those who had experience working with these key populations. Both the interviewers and supervisors were trained for 3 days in Phnom Penh on the recruitment process, informed consent procedures and the questionnaire-based interview procedure. The supervisors were responsible for ensuring that RDS sampling was properly performed, the questionnaires were properly completed, and the informed consent process was strictly followed to ensure that the participants could refuse or withdraw from the study at any time.

At VCT, HIV testing was performed using 2 rapid tests. First, blood samples were tested with Determine HIV 1/2 (*Alere HIV*). Specimens that were reactive in the first test were retested with HIV 1/2 Stat-Pak (*Chembio Diagnostic System, Inc*). This standard serial testing algorithm has been used by the national HSS for groups that have an HIV prevalence greater than 10% [2]. Then, the sera were prepared and stored before being sent to the NCHADS laboratory for quality control and storage.

All HIV-positive specimens plus a randomly selected 10% of negative specimens were tested for quality control. Serial testing was performed by the NCHADS laboratory using two ELISA tests (*Vironostika, BioMérieu; and Murex 1.2.0, Murex DiaSorin Biotech*). The Vironostika test was used first. If the result was non-reactive, the test was considered HIV negative. If the Vironostika test was reactive, the results were confirmed via the Murex test.

Statistical analysis
HIV prevalence estimates were calculated using the RDS analysis tool RDSAT 7.1 [23]. RDSAT was developed to minimize biases associated with the social network referral process by weighting the respondents' probability of being recruited into the RDS sample and recruitment patterns [21]. Individual weights generated with RDSAT for HIV status were imported into STATA to adjust for the RDS sampling process [24]. Weighted bivariable analysis and multivariate logistic regression (SVY) were used to identify factors associated with HIV prevalence. Potential confounding factors, regardless their significant level, and factors that were associated with HIV infection in the bivariable analysis at $p < 0.20$ [25] were

included in the multivariate logistic regression; the included factors were sex, age group, provincial region, marital status, education level, drug use type, number of paid sex partners, and duration of drug use.

Results
Demographic characteristics of PWUDs
Of the 1626 respondents, approximately 7.3% were PWIDs. Most of the PWUDs were men (82.0%), while women represented approximately 18.0%. The median age of the PWIDs was 28.0 years, with an interquartile range (IQR) of 24–32 years; the median age for the non-PWIDs was 24.0 years (IQR: 20–29 years). For both groups, the women were approximately 2–3 years older, and the PWIDs tended to be slightly older than the non-PWIDs (Table 1). Approximately half of the participants were un-married (i.e., single, widowed, or divorced). The median number of years of schooling was 6.0 (IQR: 3–8 years) for the PWIDs and 7.0 (IQR: 5–9 years) for the non-PWIDs. More than 40% of the PWIDs reported either living with their parents or spouse, while close to 75% of the non-PWIDs reported similar living arrangements. The PWID group was more likely to live with friends (15.3% vs. 7.8%).

Drug use behavior among PWUDs
The median duration of drug use for the PWIDs was 10.0 years (IQR: 5–13 years), compared with 4.0 years (IQR: 1–7 years) for the non-PWIDs (Table 2). Less than 20% of the PWIDs first started using drugs by injection; the rest mainly began by smoking and sniffing drugs. Both groups (91%) reported first starting drug use with friends and peers. Frequently, they were first introduced to drugs by their friends (85.9%), followed by self-initiation (8.5 and 6.6% for PWIDs and non-PWIDs, respectively). The drugs that the PWIDs most commonly reported using in the past 12 months were ice/amphetamine (78.0%) and heroin (61.9%), while the non-PWIDs reported using ice/amphetamine (81.5%) and yama (47.1%), a pill containing methamphetamine. Moreover, close to 60 and 38% of the PWIDs and non-PWIDs, respectively, reported having used at least 2 drugs in the past 12 months. In addition, 35.6% the PWIDs reported having shared needles and syringes in the past month.

Sexual behavior among PWUDs
More PWIDs (94.1%) had had sex in their lifetimes than non-PWIDs (89.7%). The women in both groups reported more sexual activity than the men (Table 3). Among those who had ever had sex in their lifetime, approximately three-quarters of both groups reported "being paid and paying for sex" in the past month. The women reported a higher proportion of paid sex

Table 1 Socio-demographic characteristics of PWUD

Variables	PWID = 119						Non PWID = 1507					
	Men		Women		Total		Men		Women		Total	
	Freq.	%	Freq.	%	Freq.	%	Freq.	%	Freq.	%	Freq.	%
Regional provinces[a]												
Low risk provinces	23	22.3	2	12.5	25	21.0	745	61.9	73	26.8	818	55.4
High risk provinces	80	77.7	14	87.5	94	**79.0**	459	38.1	199	73.2	658	**44.6**
Age, median (IQR)[b], years	28 (24–31)		30 (26–34)		28 (24–32)		23 (20–28)		27 (22–31)		24 (20–29)	
Age groups												
≤ 20 years old	12	12.1	1	6.3	13	**11.3**	351	29.6	46	17.2	397	**27.3**
21–29 years old	50	50.5	6	37.5	56	**48.7**	594	50.1	138	51.7	732	**50.4**
≥ 30 years old	37	37.4	9	59.2	46	40.0	240	20.3	83	31.1	323	22.3
Marital status												
Married	48	47.1	14	87.5	62	52.5	472	39.5	225	83.0	697	47.5
Non-married	54	52.9	2	12.5	56	47.5	723	60.5	46	17.0	769	52.5
Education, median (IQR), years	7 (3–9)		3 (1–6)		6 (3–8)		8 (6–10)		4 (0–7)		7 (5–9)	
Education level												
0–6 years in school	49	50.0	3	18.7	62	54.4	745	65.3	71	26.8	591	42.0
≥ 7 years in school	49	50.0	13	81.3	52	45.6	397	34.7	194	73.2	816	58.0
Report current living places												
Parent	36	35.3	1	6.2	36	**30.5**	708	59.3	42	15.5	763	**51.0**
Spouse	15	14.7	4	25.0	19	16.0	272	22.8	56	20.7	332	22.2
Friend	15	14.7	4	25.0	18	15.3	60	5.0	54	19.9	117	7.8
Street	5	4.9	0	0.0	5	4.3	15	1.3	20	7.4	38	2.5
Others	31	30.4	7	43.8	40	33.9	139	11.4	99	36.5	245	16.5

[a]High risk provinces: Sihanoukville, Phnom Penh, Battambang, Banteay Meanchey
Low risk provinces: Kampong Speu, Kampong Cham, Prey Veng, Svay Rieng, Siem Reap
[b]*IQR* interquartile range

than the men among both the PWIDs (85.8%) and the non-PWIDs (89.4%). However, reports of always using condoms during paid sex did not exceed 50% among the PWIDs but were greater than 60% among non-PWIDs. Condom use among the women in the PWID group was as low as 25%. In addition, reports of condom use with regular partners (spouses, intimate partners, cohabiting partners) was as low as ≤30% in both groups.

HIV prevalence among PWUDs

As shown in Table 4, the overall HIV prevalence among PWUDs was 5.1% [95% CI: 4.1–6.2]. The HIV prevalence among PWIDs was 24.8% [95% CI: 7.3–39.9]; among non-PWIDs, it was 4.0% [95% CI: 2.7–5.5]. The HIV prevalence among female PWIDs (37.5, 95% CI: 10.9–64.1) was higher than that among male PWIDs (22.5%, 95 CI: 14.0–30.9). A similar pattern was found among female non-PWIDs (11.5, 95% CI: 7.9–15.7) and male non-PWIDs (1.5, 95% CI: 0.8–2.2).

Factors associated with HIV infection in the logistic regression

The details of the bivariate analysis are presented in Table 5. The following factors were significantly associated with HIV: higher-risk province group [odds ratio (OR) = 5.2, 95% CI: 2.6–10.5] (with the lower-risk province group used as the referent group); female (males as the reference) (OR = 5.6, 95% CI: 3.0–10.6); and older age groups (aged ≤20 years as the reference) 21–29 (OR = 21.2), 30 and older (OR = 78.5). Low education level (secondary/higher education as the reference) and married PWIDs (non-married as the reference) were associated with HIV infection. The PWIDs had approximately 5 times higher odds of HIV infection than the non-PWIDs (OR = 4.6, 95% CI: 2.3–9.2). Furthermore, having had ≥2 paid sex partners in the past month and having used drugs for ≥12 months were significantly associated with HIV infection, with OR = 3.5 (95% CI: 1.6–7.5) and OR = 2.7 (95% CI: 1.3–5.6), respectively. The associations for other covariates, including reported consistent condom use with paid sex partners in the past 12 months and multiple drug use, were not statistically significant.

Table 2 Drug taking risk exposures among PWUDs

Variables	PWID = 119						Non- PWID = 1506					
	Men		Women		Total		Men		Women		Total	
	Freq.	%	Freq.	%	Freq.	%	Freq.	%	Freq.	%	Freq.	%
Duration of drug use, median (IQR)	10 (5–13)		10 (4–12)		10 (5–13)		4 (1–8)		3 (1–6)		4 (1–7)	
Duration of any drug use					n = 117						n = 1468	
Users ≤12 months	7	6.9	3	20.0	10	8.6	303	25.2	82	30.7	385	26.2
Users > 12 months	95	93.1	12	80.0	107	**91.4**	898	74.8	185	69.3	1083	**73.8**
Methods PWUDs used drugs at the first time												
Smoking	74	72.6	14	82.5	87	**73.7**	1158	96.7	254	93.7	1440	**96.1**
Sniffing/drinking	8	7.8	0	0	8	6.9	35	2.9	15	5.5	52	3.5
Injecting	20	**19.6**	2	12.5	22	**18.6**	4	0.3	2	0.7	6	0.4
Persons PWUDs used drug with at the first time												
Friends	89	87.4	13	81.3	103	**87.3**	1141	95.2	202	74.5	1370	**91.3**
Sweethearts/spouses/relatives	8	7.8	2	12.5	10	8.4	26	2.2	47	17.3	73	4.9
Alone	4	3.9	0	0.0	4	3.4	29	2.1	14	5.2	43	2.9
Others	1	0.9	1	6.2	1	0.9	3	0.3	8	3.0	15	0.9
Persons who first introduced you to use drugs												
Friends	85	83.3	12	75.0	98	**83.0**	1079	90.0	189	69.7	1292	**86.1**
Myself	8	7.8	2	12.5	10	**8.5**	73	6.1	22	8.1	99	**6.5**
Sweethearts/spouses/relatives	8	7.8	2	12.5	10	8.5	44	3.7	49	18.1	76	5.1
Others	1	1.0	0	0.0	0	0.0	3	0.2	11	4.1	34	2.3
Types of illicit drug used in the past 12 months												
Ice/amphetamine	79	77.5	14	87.5	92	**78.0**	998	82.9	203	74.6	1228	**81.5**
Yama (pill of methamphetamine)	30	29.4	7	43.8	37	**31.4**	557	46.3	148	54.4	710	**47.1**
Marijuana	16	15.7	1	6.3	17	14.4	140	11.6	13	4.8	153	10.2
Heroin	59	57.8	12	75.0	73	**61.9**	33	2.7	9	3.3	42	2.8
Ecstasy	4	3.9	3	18.8	7	5.9	54	4.5	26	9.6	80	5.3
Others (including inhalant)	13	8.1	1	1.5	19	16.1	149	12.4	17	6.3	136	5.3
Reported uses at least 2 drugs in past 12 months	58	56.8	12	75.0	70	59.3	455	37.9	107	39.4	562	38.1
Last injecting drugs with re-used syringes and needles (n = 119)	–	–	–	–	38	31.9	–	–	–	–	–	–
Reported sharing needles and syringes when injecting drugs in past month (n = 59)	–	–	–	–	21	35.6	–	–	–	–	–	–

In the final multivariable model, 4 factors were found to be independently associated with HIV infection: sex (women), older age groups, injected drug use and duration of drug use ≥12 months (Table 5). Women had higher odds of HIV infection than men, with an adjusted OR (AOR = 7.8, 95% CI: 3.0–20.4), and participants older than 20 years had a higher odds of HIV infection: age groups 21–29 (AOR = 10.3, 95% CI: 1.2–20.4) and age group ≥30 (AOR = 36.4, 95% CI: 3.6–369.4). Injected drug use remained a strong predictor of HIV infection, with AOR = 4.1 (95% CI: 1.5–10.9). Additionally, the longer a PWUD had used drugs, the higher their odds of HIV infection, with AOR = 4.0 (95% CI: 1.4–11.4).

Discussion

This study reported a high prevalence of HIV among PWIDs and a large proportion of non-PWIDs, especially ATS users. Most of the PWUDs were sexually active, and they indicated a high proportion of paid sex and low consistent condom use, especially among PWIDs. The main predictors of HIV infection included female sex, injected drug use, older age and drug use for ≥12 months.

In our study, the HIV prevalence among PWIDs was approximately 25%, which is similar to the prevalence levels for Cambodia reported a few years ago by Mathers et al., who reviewed and estimated the global HIV prevalence among drug users and the size of the

Table 3 Sexual risk exposures to HIV among PWUDs

Variables	PWID = 113						Non- PWID = 1335					
	Men		Women		Total		Men		Women		Total	
	Freq.	%	Freq.	%	Freq.	%	Freq.	%	Freq.	%	Freq.	%
Report of ever had sex	96	93.2	16	100.0	112	94.1	1063	88.6	256	94.5	1319	89.7
Age at first sex, median (IQR), years	17.5 (17–18)		18 (16–20)		18 (17–20)		18 (17–20)		18 (16–19)		18 (16–19)	
Age at first sex in years												
≤ 18 years old	73	76.0	10	62.5	83	**74.1**	557	52.5	166	64.6	723	**54.9**
> 18 years old	23	24.0	6	37.5	29	**25.9**	504	47.5	91	35.4	595	**45.1**
Ever had sex in the past month among those who ever reported sex	53	56.4	7	43.4	60	54.6	713	67.5	206	80.2	919	70.0
Report number of paid and paying sex partner in the past month					*n* = **99**						*n* = **1181**	
No sex partner	73	**79.3**	1	**14.2**	74	**74.8**	854	**82.1**	15	**10.6**	869	**73.6**
≤ 2 sex partners	11	12.0	3	42.8	14	14.1	141	13.6	45	31.9	186	15.8
≥ 3 sex partners	8	8.7	3	42.8	11	11.1	35	4.3	81	57.5	126	10.6
Always condom use with paid and paying sex partners in the past 12 months	44	43.1	4	25.0	48	**40.6**	746	62.1	165	60.7	911	**61.8**
Condom use in last sex in exchange for money	52	86.7	6	85.7	58	86.6	683	88.4	136	88.9	819	88.4
Always condom use with regular partners in the past 12 months	17	30.4	4	30.8	21	30.4	191	25.3	36	17.2	227	23.6
Condom use last time when had sex with regular partner	29	46	8	61.4	37	49	409	50.7	96	43.1	505	49.1

HIV-infected drug user population and injecting drug user population by country [26].

Despite the lower prevalence of HIV (4%) among non-PWIDs, the large non-PWUDs population (90%) remains a public health and a matter of social concern for several reasons. First, recent reports may indicate shifting patterns of HIV infection in Cambodia from non-PWIDs to PWIDs. Our findings indicated that less than 20% of PWIDs initially injected drugs. Additionally, a report from the KHANA Drop-In Center (DiC) showed that less than 5% of PWUDs who visited the center were originally injected drug users. However, in one year of the DiC implementation, approximately 3% of its visitors converted from non-PWIDs to PWIDs *(Personal communication with DiC)*.Therefore, these raise a concern what prompts PWUDs to become PWIDs and the possibility that that HIV transmission among non-PWIDs in Cambodia could increase in the future due to their related risk behaviors and the overlapping social and sexual networks among PWUDs [16, 27]. Additionally, the high proportion of transactional sex among female PWIDs in this study, particularly among non-PWID women, indicates the possibility that infection could be transmitted to non-injected drug users and then to the general population through transactional sex. Consequently, these factors potentially contribute to an increase in overall HIV prevalence in Cambodia. Therefore, it is important for HIV and drug use intervention programs to significantly target these high-risk groups.

Needle and syringe sharing among PWIDs remains high, and implements are often shared with little or no cleaning. Given that sterile needle and syringes programs (NSPs) are a key component of harm reduction and HIV prevention efforts [15, 28–30], more targeted interventions for PWIDs should be implemented continuously, without law enforcement barriers, to ensure access to adequate supplies of clean needles and syringes. Prior studies estimated that interventions (i.e., opioid substitution, needle exchange and antiretroviral therapy) that attain at least 60% coverage could cut future infections among PWIDs roughly in half, thereby decreasing the HIV epidemic among PWIDs [28]. However, the program report suggested that NSPs had very low coverage - only 16% of PWIDs reported accessing NGO drop in centers in the past 12 months [31]. Further research should include NSP assessments to improve program interventions. Additionally, the large proportion of

Table 4 HIV prevalence among PWUDs

PWID			Non-PWID		
Men	Women	Total	Men	Women	Total
% (95% CI)	% (95% CI)	% (95% CI)	% (95% CI)	% (95% CI)	% (95% CI)
22.5 (14.0–30.9)	37.5 (10.9–64.1)	24.8 (7.3–39.9)	1.5 (0.8–2.2)	11.5 (7.9–15.7)	4.0 (2.7–5.5)

Table 5 Risk factors associated with HIV in bivariate and multivariable logistic regression among drug users

Variables	N = 1583		Total sample (N = 1186)	
	OR (95% CI)	P value[b]	AOR[a] (95% CI)	P value[b]
Provincial group[a]				
Low risk provinces	Referent		Referent	
High risk provinces	5.2 (2.59–10.56)	< 0.001	1.9 (0.78–4.79)	0.154
Sex of drug users				
Men	Referent		Referent	
Women	5.6 (2.95–10.59)	< 0.001	7.8 (3.00–20.35)	**< 0.001**
Age group in years				
≤ 20	Referent		Referent	
21–29	21.2 (2.73–164.16)	0.003	10.3 (1.20–89.39)	**0.033**
≥ 30	78.5 (10.53–584. 18)	< 0.001	36.4 (3.59–369.36)	**0.002**
Marital status				
Non-married	Referent		Referent	
Married	2.9 (1.37–6.01)	0.005	0.48 (0.17–1.47)	0.205
Education level				
≤ 6 years (Primary)	2.4 (1.22–4.68)	0.011	0.92 (0.37–2.27)	0.866
> 6 years (Secondary and higher)	Referent		Referent	
Drug use type				
Non-PWID	Referent		Referent	
PWID	4.6 (2.31–9.19)	< 0.001	4.1 (1.53–10.96)	**0.005**
Number of paid and paying sex partners In past month				
< 2 partners	Referent		Referent	
≥ 2 partners	3.5 (1.64–7.48)	0.001	1.1 (0.42–2.47)	0.961
Duration of using drugs				
≤ 12 months	Referent		Referent	
> 12 months	2.7 (1.27–5.63)	0.010	4.0 (1.38–11.35)	**0.010**
Consistent condom use with casual partner in the past 12 months				
Yes	Referent			
No	1.1 (0.59–2.10)	0.735	–	–
More than one drug use in past 12 months				
One drug	Referent			
More than one drug	1.1 (0.59–2.10)	0.735	–	–

[a]High risk provinces: Sihanoukville, Phnom Penh, Battambang, Banteay Meanchey
[b]The results in this table were weighted
Low risk provinces: Kampong Speu, Kampong Cham, Prey Veng, Svay Rieng, Siem Reap

non-PWIDs, especially ATS users, is worrisome and very challenging for prevention efforts since effective prevention strategies for ATS use has little evidence base. A study of an integrated HIV and drug prevention program with conditional cash transfer was conducted in Cambodia to test the use of behavioral interventions among ATS users for improved prevention measures for this group; the results have not been published [32]. However, another formative research among study by *Carrico* et al. to reduce the risk of ATS among entertainment workers using the conditional cash transfer with behavioral intervention found the mixing results [33].

The findings of a higher risk of HIV among women who use drugs are consistent with the literature, which highlights issues associated with increased vulnerability for women (e.g., child care, concomitant sex work, lack of access to health care, mental and physical health problems, reproductive health issues, sexually transmitted infections, stigma, and violence) [8, 30]. Beyond these issues, female PWUDs with overlapping risk behaviors, such as transactional sex and drug use, often have less power to negotiate safe sex practices [8, 17, 34]. According to Azim et al., female PWUDs who were sex workers were more likely than non-drug using sex workers to engage in street-based sex work, which is associated with high-risk sex and heightened levels of violence due to different types of partners [30].

Given the high HIV prevalence among drug users with a high frequency of paid sex partners, focused intervention to assist this sub-group is an important public health goal in Cambodia. Evidence in prior studies suggests that female PWIDs who are sex workers constitute a "bridge population" [35] that can lead to a the spread of HIV epidemics from PWIDs to heterosexual populations [30, 36].

Multiple structural and behavioral interventions specifically designed for female PWUDs have been implemented globally with tailor-made interventions adapted to women's specific needs [30]. For example, a study investigating the effectiveness of HIV/STI safer sex skill-building groups for women found that these groups improved safer sex practices compared with standard HIV/STI education [37]. However, many women still struggle alone to change risky behaviors with their partners, and in these situations, it may be more effective to engage couples in harm reduction interventions [30]. Also, access to legal and heath care supports should be addressed in the multiple structural interventions.

Comprehensive interventions that address individual and socio-environmental factors are more effective than a single intervention alone [29]. Such interventions need to include many of the interventions outlined above and should also outline steps for improving understanding and sensitivity among professionals who interact with PWUDs (e.g., health care workers or NGO staff) [30]. This is particularly the case with law enforcement. As a recent study surmised, "Fear of accessing harm reduction and health services and police's negative attitudes and practices towards key populations present major barriers to HIV prevention efforts in Cambodia" [19, 38]. Efforts to reduce the fear of retaliation and/or stigma may help improve the effectiveness of broader intervention programs.

This study has several limitations. First, self-reports of sensitive information (i.e., drug use and risky sexual behaviors) and social desirability may result in the under-reporting of actual information. Second, the lifetime and 12-month recalls used in some questions may have caused recall issues. Third, although RDS was used to recruit a representative sample, we are not sure how well the seeds were represented and referred or how many PWUDs did not participate in the study (mostly PWIDs, due to self-stigma or discrimination), and we do not know the different characteristics and HIV-related risk behaviors of those who did not participate in the study. Given these factors, we may have underestimated

the HIV prevalence among PWIDs - especially female PWIDs, given the small samples - and weakened the association between the predictors and the HIV prevalence. Despite these limitations, this is the first ever large-scale survey conducted in Cambodia among PWUDs using the RDS method and involving many key stake- holders' involvement (NCHADS, NACD, UNAIDS, NGOs). It provides useful and informative findings to guide HIV and drug use program planning and policy for future interventions.

Conclusion

HIV prevalence among PWUDs remains high especially among PWIDs and women. Harm reduction programs, such as NSP, must be improved in scope and scale. Innovative strategies are needed to reach sub-groups of PWUDs, especially women who inject drugs. Furthermore, the large proportion of non-PWIDs, especially ATS users, should not be ignored; combined HIV prevention and harm reduction programs should integrate ATS users.

Abbreviations
ART: Anti-retroviral therapy;; ATS: Amphetamine-type stimulants (ATS); DiC: Drop-In Center; HSS: HIV Sentinel Surveillance; NACD: National Authority for Combating Drugs; NCHADS: National Center for HIV/AIDS, Dermatology and STIs; NSP: Needles and Syringes Program; PWIDs: People who inject drugs; PWUDs: People who use drugs; RDS: Respondent-driven sampling; VCT: HIV Voluntary Counseling and Testing Center

Acknowledgements
We would like to thank the organizations that were actively involved in the study's Technical Advisory Group (TAG): NACD, NCHADS, the National Program for Mental Health, MoEYS, MoSVY, KHANA, AusAID, UNAIDS, PSI, UNODC, Friends Int'l- Mith Samlanh, FHI 360, UNICEF and WHO. Our sincere thanks go to H.E. Meas Vyrith, Secretary General of NACD; Dr. Mean Chhi Vun (Director of NCHADS); and Dr. Oum Sopheap, KHANA Executive Director, who helped to facilitate the administrative and financial processes of the study. Special thanks to the members of the TAG, who played significant roles in the completion of this work: Mr. Kao Boumony (NACD), Dr. Mun Phalkun (NCHADS), and Dr. Suos Premprey (AusAID). We would also like to thank the GF and AusAID for the financial support through NCHADS and KHANA, respectively.

Funding
The study was supported by the Global Fund through the National Center for HIV/AIDS, Dermatology and STIs (NCHADS) and AusAID through KHANA.

Authors' contributions
HS, CC and ST conceived and designed the study. JM contributed the conceptual ideas and drafted the paper and proofreading. HS wrote the first draft of the paper, and the other coauthors contributed to the final manuscript. HS and CC were responsible for conducting the study and managing the data. HS and CC conducted the statistical analyses and the interpretation of data. All authors read and approved the final manuscript.

Competing interests
We declare that we have no competing interests.

Author details
[1]School of Public Health at the National Institute of Public Health, Lot #80, Samdech Penn Nouth Blvd. Tuol Kork District, Phnom Penh, Cambodia. [2]Center for Population and Health Research, KHANA, Phnom Penh, Cambodia. [3]Department of Epidemiology, University of Washington, Seattle, USA.

References

1. Chhea C, Saphonn V. Report on Estimation and Projections on HIV/AIDS in Cambodia 2010–2015. National Center for HIV/AIDS, Dermatology and STD: Phnom Penh; 2011.
2. Chhea C: HIV Sentinel Surveys 2010: Female Entertainment Workers (FEWs) and Antenatal Care Cinic (ANC) Attendees; Accessd on Febraury 20, 2016 at http://www.nchads.org/Publication/HSS/HSS_2010%20Report.pdf. In. Phnom Penh: National Center for HIV/AIDS, Dermatology and STIs (NCHADS); 2012.
3. Couture MC, Page K, Stein ES, Sansothy N, Sichan K, Kaldor J, Evans JL, Maher L, Palefsky J. Cervical human papillomavirus infection among young women engaged in sex work in Phnom Penh, Cambodia: prevalence, genotypes, risk factors and association with HIV infection. BMC Infect Dis. 2012;12:166.
4. NCHADS: National HIV Sero-Surveillance among ANC and MSM 2014, acceed date on October 02, 2017 at http://www.nchads.org/index.php?id=16. In. Phnom Penh: National Center for HIVAIDS, Dermatology and STIs 2014.
5. NACD: Official report (in Khmer) of the National Achievement of drug control in 2015 and Workplan 2016, National Authority for combating drug (NACD). Accessed on on December 2016 at http://www.nacd.gov.kh/images/nacd/Reports/annual/report_2015.pdf. In. Phnom Penh: NACD; 2016.
6. Klein A, Saphonn V, Reid S. Reaching out and reaching up - developing a low cost drug treatment system in Cambodia. Harm Reduct J. 2012;9:11.
7. MoEYS: Most at risk young people survey 2010. In. Phnom Penh: Ministry of Education, Youth and Sports; 2010.
8. Maher L, Phlong P, Mooney-Somers J, Keo S, Stein E, Couture MC, Page K. Amphetamine-type stimulant use and HIV/STI risk behaviour among young female sex workers in Phnom Penh, Cambodia. Int J Drug Policy. 2011;22(3): 203–9.
9. Degenhardt L, Mathers B, Guarinieri M, Panda S, Phillips B, Strathdee SA, Tyndall M, Wiessing L, Wodak A, Howard J. Meth/amphetamine use and associated HIV: implications for global policy and public health. Int J Drug Policy. 2010;21(5):347–58.
10. Colfax G, Santos GM, Chu P, Vittinghoff E, Pluddemann A, Kumar S, Hart C. Amphetamine-group substances and HIV. Lancet. 2010;376(9739):458–74.
11. Singh D, Chawarski MC, Schottenfeld R, Vicknasingam B. Substance abuse and the HIV situation in Malaysia. J Food Drug Anal. 2013;21(4):S46–51.
12. Chhea C, Sopheab H, Tuot S. National Population Size Estimation, HIV Related Risk Behaviors and HIV Prevalence among People Who Use Drugs in Cambodia in 2012. Phnom Penh: NACD, NCHADS, KHANA; 2014.
13. HIV and AIDS data hub for Asia-Pacific: Estimated size and HIV prevalence among people who inject drugs in Asia-Pacific; accessed on Jan 27, 2016 at http://www.aidsdatahub.org/people-who-inject-drugs-november-2015-slides
14. Li L, Assanangkornchai S, Duo L, McNeil E, Li J. Risk behaviors, prevalence of HIV and hepatitis C virus infection and population size of current injection drug users in a China-Myanmar border city: results from a respondent-driven sampling survey in 2012. PLoS One. 2014;9(9):e106899.
15. Mathers BM, Degenhardt L, Ali H, Wiessing L, Hickman M, Mattick RP, Myers B, Ambekar A, Strathdee SA. HIV prevention, treatment, and care services for people who inject drugs: a systematic review of global, regional, and national coverage. Lancet. 2010;375(9719):1014–28.
16. Strathdee SA, Stockman JK. Epidemiology of HIV among injecting and non-injecting drug users: current trends and implications for interventions. Curr HIV/AIDS Rep. 2010;7(2):99–106.
17. Taran YS, Johnston LG, Pohorila NB, Saliuk TO. Correlates of HIV risk among injecting drug users in sixteen Ukrainian cities. AIDS Behav. 2011;15(1):65–74.
18. Medhi GK, Mahanta J, Paranjape RS, Adhikary R, Laskar N, Ngully P. Factors associated with HIV among female sex workers in a high HIV prevalent state of India. AIDS Care. 2012;24(3):369–76.
19. Chheng K, Leang S, Thomson N, Moore T, Crofts N. Harm reduction in Cambodia: a disconnect between policy and practice. Harm Reduct J. 2012; 9(1):30.
20. Thomson N, Leang S, Chheng K, Weissman A, Shaw G, Crofts N. The village/commune safety policy and HIV prevention efforts among key affected populations in Cambodia: finding a balance. Harm Reduct J. 2012;9:31.
21. Heckathorn D. Respondent-driven sampling: a new approach to the study of hidden populations. Social Problem. 1997.
22. Chhea C, Seguy N: HIV prevalence among drug users in Cambodia 2007; accessed on Febraury 20, 2016 at www.nchads.org. In. Phnom Penh: NCHADS, NACD; 2010.
23. Volz E, Wejnert C, Degani I, Heckathorn DD. Respondent-driven sampling analysis tool (RDSAT) version 7.1. Ithaca, NY: Cornell University; 2007. p. 2012.
24. Matthew S, Heckathorn D. Sampling and estimation in hidden populations using respondent-driven sampling. Sociol Methodol. 2004.
25. Hosmer D, Lemeshow S. Applied logistic regression. 2nd ed. New York: John Wiley & Sons Inc; 2000.
26. Mathers BM, Degenhardt L, Phillips B, Wiessing L, Hickman M, Strathdee SA, Wodak A, Panda S, Tyndall M, Toufik A, et al. Global epidemiology of injecting drug use and HIV among people who inject drugs: a systematic review. Lancet. 2008;372(9651):1733–45.
27. Des Jarlais DC, Arasteh K, Perlis T, Hagan H, Abdul-Quader A, Heckathorn DD, McKnight C, Bramson H, Nemeth C, Torian LV, et al. Convergence of HIV seroprevalence among injecting and non-injecting drug users in new York City. AIDS. 2007;21(2):231–5.
28. Strathdee SA, Hallett TB, Bobrova N, Rhodes T, Booth R, Abdool R, Hankins CA. HIV and risk environment for injecting drug users: the past, present, and future. Lancet. 2010;376(9737):268–84.
29. Degenhardt L, Mathers B, Vickerman P, Rhodes T, Latkin C, Hickman M. Prevention of HIV infection for people who inject drugs: why individual, structural, and combination approaches are needed. Lancet. 2010;376(9737): 285–301.
30. Azim T, Bontell I, Strathdee SA. Women, drugs and HIV. Int J Drug Policy. 2015;26(Suppl 1):S16–21.
31. Sopheab H, Tuot S. End Project Evaluation: Changes in HIV Integrated, Prevention, Care and Impact Mitigation Efforts from 2009–2001. KHANA: Phnom Penh, Cambodia; 2012.
32. Page K, Stein ES, Carrico AW, Evans JL, Sokunny M, Nil E, Ngak S, Sophal C, McCulloch C, Maher L. Protocol of a cluster randomised stepped-wedge trial of behavioural interventions targeting amphetamine-type stimulant use and sexual risk among female entertainment and sex workers in Cambodia. BMJ Open. 2016;6(5):e010854.
33. Carrico AW, Nil E, Sophal C, Stein E, Sokunny M, Yuthea N, Evans JL, Ngak S, Maher L, Page K. Behavioral interventions for Cambodian female entertainment and sex workers who use amphetamine-type stimulants. J Behav Med. 2016;39(3):502–10.
34. Bouscaillou J, Evanno J, Proute M, Inwoley A, Kabran M, N'Guessan T, Dje-Bi S, Sidibe S, Thiam-Niangoin M, N'Guessan BR, et al. Prevalence and risk factors associated with HIV and tuberculosis in people who use drugs in Abidjan, Ivory Coast. Int J Drug Policy. 2016;30:116–23.
35. Liu H, Grusky O, Li X, Ma E. Drug users: a potentially important bridge population in the transmission of sexually transmitted diseases, including AIDS, in China. Sexually transmitted diseases. 2006;33(2):111–7.
36. Des Jarlais DC, Feelemyer JP, Modi SN, Arasteh K, Mathers BM, Degenhardt L, Hagan H. Transitions from injection-drug-use-concentrated to self-sustaining heterosexual HIV epidemics: patterns in the international data. PLoS One. 2012;7(3):e31227.
37. Tross S, Campbell AN, Cohen LR, Calsyn D, Pavlicova M, Miele GM, Hu MC, Haynes L, Nugent N, Gan W, et al. Effectiveness of HIV/STD sexual risk reduction groups for women in substance abuse treatment programs: results of NIDA clinical trials network trial. J Acquir Immune Defic Syndr. 2008;48(5):581–9.
38. Schneiders ML, Weissman A. Determining barriers to creating an enabling environment in Cambodia: results from a baseline study with key populations and police. J Int AIDS Soc. 2016;19(4 Suppl 3):20878.

23

Interferon-γ release assay as a sensitive diagnostic tool of latent tuberculosis infection in patients with HIV: a cross-sectional study

Giselle Burlamaqui Klautau[1,3*], Nadijane Valéria Ferreira da Mota[4], Mauro José Costa Salles[1*] ⓘ, Marcelo Nascimento Burattini[4] and Denise Silva Rodrigues[2,4]

Abstract

Background: In developing countries, tuberculosis (TB) is a major public health problem and the leading cause of death among patients with HIV (Human Immunodeficiency Virus). Until 2001, the tuberculin skin test (TST) was the only available tool for the diagnosis of latent tuberculosis infection (LTBI), but false-negative TST results are frequently reported. Recently, the interferon-γ (IFN-γ) release assay (IGRA) has gained ground because it can detect the IFN-γ secreted by circulating lymphocytes T cells when stimulated by specific TB antigens. However, the role of IGRA in the diagnosis of LTBI in HIV-infected patients has not been well established.

Methods: This cross-sectional study compared the accuracy of TST (performed by the Mantoux method) and IGRA (QuantiFERON-TB Gold In-Tube, Cellestis, Carnegie, Australia) on the diagnosis of LTBI among patients with HIV. LTBI is defined by LTBI risk and at least one positive test (TST or IGRA), without clinical evidence of active TB. We also assessed the accuracy of TST and IGRA among HIV patients with high and low risk for LTBI.

Results: Among 90 HIV patients, 80 met the study criteria for LTBI, fifty-nine (73.7%) patients were TST positive, 21 (26.2%) were negative, whereas 75 patients (93.7%) were IGRA positive, and five (6.2%) were negative. TST showed poor agreement with the diagnosis of LTBI (Kappa: 0.384), while IGRA demonstrated good agreement (Kappa: 0.769). Among 69 patients with high risk and 21 with low risk for LTBI, TST was positive in 48 (69.5%) and 11 (52.4%), while IGRA was positive in 68 (98.5%) and 7 (33.3%) patients, respectively. There were no association between TST and the level of risk ($P = 0,191$). Conversely, we observed a strong association between the IGRA and risk for LTBI ($p < 0.001$).

Conclusions: Compared to TST, IGRA positivity is consistent with the risk of TB infection and seems to be a better diagnostic tool for LTBI in HIV-infected patients.

Keywords: HIV, Latent tuberculosis infection, Tuberculin skin testing, Interferon-γ release assay, AIDS

Background

One-quarter of the world population is estimated to be infected with *Mycobacterium tuberculosis*, while 10.0 million cases of TB occurred worldwide in 2017 [1–3]. The best estimate is that there were 1.3 million TB deaths in 2017, with an additional 300.000 deaths resulting from TB disease among the population living with HIV [3]. TB is a major public health problem in Brazil and the leading cause of death in patients with AIDS and one of the most common opportunistic infections [4, 5]. Moreover, recently published data collected in the city of São Paulo found that among 78.6% of patients diagnosed with tuberculosis who underwent HIV testing, 9.9% were coinfected [6].

A significant number of active TB cases arise in people with LTBI within a period of 2–5 years following primary infection [7]. Between 5 and 15% of

* Correspondence: gisellebk@hotmail.com; salles.infecto@gmail.com
[1]Division of Infectious Diseases, Department of Internal Medicine Santa Casa de São Paulo School of Medical Sciences, Hospital da Irmandade da Santa Casa de Misericórdia de São Paulo, Rua Dr Cesáreo Mota Jr 112,, São Paulo, SP CEP: 01303-060, Brazil
Full list of author information is available at the end of the article

individuals with LTBI progress to active TB, and the risk of active TB increases with poor immunity, reaching 30% among individuals infected with HIV [3, 8, 9].

The available tests for the diagnosis of latent TB infection (LTBI) have limitations that pose great challenges for both the diagnosis and the treatment of these patients [10, 11]. Indeed, the diagnosis of LTBI is a worldwide problem due to the lack of a gold standard. In countries with a high incidence of tuberculosis, including Brazil, the diagnosis of LTBI has been based upon a positive TST test in individuals in whom TB disease has been ruled out [4, 5]. The TST is an easy and low-cost test to apply, although, its specificity may be affected by previous BCG (Bacillus Calmette-Guérin) vaccination or even by infection with nontuberculous mycobacteria [12]. In addition, false-negative TST results can be observed in anergic or immunodeficient patients, including individuals with AIDS [13].

Over the last years, IGRA has gained ground as an alternative to the TST because it can detect the IFN-γ secreted by circulating lymphocytes T cells when stimulated by specific TB antigens. It can be measured in the blood and used as a tool for the diagnosis of LTBI [14–17]. Studies comparing the use of the IGRA and TST for the diagnosis of LTBI have shown that the IGRA has higher specificity, especially among populations submitted to BCG vaccination [18]. Nevertheless, the TST and IGRA both have suboptimal sensitivity, and conflicting results are common. It has been described that TST have particularly low sensitivity when testing immunocompromised individuals for LTBI, and thus might not be an adequate diagnostic tool applied for patients with HIV [16]. Conversely, the IGRA seems to be highly specific for the detection of LTBI, especially in BCG-vaccinated individuals and may help to identify LTBI in HIV-infected immunosuppressed patients [17].

The detection of LTBI and the treatment of patients at increased risk for developing active TB are the only effective strategies to prevent the development of tuberculosis [3, 5, 8]. Since validated guidelines for the proper diagnosis of LTBI in HIV patients are lacking, we hypothesized that applying IGRA would improve the diagnosis of LTBI compared to that with conventional TST test in adults infected with HIV/AIDS. Furthermore, we assessed the accuracy of TST and IGRA in HIV-infected patients presenting higher and lower risk for LTBI.

Methods

This work was a cross-sectional study of 90 HIV-infected individuals older than 18 years, at risk for LTBI and recruited between March 2012 and April 2013, at the Santa Casa de São Paulo School of Medical Sciences, Clemente Ferreira Institute, and Emílio Ribas

Institute of Infectious Diseases in São Paulo, Brazil. Patients diagnosed with mycobacteria other than TB, as well as patients with other known causes of immunosuppression, including type 1 diabetes, cancer, and/or the use of immunosuppressive medications, were excluded from the study. This study was approved by the ethics committees of all three institutions involved with this study. Only those individuals who agreed to participate and who signed the informed consent form were included in the study.

Definition and risk of LTBI

Latent tuberculosis infection (LTBI) is characterized by the presence of immune response to previously acquired *Mycobacterium tuberculosis* infection without clinical evidence of active tuberculosis [19]. LTBI was defined as those with a definite risk of LTBI (high or low) with at least one positive test (TST or IGRA), in which tuberculosis disease was absent (clinical manifestations of TB and/or radiological signs suggesting TB), and with smear-negative for tuberculosis in at least two sputum samples. The LTBI risk definition was established according to previous studies [4, 20–22].

High risk patients for LTBI was defined based upon extensive period of household contact with a smear-positive pulmonary tuberculosis person, which may have occurred during nocturnal as well as extensive diurnal periods. In addition, TB index-case patients should not have started TB treatment and presented signs and symptoms of active disease, including cough longer than 3 weeks plus at least one of the following: (a) losing 10% of body weight, (b) fever (> 38 °C), and (c) night sweats. Individuals with low risk were those with outside household contact history not sharing the domicile, but instead they share the same physical space at work, during educational or social activities with the index case. In addition, index case should not have started TB therapy and presented with only one of the following signs or symptoms of the index case: cough (> 3 weeks), fever (> 38 °C), sweating or weight loss (> 10% of body weight). The principal distinction between high and low risk patients for LTBI was presence of household contact and cough in the high-risk group.

The main diagnosis criteria for active TB in the index case was microbiology; presence of sputum with positive direct bacilloscopy (by Ziehl-Neelsen staining), culture in Lowenstein-Jensen medium or an anatomopathological examination showing caseating granulomas and acid-fast bacilli in tissue specimens. The lung tissue fragments used in the anatomopathological study were obtained by means of transbronchial biopsy. Negative microbiological results on smears or lung tissue cultures were excluded despite the presence of cavities on chest x-ray. Individuals who were double-negative for TST and IGRA were considered LTBI-free.

Tuberculin skin test (TST) and interferon-γ release Assy (IGRA) with QuantiFERON®-TB gold in-tube (QFT-GIT)

Tuberculin skin test (TST)

TST was performed using the Mantoux method [23], with intradermal administration of 0.1 ml purified protein derivative (0.1 ml tuberculin PPD RT23 2 TU, SSI, Copenhagen, DK) on the middle third of the anterior face of the left forearm. The reading occurred 48–96 h after the application, using the palpation method of the maximum transverse diameter of the induration and using a ruler in millimeters for measurement according to the National Health Foundation recommendations. For all individuals who participated in the study, it was considered a reactive when the size of the induration was ≥5 mm.

Interferon-γ release assay (IGRA) with QuantiFERON®-TB gold in-tube (QFT-GIT)

The IGRA was performed according to the manufacturer's recommendations (QFT-GIT manufacturer: Cellestis, Carnegie, Australia). Blood samples for IGRA testing were collected and the blood samples were transported to the Instituto Clemente Ferreira (ICF, São Paulo, Brazil). An aliquot of 3.0 ml of blood was withdrawn by trained technicians. Three tubes were marked with the same identification number of the patient's questionnaire: negative control bottle (gray cap), vial coated with tuberculosis-specific antigens (red cap) (ESAT-6, CFP-10, TB7.7 [p4]) and positive control vial coated with phytohemagglutinin as mitogen (purple cap). After collection and homogenization, tubes containing blood were incubated at 37 °C for 16–24 h and kept upright during this period. After 16 to 24 h the tubes were centrifuged and then the plasma was separated and frozen at −70 °C. When the number of patients required to perform an ELISA plate (29 patients) or two plaques (58 patients) was reached, the ELISA assay was performed. Each patient had their plasma sample evaluated for the production of interferon gamma by lymphocytes after stimulation by specific antigens of the *M. tuberculosis*, inert antigens (negative control) and mitogens (positive control). After obtaining the ELISA crude values, these were analyzed from a specific software for QuantiFERON®-TB Gold In Tube and the results further calculated. The program evaluates the quality of the analyzes, generates a standard curve and provides a result for each individual. The final test result may be positive or negative. Those with antigen TB values minus Nil (TB Ag-Nil) greater than or equal to 0.35 IU/ml are considered positive. In the study, the "undetermined" result of the IGRA was considered as "positive".

Treatment for LTBI was recommended to individuals who were positive for either TST or IGRA and for whom TB disease was ruled out, following the standards of the Brazilian Ministry of Health [4, 5].

CD4+ and CD8+ cell counts

For this study, we considered T lymphocyte subpopulations CD4 + and CD8 + counts, obtained by flow cytometry up to three months before the data collection [24].

Statistical analysis

To investigate whether an association exists between the TST and the IGRA, we used the McNemar test. If agreement between variables was found, then we used the Kappa value to determine the level of agreement. To evaluate the values of CD4 + T cells according to the result of the TST and IGRA, we used the Mann-Whitney test. To examine the association between the test results and the risk of LTBI, we used Fisher's exact test, the McNemar test (if there was agreement), and the Kappa value, if needed, to determine the degree of agreement [25]. Receiver operating characteristic (ROC) curve was used to verify the possibility of identifying cut-off values of CD4+ T and CD8+ T cells, to optimize the sensitivity and specificity of the test results in accordance with the risk of LTBI. It was also plotted to compare the diagnostic accuracy of tests. We defined the following agreement levels: no correlation between the variables when the Kappa value was less than 0.20; poor or fair agreement for values from 0.21 to 0.40; moderate agreement for values from 0.41 to 0.60; good agreement for values from 0.61 to 0.80; and strong agreement for values from 0.81 to 1. A significance level of 5% (0.05) was adopted throughout the study. We used the statistical software Predictive Analytics Software 17.0.2 (PASW Statistics 17.0.2).

Results

Initially, 106 patients were considered eligible for the study. Of these, 16 were excluded, three for not agreeing to sign the consent form, five for not returning for TST reading and eight for lack of recent CD4 + T lymphocyte count and HIV viral load (last three months before the data collection). Therefore, 90 HIV-infected patients at risk of latent tuberculosis infection were included in the analysis, of which 56.7% were male with a mean age of 39.2 (± 10.9) years. Most of them (93.3%) were under antiretroviral therapy and 95.5% had been previously vaccinated for tuberculosis with BCG vaccine. Those classified at high and low risk for TB infection were 69 (76.6%) and 21 (23.3%) patients, respectively. Other clinical characteristics of the study population are shown on Table 1. The median values of CD4 + and CD8 + T cells, and HIV viral load are described in Table 2. Briefly, CD4 + T cells

Table 1 Demographic information of the studied population of 90 HIV-infected patients at risk of LTBI

	Frequency (n)	Percentage(%)
Sex		
Female	39	43.3
Male	51	56.7
BCG vaccination		
No	04	4.4
Yes	86	95.5
BCG scar		
No	04	4.4
Yes	86	95.5
Comorbidities		
No	36	30
Yes	54	60
ART		
No	6	6.6
Yes	84	93.3
Risk of infection for TB		
High	69	76.6
Low	21	23.3

HIV Human immunodeficiency vírus, LTBI Latent tuberculosis infection, BCG Bacillus Calmette-Guérin, ART antiretroviral therapy, TB Tuberculosis

median value was of 557.5 (± 283.89) cell /mm^3, and mean HIV viral load values was 514.5 (± 1814.02) copies/ml.

TST and IGRA results

Among 90 HIV patients, 10 patients were TST and IGRA tests negative and therefore did not meet the study criteria for LTBI. However, we could not tell whether these individuals were truly negative for LTBI or whether they were false-negative individuals. Among them, average age was 41 years, the average time of active TB exposure to infected individuals was 1.7 months, and the average CD4+ T cell count was 415 cells/mm^3. All patients were receiving ART and

Table 2 Median values of CD4+ and CD8+ T lymphocyte counts, CD4/CD8 values, HIV viral load, and log^{10} of HIV viral load in 90 patients with HIV at risk of LTBI

Variables	Median	SD	Minimun	Maximun
CD4+	557.5	283.8	114.0	1259.00
CD8+	835.4	331.7	225.0	2112.0
CD4+/CD8+	0.71	0.43	0.16	3.53
HIV (VL)	514.5	1.814	50.0	10,023.0
HIV log^{10}(VL)	1.89	0,55	1.70	4.00

CD4+ Cluster of differentiation – 4, CD8+ Cluster of differentiation – 8, HIV Human Immunodeficiency virus, VL viral load, SD Standard Deviation

had undetectable viral load, hence were most likely not to be infected with TB.

Table 3 summarizes the frequencies of TST and IGRA results in 90 HIV-infected patients included in the study. Briefly, among 80 patients who met the study criteria for LTBI, 59 (73.7%) were TST positive, while 21 (26.2%) were negative. In contrast, 75 (93.7%) patients with HIV and with LTBI were IGRA positive, and only five patients (6.2%) were negative. When assessing the level of agreement between TST and IGRA with the diagnosis of LTBI, TST showed poor agreement (Kappa: 0.384), while the IGRA showed good agreement (Kappa: 0.769).

Interestingly, only one patient presented indeterminate IGRA result, but with TST positive. This patient had a normal CD4 + T lymphocyte count (938 cels/mm^3).

Regarding discordant results between tests, 21 patients presented negative TST and positive IGRA. These patients had an average CD4 cell count of 245 cells/mm^3, while patients with both TST and IGRA positivity (n = 54) had an average CD4 cell count of 721.5 cells/mm^3. Indeed, the average CD4 cell counts in the group presenting TST negative and IGRA positive were significantly lower than in the double-positive (TST and IGRA) group (p < 0.001) (Fig. 1).

Among 69 (76.7%) patients presenting high risk for TB infection, TST was positive in 48 (69.5%), negative in 21 (30.5%), respectively. No significant association was found between the TST and the level of risk (p = 0.191). On the other hand, IGRA was positive to all but one patient (98.5%). We observed a strong association between the IGRA and risk for LTBI (p < 0.001). Low risk patients were 21 (23.3%), of which TST was positive in 11 (52.4%) and negative in 10 (47.6%), respectively. Conversely, IGRA was positive in seven (33.3%) and negative in 14 (66.7%) patients. Hence, TST results were not correlated with risk for TB infection, whereas a good correlation was found between IGRA and risk (Table 4). Using a threshold value of

Table 3 Description of frequencies related to the TST and IGRA result, according to diagnosis for LTBI in 90 HIV-infected studied

Test type	Results	Diagnosis of LTBI (n)		Total
		No	Yes	
TST	Negative	10	21	31
	Positive	0	59	59
	Total	10	80	90
IGRA	Negative	10	5	15
	Positive	0	75	75
	Total	10	80	90

TST Tuberculin Skin Test, IGRA Interferon-γ release assay, LTBI Latent tuberculosis infection, TST and LTBI (Kappa: 0.384), IGRA and LTBI (Kappa: 0.769)

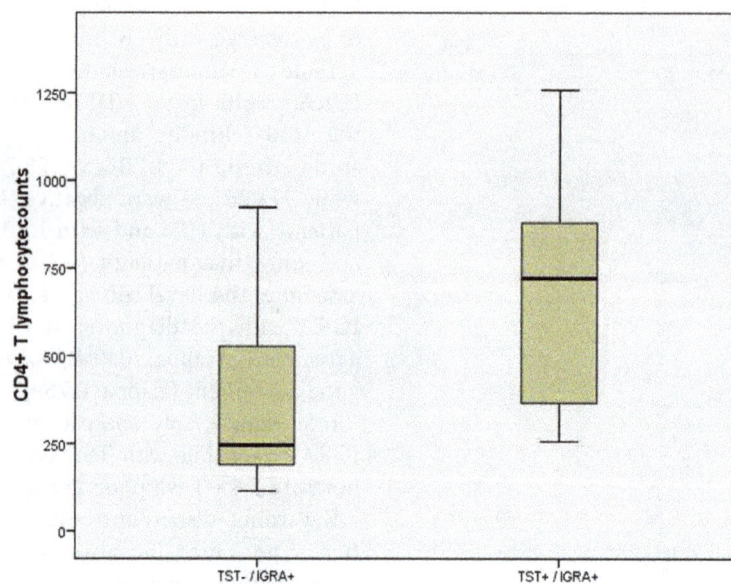

Fig. 1 CD4+ T lymphocyte counts and TST outcome in 90 HIV-infected patients with positive IGRA results and at risk of LTBI. CD4+: Cluster of differentiation – 4; HIV: Human Immunodeficiency virus; TST: Tuberculin Skin Test; IGRA: Interferon-γ release assay; LTBI: Latent tuberculosis infection

0.51UI/mL for the IGRA yielded a ROC curve with 98.6% of sensitivity and 71.4% of specificity (see Additional file 1). We observed that only six patients at low risk of LTBI were positive for both TST and IGRA, while among patients at high risk, 48 out of 69 patients (69.6%) had double-positive results (TST and IGRA). The sensitivity (Se), specificity (S), positive predictive value (PPV), and negative predictive value (NPV) were estimated for both the TST and the IGRA, considering the risk as the main criterion for a diagnosis of LTBI (Table 5).

Discordant results between TST and IGRA performed in 90 HIV-positive patients under the risk for LTBI are described in Table 6. Briefly, 21 patients presented negative TST and positive IGRA.

Table 4 Description of frequencies related to the TST and IGRA result, according to the risk for LTBI in 90 HIV-infected patients studied

Test type	Results	Risk		Total
		High	Low	
TST	Positive	48	11	59
	Negative	21	10	31
	Total	69	21	90
IGRA	Positive	68	7	75
	Negative	1	14	15
	Total	69	21	90

TST tuberculin skin test, *IGRA* Interferon-γ release assay, *LTBI* Latent tuberculosis infection; TST and risk (Fisher, $p = 0.191$). TST and risk (Kappa: 0.147, 90% CI: 0.000–0.315); IGRA and risk (Fisher, $p < 0.001$); IGRA and risk (Kappa: 0.724, 90% CI: 0.555–0.894)

Discussion

In the present study, we compared the TST with QFT-GIT (IGRA) to establish which test would be most accurate for the diagnosis of LTBI in HIV-infected adults. We acknowledge that most of HIV patients analyzed were under antiretroviral therapy (ART) and consequently had adequate immunological and virologic control of the disease showing high levels of CD4+ lymphocytes (> 500 cells/mm^3). This situation constitutes the ideal timing for the diagnosis and treatment of LTBI [26].

Nonetheless, most of the studied patients were at high risk of LTBI. Categorizing patients with HIV into high or low risk may be justified by the poor performance of the TST for the diagnosis of LTBI, although it remains an important diagnostic tool in countries with a high prevalence of TB [7]. The lack of a gold standard suitable for the diagnosis of LTBI and the difficulties in the interpretation of TST results, especially among immunocompromised patients, strongly contributed to our decision to consider risk as the main criterion for LTBI diagnosis. The classification as high or low risk for LTBI is rather arbitrary, nevertheless it was based upon clinical and epidemiological data. Additionally, we applied a scoring system to facilitate risk definition and considered the traditional concept of contact, following the definition provided by Rose [20].

In our study, we identified significantly discordant results between TST and IGRA, as it was previously shown by other authors [13]. The World Health Organization (WHO) studies concluded that TST may

Table 5 Comparison between TST and IGRA in 90 patients infected with HIV at risk of LTBI

Test	Measure	Estimate	CI 95%	
TST	Se	69.57	57.31	80.08
	S	47.62	25.71	70.22
	PPV	81.36	69.09	90.31
	NPV	32.26	16.68	51.37
IGRA	Se	98.55	92.19	99.96
	Es	66.67	43.03	85.41
	PPV	90.67	81.71	96.16
	NPV	93.33	68.05	99.83

HIV Human Immunodeficiency virus, *TST* Tuberculin Skin Test, *IGRA* Interferon-γ release assay, *CI* confidence intervals, *Se* sensitivity, *S* specificity NPV, negative predictive value, *PPV* positive predictive value

be inadequate for diagnosing LTBI in immunocompromised individuals due to HIV infection [16]. Furthermore, previous studies have also shown that the chronic state of immunosuppression in patients with HIV may lead to false TST negative results, while giving some advantage to the IGRA test, as the latter seems to suffer less influence from low CD4+ T cell counts than the TST [16]. Additionally, in immunocompromised individuals false-negative TST results may occur because late immunosuppression is directly related to T cell activities. Even though CD4+ T cell counts affect the IGRA results, this test seems to be more reliable than the TST for detecting LTBI in this population [27–31]. Another possible explanation for the discrepancy observed in the HIV patient is that the TST result may be negative within two to eight weeks after infection with TB due to a delayed-type hypersensitivity. On the other hand, it is believed that the conversion of the IGRA occurs much earlier after the infection [32].

We found no significant association between the TST and LTBI risk but rather, there were a strong association between the IGRA results and the risk of LTBI in these patients. In fact, when compared to TST, IGRA was more sensitive and specific to identify

Table 6 Description of the frequencies related to the association of the TT and IGRA results in 90 HIV-infected patients at risk of LTBI

	TST		
	Negative	Positive	Total
IGRA			
Negative	10	5	15
Positive	21	54	75
Total	31	59	90

TST Tuberculin Skin Test, *IGRA* Interferon-γ release assay, *LTBI* Latent Tuberculosis Infection, TST and IGRA (McNemar, $p = 0,003$). TST and IGRA (Kappa: 0,271, 90% IC: 0,116-0,426)

patients with LTBI. However, the specificity of IGRA observed in our study was still lower than that found in other studies (> 90%), which may reflect some intrinsic characteristics of the Brazilian population [29–31, 33]. According to our results, a negative IGRA test in the person with HIV strongly excluded LTBI. By contrast, those with positive IGRA were more likely to have LTBI. Our data suggests that, when screening HIV-infected persons for LTBI, IGRA may be a better choice than TST.

We are aware that our study presents some limitations, including the important lack of a universally accepted definition of risk of LTBI. Indeed, stratifying patients for high and low risk for LTBI is not an easy task, even with application of a scoring system and following the recommendations previously published [20]. Nevertheless, we were able to show that IGRA detected LTBI with greater reliability, especially among patients presenting lower levels of CD4 + T lymphocyte count. Another limitation is the transversal design of our study, making impossible for us to follow up patients thus assessing the possible association between positive tests and progression to TB disease. Furthermore, TST and IGRA were performed only once for each HIV patient, hindering the possibility of evaluating future tests conversion or even reversal particularly among those who had shown discordant results between tests, which could have clarified the agreement between these tests with the diagnosis of LTBI. We also argue that a longitudinal study using the TST and IGRA for the diagnosis of LTBI would better answer this question and perhaps explain the greater agreement between IGRA with diagnosis of LTBI.

Unfortunately, the definition universally accepted for diagnosing LTBI does necessarily include the performance of TST or IGRA test, which indeed may have biased our results. One attempting to assess the accuracy of a specific test for a defined disease or clinical situation, should not include the same test in the criteria for the definition. Nevertheless, our results showed a strong association between positive IGRA results and the high risk for LTBI in the HIV-positive population included in the study. Moreover, among those HIV-positive patients with lower CD_4 count, IGRA accuracy was superior when compared to TST. This may represent a strong association between IGRA and epidemiological risk factors itself [3, 8]. In this context, a recent Brazilian Ministry of Health statement recommended that for those HIV-positive patients with CD_4 count equal or lower than 350 cels/mm^3, with a defined epidemiological high risk for LTBI and when TB disease was absent should receive therapy regardless of TST or IGRA test results [8, 34]. On the other hand, World Health Organization (WHO) recently recommended that preventive TB treatment should be offered for all HIV-positive patients unlikely to have active TB with unknown or positive TST, regardless of any CD_4 count [8].

Based on these results, we may speculate that following a clinical evaluation and categorization of risk, individuals with a normal chest radiography with no signs or symptoms of TB disease should undergo IGRA. Upon positivity of IGRA, patient should start treatment as soon as possible. When IGRA is negative, LTBI would be ruled out. For the diagnosis of LTBI, the risk of infection with TB should always be considered. In developing countries with high TB-HIV coinfection burden, and limited public financial resources, TST must be considered the first choice for LTBI diagnosis due to its low cost and ease of performance.

Conclusions

In the detection of latent tuberculosis infection (LTBI) in HIV-infected individuals, IGRA showed a better performance than the TST and a better association with the risk of *M. tuberculosis* infection. Taken together, our study demonstrated that IGRA has a better performance than the TST for diagnosing infection by TB in HIV-infected individuals. Nevertheless, the challenge for a new diagnostic tool such as IGRA to become a gold standard for LTBI detection in patients with HIV.

Abbreviations
AIDS: Acquired immunodeficiency syndrome; ART: antiretroviral therapy; BCG: Bacillus Calmette-Guérin; CD4: Cluster of differentiation-4; CD8: Cluster of differentiation-8; CI: confidence intervals; HIV: Human Immunodeficiency virus; IGRA: Interferon Gamma Release Assay; INF-γ: Interferon-Gamma; LTBI: Latent Tuberculosis Infection; NPV: Negative predictive value; PPV: Positive predictive value; S: Specificity; Se: Sensitivity; TB: Mycobacterium Tuberculosis; TB: Tuberculosis; TST: Tuberculin Skin Test

Acknowledgements
This project was funded by the São Paulo Research Foundation (Fundação Amparo à Pesquisa do Estado de São Paulo - FAPESP) Process no. 2011/05805-1 (Regular Research Project) and the National Council for Scientific and Technological Development (Conselho Nacional de Desenvolvimento Científico e Tecnológico - CNPq) Process no. 141705/2011-6. Immunology Laboratory of Prof. Dr. Reinaldo Solomão - UNIFESP for technical support.

Funding
This project was funded by the São Paulo Research Foundation (Fundação Amparo à Pesquisa do Estado de São Paulo - FAPESP) Process no. 2011/05805-1 (Regular Research Project) and the National Council for Scientific and Technological Development (Conselho Nacional de Desenvolvimento Científico e Tecnológico - CNPq) Process no. 141705/2011-6. Neither FAPESP nor CNPq interfered in the study design, collection, analysis and interpretation of data and in writing this manuscript.

Authors' contributions
Conception and design: GBK, DSR. Acquisition of data: GBK. Laboratory analysis GBK, NVFM; Analysis and interpretation: GBK MJCS, MNB, DSR. All authors contributed to either drafting the manuscript and MJCS revised the manuscript and gave final approval. GBK had full access to all the data in the study and takes responsibility for the integrity of the data and the accuracy of the data analysis. All authors contributed to manuscript revisions. All authors have read and approved the final manuscript.

Competing interests
All authors declare that they have no competing interests.

Author details
[1]Division of Infectious Diseases, Department of Internal Medicine Santa Casa de São Paulo School of Medical Sciences, Hospital da Irmandade da Santa Casa de Misericórdia de São Paulo, Rua Dr Cesáreo Mota Jr 112,, São Paulo, SP CEP: 01303-060, Brazil. [2]Clemente Ferreira Institute, Rua da Consolação 717, São Paulo, SP CEP: 01221-020, Brazil. [3]Emílio Ribas Institute of Infectious Diseases, Av Dr Arnaldo 165, São Paulo, SP CEP: 01246-900, Brazil. [4]Federal University of São Paulo (UNIFESP), Rua Sena Madureira 1500, São Paulo CEP: 04021-001, Brazil.

References
1. Smith KC, Armitige L. Wanger a. a review of tuberculosis: reflections on the past, present and future of a global epidemic disease. Expert Rev Anti-Infect Ther. 2003;1:483–91.
2. Zumla A, Raviglione M, Hafner R, von Reyn CF. Tuberculosis. N Engl J Med. 2013;368:745–55.
3. World Health Organization. Global tuberculosis report 2018 (WHO/CDS/TB/2018.20). Geneva: World Health Organization; 2018. 243p. http://apps.who.int/iris/bitstream/handle/10665/274453/9789241565646-eng.pdf?ua=1. Accessed 23 Sep 2018.
4. Conde MB, Melo FA, Marques AM, Cardoso NC, Pinheiro VG, Dalcin Pde T, et al. III Brazilian thoracic association guidelines on tuberculosis. J Bras Pneumol. 2009;35:1018–48.
5. Ministério da Saúde (BR). Secretaria de Vigilância em Saúde, Departamento de Vigilância Epidemiológica. Manual de recomendações para o controle da tuberculose no Brasil. Brasília: Ministério da Saúde; 2011. 288 p. (Série A. Normas e Manuais Técnicos). http://bvsms.saude.gov.br/bvs/publicacoes/manual_recomendacoes_controle_tuberculose_brasil.pdf. Accessed 05 Apr 2014.
6. Ministério da Saúde (BR). Indicadores. Boletim Epidemiológico - Secretaria de Vigilância em Saúde - Ministério da Saúde. 2015;46(9):1–11. http://portalarquivos.saude.gov.br/images/pdf/2015/marco/25/Boletim-tuberculose-2015.pdf. Acessed 14 Jun 2018.
7. Sharma SK, Mohanan S, Sharma A. Relevance of latent TB infection in areas of high TB prevalence. Chest. 2012;142:761–73.
8. World Health Organization. Latent tuberculosis infection: updated and consolidated guidelines for programmatic management. Geneva: World Health Organization; 2018. p. 1–78p. http://apps.who.int/iris/bitstream/handle/10665/260233/9789241550239-eng.pdf;jsessionid=EF4DDEDB879F6ADF516EB46BCC4AD932?sequence=1. Acessed 14 Jun 2018.
9. Getahun H, Matteelli A, Chaisson RE, Raviglione M. Latent mycobacterium tuberculosis infection. N Engl J Med. 2015;372:2127–35.
10. Jones BE, Young SM, Antoniskis D, Davidson PT, Kramer F, Barnes PF. Relationship of the manifestations of tuberculosis to CD4 cell counts in patients with human immunodeficiency virus infection. Am Rev Respir Dis. 1993;148:1292–7.
11. Klautau GB, Kuschnaroff TM. Clinical forms and outcome of tuberculosis in HIV-infected patients in a tertiary hospital in São Paulo - Brazil. Braz J Infect Dis. 2005;9:464–78.
12. Wang L, Turner MO, Elwood RK, Schulzer M, FitzGerald JM. A meta-analysis of the effect of Bacille Calmette Guerin vaccination on tuberculin skin test measurements. Thorax. 2002;57:804–9. Erratum in: Thorax. 2003;58:188.
13. Ministério da Saúde (BR). Secretaria de Vigilância em Saúde, Departamento de DST Aids e Hepatites Virais. Protocolo clínico e diretrizes terapêuticas para manejo da infecção pelo HIV em adultos. Brasília: Ministério da Saúde; 2013. 75 p. http://bvsms.saude.gov.br/bvs/publicacoes/protocolo_clinico_manejo_hiv_adultos.pdf. Accessed 5 Apr 2014.

14. Mazurek GH, Jereb J, Vernon A, LoBue P, Goldberg S, Castro K, et al. Updated guidelines for using interferon gamma release assays to detect mycobacterium tuberculosis infection - United States. 2010 MMWR Recomm Rep. 2010;59:1–25.

15. World Health Organization Global tuberculosis control: WHO report 2011 (WHO/HTM/TB/2011.16). Geneva: World Health Organization; 2011. 246 p. http://whqlibdoc.who.int/publications/2011/9789241564380_eng.pdf. Accessed 5 Apr 2014.

16. World Health Organization. Guidelines for intensified tuberculosis case-finding and isoniazid preventive therapy for people living with HIV in resource-constrained settings. Geneva: World Health Organization; 2011. p 52. http://apps.who.int/iris/bitstream/handle/10665/44472/9789241500708_eng.pdf?sequence=1. Accessed 5 Apr 2014.

17. World Health Organization. Use of tuberculosis interferon-gamma release assays (IGRAs) in low- and middle-income countries: policy statement (WHO/HTM/TB/2011.18). Geneva: World Health Organization; 2011. 61 p. http://whqlibdoc.who.int/publications/2011/9789241502672_eng.pdf. Accessed 5 Apr 2014.

18. Menzies D, Pai M, Comstock G. Meta-analysis: new tests for the diagnosis of latent tuberculosis infection: areas of uncertainty and recommendations for research. Ann Intern Med. 2007;146:340–54.

19. World Health Organization Guidelines on the management of latent tuberculosis infection (WHO/HTM/TB/2015.01). Geneva: World Health Organization;2015,38p. http://apps.who.int/iris/bitstream/10665/136471/1/9789241548908_eng.pdf?ua=1&ua=1. Accessed 23 Feb 2016.

20. Rose CE Jr, Zerbe GO, Lantz SO, Bailey WC. Establishing priority during investigation of tuberculosis contacts. Am Rev Respir Dis. 1979;119:603–9.

21. WHO. WHO policy on collaborative TB/HIV activities. Guidelines for national programmes and other stakeholders. Geneva, 2012;1–36p. https://reliefweb.int/sites/reliefweb.int/files/resources/Full_Report_3595.pdf

22. Field SK, Escalante P, Fisher DA, Ireland B, Irwin RS. Cough due to TB and other chronic infections: CHEST guideline and expert panel report. Chest. 2018;153(2):467–97.

23. Mantoux M. La voie intradermique en tuberculinothérapie. Presse Med. 1912;20:146–8.

24. Barbesti S, Soldini L, Carcelain G, Guignet A, Colizzi V, Mantelli B, et al. A simplified flow cytometry method of CD4 and CD8 cell counting based on thermoresistant reagents: implications for large scale monitoring of HIV-infected patients in resource-limited settings. Cytometry B Clin Cytom. 2005; 68(1):43–5.

25. Agresti A. Models for matched pairs. In: John Wiley & Sons, editors. An introduction to categorical data analysis. 2nd ed. New York; 2007. p. 244–75.

26. Akolo C, Adetifa I, Shepperd S, Volmink J. Treatment of latent tuberculosis infection in HIV infected persons. Cochrane Database Syst Rev. 2010;1: CD000171.

27. Rangaka MX, Wilkinson KA, Seldon R, Van Cutsem G, Meintjes GA, Morroni C, et al. Effect of HIV-1 infection on T-cell-based and skin test detection of tuberculosis infection. Am J Respir Crit Care Med. 2007;175:514–20.

28. Kabeer BS, Sikhamani R, Raja A. Comparison of interferon gamma and interferon gamma-inducible protein-10 secretion in HIV-tuberculosis patients. AIDS. 2010;24:323–5.

29. Cattamanchi A, Smith R, Steingart KR, Metcalfe JZ, Date A, Coleman C, et al. Interferon-gamma release assays for the diagnosis of latent tuberculosis infection in HIV-infected individuals: a systematic review and meta-analysis. J Acquir Immune Defic Syndr. 2011;56:230–8.

30. Sester M, Sotgiu G, Lange C, Giehl C, Girardi E, Migliori GB, et al. Interferon-gamma release assays for the diagnosis of active tuberculosis: a systematic review and meta-analysis. Eur Respir J. 2011;37:100–11.

31. Chee CB, Sester M, Zhang W, Lange C. Diagnosis and treatment of latent infection with Mycobacterium tuberculosis. Respirology. 2013;18:205–16.

32. del Corral H, París SC, Marín ND, Marín DM, López L, Henao HM, et al. IFNgamma response to Mycobacterium tuberculosis, Risk of infection and disease in house hold contacts of tuberculosis patients in Colombia. PLoS One. 2009;4:e8257.

33. Fujita A, Ajisawa A, Harada N, Higuchi K, Mori T. Performance of a whole-blood interferon-gamma release assay with mycobacterium RD1-specific antigens among HIV-infected persons. Clin Dev Immunol. 2011;2011:325295.

34. Ministério da Saúde (BR) Secretaria de Vigilância em Saúde. Nota Informativa n° 11/2018-.DIAHV/SVS/MS. Recomendações para tratamento da Infecção Latente por Tuberculose (ILTB) em pessoas vivendo com HIV (PVHIV). 2018. 4p.https://drive.google.com/file/d/1YQuovBq8UGSJIROgw-kRD7UMeVzc2Ezz/view. Accessed 16 Jun 2018.

24

Persistent candidemia in very low birth weight neonates: risk factors and clinical significance

Jinjian Fu[1][*][†], Yanling Ding[1][†], Yongjiang Jiang[2][†], Shengfu Mo[1][†], Shaolin Xu[1] and Peixu Qin[1]

Abstract

Background: The prevalence and risk factors for persistent candidemia among very low birth weight infants are poorly understood. This study aimed to investigate the epidemiology of persistent candidemia over a 4-year period in a neonatal intensive care unit (NICU) in Liuzhou, China.

Methods: We retrospectively extracted demographic data, risk factors, microbiological results and outcomes of very low birth weight infants with candidemia in our hospital between January 2012 and November 2015. Persistent candidemia was defined as a positive blood culture for > 5 days. Logistic regression was used to identify risk factors associated with persistent candidemia.

Results: Of 48 neonates with candidemia, 28 had persistent candidemia. Both mechanical ventilation and intubation were significantly associated with increased rates of persistent candidemia ($P = 0.044$ and 0.004, respectively). The case fatality rate for the persistent candidemia group was 14.3%.

Conclusion: The rate of persistent candidemia was high among very low birth weight neonates. Mechanical ventilation and intubation were the major factors associated with the development of persistent candidemia. This study highlights the importance of intensive prevention and effective treatment among neonates with persistent candidemia.

Keywords: Persistent candidemia, Very low birth weight, Neonates, Epidemiology

Background

Candida species have emerged as important nosocomial infection pathogens associated with significant morbidity and mortality in very low birth weight (VLBW) neonates [1–4]. Candidemia is the third most common nosocomial bloodstream infection during late-onset neonatal sepsis [1]. It affects 10 to 20% of extremely low birth weight infants and 2 to 16% of very low birth weight neonates and is responsible for 25 to 30% of morbidity in neonatal intensive care units (NICUs) [2–7]. It was reported that the infants who survive candidemia frequently have long-term neurodevelopmental impairment, which occurred in 57% of these high-risk infants [7].

The contributing factors in high-risk groups include prematurity, VLBW, catheter and endotracheal tube use, prolonged NICU stay, broad-spectrum antibiotic use and total parenteral nutrition [8–10]. Lack of specific signs or symptoms in the development of candidemia among VLBW infants results were in a high risk of fatality [8]. Early diagnosis is crucial for infection control and initiating effective treatment.

Although VLBW is a well-known risk factor in the development of candidemia, it is uncertain whether this risk factor also contributes to persistent candidemia or mortality. Only a few studies have evaluated the risk factors and mortality for persistent candidemia in VLBW infants, and the results remain controversial. The potential risk factors and attributable mortality of persistent candidemia in VLBW infants in Western China are unknown. Therefore, we conducted this study to identify the incidence, risk factors, microbiological results and

* Correspondence: fujinjianaa@126.com
[†]Jinjian Fu, Yan Ling Ding, Yongjiang Jiang and Sheng Fu Mo contributed equally to this work.
[1]Department of Laboratory, Liuzhou Maternity and Child Healthcare Hospital, 50th Yingshan Road, Chengzhong District, Liuzhou 545001, China
Full list of author information is available at the end of the article

mortality associated with persistent candidemia in VLBW infants in China.

Methods

Data collection

A retrospective chart review of neonates admitted to the NICU of the Liuzhou Maternity and Child Healthcare Hospital from January 2012 to November 2015 was performed. Infants born at the hospital or transferred to the NICU at < 5 days old were included. At least one blood culture obtained by peripheral vein puncture that grew *Candida* species was defined as candidemia. Based on the study by Levy et al [11], if a single patient had a positive blood culture lasted for > 5 days starting from the first culture result indicated positive for *Candida*, the infection was considered persistent candidemia.

An electronic database was used to collect and record data. These included gestational age, birth weight, admission age, gender, delivery type, fetal membrane rupture duration, necrotizing enterocolitis, neurodevelopmental impairment, congenital diseases (such as congenital heart disease, glucose-6-phosphatedehydrogenase deficiency, and thalassemia), incidence of abdominal surgery, mechanical ventilation use, indwelling central venous catheter use, intubation > 6 days, rescue history, total parenteral nutrition status, hospitalization duration, 3rd generation cephalosporin use, carbapenem use, vancomycin use, antibiotic therapeutic duration, multiple antibiotic use (≥3 classes), *Candida* species, and mortality.

Microbiologic methods

Blood cultures were incubated using the BacT/Alert 3D system (bioMerieux). *Candida* species were cultured in CHROM Agar medium (bioMerieux) and isolates were identified using API 20C AUX (bioMerieux).

Statistical analysis

Statistical analysis was carried out using SPSS version 20.0 statistical software (SPSS Inc., Chicago, IL, USA). Potential risk factors associated with persistent candidemia were identified using logistic regression analysis. Variables with 2-tailed $P < 0.05$ were defined as statistically significant. Odds ratios (ORs) along with 95% confidence intervals (CIs) were used to assess the strength of any association.

Results

Incidence

During the 4-year period, a total of 5075 infants were admitted to the NICU, of which 484 were VLBW infants. A total of 48 cases among the VLBW infants were diagnosed with candidemia, resulting in a candidemia incidence of 9.5 per 1000 infants. Among the very low birth weight infants, the incidence of candidemia was 9.9%. For the 48 infants who suffered from candidemia, 28 experienced positive blood culture for > 5 days and were subsequently reported as having persistent candidemia. The persistent candidemia rate was 5.8% among VLBW infants.

Among the 48 *Candida* species, *Candida albicans* accounted for 39.6% of all cases (19/48), followed by *Candida glabrata* at 33.3% (16/48), and *Candida tropicalis* at 27.1% (13/48), no other *Candida* was found except *C.albicans*, *C. glabrata*, and *C. tropicalis*. *C.albicans* accounted for 25% (7/28) of cases of persistent candidemia. Non-*albicans* species were the leading causative pathogens of persistent candidemia, accounting for 75.0% of all cases, *C. glabrata* and *C. tropicalis* accounted for 42.9% (12/28) and 32.1% (9/28) of cases, respectively.

Demographics

Among the 48 VLBW infants with candidemia, 17 were males and 31 were females. The median admission age was 3.2 days (range: 1.7–4.8 days), the median birth weight was 1154.5 g (range: 950.2 g – 1358.8 g), and the median gestational age was 29.6 weeks (range: 27.6–31.6 weeks) (Table 1).

Clinical presentation

Most infants with candidemia received mechanical ventilation (70.8%, 34/48), central venous catheters (58.3%, 28/48), total parenteral nutrition (93.8%, 45/48), and had a rescue history (66.7%, 32/48) while 48% (23/48) of them received intubation for > 6 days. All of them received at least one class of antibiotics in the week before candidemia was diagnosed, and 64.6% received at least three classes of broad-spectrum antibiotics. The median antibiotic therapeutic duration was 38.9 days (range 20.7–58.0 days) while 85.4% of the neonates received prophylactic antifungal therapy with a median therapeutic duration of 10.4 days (range: 4.3–16.6 days). The median hospital length of stay was 54.9 days (range: 32.6–77.2 days).

Risk factors

Compared to the non-persistent candidemia group, the persistent candidemia cases had a significantly lower birth weight [1229.0 vs. 1097.8 g; $P < 0.001$] and significantly longer antibiotic therapeutic duration [31.1 (16.6, 55.6) days vs. 44.5 (24.3, 64.7) days; $P < 0.001$]. Persistent candidemia infants also had higher incidence of necrotizing enterocolitis (32.1% vs. 5.0%; $P < 0.001$), mechanical ventilation (85.7% vs. 50.0%; $P < 0.001$), and intubation (71.4% vs. 15.0%; $P < 0.001$) than the non-persistent cases. The non-*albicans* species were found more frequently in the persistent candidemia group (75.0% vs. 40.0%; $P < 0.001$). A logistic regression analysis using

Table 1 Clinical characteristics of neonates with and without persistent candidemia

Variable	Persistent candidemia		P value	Odds ratio (OR) (95% CI)
	Yes mean (95% CI) or n (%)	No mean (95% CI) or n (%)		
Demographics				
Gestational age (wks)	29.6 (27.3, 31.9)	29.7 (28.1, 31.2)	0.766	
Birth weight (g)	1097.8 (866.4,1309.2)	1229.0 (1051.1,1046.9)	0.029	
Male gender, n (%)	12 (42.9)	5 (25.0)	0.207	0.44 (0.13–1.57)
Admission age	1.3 (0.4, 2.2)	1.8 (2.4, 6.0)	0.611	
Risk factors				
Necrotizing enterocolitis	9 (32.1)	1 (5.0)	0.046	9.0 (1.04–78.17)
Neurodevelopmental impairment	6 (21.4)	6 (30.0)	0.501	0.64 (0.17–2.37)
Vaginal delivery	13 (46.4)	7 (35.0)	0.430	1.61 (0.49–5.25)
Fetal membrane rupture (h)	46.4 (25.1, 117.7)	18.8 (37.5, 75.1)	0.143	
Congentital diseases	15 (53.6)	10 (50.0)	0.867	1.15 (0.37–3.64)
Abdominal surgery	3 (10.7)	0 (0.0)	–	–
Mechanical ventilation	24 (85.7)	10 (50.0)	0.011	6.00 (1.52–23.70)
Central venous catheter	15 (59.6)	13 (65.0)	0.430	0.62 (0.19–2.03)
Intubation	20 (71.4)	3 (15.0)	0.000	14.17 (3.24–61.99)
Total parenteral nutrition	26 (92.9)	19 (95.0)	0.764	0.68 (0.06–8.11)
Hospitalization duration (d)	58.8 (33.8, 93.8)	49.3 (32.4, 66.2)	0.147	
3rdcephalosporins use	16 (59.3)	13 (65.0)	0.689	0.78 (0.24–2.59)
Carbapenems use	26 (92.9)	16 (80.0)	0.201	3.25 (0.53–19.82)
Vancomycin use	7 (25.0)	2 (10.0)	0.203	3.00 (0.55–16.31)
Multiple antibiotic use	18 (64.3)	13 (65.0)	0.959	0.97 (0.29–3.22)
Antibiotic therapeutic duration (d)	44.5 (24.3, 64.7)	31.1 (16.6, 55.6)	0.015	
Non-C.albicans	21 (75.0)	8 (40.0)	0.017	4.50 (1.31–15.52)
Prophylaxis antifungal therapy	25 (89.3)	16 (80.0)	0.375	2.08 (0.41–10.56)
Antifungal therapeutic duration (d)	11.3 (4.6, 18.0)	9.2 (4.6, 14.4)	0.243	
Outcome				
Death	4 (14.3)	1 (5.0)	0.320	3.17 (10.33–30.73)

backward model selection method on the 48 infants showed that candidemia cases on mechanical ventilation had a significantly increased risk of developing into persistent candidemia (OR = 5.72; 95% CI = 1.05–31.25), while intubation longer 6 days had an even higher risk (OR = 10.53; 95% CI = 2.11, 52.59) (Table 2).

Outcome

The overall mortality among 484 VLBW infants was 10.4%. The mortality for the persistent candidemia group was 14.3%, and for those who experience

Table 2 Multivariate analysis for persistent candidemia

Risk factor	Odds ratio	95% CI	P value
Intubation	10.53	2.11–52.59	0.004
Mechanical ventilation	5.72	1.05–31.25	0.044

none-persistent candidemia was 5.0%. This difference was not statistically significant (P = 0.320).

Discussion

Candidemia remains a significant cause of morbidity and mortality in premature infants. The incidence of neonatal candidemia in our NICU (9.5 per 1000 infants) was similar to those found in many other studies, which reported incidences of candidemia near 10 per 1000 patient discharges [2, 4, 10].

It was remarkable that the majority (58.3%) of VLBW neonatal candidemia cases were persistent candidemia, which was similar to one study from Israel [11] that reported persistent candidemia in 52% of infants. Hammoud et al [12] identified that 60% of neonatal blood stream infections were persistent. The definition of persistent candidemia in the current study and the investigation was conducted by Levy et al [11] Although

Robinson et al [13] reported an incidence of candidemia of 24.3% in a NICU located in the USA, their assessment of persistent candidemia incidence differed from Levy et al [11], which may explain the difference. The variation incidence highlights the importance of a consistent definition for persistent candidemia in neonates.

Many risk factors have been implicated in the pathogenesis of candidemia in infants, the most consistent one was prematurity, especially in very low birth weight groups [2, 5, 7, 8]. The results of the present study indicated that low birth weight was significantly associated with persistent candidemia, as revealed by univariate analysis, although no statistical significance was found by multivariate analysis. This finding was similar to a previous study [12], which also showed that the lower the birth weight, the greater the susceptibility to develop persistent candidemia (median birth weight, 970 and1130 g for the persistent candidemia and candidemia groups, respectively; $P = 0.04$).VLBW infants may have a higher risk of developing persistent candidemia because of their immature immune system, which may lead to an inability to eliminate pathogens from the bloodstream at the initiation of antifungal therapy.

Previous studies reported that C.albicans was the most frequent cause of candidemia in neonates, followed by C. parapsilosis [11]. Our study indicated that C.albicans was the predominant Candida species in VLBW infants, followed by Non- albicans such as C. glabrata and C. tropicalis. This pattern was consistent with previous reports conducted by Chinese, the American and Australian neonatal research groups [7, 9, 14–17], suggesting different epidemiology for neonatal candidemia around the world. A significantly higher frequency of non-albicans species (42.9 and 32.1% for C.glabrata and C.tropicalis, respectively) was found among VLBW infants with persistent candidemia compared to C.albicans (25.0%) in the current study. Published data addresses the significance of widespread implementation of prophylactic or empirical antifungal therapy in NICUs and PICUs [14–19], which may change Candida ecology. The identified risk factor for C.glabrata infection may be the result of broad-spectrum antibiotic use, particularly anti-aerobic and azole use as the empirical coverage for Gram-negative, Gram-positive and Fungal organisms in pediatric populations [2, 9, 16, 19]. One previous study identified C.glabrata as a risk factor for the development of persistent candidemia [20]. Additionally, non-albicans species themselves may also play a critical role in the pathogenesis of persistent candidemia due to their notorious capabilities of adherence to foreign surfaces, high virulence, and inherent or potential resistance to fluconazole [2, 3, 9, 19, 21–23].

Antibiotic exposure and, more importantly, the choice of an anti-aerobic spectrum of activity for routine prophylaxis or empirical therapy was the strongest risk factor for candidemia [14, 16, 24]. Our study was consistent with a previous report which showed that receipt of broad-spectrum antibiotics in the 7 days prior to candidemia diagnosis was a strong risk factor in VLBW infants [25]. A significantly longer duration of preceding antibiotic use was observed among infants with persistent candidemia when compared to infants with one episode of candidemia in the current study. This was consistent with the findings of a USA-based neonatal research group, which showed that prolonged antibiotic exposure was associated with persistent candidemia [26]. It is remarkable that the majority of infants in this study received empirical therapy (87.5%) in the preceding month. Moreover, over 85.4% of infants received multiple classes of antibiotics, either concomitantly or sequentially. Our data was consistent with the study that confirmed antibiotic prophylaxis was a common practice in many NICUs in China and around the world [9, 16, 17, 19, 27]. This finding highlights the need to reduce antibacterial exposure and employ effective medical practices for infection control.

Multiple explanations for the development of candidemia in neonatal groups have been suggested, and the most convincing explanation was the use of medical catheters and mechanical ventilation. Invasive operations provide a portal of entry and adhesion for Candida species and may be responsible for horizontal transmission [28]. It was suggested that due to the Candida species' ability to adhere to foreign materials, a residual fungal deposit might exist even after prompt removal of infected catheters or medical appliances; thus, it may take some time to eliminate the Candida species given that the antifungal therapy is effective [29]. Medical appliances, such as intubation tubes, may be the cause of persistent candidemia [18]. In the current study, both mechanical ventilation and intubation were significantly associated with persistent candidemia, as revealed by univariate and multivariate regression analysis. Previous studies have also shown that medical catheter retention increased the risk of candidemia death [30] (OR, 95% CI = 2.50, 1.06–5.91), and early removal of catheters significantly reduced candidemia-associated mortality (OR, 95% CI = 20.5, 3.9–106.5), suggesting that the implementation of appropriate medical practices, such as early removal of intubation, might improve the prognosis of VLBW infants with persistent candidemia.

Candidemia-related mortality rates in neonates range between 43 and 54% [31, 32]. The candidemia mortality rate in our study was 10.4%, and all occurred in the persistent candidemia group, which had a mortality rate of 17.9%. Our report was consistent with the investigation conducted by Levy et al [11], which showed that the crude mortality rate in newborn infants was 17.8%. However, some studies showed that persistent candidemia infections have higher mortality rates compared to non-persistent candidemia. There are several explanations about this discrepancy, one being that we failed to identify an apparent source of the persistent candidemia in the majority of cases, as only five catheter tips tested positive for Candida species (three of which had persistent candidemia). Another explanation was that we defined persistent candidemia without considering the effectiveness of the antifungal therapy, which may result in underestimation of the clinical relevance of persistent candidemia.

The present analysis was limited by the retrospective design and the study's location in a single center. Additionally, the small sample size may have compromised the statistical power of the study. A larger, multicenter prospective study is required to identify additional risk factors, ascertain the burden of persistent candidemia, and determine the antifungal susceptibility profiles to help pediatricians employ the proper intensive prevention and treatment practices.

Conclusions

In conclusion, the present data demonstrate that the incidence of persistent candidemia was high in the VLBW infants at Liuzhou Maternity and Child Healthcare Hospital, and mechanical ventilation and intubation appeared to be the crucial factors for the development of persistent candidemia. This study highlights the importance of intensive prevention and effective treatment among neonates with persistent candidemia.

Abbreviations
95%CI: 95% confidence interval; NICU: Neonatal intensive care unit; OR: Odds ratio; VLBW: Very low birth weight

Acknowledgements
Not applicable.

Funding
This manuscript was funded by Guangxi Nature Science Foundation (No. 2015GXSFBA139129), Guangxi Medical and Health Self-funding Project (No Z20170509 and No Z20180022) and the Liuzhou Science and Technology Bureau Project (No2017BD20201). The funders had no role in study design, data collection and analysis, decision to publish, or preparation of the manuscript.

Authors' contributions
YD and JF designed the study and drafted an outline. YJ and SM participated in data analysis, JF draft of initial manuscript, YJ, SX, PQ and SM participated in diagnosed and collected the data, JF revised the manuscript and all of authors approved the final content off this manuscript.

Competing interests
The authors declare that they have no competing interests.

Author details
[1]Department of Laboratory, Liuzhou Maternity and Child Healthcare Hospital, 50th Yingshan Road, Chengzhong District, Liuzhou 545001, China.

[2]Department of Neonatology, Liuzhou Maternity and Child Health Care Hospital, Liuzhou 545001, China.

References
1. Makhoul IR, Sujov P, Smolkin T, Lusky A, Reichman B. Epidemiological, clinical and microbiological characteristics of late-onset sepsis among very low birth weight infants in Israel: a national survey. Pediatrics. 2002;109:34–9.
2. Benjamin DK Jr, Stool BJ, Gantz MG, Walsh MC, Sánchez PJ, Das A, et al. Neonatal candidiasis: epidemiology, risk factors, and clinical judgment. Pediatrics. 2010;126:865–73.
3. Rodriguez D, Almirante B, Park BJ, Cuenca-Estrella M, Planes AM, Sanchez F, et al. Candidemia in neonatal intensive care units: Barcelona, Spain. Pediatr Infect Dis J. 2006;25:224–9.
4. Fridkin SK, Kaufman D, Edwards JR, Shetty S, Horan T. Changing incidence of Candida bloodstream infections among NICU patients in the United States: 1995-2004. Pediatrics. 2006;117:1680–7.
5. Kaufman D. Fungal infection in the very low birth weight infant. CurrOpin Infect Dis. 2004;17:253–9.
6. Leibovitz E. Neonatal candidosis: clinical picture, management controversies and consensus, and new therapeutic options. J Antimicrob Chemother. 2002;49Suppl 1:69–73.
7. Benjamin DK Jr, Stoll BJ, Fanaroff AA, McDonald SA, Oh W, Higgins RD, et al. Neonatal candidiasis among extremely low birth weight infants: risk factors, mortality rates, and neurodevelopmental outcomes at 18 to 22 months. Pediatrics. 2006;117:84–92.
8. Chang YJ, Choi IR, Shin WS, Lee JH, Kin YK, Park MS. The control of invasive Candida infection in very low birth weight infants by reduction in the use of 3rd generation cephalosporin. Korean J Pediatr. 2013;56:68–74.
9. Fu J, Ding Y, Wei B, Wang L, Xu S, Qin P, et al. Epidemiology of Candida albicans and non-C.albicans of neonatal candidemia at a tertiary care hospital in western China. BMC Infect Dis. 2017;17(1):329.
10. Celebi S, Hacimustafaoglu M, Koksal N, Ozkan H, Cetinkaya M, Ener B. Neonatal candidiasis: results of an 8 year study. PediatrInt. 2012;54:341–9.
11. Levy I, Shalit I, Askenazi S, Klinger G, Sirota L, Linder N. Duration and outcome of persistent Candidaemia in newborn infants. Mycoses. 2006;49:197–201.
12. Hammoud MS, Al-Taiar A, Fouad M, Raina A, Khan Z. Persistent candidemia in neonatal care units: risk factors and clinical significance. Int J Infect Dis. 2013;17:e624–8.
13. Robinson JA, Pham HD, Bloom BT, Wittler RR. Risk factors for persistent candidemia infection in a neonatal intensive care unit and its effect on mortality and length of hospitalization. J Perinatol. 2012;32:621–5.
14. Blyth CC, Chen SC, Slavin MA, Serena C, Nguyen Q, Marriott D, et al. Australian Candidemia study. Not just little adults: candidemia epidemiology, molecular characterization, and antifungal susceptibility in neonatal and pediatric patients. Pediatrics. 2009;123:1360–8.
15. Ben Abdeljelil J, Saghrouni F, Nouri S, Geith S, Khammari I, Fathallah A, et al. Neonatal invasive candidiasis in Tunisian hospital: incidence, risk factors, distribution of species and antifungal susceptibility. Mycoses. 2012;55:493–500.
16. Liu M, Huang S, Guo L, Li H, Wang F, Zhang QI, et al. Clinical features and risk factors for blood stream infections of Candida in neonates. ExpTher Med. 2015;10:1139–44.
17. Xia H, Wu H, Xia S, Zhu X, Chen C, Qiu G, et al. Invasive candidiasis in preterm neonates in China: a retrospective study from 11 NICUS during 2009-2011. Pediatr Infect Dis J. 2014;33:106–9.
18. Filioti J, Spiroglou K, Panteliadis CP, Roilides E. Invasive candidiasis in pediatric intensive care patients: epidemiology, risk factors, management, and outcome. Intensive Care Med. 2007;33:1272–83.
19. Ben-Ami R, Olshtain-Popsk KM, Oren I, Bishara J, Dan M, et al. Antibiotic exposure as a risk factor for fluconazole-resistant Candida bloodstream infection. Antimicrob Agents Chemother. 2012;56:2518–23.
20. Kovacicova G, Lovaszova M, Hanzen J, Roidova A, Mateicka F, Lesay M, et al. Persistent fungemia-- risk factors and outcome in 40 episodes. J Chemother. 2001;13:429–33.
21. Singhi S, Deep A. Invasive candidiasis in pediatric intensive care units. Indian J Pediatr. 2009;76:1033–44.
22. Jordan I, Balaguer M, López-Castilla JD, Belda S, Shuffelman C, Garcia-Teresa MA, et al. Per-species risk factors and predictors of invasive Candida infections in patients admitted to pediatric intensive care units. Development of ERICAP scoring systems. Pediatr Infect Dis J. 2014;33:e187–93.

23. Steinbach WJ, Roilides E, Berman D, Hoffman JA, Groll AH, Bin-Hussain I, et al. Results from a prospective, international, epidemiologic study of invasive candidiasis in children and neonates. Pediatr Infect Dis J. 2012;31:1252–7.

24. Kelly MS, Benjamin DK Jr, Smith PB. The epidemiology and diagnosis of invasive candidiasis among premature infants. ClinPerinatol. 2013;42:105–17.

25. Benjamin DK Jr, DeLong ER, Steinbach WJ, Cotton CM, Walsh TJ, Clark RH. Empirical therapy for neonatal candidemia in very low birth weight infants. Pediatrics. 2003;112:543–7.

26. Natarajan G, Lulic-Botica M, Aranda JV. Refractory neonatal candidemia and high-dose micafungin pharmacotherapy. J Perinatol. 2009;29:738–43.

27. Stoll BJ, Hansen N, Fanaroff AA, Wright LL, Carlo WA, Ehrenkranz RA, et al. Late-onset sepsis in very low birth weight neonates: the experience of the NICHD neonatal research network. Pediatrics. 2002;110:285–91.

28. Rolides E. Invasive candidiasis in neonates and children. Early Hum Dev. 2011;87 Suppl 1:S75–6.

29. Chapman RL, Faix RG. Persistently positive cultures and outcome in invasive neonatal candidiasis. Pediatr Infect Dis J. 2000;19:822–7.

30. Fisher BT, Vendetti N, Bryan M, Prasad PA, Russell Localio A, Damianos A, et al. Central venous catheter retention and mortality in children with candidemia: a retrospective cohort analysis. J Pediatric Infect Dis Soc. 2015;8:1–6.

31. Karadag-Oncel E, Kara A, Ozsurekci Y, Arikan-Akdagli S, Cengiz AB, Ceyhan M, et al. Candidemia in a paediatric Centre and importance of central venous catheter removal. Mycoses. 2014;58:140–8.

32. Oeser C, Lamagni T, Heath PT, Sharland M, Ladhani S. The epidemiology of neonatal and pediatric candidemia in England and Wales, 2000-2009. Pediatr Infect Dis J. 2013;32:23–6.

25

Correlation between antifungal consumption and the distribution of *Candida* species in different hospital departments of a Lebanese medical Centre

Lyn Awad[1†], Hani Tamim[2†], Dania Abdallah[3], Mohammad Salameh[4], Anas Mugharbil[5], Tamima Jisr[6], Kamal Zahran[7], Nabila Droubi[8], Ahmad Ibrahim[5] and Rima Moghnieh[9*]

Abstract

Background: In recent years, there has been a significant increase in the incidence of fungal infections attributed to *Candida species* worldwide, with a major shift toward non-*albicans Candida* (NAC). In this study, we have described the distribution of *Candida* species among different hospital departments and calculated the antifungal consumption in our facility. We also correlated the consumption of certain antifungals and the prevalence of specific *Candida species*.

Methods: This was a retrospective review of all the *Candida* isolates recovered from the computerised microbiology laboratory database of Makassed General Hospital, a tertiary care centre in Beirut, Lebanon, between January 2010 and December 2015. Data on antifungal consumption between January 2008 and December 2015 were extracted from the hospital pharmacy electronic database. We used Spearman's coefficient to find a correlation between *Candida* species distribution and antifungal consumption.

Results: Between 2008 and 2015, we observed that the highest antifungal consumption was in the haematology/oncology department (days of therapy/1000 patient days = 348.12 ± 85.41), and the lowest was in the obstetrics/gynaecology department (1.36 ± 0.47). In general, the difference in antifungal consumption among various departments was statistically significant ($P < 0.0001$). Overall, azoles were the most common first-line antifungals in our hospital. Echinocandins and amphotericin B were mostly prescribed in the haematology/oncology department. As for *Candida* species distribution, a total of 1377 non-duplicate isolates were identified between 2010 and 2015. A non-homologous distribution of *albicans* vs. non-*albicans* was noted among the different departments ($P = 0.02$). The most commonly isolated NAC was *Candida glabrata,* representing 14% of total *Candida species* and 59% of NAC. *Candida famata* (9% of NAC), *Candida parapsilosis* (3.6% of NAC) and *Candida krusei* (3% of NAC) were recovered unequally from the different departments. The total antifungal consumption correlated positively with the emergence of NAC. The use of azoles correlated positively with *Candida glabrata*, while amphotericin B formulations correlated negatively with it. None of these correlations reached statistical significance.

Conclusion: Different *Candida* species were unequally distributed among different hospital departments, and this correlated with consumption of antifungals in respective departments, highlighting the need for antifungal stewardship.

Keywords: Amphotericin B, Antifungal, Azoles, *Candida albicans*, *Candida glabrata*, *Candida famata*, Consumption, Correlation, Critical care, Echinocandins, Non-albicans *Candida*, Obstetrics, Oncology

---

* Correspondence: moghniehrima@gmail.com
[†]Lyn Awad and Hani Tamim contributed equally to this work.
[9]Head of Antimicrobial Stewardship Program, Makassed General Hospital, Beirut, Lebanon
Full list of author information is available at the end of the article

Background

In recent years, the world has witnessed a significant increase in the incidence of fungal infections due to *Candida* species [1], with *Candida albicans* (CA) being the most common causative organism [2]. However, recent studies have documented a change in this aetiology shifting toward non-*albicans Candida* (NAC) [3]. This shift has been linked to the selective pressure caused by the extensive use of broad spectrum antibiotics and antifungals [4]. For many years, azoles have been used as prophylactic agents against fungal infections in immunocompromised patients, as empiric/preemptive treatment of fungal disease in cancer or critically ill patients, in addition to their use as targeted therapy of *Candida* infections [1, 5]. However, polyenes consumption, especially lipid formulations with amphotericin B, has been used increasingly in the immunocompromised population [6], along with echinocandins, which were introduced into the market in 2002 [7].

The geographic distribution of *Candida* species may reflect the antimicrobial prescription habits in each healthcare facility [8, 9]. Multiple studies have looked at the relative distribution of *Candida* species with time [3, 8, 10]; however, few have studied its geographic distribution (i.e., in specific hospital departments along with corresponding antifungal expenditure) [8, 11]. Two studies demonstrated an increase in the incidence of *Candida parapsilosis* associated with the use of caspofungin [12, 13].

In this study, our primary aim was to calculate the consumption of each class of antifungals, and to describe the relative distribution of different *Candida* species in different hospital departments. The secondary aim was to find a correlation between the expenditure of certain antifungals and the prevalence of specific *Candida* species.

Methods

Setting and study design

This was a retrospective review of all *Candida* isolates retrieved from the computerised microbiology laboratory database at Makassed General Hospital (MGH), between January 2010 and December 2015. The MGH Institutional Review Board Committee granted this study approval. No informed consent was required due to it retrospective nature. The reporting of this study conforms to the STROBE statement [14]. MGH is a 186-bed university hospital in Beirut, Lebanon. The monthly occupancy rate ranges between 70 and 80%, with 17 beds in critical care, 71 beds in internal medicine (IM), 17 beds in haematology/oncology and bone marrow transplantation, 21 beds in surgery, 13 beds in obstetrics/gynaecology (OBGYN) and 47 beds in the paediatric departments. All *Candida* species reported in the database were selected, and non-duplicate isolates recovered during the study period were included in this study. All specimens from different culture sites, such as abscess, bronchoalveolar lavage, blood, catheter, ear, eye, fluid, sputum, deep-tracheal aspirate, throat, urine, vagina and wound were included, except for stool specimens.

Identification and speciation of Candida isolates

The identification and speciation of *Candida* isolates were performed according to the microscopic and macroscopic growth morphology and germ tube test. Isolates producing germ tubes within 3 h of incubation were further differentiated. Speciation of the *Candida* isolates was performed using the API 20 C AUX system (bio Merieux, France) [15]. Results were interpreted after 48 to 72 h of incubation at 29 °C ± 2 °C. Antifungal susceptibility testing is not available in our institution.

Protocol for antifungal use in our hospital

Broad-spectrum antifungals were prescribed on hospital setting for the management of invasive fungal infections according to institutional guidelines on antimicrobial use, which were based on international guidelines [16, 17]. Patient colonisation with *Candida spp.* such as in urine, sputum, skin or others was not usually treated with antifungals. Patients with evidence of candidemia or other invasive *Candida* infections were treated with antifungals [16]. Neutropenic patients with cancer were given prophylactic, empiric, pre-emptive or targeted antifungal therapy as per the clinical need [17]. In ICU, newly diagnosed septic patients without an evident focus of infection were evaluated by an Infectious Disease physician for the possibility of adding on systemic antifungals to their treatment regimens in the following cases: having already received broad-spectrum antibacterial therapy active against our nosocomial flora and having been colonized with *Candida species*. Systemic infections due to *C. albicans* and *C. tropicalis* were managed using fluconazole, while other NAC infections except for those caused by *C. krusei* were treated using echinocandins [16, 18]. *C. krusei*-related infections were given lipid formulation amphotericin B [16, 18].

Definitions

Non-duplicate isolates

When multiple isolates were obtained from the same patient, all species were included in the study, but only the first isolate of a given species was considered in the analysis [8].

Days of therapy (DOT)

The number of days that a patient was on an antimicrobial regardless of the dose [19].

Defined daily dose (DDD)

Corresponds to the assumed average daily dose of an antimicrobial for its main indication in adults based on the World Health Organisation Anatomical Therapeutic Chemical (WHO/ATC) classification system for each antifungal [20].

Patient days (PD)

Calculated by counting the number of patients present in any given location (e.g., hospital or ward) at a single time during a 24-h period [21].

Antifungal consumption

Data on antifungal consumption between January 2008 and December 2015 were extracted from the electronic database of the hospital pharmacy. Antifungals were categorised according to their pharmacological class: azoles (fluconazole and voriconazole), echinocandins (caspofungin, anidulafungin, micafungin) and polyenes (conventional amphotericin B and lipid formulations amphotericin B). We used two types of metrics to measure antifungal expenditure: DDD/1000 PD, and DOT/1000 PD [20, 22].

In paediatrics, the use of DOT is preferred because the antimicrobial doses are adjusted according to body weight, and there is no universal DDD [22]. In order to compare the antifungal consumption in the different hospital departments, including the paediatric department DOT/1000 PD had to be used. In the critical care and haematology/oncology departments, we used DDD/1000 PD to compare and benchmark with other studies in the published literature.

The DDD was 200 mg for fluconazole, 400 mg for voriconazole, 100 mg for anidulafungin, 50 mg for caspofungin and 100 mg for micafungin [20]. 19 There is no standardised DDD for the lipid formulations of polyenes [22, 23]. There is only a DDD for the amphotericin B deoxycholate (Fungizone®), which is 35 mg. Thus, for lipid-based formulations, we defined the DDD based on the regular daily dose used in our facility, which is 300 mg for both the liposomal and the lipid complex formulations.

Statistical analysis

The Statistical Package for Social Sciences (SPSS, version 21) program was used for data entry, management and analysis. Categorical variables are presented as number and percent, whereas continuous variables are presented as mean and standard deviation. Bivariate analysis was carried out using the chi-squared test for comparing categorical variables, whereas continuous ones were compared using the Student's t-test. The relationship between antifungal usage and the distribution of NAC was determined using the Spearman's coefficient for non-parametric correlation. A $P < 0.05$ was considered significant.

Results

Antifungal consumption

The rate of antifungal consumption in DOT/1000 PD and DDD/1000 PD are shown in Tables 1 and 2, respectively. All rates were reported as mean ± standard deviation. From 2008 to 2015, the mean total antifungal consumption, in terms of DOT/1000 PD was 180.69 ± 135.5.

Results in the two metric methods (DOT/1000 PD and DDD/1000 PD) revealed almost parallel patterns, with the exception of the azoles because the used daily doses of azoles in the hospital were much lower than the DDD, and were not consistent among different indications.

In general, the rate of antifungal consumption during the study period was not analogous among the different departments ($P < 0.0001$) (Table 1). In terms of DOT/1000 PD, total antifungal consumption was highest in the haematology/oncology department (348.12 ± 85.41), followed by critical care (73.85 ± 22.25), and was lowest in the OBGYN department (1.36 ± 0.47) (Table 1). The difference between the mean antifungal consumption in any two departments was statistically significant when compared to one another, with the exception of the consumption in the surgery department (33.56 ± 11.65) when compared to that in the paediatric department (28.70 ± 11.96), and the critical care department (73.85 ± 22.25) when compared to that in the IM department (56.48 ± 24.06), where the difference was non-significant ($P = 0.565$ and 0.23, respectively). Relative azole consumption mirrored total antifungal consumption, where the difference was statistically significant among the departments ($P < 0.0001$). Likewise, the highest consumption was seen in the haematology/oncology department (214.65 ± 47.67), and the lowest was seen in the OBGYN department (0.94 ± 1.10) (Table 1). Echinocandins

Table 1 Antifungal consumption in terms of DOT/1000 PD (mean ± SD) among different hospital departments between 2008 and 2015

Antifungal Class	Hospital Department						
	Critical care	Paediatric	Hem/Onc	OBGYN	Surgery	IM	P-value
Azoles	48.41 ± 14.58	23.29 ± 9.24	214.65 ± 47.67	0.94 ± 1.10	24.31 ± 10.24	46.44 ± 9.50	< 0.0001
Echinocandins	21.13 ± 27.26	1.35 ± 1.55	67.96 ± 19.04	0.42 ± 1.19	7.20 ± 11.25	7.69 ± 5.49	< 0.0001
Amphotericin B	4.32 ± 3.62	4.06 ± 3.36	65.50 ± 18.98	0	2.06 ± 3.62	2.34 ± 1.49	< 0.0001
Total	73.85 ± 22.25	28.70 ± 11.96	348.12 ± 85.41	1.36 ± 0.47	33.56 ± 11.65	56.48 ± 24.06	< 0.0001

KEY: *Hem/Onc* = Haematology/oncology, *IM* = Internal medicine, *OBGYN* = Obstetrics/gynaecology

Table 2 Antifungal consumption in terms of DDD/1000 PD (mean ± SD) among different hospital departments between 2008 and 2015

Antifungal Class	Hospital Department				
	Critical care	Hem/Onc	OBGYN	Surgery	IM
Azoles	33.79 (±10.98)	146.51 (±41.28)	0.56 (±1.03)	22.76 (±9.97)	39.73 (±7.25)
Echinocandins	11.36 (±8.33)	57.96 (±25.48)	0	4.38 (±8.27)	7.26 (±6.92)
Amphotericin B	4.29 (±4.36)	79.83 (±30.56)	0	0.50 (±0.98)	1.93 (±1.60)

KEY: *Hem/Onc* = Haematology/oncology, *IM* = Internal medicine, *OBGYN* = Obstetrics/gynaecology

were mostly used in oncology (67.96 ± 19.04), followed by a significantly lower consumption in critical care (21.13 ± 27.26, $P = 0.01$), and almost a null consumption in the paediatric and OBGYN departments (1.35 ± 1.55 and 0.42 ± 1.19 respectively, $P = 0.2$) (Table 1). Finally, conventional or lipid formulations of amphotericin B were mostly used in the haematology/oncology department (65.50 ± 18.98), followed by a similar distribution in critical care and paediatric departments (4.32 ± 3.62, and 4.06 ± 3.36, respectively, $P = 0.885$), then to a lesser extent in the IM and surgery departments (mean 2.34 ± 1.49, and 2.06 ± 3.62, respectively, $P = 0.840$). It was never used in the OBGYN department (Table 1). When antifungal consumption was measured in DDD/1000 PD, a similar trend was observed, excluding the paediatric department (Table 2).

Candida isolates distribution

Between 2010 and 2015, a total of 1377 non-duplicate *Candida* isolates were identified, including colonizers and pathogens. The majority of these isolates were recovered from urine (48%), followed by the respiratory tract (20% from deep-tracheal aspirate and 17% from sputum), and only 2% were from blood (Fig. 1).

The highest number of isolates was collected from the IM department (49%), followed by the critical care department (30%), the surgery (6%), paediatric (6%), haematology/oncology (5%) and OBGYN (4%) departments (Fig. 2).

General distribution of Candida species with a focus on NAC in different departments

In all departments and NAC isolation was statistically significant among hospital departments ($P = 0.02$) (Table 3).

In all departments, CA was the most commonly isolated species, representing 76% of total isolates (Fig. 3) and ranging from 91.4% in the OBGYN department to 70.8% in the surgery department (Table 4).

In terms of NAC, the OBGYN department had the lowest significant rate of NAC compared to the critical care, haematology/oncology and surgery departments ($P = 0.01$, 0.02, and 0.003 respectively).

The rate of NAC in the paediatric department was the second lowest compared to other hospital units (Table 4).

Distribution of different species of NAC

The most commonly isolated NAC in our facility was *Candida glabrata* (197 isolates), accounting for 14% of total isolates and 59% of total NAC. Non-speciated *Candida* followed, accounting for 3% of total isolates and 13.5% of total NAC. *Candida famata* came in third place, representing 2% of total isolates and 9% of total

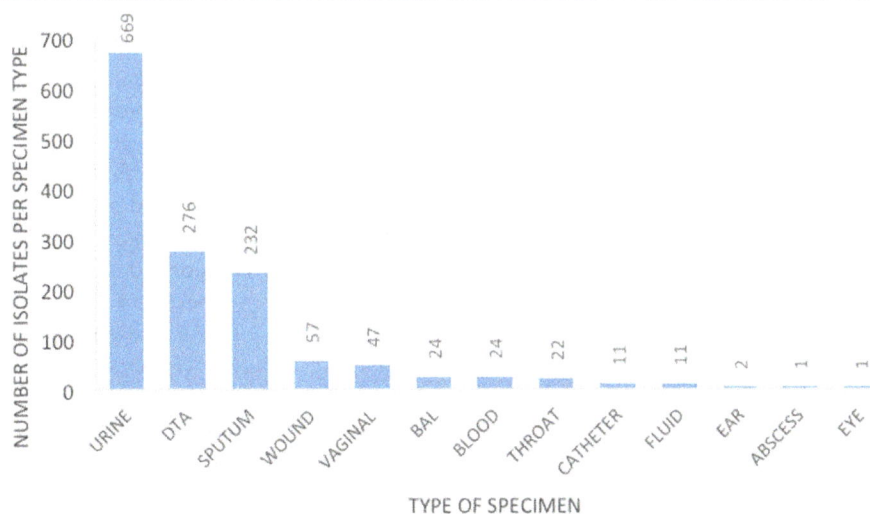

Fig. 1 Distribution of different specimens types growing *Candida* species. KEY: BAL = Bronchoalveolar lavage, DTA = Deep tracheal aspirate

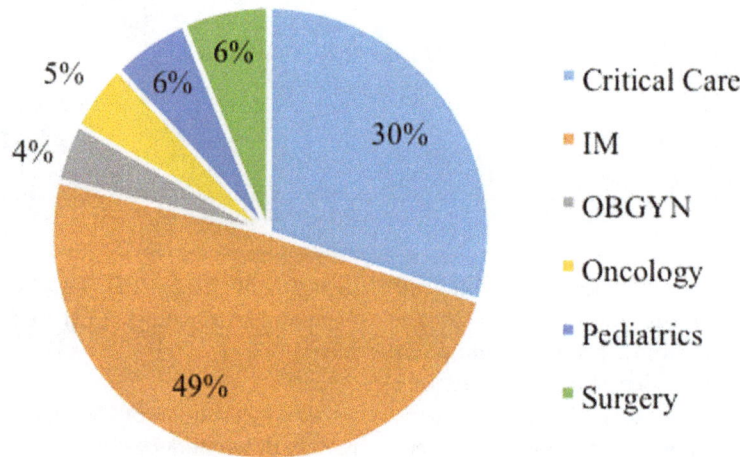

Fig. 2 Distribution of *Candida* isolates in the different hospital departments. KEY: IM = Internal medicine, OBGYN = Obstetrics/gynaecology

NAC. *Candida krusei* and *Candida tropicalis* represented 1 and 0.5% of the total isolates, respectively (Figs. 3 and 4).

Distribution of Candida glabrata in different departments
The proportion of *Candida glabrata* among NAC differed among the units. In OBGYN, *Candida glabrata* has been the only isolated NAC (100% of total NAC). The lowest rate of *Candida glabrata* among NAC was seen in the paediatric department (33% of NAC), and the haematology/oncology departments (47% of NAC) (Table 5) ($P = 0.03$).

Distribution of NAC other than Candida glabrata
The proportion of NAC other than *Candida glabrata* among different departments is presented in Table 3. There was less variability in the type of NAC in the OBGYN, haematology/oncology and paediatric departments in comparison with the IM, critical care and surgery departments.

The non-speciated *Candida* were mostly observed in the paediatric department (25% of NAC), followed by

Table 3 Distribution of *Candida albicans* versus non-albicans *Candida* among hospital departments between 2010 and 2015 and comparison between them

Department	Candida albicans (N = 1044 isolates)	Non-albicans Candida (N = 333 isolates)	P-value
Critical care	313 (76.3%)	97 (23.7%)	0.02
IM	498 (73.9%)	176 (26.1%)	
OBGYN	53 (91.4%)	5 (8.6%)	
Hem/Onc	50 (74.6%)	17 (25.4%)	
Paediatric	67 (84.8%)	12 (15.2%)	
Surgery	63 (70.8%)	26 (29.2%)	

KEY: *Hem/Onc* = Haematology/oncology, *IM* = Internal medicine, *OBGYN* = Obstetrics/gynaecology

the surgery (15% of NAC), IM (14% of NAC), critical care (12.4% of NAC) and oncology departments (6% of NAC). They were absent in the OBGYN department.

Second to *Candida glabrata* among the speciated *Candida*, *Candida famata* (9% of NAC) was the most common in all departments, with the exceptions of the paediatric and OBGYN departments.

Candida krusei (3% of NAC) was mostly recovered from the surgery and haematology/oncology departments, while it was absent from the OBGYN and paediatric departments.

Candida parapsilosis (3.6% of NAC) had the highest percentage among the speciated *Candida* isolates second to *Candida glabrata* in the paediatric department (25%).

Correlation between antifungal consumption and the isolation of specific Candida species
Using Spearman's coefficient, we observed that none of the correlations reached a statistical significance due to the limited number of hospital departments involved ($N = 5$); however, these results indicated some trends and showed clinical significance (Table 5).

The use of antifungals in general correlated positively with NAC [Spearman's Coefficient (SC) = 0.38]. The use of amphotericin B showed a similar yet weaker positive correlation for the emergence of NAC in comparison with azoles and echinocandins (SC = 0.27 vs. 0.40 and 0.39, respectively). The effect of azoles and echinocandins on recovery of NAC was almost the same.

Regarding *Candida glabrata* alone, the use of azoles correlated positively with its emergence (SC = 0.13), unlike the use of amphotericin B, which correlated negatively (SC = − 0.003).

We noticed that in wards where amphotericin B had been used (haematology/oncology and paediatrics, 19 and 14% from total antifungal consumption in each ward,

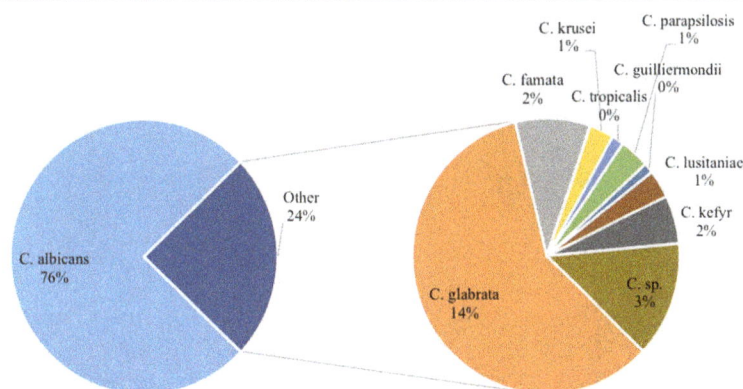

Fig. 3 Total distribution of the different *Candida* species in the hospital. KEY: C. sp. = Non-speciated *Candida*. N.B. Percentages are calculated from total *Candida* isolates recovered

respectively), there was less non-speciated *Candida* isolated from clinical specimens (Tables 1 and 5). We equally noticed less variability in the types of NAC recovered.

Discussion

The effect of antimicrobial use on the changing microbial ecology of inpatients in a specific healthcare facility is sure but slow, and the tangible consequences usually lag behind in time [24]. Accordingly, we reviewed antifungal consumption in different hospital departments from 2008 to 2015, and we studied the distribution of variable *Candida* species in the same departments during 2010 and 2015. Then, we attempted to find a correlation between the use of specific antifungals and the prevalence of specific *Candida* species.

Antifungal consumption in different departments

The discrepancies found between DOT and DDD per 1000 PD were due to the actual dosing of antifungals, especially the oral dosage form of fluconazole. The actual fluconazole doses that were used during the study period were below the DDD (200 mg actual dosing vs. 400 mg recommended dosing) for indications, including oral thrush and vaginitis.

In Lebanon, like in the Middle East and North Africa region, there are limited data about antifungal consumption. In our study, azoles were the most commonly used antifungals. Similarly, Al Othman et al. studied the burden and treatment patterns of invasive fungal infections in Lebanon and in the Kingdom of Saudi Arabia, in which they found that fluconazole was the most commonly prescribed antifungal as a first-line therapy (69%) [25]. The most common second-line antifungals were voriconazole (35%)/caspofungin (30%), followed by amphotericin B formulations in general [25]. In Europe, a multicentre French survey in 2012 involving 239 healthcare facilities similarly revealed that fluconazole

was the most frequently used antifungal agent in haematology units and intensive care units (ICUs) [26]. Antifungal expenditure recorded its highest levels in participating cancer centres, followed by university hospitals [26]. In our hospital, the haematology/oncology department showed the highest antifungal consumption.

The comparison of our antimicrobial expenditure with other studies is hindered by the fact that the metrics are not standardised across hospitals and countries. Some use the recommended daily dose (RDD)/100 PD, such as Germany [27]. Others use DDD/1000 PD as in the formerly stated French study [26]. Some use DDD/1000 inhabitants, such as the European Centre for Disease Prevention and Control [28]. In paediatrics, because the calculations become even more complicated due to weight-based dosing, we used DOT/1000 PD [22].

CA as the most commonly isolated species

CA was the most commonly isolated species (76% of total isolates) in our setting. So far in Lebanon, only two studies have described the distribution and epidemiology of variable *Candida* species in different medical institutions [10, 25]. In both of them, CA was the most commonly isolated species throughout the years (64% in 2007 [10], and 56% in 2011 [25]). In another neighbouring country, Turkey, CA was found to make up 59.5% of the total strains in various departments at the Izmir Hospital [29]. Similarly in Italy, CA was the most commonly isolated species (72.7%) in different departments of a tertiary care hospital over a three-year period [2]. These results show that, although it is clear that the rate of recovery of NAC is increasing, CA remains the most common *Candida* species in general.

Most commonly isolated NAC

The predominant speciated NAC in our study was *Candida glabrata* (59% of NAC, and 14% of total *Candida*). This finding was different from other Lebanese studies,

Table 4 Distribution of the different *Candida* species (number of isolates, %) among different wards between 2010 and 2015

Ward	Total	Total NAC	C. albicans (n = 1044)	C. glabrata (n = 197)	Non-speciated C. (n = 45)	C. famata (n = 30)	C. Kefyr (n = 19)	C. parapsilosis (n = 12)	C. lusitaniae (n = 11)	C. krusei (n = 10)	C. tropicalis (n = 5)	C. guilliermondii (n = 4)	P
Critical care	410	97	313 (76%)	60 (62%)	12 (12%)	12 (12%)	5 (5%)	3 (3%)	1 (1%)	3 (3%)	0	1 (1%)	0.005
IM	674	176	498 (74%)	106 (60%)	25 (14%)	11 (6%)	11 (6%)	5 (3%)	10 (6%)	4 (2%)	4 (2%)	0	
OBGYN	58	5	53 (91%)	5 (100%)	0	0	0	0	0	0	0	0	
Hem/Onc	67	17	50 (75%)	8 (47%)	1 (6%)	4 (23%)	0	0	0	1 (6%)	1 (6%)	2 (12%)	
Pediatrics	79	12	67 (85%)	4 (33%)	3 (25%)	1 (8%)	1 (8%)	3 (25%)	0	0	0	0	
Surgery	89	26	63 (71%)	14 (54%)	4 (15%)	2 (8%)	2 (8%)	1 (4%)	0	2 (8%)	0	1 (4%)	

KEY: *Hem/Onc* = Haematology/oncology, *IM* = Internal medicine, *NAC* = non-albicans *Candida*, *OBGYN* = Obstetrics/gynaecology
N.B. Percentages for *Candida albicans* are calculated from total isolates in each ward. Percentages for each of the non-albicans species are calculated from total NAC of each ward

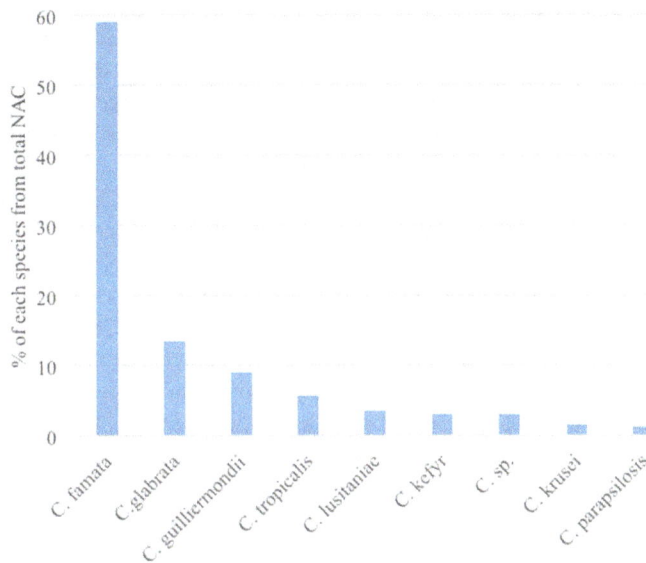

Fig. 4 Percentages of the different species of NAC from total NAC. KEY: C. sp. = Non-speciated *Candida*

in which *Candida tropicalis* was the most commonly iso-lated NAC (35–45% [10], and 20% [25], both of total iso-lates). This difference in species distribution between healthcare centres of the same country may be attributed to the selection bias used. In our study, we have included all non-faecal isolates of all departments, irrespective of their clinical significance, while in the two other studies [10, 25], the analysed isolates were retrieved from clinic-ally relevant specimens, either when speciation was per-formed based on the treating clinicians' requests [10], or in patients who warranted the use of antifungal therapy in special clinical circumstances [25].

Similar to our findings, *Candida glabrata* predomi-nated among NAC in many centres, such as in France (15% of total) [8] and in Turkey (14.4% of total) [29]. Yet, other NAC may prevail in other settings. For ex-ample, *Candida krusei* was the most common NAC

Table 5 Correlation of antifungal consumption (based on mean DOT/1000 PD) and non-albicans *Candida* isolation

		Non-albicans Candida	Candida glabrata
Total antifungals	Spearman's coefficient	0.38	0.12
	p-value	0.46	0.83
Azoles	Spearman's coefficient	0.40	0.13
	p-value	0.43	0.80
Echinocandins	Spearman's coefficient	0.39	0.18
	p-value	0.43	0.73
Amphotericin B	Spearman's coefficient	0.27	−0.003
	p-value	0.59	0.99

N.B. A positive value (Spearman's coefficient) represents a positive correlation and a negative value (Spearman's coefficient) represents a negative correlation

(12.9% of total *Candida*) in the Italian study, in which the majority of specimens were collected from patients with neutropenia [2]. Another example is the prevalence of *Candida tropicalis* in a tertiary care centre in India (46% of total) [30]. These incongruous findings of NAC distribution among different geographical zones, and even in different facilities in the same zone as in our country, highlight the importance of sample choice, anti-microbial prescription habits, the studied population, the unit(s) involved and the time frame of the study.

Distribution of different Candida species among the departments

The difference in the isolation of different *Candida* spe-cies among the departments was statistically significant in our hospital ($P = 0.005$) (Table 5). CA was the most common among all departments, with the highest pro-portion in the OBGYN department (91.4%), followed by the paediatric department (84.8%). In the Italian study, CA was found to be the most common *Candida* species (72.7%), with the following distribution among the dif-ferent departments: 64.2% in haematopoietic stem cell transplant units, 71.1% in the ICU, and 83.7% in paediat-rics ($P = 0.005$ and 0.01 when compared to paediatrics respectively) [2].

With regard to NAC in our series, *Candida glabrata* prevailed in the IM department (15.7% of total *Candida*). Likewise, in the Turkish study, investigators found *Candida glabrata* as the most common NAC in all de-partments, mostly in the infectious diseases department (40% of NAC) [29].

In critical care, the most common speciated NAC after *Candida glabrata* in our hospital was *Candida famata*

(12.4% of NAC), while in the study by Ece et al. [29], the most common NAC in the critical care/anaesthesiology department was *Candida krusei* (40% of NAC).

Candida parapsilosis is known to be a bloodstream isolate, and a common NAC in the paediatric population [31]. Our paediatric department had the highest rate of *Candida parapsilosis* (25% of NAC) compared to the other departments, but this was still less common than *Candida glabrata* (33% of NAC).

Therefore, the relative distribution of *Candida* species among different departments of the same hospital differs, with less CA in departments of the severely sick or immunocompromised patients. Among NAC, departments with critically ill and neutropenic patients had more non-*glabrata* NAC in their fungal ecology.

Correlations between antifungal consumption and Candida species distribution

The correlation between antifungal consumption and *Candida* species distribution in the literature is scarce. In a prospective multicentre French surveillance program on yeast bloodstream infections implemented in the ICU, haematology and surgery departments, involving all age groups, Lortholary et al. found that the use of echinocandins decreased CA emergence from 56 to 21% relatively to NAC [32].

Our study revealed that increasing overall consumption of antifungals and specifically azoles correlated positively with NAC, especially *Candida glabrata*. The use of azoles may exert a selection pressure, suppressing CA and fostering the growth of NAC since they are active against CA more than NAC [32].

Dagi et al. [33] determined the minimum inhibitory concentration (MIC_{90}) of different antifungals against 200 *Candida* spp. isolates from bloodstream infections between 2010 and 2013 at Selcuk University Hospital in Turkey. The MIC_{90} of antifungals against *Candida glabrata* was as such: 4 µg/mL for fluconazole, 0.12 µg/mL caspofungin and 0.06 µg/mL for anidulafungin. Based on this susceptibility of *Candida glabrata* to echinocandins, one would expect a negative correlation between them. However, our data did not show a negative correlation between the echinocandins and *Candida glabrata*. This lack of negative correlation may have been due to sampling bias whereby the majority of our specimens were from urine (Fig. 1). Despite moderate distribution of echinocandins into the kidneys, they exhibit negligible concentrations (< 2%) of intact drug in human urine. Thus, *Candida* growing in urine might not be affected by the use of echinocandins [34].

Unfortunately, antifungal susceptibility data of different *Candida* species is lacking in our study. This could have aided in interpreting Spearman's correlations, especially that reports about echinocandin resistance in

Candida glabrata have started to appear [35]. Alexander et al. tested the echinocandin susceptibility of all *Candida* species causing bloodstream infections between 2001 and 2010 at Duke University Hospital in the US and found that echinocandin resistance increased from 4.9 to 12.3% [35].

The Spearman's coefficient showed a weaker positive correlation of amphotericin B with the emergence of NAC compared to azoles (SC = 0.27 and 0.38, respectively) and a negative correlation between amphotericin B and *Candida glabrata* (SC = – 0.003). This could be explained by the fact that amphotericin B, unlike azoles, is equally active against most *Candida* species, including CA and NAC (except *Candida dubliniensis*) or more specifically *Candida glabrata* [36]. So its use in wards, such as paediatrics and oncology, might have buffered the selection pressure exerted by the azoles in promoting the growth of NAC or *Candida glabrata*.

The isolation of non-speciated *Candida* and *Candida famata* in our series (2% of total isolates, and 9% of NAC) is noteworthy. The emergence of non-classical *Candida* is increasingly reported in the literature. Between 2012 and 2015, a new species called *Candida auris* was reported from 3 continents, South East Asia (Pakistan, India), South Africa and South America (Venezuela), and has shown resistance to several classes of antifungals [37]. This change in *Candida* species epidemiology is in no doubt driven by antifungal consumption and thus highlights the importance of implementing antifungal stewardship.

Limitations and strengths

One limitation is that this study was single-centred, so our results could not be representative of the whole country. Another was the lack of antifungal susceptibility data in our facility that would have clarified the correlation between antifungal consumption and *Candida* species distribution. Another issue was that in some wards like the IM ward, some patients might have been clinically unstable necessitating ICU admission, or they might have been transferred early from the critical care unit when still unstable and on broad-spectrum antimicrobials due to shortage in ICU beds. These patients were counted as IM patients not as ICU patients. Consequently, the isolation of specific *Candida* species and antifungal consumption in the IM ward were affected by this occasional mixing of clinically stable and unstable patients. Nevertheless, this study is among the first studies in the region that describes antifungal consumption and relates it to *Candida* species distribution on hospital setting. We observed a clear difference in both elements among different wards, yet this difference would have been more significant if mixing in patient populations did not occur. In addition, this study describes overall

Candida ecology in one facility rather than being limited to *Candida*-related bloodstream infections.

Conclusion

Different *Candida* species are distributed unequally among the hospital departments of our facility, and this correlates with antifungal consumption. Our study highlights the need for benchmarking antifungal use, and standardisation of the metrics. Yet, the relationship between the changing *Candida* ecology according to the antifungal use highlights the strong need for antifungal stewardship to prevent reaching the era of predominant multi-drug resistant *Candida*.

Abbreviations

ATC: Anatomical Therapeutic Chemical; CA: *Candida albicans*; DDD: Defined Daily Dose; DOT: Days of Therapy; ICU: Intensive Care Unit; IM: Internal Medicine; MGH: Makassed General Hospital; MIC: Minimum Inhibitory Concentration; NAC: *Non-albicans Candida*; OBGYN: Obstetrics/Gynaecology; PD: Patient Days; RDD: Recommended Daily Dose; SC: Spearman's Coefficient; WHO: World Health Organisation

Acknowledgements

We would like to acknowledge Mr. Ziad Itani for providing technical assistance in data retrieval.

Funding

None.

Authors' contributions

LA, MS and KZ were responsible for data collection. HT and ND were responsible for data analysis. DA was responsible for result analysis and manuscript editing. AM and AI were in charge of study design and result analysis. TJ contributed to the microbiological analysis. RM majorly contributed to the study design and manuscript editing. All the authors have equally contributed to the drafting and reviewing of the manuscript. All authors read and approved the final manuscript.

Competing interests

The authors declare that they have no competing interests.

Author details

[1]Infectious Diseases and Antimicrobial Stewardship Clinical Pharmacist, Makassed General Hospital, Beirut, Lebanon. [2]Department of Internal Medicine, American University of Beirut, Beirut, Lebanon. [3]Pharmacy Department, Makassed General Hospital, Beirut, Lebanon. [4]Department of Internal Medicine, Makassed General Hospital, Beirut, Lebanon. [5]Division of Hematology/Oncology, Department of Internal Medicine, Makassed General Hospital, Beirut, Lebanon. [6]Department of Laboratory Medicine, Makassed General Hospital, Beirut, Lebanon. [7]Middle East Institute of Health, Bsalim, Beirut, Lebanon. [8]Pharmacy Department, Makassed General Hospital, Beirut, Lebanon. [9]Head of Antimicrobial Stewardship Program, Makassed General Hospital, Beirut, Lebanon.

References

1. Deorukhkar SC, Saini S. Non albicans Candida species: a review of epidemiology, pathogenicity and antifungal resistance. Pravara Medical Review. 2015;7(3):7–15.
2. Fadda ME, Podda GS, Pisano MB, Deplano M, Cosentino S. Prevalence of Candida species in different hospital wards and their susceptibility to antifungal agents: results of a three year survey. J Prev Med Hyg. 2008;49(2):69–74.
3. Milazzo L, Peri AM, Mazzali C, Grande R, Cazzani C, Riconi D, et al. Candidaemia observed at a university hospital in Milan (northern Italy) and review of published studies from 2010 to 2014. Mycopathologia. 2014; 178(3–4):227–41. https://doi.org/10.1007/s11046-014-9786-9.
4. Yang CW, Barkham TM, Chan FY, Wang Y. Prevalence of Candida species, including Candida dubliniensis, in Singapore. J Clin Microbiol. 2003;41(1): 472–4.
5. Ortega M, Marco F, Soriano A, Almela M, Martinez JA, Lopez J, et al. Candida species bloodstream infection: epidemiology and outcome in a single institution from 1991 to 2008. J Hosp Infect. 2011;77(2):157–61. https://doi. org/10.1016/j.jhin.2010.09.026.
6. Chandrasekar P. Management of invasive fungal infections: a role for polyenes. J Antimicrob Chemother. 2011;66(3):457–65. https://doi.org/10.1093/jac/dkq479.
7. Krcmery V, Kalavsky E. Antifungal drug discovery, six new molecules patented after 10 years of feast: why do we need new patented drugs apart from new strategies? Recent Pat Antiinfect Drug Discov. 2007;2(3):182–7.
8. Fournier P, Schwebel C, Maubon D, Vesin A, Lebeau B, Foroni L, et al. Antifungal use influences Candida species distribution and susceptibility in the intensive care unit. J Antimicrob Chemother. 2011;66(12):2880–6. https://doi.org/10.1093/jac/dkr394.
9. Falagas ME, Roussos N, Vardakas KZ. Relative frequency of albicans and the various non-albicans Candida spp among candidemia isolates from inpatients in various parts of the world: a systematic review. Int J Infect Dis. 2010;14(11):e954–66. https://doi.org/10.1016/j.ijid.2010.04.006.
10. Araj GF, Asmar RG, Avedissian AZ. Candida profiles and antifungal resistance evolution over a decade in Lebanon. J Infect Dev Ctries. 2015;9(9):997–1003. https://doi.org/10.3855/jidc.6550.
11. Guinea J. Global trends in the distribution of Candida species causing candidemia. Clin Microbiol Infect. 2014;20(Suppl 6):5–10. https://doi.org/10. 1111/1469-0691.12539.
12. Forrest GN, Weekes E, Johnson JK. Increasing incidence of Candida parapsilosis candidemia with caspofungin usage. J Inf Secur. 2008;56(2):126– 9. https://doi.org/10.1016/j.jinf.2007.10.014.
13. Paugam A, Baixench MT, Taieb F, Champagnac C, Dupouy-Camet J. Emergence of Candida parapsilosis candidemia at Cochin hospital. Characterization of isolates and search for risk factors. Pathol Biol (Paris). 2011;59(1):44–7. https://doi.org/10.1016/j.patbio.2010.08.009.
14. Von Elm E, Altman DG, Egger M, Pocock SJ, Gøtzsche PC, Vandenbroucke JP, Strobe Initiative. The Strengthening the Reporting of Observational Studies in Epidemiology (STROBE) statement: guidelines for reporting observational studies. PLoS medicine. 2007;4(10):e296.
15. Agha M, Agha SA, Sharafat S, Barakzai R, Zafar NU, Khanani MR, Mirza MA. API 20C: a reliable and rapid diagnostic tool for fungal infections. Gomal J Med Sci. 2012;10:237–40.
16. Pappas PG, Kauffman CA, Andes DR, Clancy CJ, Marr KA, Ostrosky-Zeichner L, Reboli AC, Schuster MG, Vazquez JA, Walsh TJ, Zaoutis TE. Clinical practice guideline for the management of candidiasis: 2016 update by the Infectious Diseases Society of America. Clin Infect Dis. 2015;62(4):e1–50.
17. Freifeld AG, Bow EJ, Sepkowitz KA, Boeckh MJ, Ito JI, Mullen CA, Raad II, Rolston KV, Young JA, Wingard JR. Clinical practice guideline for the use of antimicrobial agents in neutropenic patients with cancer: 2010 update by the Infectious Diseases Society of America. Clin Infect Dis. 2011;52(4):e56–93.
18. Lewis RE. Current concepts in antifungal pharmacology. Mayo Clin Proc. 2011;86(8):805–17.
19. Griffith M, Postelnick M, Scheetz M. Antimicrobial stewardship programs: methods of operation and suggested outcomes. Expert Rev Anti-Infect Ther. 2012;10(1):63–73. https://doi.org/10.1586/eri.11.153.
20. WHO Collaborating Centre for Drug Statistics Methodology. Guidelines for ATC classification and DDD assignment, vol. 2012. Oslo: World Health Organization; 2013. p. 250.
21. Ibrahim OM, Polk RE. Antimicrobial use metrics and benchmarking to improve stewardship outcomes: methodology, opportunities, and challenges. Infect Dis Clin N Am. 2014;28(2):195–214. https://doi.org/10. 1016/j.idc.2014.01.006.
22. Guillot J, Lebel D, Roy H, Ovetchkine P, Bussieres JF. Usefulness of defined daily dose and days of therapy in pediatrics and obstetrics-gynecology: a comparative analysis of antifungal drugs (2000-2001, 2005-2006, and 2010- 2011). J Pediatr Pharmacol Ther. 2014;19(3):196–201. https://doi.org/10.5863/ 1551-6776-19.3.196.
23. Valerio M, Munoz P, Rodriguez CG, Caliz B, Padilla B, Fernandez-Cruz A, et al. Antifungal stewardship in a tertiary-care institution: a bedside intervention. Clin Microbiol Infect. 2015;21(5):492 e1–9. https://doi.org/10.1016/j.cmi.2015.01.013.
24. Singer AC, Shaw H, Rhodes V, Hart A. Review of antimicrobial resistance in the environment and its relevance to environmental regulators. Front Microbiol. 2016;7:1728. https://doi.org/10.3389/fmicb.2016.01728.

25. Alothman AF, Althaqafi AO, Matar MJ, Moghnieh R, Alenazi TH, Farahat FM, et al. Burden and treatment patterns of invasive fungal infections in hospitalized patients in the Middle East: real-world data from Saudi Arabia and Lebanon. Infect Drug Resist. 2017;10:35–41. https://doi.org/10.2147/IDR.S97413.

26. Dumartin C, Rogues AM, Heriteau F, Pefau M, Bertrand X, Jarno P, et al. Antifungal use in France: first multicentre survey in haematology, intensive care units and at hospital level in 2012.Presented at ESCMID in 2016.

27. Gross BN, Steib-Bauert M, Kern WV, Knoth H, Borde JP, Krebs S, et al. Hospital use of systemic antifungal drugs: a multi-center surveillance update from Germany. Infection. 2015;43(4):423–9. https://doi.org/10.1007/s15010-015-0742-5.

28. European Centre for Disease Prevention and Control. Surveillance of antimicrobial consumption in Europe 2012. Stockholm: ECDC. p. 2014.

29. Ece G. Distribution of yeast-like fungi at a university hospital in Turkey. Jundishapur J Microbiol. 2014;7(12):e13141. https://doi.org/10.5812/jjm.13141.

30. Rajeevan S, Thomas M, Appalaraju B. Characterisation and antifungal susceptibility pattern of Candida species isolated from various clinical samples at a tertiary care Centre in South India. Indian J Microbiol Res. 2016; 3(1):53–7. https://doi.org/10.5958/2394-5478.2016.00014.5.

31. van Asbeck EC, Clemons KV, Stevens DA. Candida parapsilosis: a review of its epidemiology, pathogenesis, clinical aspects, typing and antimicrobial susceptibility. Crit Rev Microbiol. 2009;35(4):283–309. https://doi.org/10.3109/10408410903213393.

32. Lortholary O, Desnos-Ollivier M, Sitbon K, Fontanet A, Bretagne S, Dromer F, et al. Recent exposure to caspofungin or fluconazole influences the epidemiology of candidemia: a prospective multicenter study involving 2,441 patients. Antimicrob Agents Chemother. 2011;55(2):532–8. https://doi.org/10.1128/AAC.01128-10.

33. Dagi HT, Findik D, Senkeles C, Arslan U. Identification and antifungal susceptibility of Candida species isolated from bloodstream infections in Konya. Turkey Ann Clin Microbiol Antimicrob. 2016;15(1):36. https://doi.org/10.1186/s12941-016-0153-1.

34. Stone JA, Xu X, Winchell GA, Deutsch PJ, Pearson PG, Migoya EM, et al. Disposition of caspofungin: role of distribution in determining pharmacokinetics in plasma. Antimicrob Agents Chemother. 2004;48(3):815–23.

35. Alexander BD, Johnson MD, Pfeiffer CD, Jimenez-Ortigosa C, Catania J, Booker R, et al. Increasing echinocandin resistance in Candida glabrata: clinical failure correlates with presence of FKS mutations and elevated minimum inhibitory concentrations. Clin Infect Dis. 2013;56(12):1724–32. https://doi.org/10.1093/cid/cit136.

36. Sabatelli F, Patel R, Mann PA, Mendrick CA, Norris CC, Hare R, et al. In vitro activities of posaconazole, fluconazole, itraconazole, voriconazole, and amphotericin B against a large collection of clinically important molds and yeasts. Antimicrob Agents Chemother. 2006;50(6):2009–15. https://doi.org/10.1128/AAC.00163-06.

37. Lockhart SR, Etienne KA, Vallabhaneni S, Farooqi J, Chowdhary A, Govender NP, et al. Simultaneous emergence of multidrug-resistant Candida auris on 3 continents confirmed by whole-genome sequencing and epidemiological analyses. Clin Infect Dis. 2017;64(2):134–40. https://doi.org/10.1093/cid/ciw691.

26

Immunohistochemical characterization of the M4 macrophage population in leprosy skin lesions

Jorge Rodrigues de Sousa[1,2], Francisco Dias Lucena Neto[3], Mirian Nacagami Sotto[4,5] and Juarez Antonio Simões Quaresma[1,2,3,5,6*] (iD)

Abstract

Background: Since macrophages are one of the major cell types involved in the *Mycobacterium leprae* immune response, roles of the M1 and M2 macrophage subpopulations have been well defined. However, the role of M4 macrophages in leprosy or other infectious diseases caused by mycobacteria has not yet been clearly characterized. This study aimed to investigate the presence and potential role of M4 macrophages in the immunopathology of leprosy.

Methods: We analyzed the presence of M4 macrophage markers (CD68, MRP8, MMP7, IL-6, and TNF-α) in 33 leprosy skin lesion samples from 18 patients with tuberculoid leprosy and 15 with lepromatous leprosy by immunohistochemistry.

Results: The M4 phenotype was more strongly expressed in patients with the lepromatous form of the disease, indicating that this subpopulation is less effective in the elimination of the bacillus and consequently is associated with the evolution to one of the multibacillary clinical forms of infection.

Conclusion: M4 macrophages are one of the cell types involved in the microbial response to *M. leprae* and probably are less effective in controlling bacillus replication, contributing to the evolution to the lepromatous form of the disease.

Keywords: Macrophage, Immunohistochemistry, Mycobacteria, Immunology

Background

Leprosy is a chronic infectious disease caused by *Mycobacterium leprae*, an obligate intracellular bacillus that infects macrophages, dendritic cells, and Schwann cells [1, 2]. Leprosy is considered a neglected disease that represents a serious public health problem in developing countries [3, 4].

Clinically, leprosy shows spectral behavior in which the clinical evolution of the disease and associated histopathological changes are dependent on the host immune response. According to the Ridley-Jopling classification based on clinical, histopathological, immunological, and bacilloscopic criteria, leprosy presents in five main clinical forms: tuberculoid leprosy (TT), borderline-tuberculoid leprosy (BT), borderline-borderline leprosy (BB), borderline-lepromatous leprosy (BL), and lepromatous leprosy (LL) [5, 6].

The clinical evolution of the disease is closely related with the immune response triggered in the host. Given the spectral nature of the disease, with well-defined clinical and immunological presentations at each stage, leprosy represents an efficient model for investigating the host–parasite relationship [7, 8]. In the TT form, the cellular response is mediated by T helper (Th)1 lymphocytes, which produce cytokines that induce a pro-inflammatory response. In the LL form, the cellular immune response is characterized by the predominance of Th2 lymphocytes, which trigger a suppressive response. In the forms BT, BB, and BL, the cellular response presents a heterogeneous differentiation pattern that varies between the cellular responses in the TT and LL forms [1, 7, 8].

* Correspondence: juarez.quaresma@gmail.com
[1]Instituto Evandro Chagas, Secretaria de Vigilância em Saúde, Ministério da Saúde, Ananindeua, PA, Brazil
[2]Núcleo de Medicina Tropical, Universidade Federal do Pará, Belém, PA, Brazil
Full list of author information is available at the end of the article

Previous studies have shown that according to the evolution or chronicity of spectral diseases, certain cell groups show a response that polarizes between pro- and anti-inflammatory activities. In this context, macrophages belong to a group of cells associated with the innate immune response that undergo phenotypic modification and produce receptors, co-stimulatory molecules, enzymes, and cytokines that induce the development of the suppressive or inflammatory response [9–11].

In the TT form of leprosy, activation of the classical pathway by M1 macrophages induces the production of tumor necrosis factor-alpha (TNF-α), interferon-gamma (IFN-γ), and induced nitric oxide synthase (iNOS), which induce the generation of free radicals that destroy the bacillus [12]. Moreover, the LL form shows a predominance of M2 macrophages that induce the production of interleukin (IL)-10, transforming growth factor (TGF)-β, fibroblast growth factor (FGF)-β, arginase 1, CD209, CD163, and IDO, which contribute to the immunosuppressive response as well as tissue repair [13, 14].

There is growing evidence pointing to a new subpopulation of macrophages known as M4, which arise from M0 macrophages that change their behavior in the presence of CXCL4 to differentiate into M4 macrophages and produce CD68, IL-6, TNF-α, MRP8, matrix metalloproteinase (MMP)7, and MMP12 [15–17]. The first study on M4 macrophages showed their predominance in atherosclerotic lesions, which increase the expression of receptors for low-density lipoprotein (LDL), thereby provoking the accumulation of oxidized LDL in phagocytes and ultimately causing the development of atheroma plaques and oxidative lesions [18].

Although it is known that macrophages are the main cells participating in the host immune response against *M. leprae* infection, the behavior of this new M4 subtype of macrophages and their potential influence on the development of the in-situ immune response in the leprosy spectrum remain unknown. Such information could help broaden the discussion about the immunopathogenesis of the disease. Therefore, we investigated the responses of M4 macrophages in the polar forms of leprosy.

Materials and methods
Study design and participants
Biopsy samples of 33 untreated patients (25 men and 8 women) at the Center of Tropical Medicine, Federal University of Para, and Dermatology Department of State University of Para with a confirmed diagnosis of leprosy that was made according to the classification of Ridley-Joplin were analyzed in this study; 18 patients had tuberculoid leprosy (TT) and 15 had lepromatous leprosy

(LL). All patients were from the state of Para, Brazil, and their mean age was 25.6 years.

Histopathology and immunohistochemistry
For histopathological analysis, 5-μm thick slices were prepared from tissue biopsies, embedded in paraffin, and stained with hematoxylin and eosin.

Tissue-specific staining was achieved through immunohistochemistry using the biotin-streptavidin-peroxidase method with antibodies against CD68 (CM033C; Biocare Medical, Pacheco/CA, USA), MRP8 (ab92331; Abcam, Cambridge/MA, USA), MMP7 (ab205525; Abcam, Cambridge/MA, USA), IL-6 (ab154367; Abcam, Cambridge/MA, USA), and TNF-α (ab6671; Abcam, Cambridge/MA, USA). First, the tissue samples were deparaffinized in xylene and hydrated in a decreasing alcohol series. Endogenous peroxidase was blocked by incubating the sections in 3% hydrogen peroxide for 45 min. For antigen retrieval, the sections were incubated in citrate buffer (pH 6.0) at 90 °C for 20 min. Next, non-specific proteins were blocked by incubating the sections in 10% skim milk for 30 min. The histological sections were then incubated with the primary antibodies diluted in 1% bovine serum albumin for 14 h. Then, the slides were immersed in 1× phosphate-buffered saline (PBS) and incubated with the secondary biotinylated antibody [labeled streptavidin biotin (LSAB), Dako Cytomation] in an oven for 30 min at 37 °C. The slides were again immersed in 1× PBS and incubated with streptavidin peroxidase (LSAB) for 30 min at 37 °C. The reaction was developed with the addition of 0.03% diaminobenzidine plus 3% hydrogen peroxide as the chromogen solution. The slides were stained with Harris hematoxylin for 1 min, dehydrated in an increasing alcohol series, and cleared in xylene. CD68 and MRP8 double staining was conducted on the same histological sections, using streptavidin alkaline phosphatase and diaminobenzidine and as a chromogenic substrate (yielding a pink reaction product), according to the protocol described by Azevedo et al. [19].

Quantitative analysis and photodocumentation
The immunohistochemical staining-positive areas were quantified using as a criterion of positivity the brownish deposit to coincide with macrophage morphology in the granulomatous infiltrate in the dermis. Immunostaining was quantified in five randomly selected fields that were visualized under an Axio Imager Z1 microscope (model 4,560,006; Zeiss) at a magnification of 400× using a 0.0625-mm^2 grid with 10 × 10 subdivisions in the granulomatous inflammatory infiltrate, according to a previously described protocol [20–22].

Statistical analysis

Data were stored in electronic spreadsheets of the Excel 2007 program. Statistical analysis was performed using GraphPad Prism V.5.0. In univariate analysis, frequencies and measures of central tendency and dispersion were obtained. The Mann-Whitney t-test and Spearman correlation test were applied to test the hypotheses. A threshold significance level of 5% ($p \leq 0.05$) was adopted for all tests.

Results

Characteristics of the study subjects

The patients had altered tactile and thermal, and/or painful sensations on dermatoneurological examination. Patients with the TT form had cutaneous lesions consisting of erythematous or erythematous-hypochromic plaques with sharp edges and most anesthetic. Patients with the LL form had hypochromic spots and diffuse erythematous plaques and erythematous-violet or nodules that were infiltrated, bright, and sometimes coalescing. Histopathologically, the TT form was characterized by the presence of granulomas constituted of groups of epithelioid cells and sometimes surrounded by a dense or mild lymphocytic halo, with bacillus-negative status.

In the LL form, we observed granulomatous infiltrate consisting of histiocytes and plasma cells, extending along the entire upper dermis and surrounding the nerves and blood vessels, which could involve the deep dermis to the hypodermis and had bacillus positive status.

Immunohistochemical characterization of M4 macrophages

In tissue immunostaining, M4 macrophages were visible as depositions of brown-stained material in the cytoplasm or around cells, contrasting with the immunostaining-negative blue background (hematoxylin counterstaining). The presence of brown-stained areas coinciding with cell morphology was defined as a positive event. In the double staining experiment, brown-stained areas associated with pink-stained areas were areas positive for CD68 and MRP8. These criteria were adopted to minimize the counting of nonspecific staining, resulting in more accurate quantification.

Immunostaining for CD68 differed between the groups studied, with a significantly ($p < 0.0001$) lower median number of stained cells observed in the TT group (22.00 $\pm$ 3.55 cells/field) than in the LL group (61.00 $\pm$ 6.58 cells/field) (Figs. 1a, 2a and b). The median immuno-expression

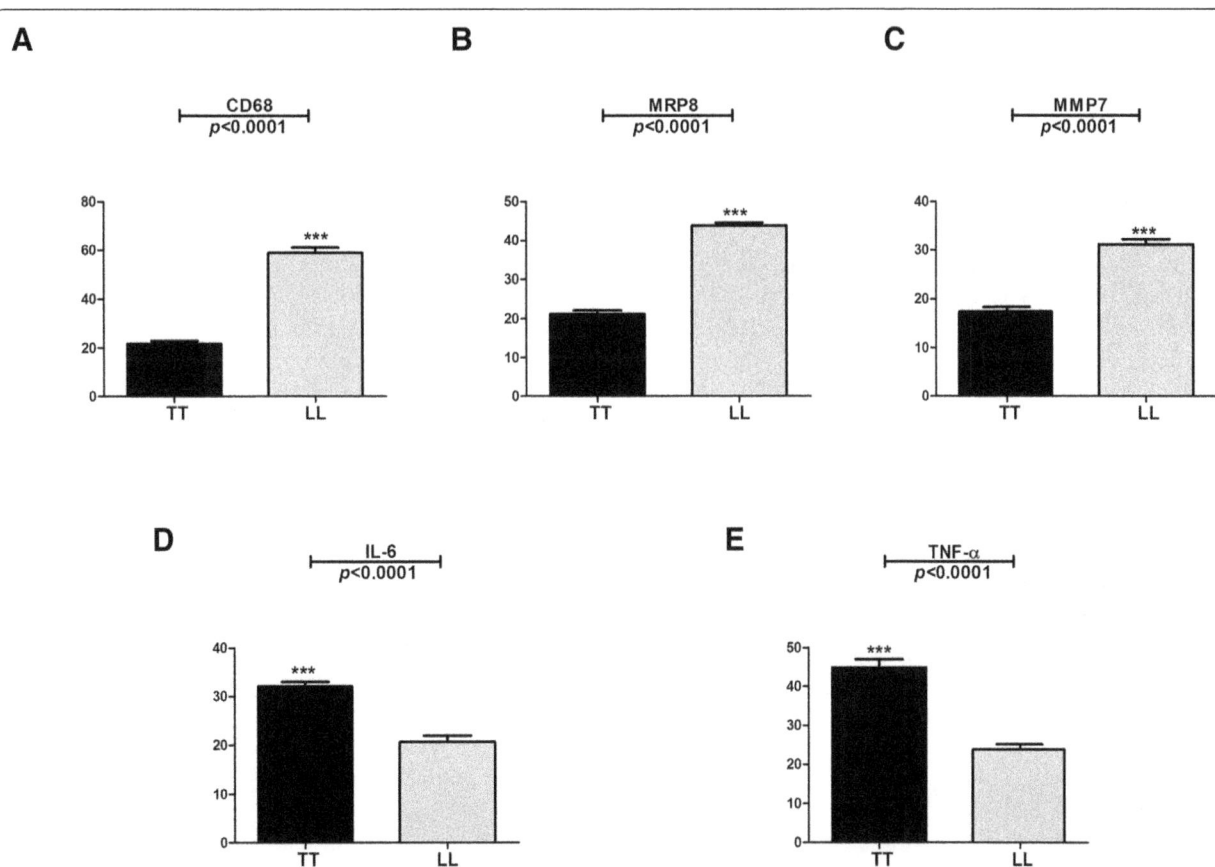

Fig. 1 Quantitative analysis for the immunostaining of CD68 (a), MRP8 (b), MMP7 (C) and IL-6 (d) and TNF-α (e) in TT and LL forms of leprosy

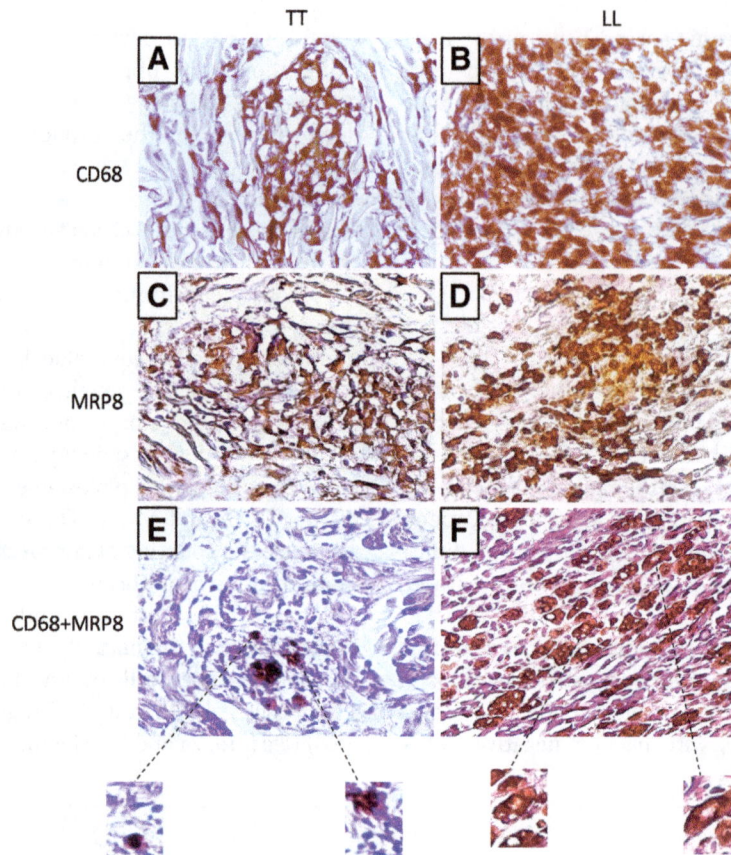

Fig. 2 Positive immunohistochemistry for CD68 (**a**: TT, **b**: LL), MRP8 (**c**: TT, **d**: LL) and double labeling for CD68/MRP8 (**e**: TT, **f**: LL) in TT and LL forms of leprosy

of MRP8 (Figs. 1b, 2c and d) and MMP7 (Figs. 1c, 3a and b) was also significantly (both $p < 0.0001$) lower in the TT group (MRP8: 21.50 ± 2.82 cells/field, MMP7: 17.00 ± 2.98 cells/field) than in the LL group (MRP8: 44.50 ± 2.57 cells/field, MMP7: 31.50 ± 3.44 cells/field). However, the immuno-expression of IL-6 and TNF-α was significantly (both $p < 0.0001$) higher in the TT group (IL-6: 32.00 ± 2.76 cells/field, TNF-α: 43.00 ± 6.81 cells/ field) than in the LL group (IL-6: 21.00 ± 4.30 cells/field, TNF-α: 24.00 ± 4.21 cells/field) (Figs. 1d, e, 3c-f). The double positive labeling for CD68 and MRP8 confirmed the presence of M4 macrophages in leprosy skin lesions (Figs. 2e and f).

Linear correlation analysis of immuno-expression in lesions of the TT and LL patients showed several positive associations, highlighting synergistic effects among CD68, MRP8, and MMP7 in the TT and LL forms (Table 1).

Discussion

Leprosy is an intriguing immunologic complex disease in which *M. leprae* causes granulomatous lesions and demyelination in the peripheral nerves [23, 24].

Leprosy is considered a spectral disease, with clinical and histopathological changes showing strong relationships with the pattern of the immune response triggered in the host [6, 25].

Macrophages belong to a select group of cells that differentiate, go through phenotypic modification, and participate in the microbicidal response in the activation of the classical pathway by M1 macrophages or in tissue repair in response to the action of M2 macrophages [26, 27]. Recently, the involvement of M4 macrophages in the pathogenesis of atherosclerosis has been recognized; however, the role of this new subtype in leprosy has not yet been investigated [28, 29].

The results obtained in the present study suggest that M4 macrophages have characteristics that imply they are probably ineffective in the microbicidal response to *M. leprae*, thus contributing to the development of clinical forms with more lesions and enhanced bacillary proliferation, as observed in the LL form. Within this context, the immunosuppressive behavior of M4 macrophages in inhibiting the microbicidal response [30, 31] strongly suggests a possible

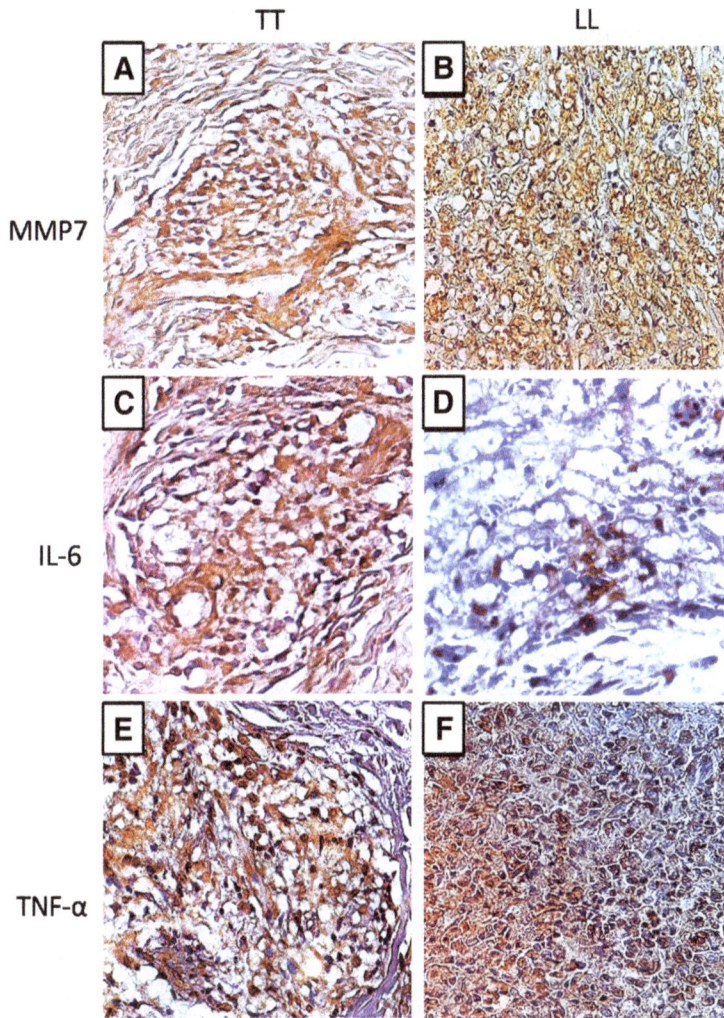

Fig. 3 Positive immunohistochemistry for MMP7 (**a**: TT, **b**: LL), IL-6 (**c**:TT, **d**: LL) and TNF-α (**e**: TT, **f**: LL) in TT and LL forms of leprosy

role in mediating the immune response in the LL form of disease.

The first report of the emergence of M4 macrophages showed that phagocytosis might be completely suppressed in these macrophages, which is likely directly related to the low expression of CD163, a scavenger receptor that recognizes hemoglobin/haptoglobin complexes [32]. In the LL form, this problematic characteristic of M4 macrophages might be crucial for maintaining the survival of the bacillus in the phagocytes owing to pathogen-triggered immune evasion. Therefore, the response of M4 macrophages as well as that of M2 macrophages suggests that the immunosuppressive environment established in the LL form of leprosy can restrict the microbicidal response to facilitate bacillus proliferation, resulting in more numerous lesions [13, 14].

Considering the cellular infiltrates, it is worth mentioning that the predominance of M4 macrophages in diseases such as atherosclerosis demonstrates that cells change their behavior favoring the appearance of foam cells and the development of an oxidative stress response inducing chemokine production and monocyte recruitment, thereby facilitating the accumulation of macrophages that express large amounts of LDL receptors [33, 34]. One of the greatest challenges associated with immunopathological studies of the LL form lies in understanding the activity of macrophages and the differentiation mechanisms that influence their morphological patterns [35]. Through the numerous changes that occur in the tissue environment, Virchow's cells emerge as part of the adaptive process, which demonstrates that in the chronicity of the inflammatory response, macrophages lose the ability to destroy the bacillus, and lipid degeneration caused by the oxidative stress favors the appearance of foamy macrophages with vacuoles containing large numbers of bacilli [35–37]. Through the immunolabeling of markers that

Table 1 Linear correlation analysis between markers that characterize the response of M4 macrophages in polar forms of leprosy

Correlation	TT	LL
CD68 x MRP8	$r = 0.7796$ $p = 0.0078$**	$r = 0.6821$ $p = 0.0298$*
CD68 x MMP7	$r = 0.6895$ $p = 0.0312$*	$r = 0.7222$ $p = 0.0183$*
CD68 x IL-6	$r = 0.6364$ $p = 0.0479$*	$r = 0.0615$ $p = 0.8993$
CD68 x TNF-α	$r = 0.6771$ $p = 0.0315$*	$r = 0.7477$ $p = 0.0129$*
MRP8 x MMP7	$r = 0.6895$ $p = 0.0312$*	$r = 0.6604$ $p = 0.0377$*
MRP8 x IL-6	$r = 0.4458$ $p = 0.1966$	$r = 0.2609$ $p = 0.4666$
MRP8 x TNF-α	$r = 0.2883$ $p = 0.4191$	$r = 0.2050$ $p = 0.5700$
MMP7 x IL-6	$r = 0.1734$ $p = 0.6319$	$r = 0.1486$ $p = 0.6820$
MMP7 x TNF-α	$r = 0.4939$ $p = 0.1468$	$r = 0.2724$ $p = 0.4463$
TNF-α x IL-6	$r = 0.4644$ $p = 0.1763$	$r = -0.1111$ $p = 0.7599$

characterize the response of M4 macrophages (CD68, S100A8, and MMP7), we observed a statistically significant difference in M4 macrophages in the LL form compared to the TT form.

Moreover, correlation analysis revealed an association between the expression of CD68, S100A8, and MMP7, which probably results in increased cellular activity in the polar disease forms. Of note, in the LL form, the expression of CD68, S100A8, and MMP7 was predominant in the inflammatory infiltrate composed of numerous foamy macrophages. The predominance of CD68 in the LL form of leprosy has been previously reported. Furthermore, the CD68 level is positively correlated with the production of iNOS in the microbicidal response in TT form of leprosy, which is one of the main enzymes that induce the production of NO and free radicals [38].

MRP8 (also known as S100A8 or calgranulin A) has been linked to numerous regulatory functions that modulate cell differentiation as well as phagocyte recruitment and activity [39, 40]. MRP8 exhibits ambiguous behavior in response to *Mycobacterium tuberculosis* infection. In macrophages infected with *M. tuberculosis*, MRP8 formed a complex with MRP14 that facilitated bacillus survival [41]. In contrast, other studies have shown that macrophages infected with *M. tuberculosis* or *M. leprae* had increased MRP8 activity of the phagolysosome, mainly due to the response of IL-22 [42, 43].

MMP7 (also known as matrilisin) is a zinc- and calcium-dependent endopeptidase that degrades the extracellular matrix and regulates various cellular processes, including cellular proliferation, tissue remodeling, the inflammatory response, and apoptosis [44, 45]. In an attempt to control the environment of tissue stress, increased MMP7 expression may mediate the tissue repair response by acting together with other cytokines, such as TGF-β and NGF, to promote tissue regeneration, and thus avoid the development of multiple lesions that are characteristic of LL clinical form [46, 47].

Finally, we investigated the expression levels of IL-6 and TNF-α in the TT and LL forms of the disease, and we found that both IL-6 and TNF-α are increased in the TT form. Classically, IL-6 and TNF-α are considered to be cytokines that are strongly associated with the development of the M1 macrophage response and induction of the microbicidal response. In the TT form, these cytokines also participate in the responses of the lymphocytes Th1, Th17, and Th22, thereby aggravating the tissue damage [43, 46, 47].

Conclusion

Our study demonstrated that the presence of M4 macrophages in the LL skin lesions may be involved in an infective immune response and consequently the survival of *M. leprae*. Previous findings on the pathogenesis of atherosclerosis and the formation of vacuolated macrophages morphologically similar to Virchow's cells support our immunohistopathological findings in the LL form of leprosy. Our data also suggest that these cells can induce the establishment of a regenerative environment and remodeling of the extracellular matrix, which are important for the pathogen–host interaction during infection by *M. leprae*. Further studies in experimental models are needed to elucidate the detailed mechanisms underlying the roles of M4 macrophages in the pathogenesis of leprosy lesions and provide further insights into the disease spectrum.

Acknowledgements
We thank the Department of Dermatology and Leprosy Service of Para State University for support in this study.

Funding
Dr. Juarez A. S. Quaresma is a Research Productivity Fellow and Senior Postdoctoral Fellow at the Brazilian National Council for Scientific and Technological Development – CNPq/Brazil (grants number 302553/2015–0 and 116427/2016–7).

Authors' contributions
JRS, FDLN, MNS, and JASQ contributed to research design, JRS and FDLN were involved in data acquisition and JRS, MNS, and JASQ were involved in data analysis and interpretation. All authors were involved in drafting and/or critically revising of the manuscript, and all authors approved the submitted final version.

Competing interests

The authors declare that they have no competing interests.

Author details

[1]Instituto Evandro Chagas, Secretaria de Vigilância em Saúde, Ministério da Saúde, Ananindeua, PA, Brazil. [2]Núcleo de Medicina Tropical, Universidade Federal do Pará, Belém, PA, Brazil. [3]Centro de Ciências Biológicas e da Saúde, Universidade do Estado do Pará, Belém, PA, Brazil. [4]Faculdade de Medicina, Universidade de São Paulo, São Paulo, SP, Brazil. [5]Instituto de Medicina Tropical de São Paulo, Universidade de São Paulo, São Paulo, SP, Brazil. [6]Núcleo de Medicina Tropical, UFPA, Av. Generalíssimo Deodoro 92, Umarizal, Belém, Pará 66055-190, Brazil.

References

1. Sousa JR, Pagliari C, de Almeida DS, Barros LF, Carneiro FR, Dias LB Jr, Souza Aarão TL, Quaresma JA. Th9 cytokines response and its possible implications in the immunopathogenesis of leprosy. J Clin Pathol. 2017;70:521–7.
2. Ogawa R, Hsu CK. Mechanobiological dysregulation of the epidermis and dermis in skin disorders and in degeneration. J Cell Mol Med. 2013;17:817–22.
3. Global leprosy update. 2016: accelerating reduction of disease burden. Wkly Epidemiol Rec. 2017;92:501–19.
4. Assembly WH. Global leprosy update, 2015: time for action, accountability and inclusion. Wkly Epidemiol Rec. 2015;91:405–20.
5. Talhari C, Talhari S, Penna GO. Clinical aspects of leprosy. Clin Dermatol. 2015;33:26–37.
6. Ridley DS, Jopling WH. Classification of leprosy according to immunity: a five-group system. Int J Lepr Other Mycobact Dis. 1966;34:255–73.
7. Aarão TL, Esteves NR, Esteves N, Soares LP, Pinto Dda S, Fuzii HT, Quaresma JA. Relationship between growth factors and its implication in the pathogenesis of leprosy. Microb Pathog. 2014;77:66–72.
8. Aarão TL, de Sousa JR, Botelho BS, Fuzii HT, Quaresma JA. Correlation between nerve growth factor and tissue expression of IL-17 in leprosy. Microb Pathog. 2016;90:64–8.
9. Mills CD. M1 and M2 macrophages: oracles of health and disease. Crit Rev Immunol. 2012;32:463–88.
10. Ouedraogo R, Daumas A, Ghigo E, Capo C, Mege JL, Textoris J. Whole-cell MALDI-TOF MS: a new tool to assess the multifaceted activation of macrophages. J Proteome. 2012;75(18):5523–32.
11. Mosser DM, Edwards JP. Exploring the full spectrum of macrophage activation. Nat Rev Immunol. 2008;8:958–69.
12. Simoes Quaresma JA, de Almeida FA, de Souza Aarao TL, de Miranda Araujo Soares LP, Nunes Magno IM, Fuzii HT, Feio Libonati RM, Xavier MB, Pagliari C, Seixas Duarte MI. Transforming growth factor β and apoptosis in leprosy skin lesions: possible relationship with the control of the tissue immune response in the Mycobacterium leprae infection. Microbes Infect. 2012;14:696–701.
13. Sousa JR, Sousa RP, Aarão TL, Dias LB Jr, Carneiro FR, Fuzii HT, Quaresma JA. In situ expression of M2 macrophage subpopulation in leprosy skin lesions. Acta Trop. 2016;157:108–14.
14. Moura DF, de Mattos KA, Amadeu TP, Andrade PR, Sales JS, Schmitz V, Nery JA, Pinheiro RO, Sarno EN. CD163 favors Mycobacterium leprae survival and persistence by promoting anti-inflammatory pathways in lepromatous macrophages. Eur J Immunol. 2012;42:2925–36.
15. Chistiakov DA, Bobryshev YV, Orekhov AN. Changes in transcriptome of macrophages in atherosclerosis. J Cell Mol Med. 2015;19:1163–73.
16. Butcher MJ, Galkina EV. Phenotypic and functional heterogeneity of macrophages and dendritic cell subsets in the healthy and atherosclerosis-prone aorta. Front Physiol. 2012;3:44.
17. de Paoli F, Staels B, Chinetti-Gbaguidi G. Macrophage phenotypes and their modulation in atherosclerosis. Circ J. 2014;78:1775–81.
18. Erbel C, Tyka M, Helmes CM, Akhavanpoor M, Rupp G, Domschke G, Linden F, Wolf A, Doesch A, Lasitschka F, Katus HA, Gleissner CA. CXCL4-induced plaque macrophages can be specifically identified by co-expression of MMP7+S100A8+ in vitro and in vivo. Innate Immun. 2015;21:255–65.
19. Azevedo RSS, de Sousa JR, Araujo MTF, Martins Filho AJ, de Alcantara BN, Araujo FMC, Queiroz MGL, Cruz ACR, Vasconcelos BHB, Chiang JO, Martins LC, Casseb LMN, da Silva EV, Carvalho VL, Vasconcelos BCB, Rodrigues SG, Oliveira CS, Quaresma JAS, Vasconcelos PFC. In situ immune response and

20. de Lima Silveira E, de Sousa JR, de Sousa Aarão TL, Fuzii HT, Dias Junior LB, Carneiro FR, Quaresma JA. New immunologic pathways in the pathogenesis of leprosy: role for Th22 cytokines in the polar forms of the disease. J Am Acad Dermatol. 2015;72:729–30.
21. Kibbie J, Teles RM, Wang Z, Hong P, Montoya D, Krutzik S, Lee S, Kwon O, Modlin RL, Cruz D. Jagged1 instructs macrophage differentiation in leprosy. PLoS Pathog. 2016;12:e1005808.
22. Sousa JR, Sotto MN, Simões Quaresma JA. Leprosy as a complex infection: breakdown of the Th1 and Th2 immune paradigm in the immunopathogenesis of the disease. Front Immunol. 2017;8:1635.
23. Gimblet C, Loesche MA, Carvalho L, Carvalho EM, Grice EA, Artis D, Scott P. IL-22 protects against tissue damage during cutaneous leishmaniasis. PLoS One. 2015;10:e0134698.
24. Neal JW, Gasque P. The role of primary infection of Schwann cells in the aetiology of infective inflammatory neuropathies. J Inf Secur. 2016;73:402–18.
25. Zhu TH, Kamangar F, Silverstein M, Fung MA. Borderline Tuberculoid leprosy masquerading as granuloma Annulare: a clinical and histological pitfall. Am J Dermatopathol. 2017;39:296–9.
26. Sica A, Mantovani A. Macrophage plasticity and polarization: invivoveritas. J Clin Invest. 2012;122:787–95.
27. Wang N, Liang H, Zen K. 2014. Molecular mechanisms that influence the macrophage M1–M2 polarization balance. Front Immunol. 2014;5:614.
28. Oksala NKJ, Seppälä I, Rahikainen R, Mäkelä KM, Raitoharju E, Illig T, Klopp N, Kholova I, Laaksonen R, Karhunen PJ, Hytönen VP, Lehtimäki T. Synergistic Expression of Histone Deacetylase 9 and Matrix Metalloproteinase 12 in M4 Macrophages in Advanced Carotid Plaques. Eur J Vasc Endovasc Surg. 2017;53:632–40.
29. Liberale L, Dallegri F, Montecucco F, Carbone F. Pathophysiological relevance of macrophage subsets in atherogenesis. Thromb Haemost. 2017;117:7–18.
30. Nikiforov NG, Kornienko VY, Karagodin VP, Orekhov AN. Macrophage activation in atherosclerosis. Message 1: Activation of macrophages normally and in atherosclerotic lesions. Patol Fiziol Eksp Ter. 2015;3:128–31.
31. Lu X. Impact of macrophages in atherosclerosis. Curr Med Chem. 2016;23:1926–37.
32. Colin S, Chinetti-Gbaguidi G, Staels B. Macrophage phenotypes in atherosclerosis. Immunol Rev. 2014;262:153–66.
33. Erbel C, Wolf A, Lasitschka F, Linden F, Domschke G, Akhavanpoor M, Doesch AO, Katus HA, Gleissner CA. Prevalence of M4 macrophages within human coronary atherosclerotic plaques is associated with features of plaque instability. Int J Cardiol. 2015;186:219–25.
34. Ley K, Miller YI, Hedrick CC. Monocyte and macrophage dynamics during atherogenesis. Arterioscler Thromb Vasc Biol. 2011;31:1506–16.
35. Elamin AA, Stehr M, Singh M. Lipid Droplets and Mycobacterium leprae Infection. J Pathol 2012;2012:361374.
36. Kaur G, Kaur J. Multifaceted role of lipids in Mycobacterium leprae. Future Microbiol. 2017;12:315–35.
37. Mattos KA, Lara FA, Oliveira VG, Rodrigues LS, D'Avila H, Melo RC, Manso PP, Sarno EN, Bozza PT, Pessolani MC. Modulation of lipid droplets by Mycobacterium leprae in Schwann cells: a putative mechanism for host lipid acquisition and bacterial survival in phagosomes. Cell Microbiol. 2011;13:259–73.
38. Sousa JR, Sousa RPM, Souza Aarão TL, Dias LB Jr, Oliveira Carneiro FR, Simões Quaresma JA. Response of iNOS and its relationship with IL-22 and STAT3 in macrophage activity in the polar forms of leprosy. Acta Trop. 2017;171:74–9.
39. Schrezenmeier EV, Barasch J, Budde K, Westhoff T, Schmidt-Ott KM. Biomarkers in acute kidney injury - pathophysiological basis and clinical performance. Acta Physiol. 2017;219:554–72.
40. Pruenster M, Vogl T, Roth J, Sperandio M. S100A8/A9: From basic science to clinical application. Pharmacol Ther. 2016;167:120–31.
41. Pechkovsky DV, Zalutskaya OM, Ivanov GI, Misuno NI. Calprotectin (MRP8/14 protein complex) release during mycobacterial infection in vitro and in vivo. FEMS Immunol Med Microbiol. 2000;29:27–33.
42. Dhiman R, Venkatasubramanian S, Paidipally P, Barnes PF, Tvinnereim A, Vankayalapati R. Interleukin 22 inhibits intracellular growth of

Mycobacterium tuberculosis by enhancing calgranulin A expression. J Infect Dis. 2014;209:578–87.

43. Gimblet C, Loesche MA, Carvalho L, Carvalho EM, Grice EA, Artis D, Scott P. IL-22 protects against tissue damage during cutaneous leishmaniasis. PLoS One.. 2015;10:e0134698.

44. He W, Tan RJ, Li Y, Wang D, Nie J, Hou FF, Liu Y. Matrix metalloproteinase-7 as a surrogate marker predicts renal Wnt/β-catenin activity in CKD. J Am Soc Nephrol. 2012;23:294–304.

45. Chakraborti S, Mandal M, Das S, Mandal A, Chakraborti T. Regulation of matrix metalloproteinases: an overview. Mol Cell Biochem. 2003;253:269–85.

46. Saini C, Siddiqui A, Ramesh V, Nath I. Leprosy Reactions Show Increased Th17 Cell Activity and Reduced FOXP3+ Tregs with Concomitant Decrease in TGF-β and Increase in IL-6. PLoS Negl Trop Dis. 2016;10:e0004592.

47. Quaresma JAS, Almeida FA, Aarao TLS, Soares LPMA, Magno IMN, Fuzii HT, Libonati RMF, Xavier MB, Pagliari C, Duarte MIS. Transforming growth factor β and apoptosis in leprosy skin lesions: possible relationship with the control of the tissue immune response in the Mycobacterium leprae infection. Microbes Infect. 2010;14:696–701.

27

Seroprevalence and distribution of leptospirosis serovars among wet market workers in northeastern, Malaysia: a cross sectional study

Mas Harithulfadhli Agus Ab Rahman[1], Suhaily Mohd Hairon[1], Rukman Awang Hamat[2],
Tengku Zetty Maztura Tengku Jamaluddin[2], Mohd Nazri Shafei[1], Norazlin Idris[1], Malina Osman[2], Surianti Sukeri[1],
Zainudin A. Wahab[3], Wan Mohd Zahiruddin Wan Mohammad[1], Zawaha Idris[4] and Aziah Daud[1*]

Abstract

Background: Leptospirosis is a zoonotic disease associated with occupations which exposed workers to environments contaminated with urine of infected animals. The objective of this study was to determine the seroprevalence of leptospirosis among wet market workers in Kelantan.

Methods: A cross sectional study was conducted in two main wet markets in Kelantan and 232 wet market workers were randomly selected. Blood samples were analysed for microscopic agglutination test (MAT) against 20 live leptospirosis reference serovars. MAT titres of 1:100 or more were considered as seropositive.

Results: It was found that the overall seroprevalence for leptospirosis among the respondents was 33.6% (95% CI = 27.5, 39.7). The samples were tested positive against serovars *Melaka* (IMR LEP 1), *Terengganu* (IMR LEP 115), *Sarawak* (IMR LEP 175), *Copenhageni* (IMR LEP 803/11), *Hardjobovis* (IMR LEP 27), *Australis, Autumnalis, Bataviae, Canicola, Grippotyphosa, Hardjoprajitno, Icterohaemorrhagiae, Javanica, Pyrogenes, Terrasovi, Djasiman, Patoc* and *Pomona*. The predominant serovars was *Autumnalis* (18.2%).

Conclusion: Wet markets workers were at risk for leptospirosis infection evidenced by high seroprevalence of leptospirosis in this study. Further research need to be conducted to determine factors that favours infection in this groups.

Keywords: Leptospirosis, Seroprevalence, Wet market workers, High risk group

Background

Leptospirosis is a worldwide zoonotic disease caused by spiral-shaped bacteria of the genus *Leptospira* which can be categorized into pathogenic and saprophytic groups. The pathogenic groups caused disease in human and become the concern of health authority. More than 250 *Leptospira* serovars have been recognized all over the world [1]. *In Malaysia, 37 serovars of Leptospira have been identified from human and animal samples* [2].

Human leptospirosis is acquired through contact with urine of infected animals, either directly or indirectly. Rodents were the natural reservoirs for the bacteria. Other infected animals including horses, cows, goats, pigs, cats and dogs can be carriers for the bacteria if they are not treated. These animals can excrete leptospires through urine during their lifetime and contaminate the environment. The bacteria can gain entry into the human ecosystem through cuts in skin and mucous membranes [3]. Infected humans develop a spectrum of symptoms that can mimic other febrile illnesses including dengue, malaria and typhoid [4].

Leptospirosis causes significant morbidity and mortality with an estimation of more than one million cases and

* Correspondence: aziahkb@usm.my
[1]Department of Community Medicine, School of Medical Sciences, Universiti Sains Malaysia, 16150 Kubang Kerian, Kelantan, Malaysia
Full list of author information is available at the end of the article

58,900 deaths worldwide on an annual basis. The majority of the cases happen in tropical and the world's poorest regions such as South and Southeast Asia [5]. Figures on leptospirosis can potentially be higher than reported since the true extent of cases remains unknown due to difficulty in diagnosing the condition and lack of systematic surveillance [6]. In Malaysia, leptospirosis is endemic, and the number of cases showed an increasing trend over the years and is becoming a genuine public health challenge [7].

Certain groups have been recognized to have a higher risk of infection due to the increased likelihood of contact with contaminated animals or environments [4]. Leptospirosis has been recognized as a hazard in certain occupations with increased exposure to infected animal such as agricultural workers, sewage workers, military personnel, veterinary and animal handlers [8, 9].

Another potential group at risk are wet market workers. Wet markets are places where people sell fresh meat and produce. Human activities at wet markets can provide a suitable environment and a rich source of food favouring the presence of rodents. Studies on rodents and environmental samples at wet market areas showed presence of pathogenic *Leptospira species* [10–12]. Hence, the aim of this study was to determine the seroprevalence of leptospirosis among wet market workers in Kelantan, Malaysia.

Methods

A cross sectional study was conducted in two main wet markets in Kelantan, which is in the northeastern part of Peninsular Malaysia. This study was carried out from January to June 2017. Two main wet markets selected for this study were Siti Khadijah Market in the Kota Bharu district and Pasir Mas Market in Pasir Mas district. In 2014, Kota Bharu and Pasir Mas districts had recorded the highest number of leptospirosis cases in Kelantan and these wet markets were selected as they were the largest wet markets in the areas. Systematic random sampling was used to select participants from list of wet market workers obtained from the local municipals. A total of 232 workers from those wet markets were selected in this study. Sample size was calculated using one proportion formula and $p = 0.35$ [13] was used as a reference. Workers who were at the age of 18 years or above and worked for at least three months at the wet markets were eligible for inclusion in the study. Non-citizen and workers who were not available during the study period were excluded from the study.

Before the conduct of the study, ethical clearance was obtained from Research and Ethic Committee (Human), School of Medical Sciences, Health Campus, Universiti Sains Malaysia (USM/JEPeM/15120552). The study was explained in sufficient detail and written consent was obtained from all participants. A proforma was used to gather information on sociodemographic and professional information of the participants. Venous blood samples were collected from the participants using standard procedures [14]. The blood samples were then centrifuged for 10 min at 1300 to 2000 rpm. The separated serum was kept in a plastic screw-cap vial and stored at -20 °C until MAT was performed.

A microscopic agglutination test (MAT) was carried out at the Microbiology Laboratory of Universiti Putra Malaysia following standard methods. Serum samples were serially diluted in microtiter plates and live leptospires representing 20 reference serovars were added to each well. The plates were then incubated for two hours at 30 °C and examined using dark field microscope. The mixture was considered as positive when it showed 50% agglutination leaving 50% free cells compare to the control culture. MAT titre of 1:100 or more was used as cut off point for seropositive result [4]. This cut off point had also been used in other seroprevalence studies [13, 15].

The samples were tested for leptospiral antibodies against 20 live reference serovars as recommended by the Institute for Medical Research (IMR), Malaysia. The types of *Leptospira* tested for this study were from serovars *Melaka* (IMR LEP 1), *Terengganu* (IMR LEP 115), *Sarawak* (IMR LEP 175), *Copenhageni* (IMR LEP 803/11), *Hardjobovis* (IMR LEP 27), *Lai, Australis, Autumnalis, Bataviae, Canicola, Celledoni, Grippotyphosa, Hardjoprajitno, Icterohaemorrhagiae, Javanica, Pyrogenes, Terrasovi, Djasiman, Patoc* and *Pomona* [16].

Data were analysed using IBM SPSS statistics version 24.0. Numerical variables were presented as means and standard deviations (SD) whereas categorical data were presented as frequencies and percentages. The seroprevalence was calculated by dividing number of positive MAT over total samples and presented as percentage with 95% confidence interval (CI).

Results

A total of 232 wet market workers participated in this study. Table 1 shows the characteristics of the participants. All of them were Malays. The mean (SD) age was 42.6 (14.7) years old with the age range of 18 to 79 years old. Majority of them were female and 77.2% were married. Regarding level of education, more than half of the participants had at least attended secondary school. Out of 232 blood samples tested for antibodies against leptospirosis, 78 samples were positive, defining the overall seroprevalence of leptospirosis among wet market workers at 33.6% (95% CI = 27.5, 39.7). Both markets had similar results with 39 out of 116 workers were tested positive (33.6%).

Table 2 shows the distribution of positive leptospirosis serovars tested in this study. Respondents in this study

Table 1 Socio-demographic characteristics of respondents (n = 232)

Variables	Frequency (%)		
	Overall n = 232	Siti Khadijah market n = 116	Pasir mas market n = 116
Age	42.6 (14.7) [a]	42.0 (15.5)[a]	43.0 (13.8)[a]
Gender			
Male	83 (35.8)	34 (29.3)	51 (44.0)
Female	149 (64.2)	82 (70.7)	65 (56.0)
Ethnicity			
Malay	232 (100)	116 (100)	116 (100)
Marital Status			
Single/widower	53 (19.0)	30 (25.8)	23 (19.8)
Married	179 (77.2)	86 (74.2)	93 (80.2)
Educational Level			
No formal education	19 (8.2)	8 (6.9)	11 (9.5)
Primary school	30 (12.9)	14 (12.1)	16 (13.8)
Secondary school	137 (59.1)	64 (55.2)	73 (62.9)
Form 6/Diploma/Others	46 (19.8)	30 (25.9)	16 (13.8)

[a]Mean (SD)

Table 2 Serovars distribution among positive MAT results on all serovars (n = 137)

Serovars	Overall		Siti Khadijah market		Pasir mas market	
	Frequency (n = 137)	Percentage (%)	Frequency (n = 68)	Percentage (%)	Frequency (n = 69)	Percentage (%)
Autumnalis	25	18.2	8	11.8	17	24.6
Sarawak (IMR LEP 175)	21	15.4	13	19.1	8	11.6
Copenhageni (IMR LEP 803/11)	12	8.8	8	11.8	4	5.8
Canicola	10	7.3	8	11.8	2	2.9
Djasiman	9	6.6	5	7.4	4	5.8
Australis	8	5.8	2	2.9	6	8.7
Patoc	8	5.8	3	4.4	5	7.2
Hardjoprajitno	7	5.1	1	1.5	6	8.7
Pyrogenes	7	5.1	4	5.8	3	4.3
Tarassovi	6	4.4	6	8.8	0	0.0
Pomona	6	4.4	4	5.8	2	2.9
Javanica	5	3.6	1	1.5	4	5.8
Icterohaemorrhagiae	4	2.9	0	0.0	4	5.8
Grippotyphosa	3	2.2	2	2.9	1	1.5
Hardjobovis (IMR LEP 27)	2	1.5	1	1.5	1	1.5
Bataviae	2	1.5	0	0.0	2	2.9
Melaka (IMR LEP 1)	1	0.7	1	1.5	0	0.0
Terengganu (IMR LEP 115)	1	0.7	1	1.5	0	0.0

Respondents can be positive to more than one serovars
Total of 137 positive MAT results on all serovars

can be positive to more than one leptospiral serovars. Out of 20 live reference serovars used for MAT analysis, 18 serovars were tested positive to at least one serum sample. Serovars *Autumnalis, Sarawak* (IMR LEP 175) and *Copenhageni* (IMR LEP 803/11) were the most common serovars to be positive by MAT which contributed more than one third of positive MAT results. No samples were positive for serovars *Lai* and *Celledoni*.

Table 3 shows the MAT results according to products sold by the participants. The highest seroprevalence was noted in participants who sold processed food (36.4%). It was followed by other products (34.7%), fresh meat and fish (31.6%) and fruits and vegetables (25.7%).

Discussion

Leptospirosis has long been associated with occupations and activities that increase interactions between humans, animals and contaminated environments. Both wild and domestic animals can spread *Leptospira* through their urine. However, most human infections have been attributed to rodents [2]. Environments at wet market areas have provided a favourable condition for rodents' infestation due to availability of foods and breeding place. Unhygienic conditions, open sewers and poor drainage at wet markets further attract these pests to populate the areas. The wet and moist conditions which are common in wet markets are also suitable for survival of *Leptospira* where they can survive for several weeks in stagnant water and wet soil [17].

The result of this study showed high seroprevalence of leptospirosis among wet market workers in Kelantan. This outcome supports the suspicion on risk of leptospirosis to wet market workers as they are exposed to contaminated environments and rodents at their workplace. These are supported by previous studies which noted the presence of pathogenic *Leptospira spp* in soil and water samples taken from wet markets areas [10, 11]. Azali et al. (2016) reported that 19.4% water samples taken from market areas were positive for *Leptospira spp* [10] whereas Benacer et al (2013) found that 23.1% of water and 23.3% of soil cultures were positive for *Leptospira spp* [11]. Study on rodents from wet

market areas in Kuala Lumpur by Benacer et al. (2013) also noted the presence of pathogenic *Leptospira spp* in the animal samples [12].

Studies on high risk groups showed a wide range of seroprevalence for leptospirosis. This indicates different degrees of exposure to contaminated environments and animals. Shafei et al. (2012) reported overall seroprevalence of 24.7% among town service workers in a study done in Kota Bharu, Kelantan [15]. The seroprevalence varies according to job categories which were garbage collector (27.4%), landscaper (23.8%), town cleaner (26.0%) and lorry driver (17.9%). Work activities and duration of exposure to contaminated environments have contribute to high seroprevalence among garbage collectors. Another study which was conducted among 350 high-risk palm oil planters in the southern state of Malaysia showed an overall seroprevalence of 28.6%. The seroprevalence ranged from 21.1 to 59.2% between different job categories. Fruit collectors, harvesters and pesticide applicators were job categories with the highest seroprevalence due to longer contact with polluted soil and water [18]. In our study, the seroprevalence varies from 25.7 to 36.4% between workers and their type of product sold. Workers who sell processed food had the highest seroprevalence. This can be due to availability of food that were stored in their shop which can lead to rodents' infestation. These workers shared similar workplace in a confined area and rodents can move and excrete the bacteria through their urine into the environment at the wet market. This factor might explain the seroprevalence level of workers who sell fruits, vegetables, fresh meat, fish and other products.

The predominant serovars detected in this study were *Autumnalis, Sarawak* (IMR LEP 175) and *Copenhageni* (IMR LEP 803/11) which constituted more than 40% of the immune responses among the participants. Out of 20 serovars tested, 18 serovars were tested positive with the blood samples from wet market workers. Other studies among high risk groups in Malaysia demonstrated several types of serovars detected. Ridzuan et al. (2016) reported 9 types of serovars tested positive with samples from high risk planters with the *Sarawak* (IMR LEP 175), *Patoc* and *Celledoni* were found to be the predominant serovars [18]. A study among town service workers by Shafei et al. (2012) noted 12 types of serovars were positive with the *Patoc, Bataviae* and *Javanica* were predominant [15]. A review on leptospirosis cases in Malaysia noted about 37 serovars had been isolated from animals and human. The wet and warm climate in this region provides suitable conditions for *Leptospira* to be firmly established in the diverse environments [2].

Table 3 Seroprevalence of leptospirosis according types of product sold (n = 232)

Type of product	No. of workers	MAT 1 ≥ 100	
		Frequency (%)	95% CI
Processed food	77	28 (36.4)	25.7, 48.1
Fruits and vegetables	35	9 (25.7)	12.5, 43.3
Fresh meat and fish	19	6 (31.6)	12.6, 56.6
Others (kitchen utensils, toys)	101	35 (34.7)	25.5, 44.8

Conclusion

The findings in this study demonstrates high seroprevalence of leptospirosis among wet market workers in Kelantan. As wet markets are places where buyers and sellers meet, the risk of infection may also be shared by the public. Thus, further assessment should be carried out to determine factors that contribute to increase risk to leptospirosis infection in wet market places which will assist in the development of preventive measures for workers as well as to the public.

Abbreviations

IMR: Institute for Medical Research; MAT: Microscopic agglutination test

Acknowledgements

We would like to express our sincere thanks to all participants, Ministry of Higher Education Malaysia for funding the study using Long Term Research Grant Scheme (203/PPSP/6770003) and all others who were directly and indirectly involved in this study.

Funding

This study was funded by Ministry of Higher Education Malaysia for funding the study using Long Term Research Grant Scheme (203/PPSP/6770003). The funding body did not involve in the design of the study and collection, analysis, and interpretation of data and in writing the manuscript.

Authors' contributions

AD, SMH, MNS, MO, SS, ZAW and WMZWM involved in conceptualization of the study, SMH, MHAAR, RAH, TZMTJ, MO, SS, ZAW and ZI involved in planning the methodology of this study, MHAAR and SMH involved in analyzing data, MHAAR and NI involved in collecting data, RAH, TZMTJ, MNS, MO, SS, ZAW, WMZWM and ZI involved in managing resources, AD involved in supervision and funding acquisition. All authors read and approved the final manuscript.

Competing interests

The authors declare that they have no competing interests.

Author details

[1]Department of Community Medicine, School of Medical Sciences, Universiti Sains Malaysia, 16150 Kubang Kerian, Kelantan, Malaysia. [2]Department of Medical Microbiology and Parasitology, Faculty of Medicine and Health Sciences, Universiti Putra Malaysia, UPM, 43400 Serdang, Selangor, Malaysia. [3]Health Department of Federal Territory Kuala Lumpur & Putrajaya, Jalan Cenderasari, 50590 Kuala Lumpur, Malaysia. [4]Health Promotion Unit, Penang State Health Department, Floor 7, Bangunan Persekutuan, Jalan Anson, 10400 Penang, Malaysia.

References

1. Lehmann JS, Matthias MA, Vinetz JM, Fouts DE. Leptospiral Pathogenomics. Pathogens. 2014;3(2):280–308. https://doi.org/10.3390/pathogens3020280.
2. El Jalii IM, Bahaman AR. A review of human leptospirosis in Malaysia. Trop Biomed. 2004;21(2):113–9.
3. Victoriano AFB, Smythe LD, Gloriani-Barzaga N, Cavinta LL, Kasai T, Limpakarnjanarat K, et al. Leptospirosis in the Asia Pacific region. BMC Infect Dis. 2009;9(1):147. https://doi.org/10.1186/1471-2334-9-147.
4. WHO (2003) Human leptospirosis: guidance for diagnosis, surveillance and control. http://www.who.int/iris/handle/10665/42667. Accessed 5 June 2016.
5. Costa F, Hagan JE, Calcagno J, Kane M, Torgerson P, Martinez-Silveira MS, et al. Global morbidity and mortality of leptospirosis: a systematic review. PLoS Negl Trop Dis. 2015;9(9):e0003898. https://doi.org/10.1371/journal.pntd.0003898.
6. Hartskeerl RA. Leptospirosis: current status and future trends. Indian J Med Microbiol. 2006;24(4):309.
7. Benacer D, Thong KL, Verasahib KB, Galloway RL, Hartskeerl RA, Lewis JW, et al. Human leptospirosis in Malaysia: reviewing the challenges after 8 decades (1925-2012). Asia Pac J Public Health. 2016;28(4):290–302. https://doi.org/10.1177/1010539516640350.
8. Centre for Disease Control and Prevention (2014) Leptospirosis. https://www.cdc.gov/leptospirosis/. Accessed 10 September 2016.
9. Schneider MC, Jancloes M, Buss DF, Aldighieri S, Bertherat E, Najera P, et al. Leptospirosis: a silent epidemic disease. Int J Environ Res Public Health. 2013;10(12):7229–34. https://doi.org/10.3390/ijerph10127229.
10. Azali MA, Yean Yean C, Harun A, Aminuddin Baki NN, Ismail N. Molecular characterization of Leptospira spp. in environmental samples from north-eastern Malaysia revealed a pathogenic strain, Leptospira alstonii. J Trop Med. 2016, 2016:2060241. https://doi.org/10.1155/2016/2060241.
11. Benacer D, Woh PY, Mohd Zain SN, Amran F, Thong KL. Pathogenic and saprophytic Leptospira species in water and soils from selected urban sites in peninsular Malaysia. Microbes Environ. 2013;28(1):135–40. https://doi.org/10.1264/jsme2.ME12154.
12. Benacer D, Zain SNM, Amran F, Galloway RL, Thong KL. Isolation and molecular characterization of Leptospira interrogans and Leptospira borgpetersenii isolates from the urban rat populations of Kuala Lumpur, Malaysia. Am J Trop Med Hyg. 2013;88(4):704–9. https://doi.org/10.4269/ajtmh.12-0662.
13. Samsudin S, Masri SN, Tengku-Jamaluddin TZM, Saudi SNS, Md-Ariffin UK, Amran F, et al. Seroprevalence of Leptospiral antibodies among healthy municipal service workers in Selangor. Advances in Public Health. 2015;2015. https://doi.org/10.1155/2015/208145.
14. WHO. WHO guidelines on drawing blood: best practices in phlebotomy. Geneva: Switzerland; 2010.
15. Shafei MN, Sulong MR, Yaacob NA, Hassan H, Wan Mohd Zahiruddin W, Aziah D, et al. Seroprevalence of leptospirosis among town service workers on northeastern state of Malaysia. International Journal of Collaborative Research on Internal Medicine & Public Health. 2012;4:395–403.
16. WCO India (2007) Leptospirosis Laboratory Manual. http://www.who.int/iris/handle/10665/205429. Accessed 2 June 2015.
17. Wynwood SJ, Graham GC, Weier SL, Collet TA, McKay DB, Craig SB. Leptospirosis from water sources. Pathogens and Global Health. 2014;108(7):334–8. https://doi.org/10.1179/2047773214Y.0000000156.
18. Ridzuan JM, Aziah D, Zahiruddin WM. Study on Seroprevalence and Leptospiral antibody distribution among high-risk planters in Malaysia. Osong Public Health Res Perspect. 2016;7(3):168–71. https://doi.org/10.1016/j.phrp.2016.04.006.

28

Analysis of sero-epidemiological characteristics of varicella in healthy children in Jiangsu Province, China

Lei Zhang[1], Wang Ma[3†], Yuanbao Liu[2†], Yong Wang[1], Xiang Sun[2], Ying Hu[2], Xiuying Deng[2], Peishan Lu[2], Fenyang Tang[2], Zhiguo Wang[2*] and Minghao Zhou[1,2*]

Abstract

Background: In recent years, outbreaks of varicella have continued to occur, and the coverage rate of varicella vaccine in Jiangsu Province, China, remains unclear. This study aims to analyse the levels of immune antibody against varicella and obtain a comprehensive understanding of the varicella attenuated live vaccine (VarV) coverage rate in children aged 1–9 years in Jiangsu Province.

Methods: From June to October 2016, a cross-sectional survey was conducted to collect 3631 serum samples from healthy children aged 1–9 years in Jiangsu Province. The immunoglobulin G (IgG) antibody levels of varicella were detected by enzyme-linked immunosorbent assay (ELISA).

Results: The VarV coverage rate of healthy children was only 43.1% (95% CI: 41.1–44.7%). The seroprevalence after vaccination with a single dose of VarV was only 57.1%, and the overall seropositivity and geometric antibody titre (GMC) were 43.5% and 225.4 mU/ml, respectively. The seropositivity was significantly higher in girls than in boys ($x^2 = 18.82$, $P < 0.001$). The difference in seropositivity between the 5–9 age group and 1–4 age group was statistically significant ($x^2 = 84.31$, $P < 0.001$). The difference in seropositivity between different regions was statistically significant, with the highest seropositivity in the northern area, 53.7% ($x^2 = 35.64$, $P < 0.001$). The seropositivity in the group receiving one dose of VarV was significantly higher than that of the unvaccinated group ($x^2 = 205.16$, $P < 0.001$). Linear regression analysis suggested that the GMC of varicella antibodies wanes with the time since vaccination ($F = 65.01$, $P = 0.002$).

Conclusion: The VarV coverage rate of healthy children in Jiangsu Province was low. Sero-conversion rates were also low after one dose of VarV, and the immune effectiveness of a single dose of VarV was limited. To control the spread of varicella, VarV should be included in the routine immunization program, and strengthened immunization measures for the varicella-susceptible population warrant additional consideration.

Keywords: Varicella, Geometric antibody concentrations, Seroprevalence

Background

Varicella is a highly contagious disease caused by initial infection by the varicella-zoster virus [1]. Varicella is prone to spread in collective institutions, such as kindergartens and primary and secondary schools. The most effective way to reduce the incidence of varicella in children is through vaccinations with the varicella attenuated live vaccine (VarV) [2, 3]. Until recently, the coverage rate of one-dose varicella vaccine was low because it is still a voluntarily self-funded vaccine and has not been introduced to the Expanded Programme of Immunization in Jiangsu Province, China. Unvaccinated students can receive emergency vaccination for free when a varicella outbreak occurs in school [4]. Individuals aged 12 months to 12 years old are recommended

* Correspondence: 1020389031@qq.com; zmhjscdc@126.com
†Wang Ma and Yuanbao Liu contributed equally to this work.
[2]Department of Expanded Programme on Immunization, Jiangsu Provincial Center for Disease Control and Prevention, Nanjing 210009, Jiangsu Province, China
[1]Department of Epidemiology, School of Public Health, Nanjing Medical University, Nanjing 211166, Jiangsu Province, China
Full list of author information is available at the end of the article

to receive 1 dose of VarV by private purchase [4, 5]. Of the varicella cases in Jiangsu Province in 2016, 76.5% were among children aged 1–9 years old. Most recently, outbreaks of varicella have continued to occur, and breakthrough cases of varicella have received increasing attention and are becoming a serious public health problem [6].

To gain a comprehensive understanding of the vaccination coverage rate of children's VarV in Jiangsu Province and to describe the profile of immunoglobulin G (IgG) levels of varicella antibodies among children, a sero-survey of varicella was conducted in healthy children in Jiangsu Province, China.

Materials and methods

Varicella surveillance

Surveillance and management of varicella are based on its designation as a class C infectious disease in China. All patients diagnosed with varicella by a hospital or laboratory need to be recorded in the National Notifiable Disease Reporting System, a web-based computerized reporting system. Demographic data were provided by the Jiangsu Provincial Bureau of Statistics.

Serological survey

A cross-sectional survey was conducted by stratified cluster random sampling from June to October 2016. In the first stage, the province was divided into three regions, namely, south, central and north, according to socio-economic level and geographical location. One city was randomly selected from each region as a research site: Changzhou, Taizhou and Huaian (see Fig. 1). In the second stage, the random number table method was used to select 3–5 townships in each city. In the third stage, children were recruited from the townships included in the sample. The inclusion criteria for children were as follows: (1) aged 1–9 years and had consent from a guardian for blood collection; (2) had been a local resident for at least 3 months; and (3) were in good physical health (with axillary temperature < 38 °C and without acute or chronic diseases). The exclusion criteria were as follows: (1) refused collection of venous blood; or (2) had a serious illness or other medical reasons for not participating in the study after clinical evaluation.

A total of 3709 eligible children were recruited in this study. Seventy-eight children refused to donate venous blood for unknown reasons, resulting in a total of 3631

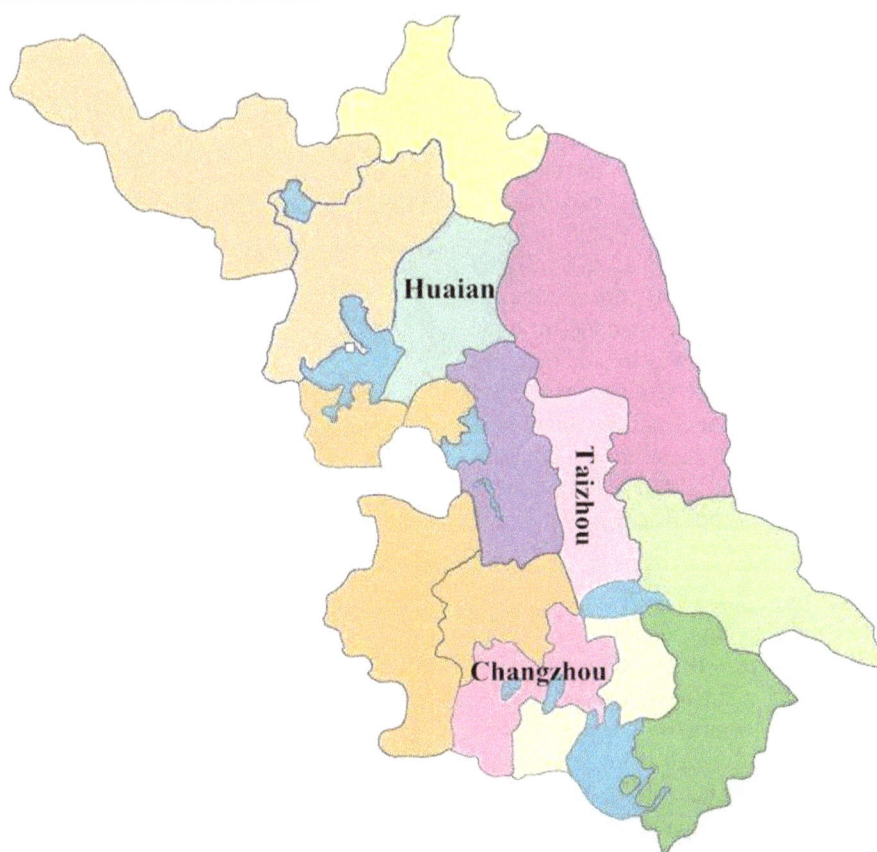

Fig. 1 Map of Jiangsu Province; the cities randomly selected based on geographical location and economic situation are Huaian, Taizhou and Changzhou

serum samples from individuals aged 1–9 collected from January to November 2016. The study was approved by the Medical Ethics Committee of the Jiangsu Provincial Center for Disease Control and Prevention (No: SL2015-B015–02). Written informed consent was obtained from the parents/guardians of the children before enrolment. Guardians of the children were required to complete a questionnaire regarding their children's information and immunization history, such as age, gender, date of birth, date of vaccination, and date of sampling. If the entire immunization history of a child was missing, we looked for it on the Jiangsu Provincial Immunization Information System.

Laboratory assay

Serum samples were collected and frozen at − 70 °C until testing. Enzyme-linked immunosorbent assay (ELISA) was used to detect varicella-specific IgG antibodies; all the experiments were performed at the laboratory of the Department of the Expanded Programme on Immunization at the Jiangsu Provincial Center for Disease Control and Prevention. To avoid test bias, all detection tests were conducted by the same staff members using commercial ELISA kits from Institut Virion\Serion GmbH (SERION ELISA classic anti-varicella virus IgG, batch number: SLF.CL). The ELISA results were first expressed as optical density (OD) measurements at 402 nm and later converted to the antibody concentration values (U/ml) using software from SERIO, according to the product instructions. According to the kit instructions, the serum antibody concentration ranged from 15 to 2000 mIU/ml, the samples with an antibody concentration > 2000 mIU/ml were labelled as 2000 mIU/ml, and samples < 15 mIU/ml were labelled as 15 mIU/ml. An antibody concentration ≥ 100 mIU/ml was considered positive, and a concentration < 80 mIU/ml was considered negative. In addition, we used commercial ELISA kits from the same company, and all tests were conducted by the same staff members with strict quality control under similar laboratory conditions. Furthermore, equivocal samples (80–100 mIU/ml) were retested prior to categorization as positive or negative.

Statistical analysis

EpiData software was used to input information from the questionnaires in duplicate, with suitable edits and validations. Geometric antibody titres (GMCs) in different groups were compared by one-way ANOVA, and multiple comparisons were performed using the SNK-q test. The antibody seroprevalence in different age groups, gender groups, region groups and immune status was compared by Pearson's χ^2 test. The relationship between the GMC value and vaccination duration was analysed by linear regression. All statistical tests used a two-sided $\alpha = 0.05$ as the significance threshold and were performed using R 2.10.0 statistical software.

Results

Sero-survey of varicella in children aged 1–9 years in 2016

A total of 3631 serum samples from healthy children in Changzhou, Taizhou and Huaian were collected. Among them, 1563 children had a history of VarV vaccination, resulting in a vaccination coverage rate of 43.1% (95% CI: 41.4–44.7%). See Table 1 for details. The antibody sero-conversion rate was 57.1% (95 CI: 54.6–59.5%) after one dose of VarV. The overall seroprevalence of varicella antibodies was only 43.5% (95% CI 41.9–45.1%). The seroprevalence of varicella antibodies in the 1–4-year age group was significantly higher than that in the 5–9-year age group (52.3% vs 37.0%, $P < 0.001$). The positive rate of varicella antibodies in girls was significantly higher than that in boys (47.3% vs. 40.1%, $P < 0.001$). The seroprevalence of children with a history of immunization was significantly different from that of children without immunization (57.1% vs. 33.3%, $P < 0.001$). The positive rate of virus antibody was the highest in children in northern Jiangsu (53.7, 95% CI: 50.8–56.5%) and was significantly higher than the rates in southern Jiangsu and Suzhong ($P < 0.001$); See Table 2.

Among children with a history of VarV vaccination, the longer it had been since they had received the VarV, the lower their antibody GMC value was, suggesting that the varicella antibody titre has a tendency to wane with time (F = 69.01, $P = 0.003$); See Table 3.

In addition to the incidence of varicella and the seroprevalence of antibodies in 2016, the reported incidence of varicella was the lowest and the seroprevalence was the highest in northern Jiangsu Province. The reported incidence rate decreased with increases in the antibody positive rate.

Discussion

Varicella is a highly contagious disease that can be transmitted through daily contact [7]. The susceptible population is concentrated in children, particularly those in nurseries, kindergartens, primary and secondary schools and other collective units [7–9]. Immunocompromised adults with varicella are more likely to experience a severe course and have serious complications [10]. Since 2015, reported varicella cases have increased in number and have become a serious public health problem, and outbreaks of varicella have been reported among highly vaccinated preschool children [5, 6, 11, 12]. The increasing number of varicella cases between 2016 and 2017 in Jiangsu Province may be the result of the continuing low vaccination coverage, which leads to an accumulation of susceptible persons. There have been many studies to

Table 1 Characteristics of coverage of varicella vaccine for healthy children in some areas of Jiangsu Province in 2016

Characteristics		Sample size	Number of children vaccinated	Coverage rate(%,95 CI)	χ^2 value	P value
Age (year)	1–4	1543	740	47.1(44.5–49.5)	2.98	0.084
	5–9	2088	941	45.1(42.9–47.2)		
Gender	Boy	1898	1080	56.9(54.6–59.1)	60.07	< 0.001[a]
	Girl	1733	763	44.1(41.7–46.4)		
Area	Changzhou	1249	590	47.2(44.4–50.1)	107.18	< 0.001[a]
	Taizhou	1178	609	51.7(48.8–54.6)		
	Huaian	1204	582	31.7(29.1–34.4)		
Total		3631	1581	43.1(41.4–44.7)		

Attention: [a] means P value≤0.05

date on antibody levels in varicella, but few studies on the VarV coverage rate and the attenuation of antibody levels in healthy children, which could help optimize immunization programs in China, have been performed [13]. This study conducted a cross-sectional survey on varicella IgG antibody levels in 2016 to understand the actual vaccination coverage rate of healthy children in Jiangsu Province, to comprehensively describe the immunization profile of children aged 1–9 years old based on varicella surveillance data, and to provide an immunological basis for VarV to be included in the routine immunization program.

This study found that the vaccination coverage rate of healthy children in Jiangsu Province was low (43.1%), and it was lower than the estimated coverage rate of varicella in Jiangsu Province's vaccine management system (approximately 55–65%). The overall antibody positive rate (43.5%)

and antibody GMC (225.4 mU/ ml) were lower than those reported in relevant studies in Beijing city and Shanghai city [14–16]. According to several clinical trial and observational studies in the domestic and foreign literature, relatively low vaccination rates and sero-conversion rates will lead to an increase in varicella outbreaks [17–19]. This study's findings confirm previous reports that single-dose varicella vaccine is insufficient to provide the population with an immune barrier. Based on varicella surveillance and seroprevalence data, it was found that there was a negative correlation between the reported incidence and seroprevalence among regions, which indirectly indicated that the immunization effect of varicella vaccine could prevent the spread of varicella to a certain extent [20]. The state of the varicella epidemic is the most serious and the seroprevalence of antibody in children is the lowest in the southern Jiangsu region, meaning that the occurrence of

Table 2 Analysis of IgG antibody levels of varicella in children aged 1–9 years in Jiangsu Province in 2016

Characteristics		Sample size	N	Seroprevalence(%, 95 CI)	GMC(mU/ml, 95 CI)
Age(year)	1–4	1543	807	52.3(49.7–54.8)	275.2(235.4–297.6)
	5–9	2088	773	37.0(34.9–39.1)	183.7(153.2–207.9)
χ^2/t value			84.31	3.65	
P value			< 0.001	< 0.001	
Gender	Boy	1898	761	40.1(37.9–42.3)	212.6(175.2–236.5)
	Girl	1733	819	47.3(44.9–49.6)	260.4(240.3–295.2)
χ^2/t value			18.92	2.52	
P value			< 0.001	< 0.001	
Area	South	1249	438	35.1(32.4–37.8)	216.2(198.7–232.4)
	North	1204	646	53.7(50.8–56.5)	191.8(178.5–221.2)
	central	1178	496	42.1(39.3–44.9)	298.1(273.1–321.6)
χ^2/F value			35.64	24.21	
P value			< 0.001	< 0.001	
Immune history	1 dose	1563	892	57.1(54.6–59.5)	294.9(265.2–330.4)
	0 dose	2068	688	33.3(30.9–35.1)	120.2(97.5–153.6)
χ^2/t value			205.16	5.36	
P value			< 0.001	< 0.001	
Total		3631	1580	43.5(41.9–45.1)	225.4(185.4–247.6)

Table 3 Relationship between GMCs, seroprevalence and time since vaccination before the sero-survey

Time since vaccination (year)	Sample size	N	Seroprevalence(%, 95 CI)	GMC(95% CI, mU/ml)	Statistics	P value
1	48	29	60.4(45.3–74.2)	298.6 (275.2–313.5)	F = 65.01	0.002
2	130	74	56.9(47.9–65.6)	263.5(243.4–280.6)		
3	415	211	50.8(45.9–55.8)	218.7(198.6–234.7)		
4	111	52	46.8(37.3–56.6)	224.8(205.1–239.8)		
5	185	91	49.2(41.8–56.6)	164.2(124.1–185.4)		
6	604	224	37.1(33.2–41.1)	155.6(134.2–177.9)		
7	70	27	38.6(27.2–50.9)	165.3(144.2–188.9)		

varicella virus infection in this region can easily cause an epidemic outbreak of varicella. This study shows that the seroprevalence is significantly higher in girls than in boys, and the reported incidence rate is lower in girls than in boys. The reasons for this finding may be complicated and may include the different contact rate, different exposure levels and different asymptomatic infection rate of these children [21, 22]. By contrast, a German study showed that there was no difference between boys and girls, which may indicate cultural differences, and in-depth reasons for this discrepancy should be further explored [23].

The study showed that among 1563 children with a history of VarV vaccination, the seroprevalence of varicella antibodies was only 57.1%, which may be one of the reasons for the increase in breakthrough cases, and it also indicates that the effect of a single dose of VarV is limited. This study found that the antibody GMC values tend to wane with the time since vaccination. Several studies on school outbreaks have suggested that extended time since vaccination may be associated with the possibility of breakthrough varicella [18, 24, 25]. To better control the varicella epidemic, the need to increase immunization coverage rates with varicella vaccine among children in Jiangsu Province has also been suggested. The US Advisory Committee on Immunization Practices issued the following regulations on the second dose of varicella vaccination in 2006: it is recommended that children aged 4–6 who have received one dose of varicella vaccine be vaccinated once more. The surveillance and investigation results show that two doses of varicella vaccine are more effective in controlling the occurrence of varicella breakthrough cases [26, 27]. It is suggested that Jiangsu Province implement a two-dose varicella vaccine schedule for children and maintain high coverage of two-dose varicella vaccine for children enrolled in kindergartens and primary schools; this approach could improve protection from both primary vaccine failure and waning vaccine-induced immunity [18].

This study described the VarV coverage rate and immunization level of healthy children aged 1–9 years in some areas of Jiangsu Province using a large sample size. One limitation of this study is that it is a cross-sectional

study, which provides insight only regarding the immunization strategy of varicella; evidence from prospective studies is still needed. Another limitation is that seropositivity is only a reference range for preventing varicella infection. The seropositivity can only roughly reflect the susceptibility of children to varicella virus, and the optimal age for the second varicella vaccine warrants further exploration.

Conclusions

Overall, this study summarizes the findings of an observational population-based study of varicella immunity in children aged 1–9 years and shows that these children were at high risk of varicella infection. Waning immunity in terms of seroprevalence and GMCs was observed. The VarV coverage rate of healthy children in Jiangsu Province was low. Sero-conversion was also low after one dose of VarV was administered, and the immune effect of a single dose of VarV was limited. To better control varicella spread, VarV should be included in an expanded immunization program, and a second dose of varicella vaccine should be recommended for all children, which could compensate for the first immune failure and waning-induced immunity.

Abbreviations
ELISA: Enzyme-linked immunosorbent assay; GMCs: Geometric antibody titres; IgG: Immunoglobulin G; VarV: Varicella attenuated live vaccine

Acknowledgements
We would like to thank all the following CDCs in Jiangsu Province for their field work: Changzhou Center for Disease Control and Prevention (CDC), Huaian CDC, Lianyungang CDC, Taizhou CDC, Zhenjiang CDC, Xuzhou CDC, Wujin district CDC, and Lianshui county CDC.

Funding
This work was supported by the National Natural Science Foundation of China under grant number 81502860; the Jiangsu Provincial Medical Youth Talent under grant number QNRC2016547; the "333" Project of Jiangsu Province under grant number BRA2017538.

Authors' contributions
Conceived and designed the experiments: MZ, LZ, YL. Performed the experiments: LZ, YW, WM, ZW, PL, YH, FT. Analysed the data: LZ, WM, YL, XS.

Contributed reagents/materials/analysis tools: QZ, WL, YW, YL, SL, XD. Wrote the paper: LZ, WM, MH. All authors read and approved the final manuscript.

Competing interests

The authors declare that they have no competing interests.

Author details

[1]Department of Epidemiology, School of Public Health, Nanjing Medical University, Nanjing 211166, Jiangsu Province, China. [2]Department of Expanded Programme on Immunization, Jiangsu Provincial Center for Disease Control and Prevention, Nanjing 210009, Jiangsu Province, China. [3]First Affiliated Hospital of Nanjing Medical University, Nanjing 211166, Jiangsu Province, China.

References

1. Chan DYW, Edmunds WJ, Chan HL, Chan V, Lam YCK, Thomas SL, et al. The changing epidemiology of varicella and herpes zoster in Hong Kong before universal varicella vaccination in 2014. Epidemiol Infect. 2018;146(6):723–34.
2. Smith-Norowitz TA, Saadia TA, Norowitz KB, Joks R, Durkin HG, Kohlhoff S. Negative IgG varicella zoster virus antibody status: immune responses pre and post re-immunization. Infect Dis Ther. 2018;7(1):175–81.
3. Melegaro A, Marziano V, Del Fava E, Poletti P, Tirani M, Rizzo C, et al. The impact of demographic changes, exogenous boosting and new vaccination policies on varicella and herpes zoster in Italy: a modelling and cost-effectiveness study. BMC Med. 2018;16(1):117.
4. Fu C, Wang M, Liang J, Xu J, Wang C, Bialek S. The effectiveness of varicella vaccine in China. Pediatr Infect Dis J. 2010;29(8):690–3.
5. Fu J, Wang J, Jiang C, Shi R, Ma T. Outbreak of varicella in a highly vaccinated preschool population. Int J Infect Dis. 2015;37:14–8.
6. Suo L, Lu L, Wang Q, Yang F, Wang X, Pang X, et al. Varicella outbreak in a highly-vaccinated school population in Beijing, China during the voluntary two-dose era. Vaccine. 2017;35(34):4368–73.
7. World Health Organization. Varicella and herpes zoster vaccines: WHO position paper, June 2014. Wkly Epidemiol Rec. 2014;89:265–88.
8. Lee H, Cho HK, Kim KH. Seroepidemiology of varicella-zoster virus in Korea. J Med Sci. 2013;28(2):195–9.
9. Oh HS, Bae JM. Vaccination history in elementary school children enrolled in the varicella epidemic investigations held in Jeju-si, Korea in the first half of 2017. Epidemiol Health. 2017;39:e2017053.
10. Zhang X, Yu Y, Zhang J, Kwan EP, Huang S, Wang Z, et al. One-dose vaccination associated with attenuated disease severity of adolescent and adult varicella cases in Beijing's Fengtai District. Hum Vaccin Immunother. 2014;10(8):2417–20.
11. Vaidya SR, Tilavat SM, Kumbhar NS, Kamble MB. Chickenpox outbreak in a tribal and industrial zone from the union territory of Dadra and Nagar Haveli. India Epidemiol Infect. 2018;146(4):476–80.
12. Vairo F, Di Bari V, Panella V, Quintavalle G, Torchia S, Serra MC, et al. An outbreak of chickenpox in an asylum seeker centre in Italy: outbreak investigation and validity of reported chickenpox history, December 2015–May 2016. Euro Surveill. 2017; 22(46).
13. Ihara H, Miyachi M, Imafuku S. Relationship between serum anti-varicella zoster virus antibody titer and time from onset of herpes zoster. J Dermatol. 2018;45(2):189–93.
14. Zhang X, Yu Y, Zhang J, Huang S, Wang Z, Zhang J, et al. The epidemiology of varicella cases among children in Beijing's Fengtai District from 2008 to 2012. Vaccine. 2014;32(29):3569–72.
15. Suo L, Lu L, Chen M, Pang X. Antibody induced by one-dose varicella vaccine soon became weak in children: evidence from a cross-sectional seroepidemiological survey in Beijing, PRC. BMC Infect Dis. 2015;15:509.
16. Wu QS, Liu JY, Wang X, Chen YF, Zhou Q, Wu AQ, et al. Effectiveness of varicella vaccine as post-exposure prophylaxis during a varicella outbreak in Shanghai, China. Int J Infect Dis. 2018;66:51–5.
17. Min SW, Kim YS, Nahm FS, Yoo da H, Choi E, Lee PB, et al. The positive duration of varicella zoster immunoglobulin M antibody test in herpes zoster. Medicine (Baltimore). 2016; 95(33):e4616.
18. Chaves SS, Gargiullo P, Zhang JX, Civen R, Guris D, Mascola L, et al. Loss of vaccine-induced immunity to varicella over time. N Engl J Med. 2007; 356(11):1121–9.
19. Schwarz TF, Volpe S, Catteau G, Chlibek R, David MP, Richardus JH, et al. Persistence of immune response to an adjuvanted varicella-zoster virus subunit vaccine for up to year nine in older adults. Hum Vaccin Immunother. 2018;14(6):1370-77.
20. Amjadi O, Rafiei A, Haghshenas M, Navaei RA, Valadan R, Hosseini-Khah Z, et al. A systematic review and meta-analysis of seroprevalence of varicella zoster virus: a nationwide population-based study. J Clin Virol. 2017;87:49–59.
21. Suo LD, Lu L, Wu J, Liu DL, Pang XH. The epidemiological impact of varicella vaccination in kindergartens, primary and secondary schools. Chin J Prev Med. 2012;46(1):46–9.
22. Ferreira CSM, Perin MCAA, Moraes-Pinto MI, Simão-Gurge RM, Goulart AL, Weckx LY, et al. Humoral immune response to measles and varicella vaccination in former very low birth weight preterm infants. Braz J Infect Dis. 2018; 22(1):41-46.
23. Wiese-Posselt M, Siedler A, Mankertz A, Sauerbrei A, Hengel H, Wichmann O, et al. Varicella-zoster virus seroprevalence in children and adolescents in the pre-varicella vaccine era, Germany. BMC Infect Dis. 2017;17(1):356.
24. Miyachi M, Ihara H, Imafuku S. Incidence of serum antibody titers against varicella zoster virus in Japanese patients with herpes zoster. J Dermatol. 2017; 44(6);656-9.
25. Andrade AL, da Silva Vieira MA, Minamisava R, Toscano CM, de Lima Souza MB, Fiaccadori F, et al. Single-dose varicella vaccine effectiveness in Brazil: A case-control study. Vaccine. 2018;36(4):479–83.
26. Henry O, Brzostek J, Czajka H, Leviniene G, Reshetko O, Gasparini R, et al. One or two doses of live varicella virus-containing vaccines: efficacy, persistence of immune responses, and safety six years after administration in healthy children during their second year of life. Vaccine. 2018;36(3):381–7.
27. Michalik DE, Steinberg SP, Larussa PS, Edwards KM, Wright PF, Arvin AM, et al. Primary vaccine failure after 1 dose of varicella vaccine in healthy children. J Infect Dis. 2008;197(7):944–9.

29

Utilization of "prevention of mother-to-child transmission" of HIV services by adolescent and young mothers in Mulago Hospital, Uganda

Mariama Mustapha[1,2]* (iD), Victor Musiime[1,3], Sabrina Bakeera-Kitaka[1], Joseph Rujumba[1] and Nicolette Nabukeera-Barungi[1]

Abstract

Background: Prevention of mother to child transmission (PMTCT) has lowered the incidence of paediatric HIV globally. The risk of mother-to-child transmission of HIV (MTCT) remains high in Africa, where there is a high prevalence of pregnancy and poor health-seeking behaviour among young girls and women.

Methods: In this cross-sectional, mixed-methods study, we evaluated the utilization of PMTCT services and associated factors among adolescent and young postpartum mothers aged 15 to 24 years at a public urban referral hospital in Uganda. Both HIV-positive and HIV-negative participants were recruited. Utilization of PMTCT services was defined as use of the PMTCT cascade of services including ever testing for HIV, receiving HIV test results; If tested negative, subsequent retesting up to 14 weeks; If tested positive, Antiretroviral drugs (ARVs) for the mother, ARVs and septrin prophylaxis for infant, safe delivery, safer infant feeding, early infant diagnosis within 6 weeks, and linkage to treatment and care. Optimal utilization of PMTCT was defined as being up to date with utilization of PMTCT services for reported HIV status at the time of being interviewed. The overall proportion of participants who optimally utilized PMTCT services was determined using descriptive statistics. Qualitative data was analyzed manually using the content thematic approach.

Results: Of the 418 participants, 65 (15.5%) were HIV positive. Overall, only 126 of 418 participants (30.1%) had optimally utilized PMTCT services. However, utilization of PMTCT services was better among HIV positive mothers, with 83% (54/65) having utilized the services optimally, compared to only 20% (72/353) of the HIV negative mothers (OR 18.2 (95% CI; 9.0–36.7)). The benefits of knowing ones HIV status, health of the unborn child, and counseling and support from health workers and peers, were the major factors motivating adolescent and young mothers to utilize PMTCT services, while stigma, financial constraints, non-disclosure, and lack of partner and family support were key demotivating factors.

Conclusion: Utilization of PMTCT services by these adolescent and young mothers was suboptimal. Special consideration should be given to adolescents and young women in the design of elimination of mother to child transmission (EMTCT) programs, to improve the utilization of PMTCT services.

Keywords: Adolescents, HIV, PMTCT, Utilization, Uganda

* Correspondence: mamspha@yahoo.com
[1]Department of Paediatrics and Child Health, School of Medicine, Makerere University College of Health Sciences, Kampala, Uganda
[2]Ministry of Health and Sanitation, Freetown, Sierra Leone
Full list of author information is available at the end of the article

Background

In 2016, there were 1.8 million new HIV infections, with a total of 36.7 million people living with HIV worldwide [1]. In high-prevalence settings, young women remain at unacceptably high risk of HIV infection [1]. In eastern Africa, young women (aged 15–24 years) accounted for 26% of new HIV infections in 2016 despite making up just 10% of the population [1].

Adolescents and young people remain extremely vulnerable to acquiring HIV infection, especially girls who live in settings with a generalized HIV epidemic or who are members of populations at high risk for HIV acquisition or transmission [2]. Although early diagnosis and treatment reduce HIV progression and prevent transmission, adolescents are less likely than adults to be tested, access care, remain in care and achieve viral suppression [2]. The Ministry of Health conducted an assessment of adolescent HIV and sexual and reproductive health care and treatment services at 30 health facilities in Uganda. This study found that pregnant adolescents (10–19 years) had less coverage of PMTCT services compared to mothers aged 20 years and above [3]. This study also found that 90% of pregnant adolescents attending antenatal care (ANC) took an HIV test but only 94% of those positive received ARVs [3]. This was in contrast with the adult mothers of whom 99% received ARVs for PMTCT [3].

Pregnant adolescent and young mothers have unique challenges that would hinder them from accessing HIV care [4]. For pregnant adolescents; obtaining access to relevant services, such as prenatal care, skilled attendants during birth, and PMTCT services, is more difficult [5]. Due to their young age, teenage mothers have to deal with disapproving health care providers. In addition, those living with HIV may face stigma and discrimination in health care settings [5].

PMTCT covers a package of interventions summarized as 4 prongs, which should be implemented simultaneously: Primary prevention of HIV infection among women of childbearing age, preventing unintended pregnancies among women living with HIV, preventing HIV transmission from a woman living with HIV to her infant using option B+ approach, and providing appropriate treatment, care and support to mothers living with HIV and their children and families [6]. The PMTCT cascade is a series of key stepwise activities that begins with all pregnant women and ends with the detection of a final HIV status in HIV-exposed infants [7]. The cascade comprises 18 months of care and includes attending antenatal care (ANC), HIV testing and counselling during ANC, receiving HIV test results; If tested negative, subsequent retesting; If tested positive, antiretroviral drugs (ARVs) for the mother, ARVs and septrin prophylaxis for the infant(s), safe delivery, safer infant feeding, early infant diagnosis within 6 weeks, second DNA PCR test done 6 weeks after cessation of the breastfeeding, serology at 18 months if DNA PCR negative, and linkage to treatment and care [7]. Optimal utilization of the PMTCT cascade of services has not been previously described in the literature.

Initiation and completion of the PMTCT cascade is important for elimination of paediatric HIV [8]. Adolescents have poor health seeking behaviour if services are not adolescent friendly, and few facilities in Uganda were found to be adolescent friendly in a 2007 study [9]. Since over 90% of new HIV infections among infants and young children occur through MTCT, it is certain that PMTCT remains the top priority. A focus on women is a key strategy to preventing/reducing HIV infection among children [10]. PMTCT programs not only reduce transmission of HIV, but if well implemented as part of a full continuum of care, they can result in HIV-free survival, meaning that infants are protected from other causes of death as well.

Thirty percent of Uganda's 35 million people is comprised of adolescents and young people aged 10–24 years [11], with a birth rate of 140 per 1000 among adolescents by age 19 years [12]. This group may need PMTCT services and messages that are different from those which target older women. Although adolescent and young mothers have been noted to have poor utilization of health services (6), there is limited data on the utilization of PMTCT of HIV services by adolescent and young mothers in Uganda. Identifying the gaps in the utilization of PMTCT services and the associated factors will contribute to the development of practical strategies in policy and practice to improve utilization of PMTCT services by these young mothers, and hence achieve elimination of paediatric HIV infection.

We described the utilization of PMTCT of HIV services and the associated factors among adolescent and young mothers at a public urban referral hospital in Uganda.

Methods

Study design

This was cross-sectional and mixed methods study which employed both quantitative and qualitative methods.

Study site

This study was conducted at the immunization, postnatal and family planning clinics at Mulago National Referral Hospital, located in Kampala, the capital city of Uganda. Mulago Hospital serves about 115, 000 inpatients (including 30, 000 children) per year. These clinics are located in the same building in upper Mulago Hospital, work hand-in-hand, and run Mondays through Fridays. The median number of postpartum mothers seen in the clinics daily is 80. Of these 80 women, 5–10 (6–13%) are adolescent and young women. Routine HIV testing is performed by a trained counsellor, and those who test positive are linked either to Baylor-Uganda Clinical

Centre of Excellence or to the PMTCT follow-up clinic, both within a 200 m radius.

Quantitative component
Study population

The study population for the quantitative component of the study was all postpartum mothers (HIV positive and negative) aged 15–24 years attending the clinics who: provided written informed consent, and had a child or children aged 9 months and below. Age 9 months and below was chosen for the infants' age in order to include mothers whose pregnancy was therefore recent, and hence minimize recall bias.

Sample size estimation

Utilization of PMTCT services is use of the PMTCT cascade of services including testing for HIV, receiving HIV test results; If tested negative, subsequent retesting up to 14 weeks; If tested positive, Antiretroviral drugs (ARVs) for the mother, ARVs and septrin prophylaxis for infant, safe delivery, safer infant feeding, early infant diagnosis within 6 weeks, and linkage to treatment and care. Optimal utilization of PMTCT is being up to date with utilization of PMTCT services for reported HIV status at the time of being interviewed. Testing for HIV is a crucial first step in utilization of the PMTCT cascade of services for both HIV negative and HIV positive women. Using an HIV testing rate of 61.7 [13], a sample size of 363 participants, provided 90% power to assess the optimal utilization of PMTCT services in this population allowing for a 10% data loss through data collection constraints and errors.

Quantitative data collection

Two interviewers (nurses) received a two-day training by the researcher on the questionnaire, data collection procedures and sampling methods. They were available at the clinics on all clinic days and were supervised by the researcher. A pre-tested structured questionnaire was used to obtain information on the participants' socio-demographic characteristics, HIV/AIDS and PMTCT-related knowledge, PMTCT utilization, and factors influencing utilization of PMTCT services. The nurses administered the questionnaire using face-to-face exit interviews from March–June 2015. All postpartum mothers attending the clinics were invited to participate. A woman was eligible if she was 15–24 years old, had a child aged 9 months and below, and consented for interview.

Quantitative data management and analysis

Completed questionnaires were scrutinized by the researcher on the spot for immediate correction of erroneous entry, and feedback given to the research assistants. After data collection, all questionnaires were stored in a safe that was accessible only to the researcher. Data was cleaned, coded, and double-entered into Epidata version 3.1. Range, consistency and validity checks were built in to minimize errors. A back up copy of the data was kept on an external hard drive. Data was exported and analyzed using STATA version 12.0 (STATA Corporation, Houston, Texas). A descriptive analysis was done so as to depict the baseline characteristics of the study population. The distribution of the participants' characteristics was presented as frequencies with respective proportions.

The primary outcome of the study was optimal utilization of PMTCT services as defined by being up to date with utilization of PMTCT services. This meant that at that particular point in time when the mother was interviewed during the study, she was where she was supposed to be at the PMTCT cascade for her reported HIV status.

A logistic regression model was used to assess the association of selected variables with the overall optimal utilization of PMTCT services. Bivariate factors with a p-value < 0.2 were considered for multivariate analysis. The distribution of each selected variable was compared between those who optimally utilized PMTCT services and those who did not. In all analyses, a p-value of < 0.05 was taken as statistically significant.

Qualitative component
Study population

To complement the quantitative findings, interviews were held with purposively selected health workers involved in the provision of PMTCT services at Mulago Hospital, and purposively selected adolescent and young mothers (HIV positive and negative) with either good or poor utilization of PMTCT services.

Qualitative data collection
In-depth interviews (IDI)

During the study, after administration of the questionnaire, adolescent and young mothers for participation in the qualitative component were identified. IDIs were conducted with mothers who provided consent. Twenty adolescent and young mothers (10 HIV positive and 10 HIV negative) were interviewed. After the 20 interviews, no further interviews were conducted since no new information was being generated. IDIs were aimed at obtaining an in-depth understanding of the facilitators and barriers to utilization of PMTCT services by adolescent and young mothers. In-depth interviews were chosen to allow free and confidential interaction between researchers and adolescent mothers. The interviews took the form of informal conversations and were conducted in the local language, *Luganda*, which was the language preferred by the mothers. The interviews were conducted by a research assistant with experience in qualitative studies involving adolescents and young people. A pre-tested flexible interview guide with probes was used to explore the ideas and experiences of the participants regarding HIV testing among adolescent and young mothers, and the factors that influence the utilization of PMTCT services, and suggestions for improving utilization of PMTCT services by this group. The interviews were audio recorded (except for 3 mothers who were not comfortable with being recorded), transcribed and translated by the research assistant. Each interview took an average of 35 min.

Key-informant interviews (KII)

KIIs were held on appointment with selected participants at the health facility during the study. Nine key informant interviews were conducted, and these included 2 nurses, 2 counsellors, 3 peer educators, and 2 doctors who were both PMTCT coordinators. Key informants were selected based on their involvement in the provision of PMTCT services and were intended to contribute to a better understanding of adolescent and young mothers' experiences with PMTCT services. The interviews were guided by a pre-tested flexible interview guide with probes to identify the characteristics of the health workers, their role in providing PMTCT services, their views on the motivators and barriers to the utilization of PMTCT services by adolescent and young mothers, and their suggestions for improving utilization of PMTCT services by this group. Interviews were conducted in English, audio recorded, and transcribed by the research assistant experienced in conducting qualitative research. Each interview lasted about 35 min.

Qualitative data management and analysis

Qualitative data was analysed manually using the content thematic approach [14]. Data analysis was done by the first author in collaboration with the fourth author (an experienced qualitative researcher). This involved reading scripts several times, identifying themes and sub-themes, and grouping data according to these themes for interpretation. The main study themes were; motivators and barriers to utilization of PMTCT services. All co-authors were involved in discussions of study themes, sub-themes and interpretation of findings. This process facilitated researcher triangulation [15] to attain a broader understanding of adolescent and young mothers motivators and barriers to utilization of PMTCT services. Direct quotations from study participants reflecting motivators and barriers to use of PMTCT services were identified and used in the presentation of the study findings.

Ethical considerations

Ethical approval for the study was obtained from the Makerere University College of Health Sciences School of Medicine Research Ethics Committee. Written informed consent was obtained from eligible mothers and health workers who agreed to participate in the study. Study participants below 18 years of age independently provided informed consent as emancipated minors, due to them having children, under the Uganda National Council for Science and Technology (UNCST) National Guidelines for Research [16]. The interviewers were instructed on how to comply with strict confidentiality practices for all clients both during and after data collection. For purposes of confidentiality only study specific serial numbers were used in data entry and analysis and the data was only accessible to the research team.

Results
Characteristics of the study population

We screened 453 adolescent and young postpartum mothers attending the Mulago Hospital immunization, postnatal and family planning clinics during the study period (March to June 2015). Of these, 418 were enrolled and interviewed. Out of 35 mothers not enrolled, 25 declined consent for participation, and 10 had children older than 9 months of age.

The median age of the participants was 22 years (IQR 15–24 years). Of the 418 participants, 65 (15.5%) were HIV positive, and 353 (84.5%) were HIV negative.

The majority of the 418 participants were married (76.6%), had a secondary education (62.0%), not employed (66.3%), had a monthly household income between 50,000 and 200,000 Ugandan shillings (15–59 USD) (70.1%), used public transport to get to the facility (71.0%), and attended antenatal care at least once during their most recent pregnancy (98.6%). Only 81 mothers (19.7%) had attended ANC four or more times as shown in Table 1.

Utilization of PMTCT services

Of the 418 participants, all of them (100%) had ever tested for HIV and received their test results. Of these, 400 (95.7%) tested during their most recent pregnancy, while 18 (4.3%) tested prior to their most recent pregnancy. Of the 400 mothers who tested for HIV during their most recent pregnancy, 395 (98.7%) tested in ANC, while 5 (1.3%) tested out of ANC.

Of the 418 participants, 65 (15.5%) reported that they tested HIV positive, and 353 (84.5%) reported that they tested HIV negative. The participants' self-reported HIV status was verified from clinic records.

Of the 353 participants who tested HIV negative, 154 (43.6%) did not retest after receiving their first test results and hence were not retained in the HIV negative PMTCT cascade. Of the 199 who retested for HIV, 97 (49%)

Table 1 Characteristics of 418 mothers attending immunization, postnatal, and family planning clinics of Mulago Hospital, Kampala in 2015

Variable	Distribution of participants	
	Number	Percentage
Age categories (years)		
15–19	76	18.2
20–24	342	81.8
Marital status		
Single	67	16.0
Married	320	76.6
Co-habiting	23	5.5
Separated	8	1.9
Education		
Primary	107	25.6
Secondary	259	62.0
Tertiary	47	11.2
Never	5	1.2
Employment status		
Employed	141	33.7
Not employed	277	66.3
Religion		
Christian	335	80.1
Moslem	83	19.9
Combined Monthly income[a]		
< 50,000	20	4.8
50,000-200,000	293	70.1
200,001-500,000	100	23.9
> 500,000	5	1.2
Travel means to the clinic		
Walk	114	27.3
Public transport	297	71.0
Private transport	7	1.7
Attend ANC for most recent pregnancy		
No	6	1.4
Yes	412	98.6
Number of ANC attendances		
< 4	331	80.3
≥ 4	81	19.7
Parity		
One	294	70.3
Two	101	24.2
Three	20	4.8
Four	3	0.7
Reported HIV status[b]		
Positive	65	15.5
Negative	353	84.5

[a]Combined monthly income in Ugandan Shillings
[b]Reported HIV Status: As was reported by the mothers

retested during the third trimester of their pregnancy, and 30 (15%) retested during labour/delivery, but were not up to date with retesting for HIV, resulting in delays in retesting for HIV after the first negative test. Of the 199 who retested for HIV, only 72 (36%) were up to date with retesting for HIV as was recommended.

Of the 65 mothers who tested HIV positive, 64 (98.5%) were enrolled in HIV care and used PMTCT ARVs. One mother was not enrolled in care because she declined enrolment and was not retained in the PMTCT cascade. Three of the 64 mothers who were enrolled in HIV care reported that their babies tested HIV positive by DNA PCR done at 6 weeks of age, giving an HIV transmission rate of 4.7%. The reported HIV status of the babies was verified from clinic records. The characteristics of the mothers of these 3 babies were similar to those of the other mothers whose babies were reportedly HIV negative. Among the infants of the 64 mothers who were enrolled in care, one was not started on ARV prophylaxis at birth for unknown reasons. There were delays in the utilization of the PMTCT cascade for four mothers whose infants were not started on septrin prophylaxis at 6 weeks, and 8 infants whose DNA PCR was not done at 6 weeks of age.

The details of the utilization of the early PMTCT cascade for 418 adolescent and young mothers attending Mulago Hospital are shown in Fig. 1.

Optimal utilization of PMTCT services

Utilization of PMTCT services was higher among HIV positive mothers, with 54 of the 65 (83.1%) HIV positive mothers having utilized the services optimally, compared to only 72 of the 353 (20.4%) HIV negative mothers (OR 18.2 (95% CI: 9.0–36.7)).

A higher proportion of mothers aged 20–24 years (32.5%), regardless of HIV status, had optimally utilized the services compared to only 19.7% of mothers aged 15–19 years (OR 1.9 (95% CI: 1.1–3.6)).

Factors associated with optimal utilization of PMTCT services

Age and reported HIV status were significantly associated with optimal utilization of PMTCT services at bivariate analysis. Compared to women in the age group 15–19 years, women in the age group 20–24 years were more likely to optimally utilize PMTCT services (OR 1.9 (95% CI: 1.1–3.6); p-value = 0.031).

The factors at bivariate analysis with a p-value < 0.2 which were considered for multivariate analysis, included: age, reported HIV status, and attendance of ANC. Of these 3 variables, only reported HIV status was significantly associated with optimal utilization of

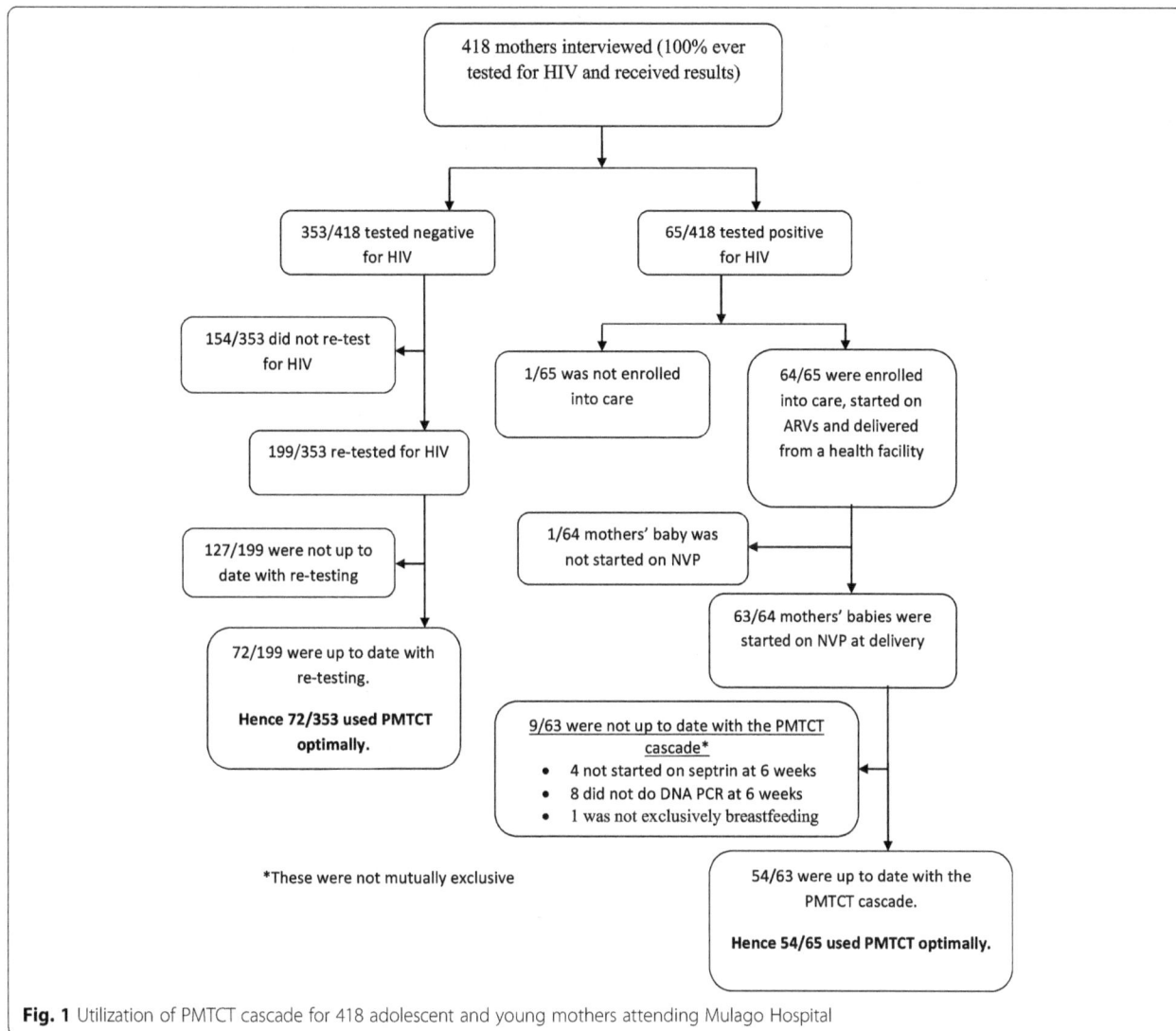

Fig. 1 Utilization of PMTCT cascade for 418 adolescent and young mothers attending Mulago Hospital

PMTCT services at multivariate analysis, (OR 18.2 (95% CI: 9.0–36.7)), as shown in Table 2.

Motivators for utilization of PMTCT services
The benefits of knowing HIV status (90.2%) was the commonest reported motivating factor for utilizing PMTCT services. Other reported motivating factors included health of unborn child (81.3%), responsibility to prevent spread of HIV (73.2%), desire to know ones' status (72.97%), counselling by health care staff (69.1%), perception of need (61.7%), and peer and family support (34.9%), as shown in Table 3.

Barriers to utilization of PMTCT services
Stigma (56.7%) was the commonest reported barrier to adolescent and young mothers' utilization of PMTCT services. Other commonly reported barriers included lack of confidentiality in the clinics (29.4%), long waiting times at the clinics (25.9%), poor health worker

Table 2 Adjusted analysis of factors independently associated with optimal utilization of PMTCT services by adolescent and young mothers attending Mulago Hospital

Variable	Adjusted odds ratio (95% CI)	P value
Age category		
15–19	1.0	
20–24	1.8 (0.9–3.5)	0.110
Reported HIV status		
Negative	1.0	
Positive	18.2 (9.0–36.7)	0.001
Attended ANC		
No	1.0	
Yes	0.3 (0.04–2.6)	0.299

Table 3 Perceived motivators of utilization of PMTCT services by adolescent and young mothers attending Mulago Hospital

Motivating Factor	Percentage[a] ($N = 418$)
Benefits of knowing HIV status	90.19
Health of unborn child	81.34
Responsibility to prevent spread of HIV	73.21
Desire to know ones status	72.97
Counselling by health care staff	69.14
Perception of need	61.72
Peer and family support	34.93

[a]Percentages add up to > 100% given non-mutually exclusive answer count

and client interaction (18.9%), financial constraints (16.7%), and limited information (15.1%), as shown in Fig. 2.

Qualitative study findings

Of the 20 mothers involved in the IDIs, 6 were aged 15–19 years (2 HIV positive and 4 HIV negative), while 14 were aged 20–24 years (8 HIV positive and 6 HIV negative). A total of 9 key informants were interviewed. All of the key informants were females (only females were found to be involved in the provision of the PMTCT

services), 4 out of 9 were aged 30 years or less. Three of the KIs had been involved in providing PMTCT services for less than 5 years, four had been involved in providing PMTCT services between 5 and 10 years, and two had been involved in providing PMTCT services for more than 10 years.

HIV testing knowledge and practices

Data from both IDIs and KIIs showed that most mothers had heard about HIV testing prior to their coming to Mulago Hospital. Most mothers had learnt about HIV testing from the media, friends, and from ANC for previous pregnancies.

HIV testing as part of ANC was not a surprise for the adolescent and young mothers, yet many found it a difficult step to take. Most believed that HIV testing was only necessary when a woman is sick or pregnant as one participant noted:

It is not easy because some young mothers say they cannot look for trouble by coming to test for HIV. They wait to get a reason for testing such as pregnancy or sickness and then they will be forced to test because during antenatal it is a must to test... (Single, 23 years, HIV positive).

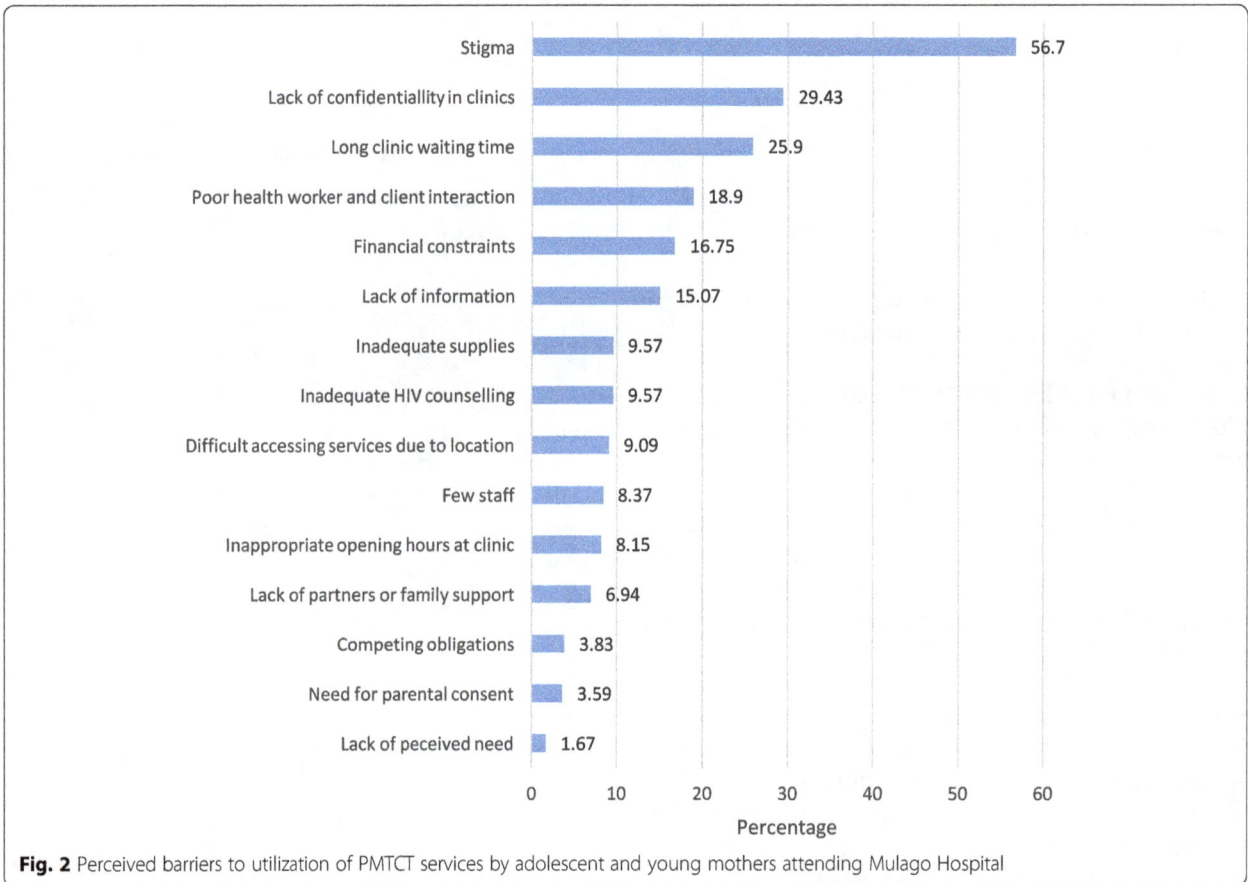

Fig. 2 Perceived barriers to utilization of PMTCT services by adolescent and young mothers attending Mulago Hospital

Consistent with quantitative findings, qualitative interviews revealed that all of the study participants had tested for HIV, mainly during pregnancy.

Generally, the HIV negative participants thought retesting for HIV after a first negative test was easy, although not many go back to retest. The HIV positive participants however thought that retesting was not easy for HIV negative women, for fear of the results turning positive, and the fact that they saw it as unnecessary. This sentiment was also shared by the health workers, who thought that the women see no need to retest after testing HIV negative the first time.

However, many narratives of HIV positive mothers indicated that they had at onetime tested HIV negative, and later tested HIV positive.

During the time I used to go for antenatal, I was tested and on all occasions my results showed that I was HIV negative... However, when I was tested again after delivery I was found to be positive... (Separated, 21 years, HIV positive).

Motivators for utilization of PMTCT services

In the IDIs, the participants revealed that services were better for HIV positive women as compared to HIV negative ones which could influence their utilization of PMTCT services. HIV positive women had more services available to them such as income generation activities and peer support.

The care and attention that health workers give us is very encouraging and can motivate other mothers to also utilize the services... (Married, 23 years, HIV positive).

This was further highlighted by the health workers in the KI interviews.

Consistent with quantitative findings, most participants in the IDIs mentioned the benefits of knowing their HIV status, such as getting access to free treatment and services, as a strong motivator for utilization of PMTCT services. This view was also shared by the health workers.

The desire to protect their unborn children from acquiring HIV infection was another dominant motivator for these women.

Most young mothers who utilize PMTCT services are driven by the desire to protect their children from infection. Sometimes a young mother could have given up on themselves but when they teach them that their babies can be HIV negative, they begin to use the service for the sake of the baby.. (Separated, 21 years, HIV positive).

In-depth and KI interviews further revealed that counselling and support by health care staff and peer educators were strong motivators for mothers to utilize PMTCT services.

The health workers and peer educators are actually good because they take the initiative and call you in case you default on your refills for the baby. They call and remind you to come for your drugs or send someone to pick them for you in case you are unable to. (Cohabiting, 22 years, HIV positive).

At the PMTCT clinic the peer educators who are also HIV positive share their testimonies with these mothers to encourage them and help them understand that one can live positively and live healthy. Most of the peer educators have been beneficiaries of PMTCT and their children are negative. This encourages mothers to adhere to treatment as well as to continue coming for the services.. (Peer educator).

The personal experiences of these mothers further highlighted the different factors that motivated them to utilize PMTCT services. Such motivators were; a longing to learn about HIV, fear of death, and desire to protect the baby from getting infected with HIV.

Barriers to utilization of PMTCT services

Consistent with quantitative findings, individual factors, health services related factors, as well as societal factors came up as barriers to utilization of PMTCT services in both the in-depth interviews and the KI interviews.

Stigma

Stigma emerged as a major barrier to the participants' utilization of PMTCT services as noted by one mother:

Stigma is a major issue. Young mothers fear that their results will be shared or discovered by other people especially if they test positive.. (Cohabiting, 23 years, HIV negative).

Similarly, key informants stressed the role of stigma as a barrier to utilization of PMTCT services by was noted by one key informant:

Stigma is the biggest challenge adolescent mother's face. They first of all stigmatize themselves and then the stigma that comes from the community. Young mothers think that when one is tested positive, they are going to die and they lose hope in themselves... (Peer educator).

Individual level barriers

At the individual level, financial constraints, competing obligations, non-disclosure, lack of symptoms, lack of partner and family support, lack of information, and fear of drugs stood out as factors that prevent adolescent and young mothers from utilizing PMTCT services.

I am not ready to disclose to my parents yet...It was impossible for me to practice exclusive breast feeding because each time the baby cried, my grandmother and the people around would tell me to give him food and then breastfeed him.. (Married, 23 years, HIV positive).

Fear to swallow drugs for a long period of time was another factor hindering adolescent and young mothers from utilizing PMTCT services.

Young mothers fear to swallow drugs. When they are told that they have to take the drugs every day for their life time, they become tired even before starting... (Peer educator).

Health services barriers

At the health services level, negative attitude of health workers stood out as a barrier to utilization of PMTCT services.

There is a particular health worker who abuses young girls a lot for being pregnant. Some mothers used to run away before being attended to... (Cohabiting, 20 years, HIV negative).

Some nurses are very harsh to mothers especially when they are tired. They become very rude, and this can discourage the mothers from coming back to the clinics .. (Single, 23 years, HIV positive).

Long waiting time at the clinic, long distance to the health facility, and lack of adolescent specific clinics were also mentioned as barriers to utilization of PMTCT services. Waiting time was related to the high number of clients compared to health workers.

The clinic receives very many mothers, and this increases their waiting time...Considering the fact that they are either pregnant or nursing babies, they don't like waiting for a long time (Counsellor).

When mothers stay far from the hospital and need to pay for transport, they could be discouraged especially if they are not working and have no one giving them financial support... (Single, 21 years old, HIV positive)

Discussion

The key finding in this study is that the proportion of adolescent and young mothers who had optimally utilized PMTCT services was low. Optimal utilization of PMTCT services was defined as being up to date with utilization of the PMTCT cascade of services for reported HIV status at the time the interview was conducted. There is limited information on optimal utilization of the PMTCT cascade of services as defined in this study, as most studies only looked at one step or the other of the cascade, and not the entire cascade as a whole [17, 18]. Optimal utilization of PMTCT services was significantly associated with reported positive HIV status. One explanation could be that programs in the hospital designed to improve PMTCT uptake have been focussing on HIV positive mothers. These programs use highly motivated peer educators to counsel and follow up the HIV positive mothers, and also have income generating and psychosocial support activities for them further encouraging their utilization of the services. Overall, the support for HIV negative adolescent and young women seem to end after communicating negative results. This emphasizes the need for sustained HIV prevention efforts to scale up primary prevention among young HIV negative women. Another explanation could be that the HIV positive mothers included in this study formed the population of HIV positive women who came back for clinic services, and so are better at utilizing PMTCT services compared to the population who do not come back. Hence there is a potential for overestimation of retention in the PMTCT cascade among this population of HIV positive mothers included in this study.

In this study, only 20% of HIV negative mothers had optimally utilized PMTCT services. As much as 43.6% of them did not retest for HIV after the first test, and of those who retested, more than 60% were not up to date with retesting for HIV. Whereas it is understandable for more support to be accorded to women who test HIV positive, the apparent inattention given to those who tested HIV negative the first time could explain their poor utilization of PMTCT services. It is however important to note that some mothers who test HIV negative the first time could test HIV positive later on in the pregnancy or after delivery. New HIV infections could remain undetected in previously HIV negative mothers due to their low rates of retesting, leading to undiagnosed maternal infection, and hence mother-to-child transmission of HIV [7]. This highlights the importance of retaining HIV-negative women in the PMTCT cascade.

This study found a high uptake of PMTCT services (98.5%) among HIV positive participants including enrolment into care, taking ARVs and delivering from a health facility. These findings closely align with the report by the Uganda's Ministry of Health (MOH) that more than 90% of HIV positive pregnant women were enrolled in care, received ARVs for themselves and their babies, and exclusively breastfed their babies in Uganda in 2013 [19]. Other African studies have reported similar findings [20, 21]. Given the efficacy of Antiretroviral Therapy (ART) in HIV-infection control, and especially where adherence to treatment is good, high program uptake can translate into a significant reduction in the burden of HIV infections in the paediatric population. The MTCT rate of 4.7% found among the participants is lower than that reported previously [22], prior to introduction of the World Health Organization (WHO) option B- plus strategy in Uganda, but it still falls below the elimination target of < 2% [23].

This study highlights a number of issues useful for understanding factors influencing the utilization of PMTCT services. The study also documented potential areas for improving PMTCT interventions.

Adolescents had less utilization than young women, and this was significant at bivariate analysis. Although this significance fell out at multivariate analysis, adolescents have been noted to have less utilization of PMTCT services (4).

Health workers in this study recognized that psychosocial support and the engagement of peer educators encouraged adolescent and young mothers to utilize PMTCT services. Studies in Uganda have shown that adolescents experience a lot of psychosocial challenges especially when pregnant [4, 9], hence it is no surprise that continuous support and counselling of these mothers would increase their utilization of these services. Peer support should be maximized in all centres offering PMTCT services in order to improve utilization of these services.

This study further emphasizes the fact that the desire to protect the baby from becoming infected with HIV is a strong motivator for young mothers' utilization of PMTCT services. This implies that focussing on the baby in prevention messages could improve utilization of PMTCT services in this vulnerable group.

This study has revealed multiple social, cultural, economic and physical barriers that might hinder the success of PMTCT interventions. Stigma was found to be a key demotivating factor for adolescent and young mothers' utilization of PMTCT services. A study in Kenya found that stigma and health system factors were barriers to utilization of PMTCT services [21]. Stigma remains a major concern with women not wishing to have their HIV status disclosed. Many women are therefore reluctant to utilize PMTCT services for fear of being stigmatized and discriminated against, emphasizing the importance of addressing stigma as a barrier, if EMTCT is to be realized.

This study has several strengths: The study contributes to the literature by identifying some of the gaps in the utilization of PMTCT services which were not previously described. The study had both quantitative and qualitative aspects. Qualitative interviews involving use of probes and triangulation of data from different sources helped to improve the trustworthiness of the study findings. Furthermore, the inclusion of HIV positive and HIV negative mothers in the study provided an opportunity to uncover the unique experiences and support needs for each of the two groups of adolescent and young women.

The findings of this study should however be interpreted in view of the following limitations:

Recall bias cannot be excluded. However, analysis was limited to mothers whose infants were 9 months old or younger and whose pregnancy was therefore recent. The fact that quantitative interviews were conducted by nurses may have affected participants' response to perceived barriers to utilization of PMTCT services. The study was conducted at the National Referral Hospital, a public hospital characterized by congestion and delays at the clinics. It is possible that women with higher incomes obtain care from private clinics and may thus be under-represented in this study. Optimal utilization of PMTCT services in this study was determined for the first 9 months of the recommended PMTCT cascade (in order to minimize recall bias), instead of the entire PMTCT cascade of 18 months. The relatively smaller number of HIV positive women included in the study ($N = 65$), and their unequal distribution (only 7 were adolescents aged 15–19 years) could have affected the results of this study. However, these HIV positive mothers provided very useful information with regards to the motivators and barriers of their utilization of PMTCT services.

Conclusions

Optimal utilization of PMTCT services among adolescent and young mothers at 30% was low. However, optimal utilization of PMTCT services was better among the HIV positive women as majority (83%) of them had optimally utilized the services, compared to only 20% of the HIV negative mothers. The study further demonstrated losses and delays throughout the PMTCT cascade. Reported positive HIV status was significantly associated with optimal utilization of PMTCT services. The major factors motivating adolescent and young mothers to utilize PMTCT services included: the benefits of knowing ones' HIV status, health of the unborn child, and counselling and support by health care staff. Stigma was a key demotivating factor for the adolescent and young mothers' utilization of PMTCT services.

We recommend that special consideration should be given to adolescents and young women in the design of EMTCT programs, to improve the utilization of PMTCT services particularly among those found HIV negative at the first HIV test to support them to remain HIV negative. In addition, we recommend that stigma as a barrier to the utilization of PMTCT services should be addressed by PMTCT service providers and policy makers, and that counselling and health care support should emphasize on the benefits of PMTCT services since they motivate adolescent and young mothers to utilize the services.

Abbreviations
AIDS: Acquired immunodeficiency syndrome; ANC: Antenatal care; ART: Antiretroviral Therapy; ARV: Antiretroviral drug; DNA PCR: Deoxyribonucleic acid polymerase chain reaction; EMTCT: Elimination of mother-to-child transmission (of HIV); HIV: Human immunodeficiency virus; IDI: In-depth interviews; KII: Key-informant interviews; MOH: Ministry of Health; MTCT: Mother-to-child transmission (of HIV); NVP: Nevirapine syrup; PMTCT: Prevention of mother-to-child transmission (of HIV); UNCST: Uganda National Council for Science and Technology; WHO: World Health Organization

Acknowledgments
Our special thanks go to the mothers at Mulago Hospital who consented to participate in this study.

Funding
Ministry of Health and Sanitation, Sierra Leone, and the Makerere University School of Public Health Centre for Excellence for Maternal and Newborn through training of the principal investigator. The above institutions played no role in the design of the study and collection, analysis, and interpretation of data and in writing the manuscript.

Authors' contributions
MM conceived of the study and drafted the manuscript. VM, SBK, JR, and NNB participated in its design and coordination, read, revised and approved the final manuscript. All authors read and approved the final manuscript.

Competing interests
The authors declare that they have no competing interests.

Author details
[1]Department of Paediatrics and Child Health, School of Medicine, Makerere University College of Health Sciences, Kampala, Uganda. [2]Ministry of Health and Sanitation, Freetown, Sierra Leone. [3]Joint Clinical Research Centre, Kampala, Uganda.

References
1. Joint United Nations Programme on HIV/AIDS (UNAIDS), UNAIDS data 2017. 2017.
2. Joint United Nations Programme on HIV/AIDS. World AIDS day report 2011. How to get to zero: faster. Smarter. Better. Geneva: Joint United Nations Programme on HIV/AIDS; 2011. p. 6–7.
3. Ministry of Health Kampala Uganda, Assessment of adolescent HIV care and treatment services. 2014.
4. Atuyambe L, et al. Adolescent and adult first time mothers' health seeking practices during pregnancy and early motherhood in Wakiso district, Central Uganda. Reprod Health. 2008;5(1):13.
5. Birungi H, et al. Maternal health care utilization among HIV-positive female adolescents in Kenya. Int Perspect Sex Reprod Health. 2011;37(3):143–9.
6. The Global Fund, Scaling up prevention of mother-to-child transmission of HIV (PMTCT) information note. 2010.
7. Hamilton E, et al. Using the PMTCT cascade to accelerate achievement of the global plan goals. J Acquir Immune Defic Syndr. 2017;75(1):S27–35.
8. Mbonye A, et al. Barriers to prevention of mother-to-child transmission of HIV services in Uganda. J Biosoc Sci. 2010;42(02):271–83.
9. Atuyambe L, et al. Experiences of pregnant adolescents-voices from Wakiso district, Uganda. Afr Health Sci. 2007;5(4):304–9.
10. Joint United Nations Programme on HIV/AIDS (UNAIDS), A focus on women: a key strategy to preventing HIV among children. 2014.
11. Uganda Bureau Of Statistics, National population and housing census 2014. 2014.
12. World Health Organization. Global Health Observatory data repository. http://apps.who.int/gho/data/node.main.REPADO39?lang=en. [Accessed 7 Mar 2018].
13. Ministry of Health Kampala Uganda, Uganda AIDS Indicator Survey 2011. 2012.
14. Graneheim UH. L.B.Q.c.a.i.n.r.c, procedures and measures to achieve trustworthiness. Nurse Educ Today. 2004;24(2):105–12.
15. Tong A, Sainsbury P, Craig J. Consolidated criteria for reporting qualitative research (COREQ): a 32-item checklist for interviews and focus groups. Int J Qual Health Care. 2007;19(6):349–57.
16. Uganda National Council for Science and Technology (UNCST). National guidelines for research involving humans as research participants. Kampala: UNCST; 2014.
17. Amoran OE, Salami OF, Oluwole FA. A comparative analysis of teenagers and older pregnant women in the utilization of prevention of mother to child transmission [PMTCT] services in, Western Nigeria. BMC Int Health Hum Rights. 2012;12(1):1.
18. Deressa W, et al. Utilization of PMTCT services and associated factors among pregnant women attending antenatal clinics in Addis Ababa, Ethiopia. BMC Pregnancy Childbirth. 2014;14(1):1.
19. United States Agency International Development (USAID), USAID strengthening Uganda's systems for treating AIDS nationally quarterly report April–June 2013. 2013.
20. Ajewole OJ, Sparks BL, Omole OB. Uptake and factors that affect enrolment into the prevention of mother-to-child transmission of human immunodeficiency virus programme in rural Limpopo Province. S Afr Fam Pract. 2013;55(6):555–60.
21. Kinuthia J, et al. Uptake of prevention of mother to child transmission interventions in Kenya: health systems are more influential than stigma. J Int AIDS Soc. 2011;14(1):1.
22. Uganda AIDS Commission. Global AIDS response progress report; country progress report Uganda. Kampala: UAC; 2012.
23. The United Nations Children's Fund and World Health Organization, Towards the elimination of mother-to-child transmission of HIV: report of a WHO technical consultation, 9-11 November 2010, Geneva, Switzerland. 2011.

30

Soluble fibrinogen-like protein 2 levels in patients with hepatitis B virus-related liver diseases

Hoang Van Tong[1,2,3*†], Nguyen Van Ba[1†], Nghiem Xuan Hoan[3,4,5], Mai Thanh Binh[3,4,5], Dao Thanh Quyen[3,4,5], Ho Anh Son[1,2], Hoang Van Luong[1], Do Quyet[1], Christian G. Meyer[3,5,6], Le Huu Song[4,5], Nguyen Linh Toan[2] and Thirumalaisamy P. Velavan[3,5,6*]

Abstract

Background: Clinical progression of HBV-related liver diseases is largely associated with the activity of HBV-specific T cells. Soluble fibrinogen-like protein 2 (sFGL2), mainly secreted by T cells, is an important effector molecule of the immune system.

Methods: sFGL2 levels were determined by ELISA assays in sera of 296 HBV patients clinically classified into the subgroups of acute hepatitis B (AHB), chronic hepatitis B (CHB), liver cirrhosis (LC), hepatocellular carcinoma (HCC) and patients with LC plus HCC. As control group, 158 healthy individuals were included. FGL2 mRNA was quantified by qRT-PCR in 32 pairs of tumor and adjacent non-tumor liver tissues.

Results: sFGL2 levels were elevated in HBV patients compared to healthy controls ($P < 0.0001$). In the patient group, sFGL2 levels were increased in AHB compared to CHB patients ($P = 0.017$). sFGL2 levels were higher in LC patients compared to those without LC ($P = 0.006$) and were increased according to the development of cirrhosis as staged by Child-Pugh scores ($P = 0.024$). Similarly, HCC patients had increased sFGL2 levels compared to CHB patients ($P = 0.033$) and FGL2 mRNA was up-regulated in tumor tissues compared to adjacent non-tumor tissues ($P = 0.043$). In addition, sFGL2 levels were positively correlated with HBV-DNA loads and AST (Spearman's rho = 0.21, 0.25 and $P = 0.006, 0.023$, respectively), but reversely correlated with platelet counts and albumin levels (Spearman's rho = − 0.27, − 0.24 and $P = 0.014, 0.033$, respectively).

Conclusions: sFGL2 levels are induced by HBV infection and correlated with the progression and clinical outcome of HBV-related liver diseases. Thus, sFGL2 may serve as a potential indicator for HBV-related liver diseases.

Keywords: sFGL2 levels, HBV infection, Viral hepatitis, Liver cirrhosis, Hepatocellular carcinoma

Background

Hepatitis B virus (HBV) infection is a major health problem with approximately 257 million people infected and 887,000 deaths annually due to complications [1]. HBV is highly prevalent in sub-Saharan Africa, Asia and parts of America with infection rates ranging from 8 to 20% of the populations [1]. Vietnam is a highly endemic country for HBV infection with a prevalence of up to 20%. In spite of the effective coverage of anti-HBV vaccination in Vietnam, HBV-related liver diseases are foreseen to be an important public health problem in the next decades due to the long latency of chronic hepatitis, liver cirrhosis, and hepatocellular carcinoma [2]. Estimations made in 2012 have indicated that up to 10 million people are living with chronic hepatitis B in Vietnam with 23,300 deaths annually due to the infection [3].

* Correspondence:
hoangvantong@vmmu.edu.vn; velavan@medizin.uni-tuebingen.de
†Hoang Van Tong and Nguyen Van Ba contributed equally to this work.
[1]Institute of Biomedicine and Pharmacy, Vietnam Military Medical University, 222 Phung Hung, Ha Dong, Hanoi, Vietnam
[3]Institute of Tropical Medicine, University of Tübingen, Wilhelmstrasse 27, 72074 Tübingen, Germany
Full list of author information is available at the end of the article

HBV infection leads to a wide spectrum of liver diseases, including an asymptomatic carrier status, acute self-limiting and fulminant hepatitis, chronic hepatitis B (CHB), liver cirrhosis (LC) and hepatocellular carcinoma (HCC) [1]. CHB is the most important risk factor for the development of HCC with a 100-fold increase in chronic HBV carriers compared to non-carriers [4]. HCC is the third leading cause of cancer-related deaths and more than 500,000 new cases are diagnosed worldwide annually [4]. HBV stimulates both the innate and adaptive immune systems to establish persistent infections and the liver injuries in chronic infection are associated with the activity of HBV-specific T cells [5]. The mechanism of hepatocellular injury is immune-mediated and strongly dependent on the interaction between distinct viral factors and host immune responses [5]. Sequential transformation of normal hepatocytes to malignant cells during HCC development is associated with the immune response to HBV-infected liver cells, accumulated genetic alterations, and the interaction between the viral HBx protein with host signaling proteins [6].

Fibrinogen-like protein 2 (FGL2), also known as fibroleukin, belongs to the fibrinogen-associated superfamily of proteins and is homologous to the β and γ chains of fibrinogen [7]. FGL2 is encoded by the *FGL2* gene, which contains two exons and is localized to the proximal region of chromosome 7q11.23 (NC_000007.14) [8]. There are two different forms of FGL2, namely the type II transmembrane FGL2 (mFGL2) and the soluble FGL2 (sFGL2). mFGL2 has prothrombinase activity to cleave thrombin from prothrombin and is expressed on the surface of different cell types such as macrophages, endothelial and dendritic cells [8, 9], while sFGL2 is mainly secreted by CD4+, CD8+ and regulatory T cells, and has immune regulatory activity [10, 11]. sFGL2 is an important effector molecule involved in various processes of immunity, including antigen presentation, immunosuppression and apoptosis [7]. It is also part of various signaling pathways such as ITAM/ITIM (immunoreceptor tyrosine-based activating motif/ immunoreceptor tyrosine-based inhibitory motif), NF-κB (nuclear factor kappa-light-chain-enhancer of activated B cells) and MAPK (mitogen-activated protein kinases) [7, 12].

Clinically, sFGL2 plays an important role in organ transplantation through regulation of T and B cell mediated immunity. Increased sFGL2 levels have been observed in recipients with acute allograft rejection [12, 13]. sFGL2 has been implicated in different types of diseases, including cancer, autoimmune and infectious diseases [7, 14–16]. In viral hepatitis, sFGL2 is involved in the immune responses against HBV and HCV infections. Expression of FGL2 was associated with susceptibility to murine hepatitis virus strain 3 (MHV-3) infection in vivo [11], and the *FGL2* gene has been

suggested as a potential target for treatment of fulminant viral hepatitis [11, 17, 18]. In a clinical study, plasma sFGL2 levels were significantly increased and correlated with clinical progression of HCV infection and antiviral therapy [19]. In addition, sFGL2 regulates the T-cell function in cirrhotic patients with HCC [14], and plasma sFGL2 levels are positively associated with the severity of non-alcoholic fatty liver disease (NAFLD) [16]. The present study investigates plasma levels of sFGL2 in Vietnamese patients with HBV-related liver diseases and their correlation with clinical progression of HBV infection.

Methods
Patients and controls

Two hundred and ninety-six Vietnamese patients ($n = 296$) with HBV infections were recruited from the 108 Military Central Hospital and 103 Military Hospital, Hanoi, Vietnam between the years 2014 and 2016 [20]. All recruited HBV patients were negative for HCV and HIV. The recruited chronic HBV patients were diagnosed based on the guidelines of European Association for the Study of the Liver (EASL) [21], and the HCC patients based on the guidelines from American Association for the Study of Liver Diseases (AASLD) [22]. The patients were further sub-classified into five groups based on the clinical manifestations, biochemical and serological parameters. The patient groups were acute hepatitis B (AHB; n = 29), chronic hepatitis B (CHB; $n = 73$), patients with only liver cirrhosis (LC; $n = 70$), patients with only hepatocellular carcinoma (HCC; $n = 99$) and patients with both liver cirrhosis and hepatocellular carcinoma (HCC + LC, $n = 25$). In addition, patients with LC were further classified either as Child-A, Child-B or Child-C according to Child-Pugh scores [23]. Laboratory and clinical parameters such as blood counts, total and direct bilirubin, prothrombin, albumin, alanine transaminase (ALT), aspartate transaminase (AST), alpha-fetoprotein (AFP) and HBV-DNA loads were measured by routine laboratory tests. As control group, we recruited one hundred and fifty-eight healthy Vietnamese blood donors (HC; $n = 158$) who were confirmed negative for HBsAg, anti-HCV and anti-HIV antibodies [20]. All control individuals had no history of alcohol or drug use. Approximately five milliliters of venous blood was collected and respective serum and/or plasma was separated from whole blood immediately and stored at – 20 °C until further use. In addition, 32 pairs of tumor and adjacent non-tumor tissues were collected from HCC patients who underwent surgery at the 108 Military Central Hospital. The clinical profiles of the HCC patients have been described in our previous published study [20] [24].

Ethics approval and consent to participate

Informed written consent was received from all participants after detailed explanation of the study at the time of blood sampling. The study was approved by the Institutional Review Board of the Vietnam Military Medical University (VMMU) and the 108 Military Central Hospital, Hanoi, Vietnam. All experiments were performed in accordance with relevant guidelines and regulations.

Quantification of sFGL2 levels by ELISA

Soluble FGL2 levels were measured in the plasma samples from the patients with HBV-related liver diseases and in healthy controls using a commercially available Fibrinogen-Like 2 (FGL2) ELISA kit (Wuhan USCN Business Co., Ltd., Wuhan, China) following the manufacturer's instructions. The microtiter plate provided of the kit was delivered already coated with a specific FGL2 monoclonal antibody. 100 µL of the FGL2 standard and the study samples were added to the wells of the coated ELISA plate and incubated for 2 h at 37 °C. The liquid of each well was removed and 100 µL of the first detection solution with a biotin-conjugated antibody preparation specific for FGL2 was added and incubated for 1 h at 37 °C. After washing with wash solution, the second detection solution with avidin conjugated to Horseradish Peroxidase (HRP) was added to each microplate well and incubated for 30 min at 37 °C. After washing again, TMB substrate solution was added and incubated for 15–25 min at 37 °C. Subsequently, stop solution was added and the plates were immediately read at a wavelength of 450 nm by an ELISA reader. The standard curve was plotted based upon the mean of O.D. (optical density) value and the known concentration of the standard. The concentrations of sFGL2 protein were calculated based upon the standard curve. The minimum detectable limit of sFGL2 proteins was less than 0.19 ng/mL.

Quantification of FGL2 mRNA by RT-PCR

Total RNA was extracted from the 32 tumour and adjacent non-tumour tissues using Trizol reagent (Life Technologies, Carlsbad, CA, USA) and was reverse transcribed into cDNA by using QuantiTect Reverse Transcription Kit (Qiagen, Hilden, Germany) [20]. Quantification of cDNA was performed by quantitative real-time PCR with GAPDH (glyceraldehyde-3-phosphate dehydrogenase) as a reference gene. Primer sequences were FGL2_F: 5'-AGG CAG AAA CGG ACT GTT GT-3' and FGL2_R: 5'-CCA GGC GAC CAT GAA GTA CA-3', GAPDH_F: 5'-TGC ACC ACC AAC TGC TTA GC-3' and GAPDH_R: 5'-GGC ATG GAC TGT GGT CAT GAG-3' [25]. In brief: real-time PCR amplification was carried out in a reaction volume of 25 µl containing 12.5 µl 2X SYBR Green PCR master mix (Bioline, Luckenwalde, Germany),

0.5 µM specific primer pairs for target gene or reference gene, 5 ng cDNA and RNase-free water up to 25 µl of reaction volume. Thermal conditions were initial denaturation at 95 °C for 2 min followed by 45 cycles of denaturation at 95 °C for 5 s, primer specific annealing and an extension step at 58 °C for 20 s. Melting curve analyses starting from 58 °C to 85 °C were performed after each run to confirm the presence of specific PCR products [20]. All reactions were performed in duplicates and each run was repeated twice using the LightCycler® 480 real-time PCR system (Roche, Basel, Switzerland). The relative expression of FGL2 mRNA was calculated based on the ΔCt algorithm and by normalizing the expression of the house keeping gene GAPDH.

Statistical analysis

Quantitative variables were tested for normality and were presented as mean and standard deviation if the data are normally distributed. Normally distributed data were compared using Student's t-test and ANOVA for two and/or more than two groups, respectively. If the data are not normally distributed, quantitative variables were presented as medians with range and were compared using Mann Whitney Wilcoxon and Kruskal-Wallis test for two and more than two groups, respectively. Parametric Pearson's correlation coefficient or non-parametric Spearman's rank correlation coefficient were used to correlate the given two variables, where appropriate. Paired-samples t test was used to compare the relative expression of FGL2 mRNA between tumour and adjacent non-tumour tissues. The SPSS software (SPSS Statistics, IBM, Armonk, NY, the USA) was used for all statistical analyses and the significant level was set at $P < 0.05$.

Results

Baseline characteristics of study participants

The demographic characteristics such as age, gender and clinical parameters such as blood counts, liver function tests, HBV-DNA load and the tumor marker alpha-feto protein (AFP) of all investigated Vietnamese hepatitis B patients and healthy controls are presented in Table 1. Red blood cell counts was observed to be lowest among patients with HCC followed by patients with LC + HCC, LC and CHB patients ($P < 0.01$). White blood cell counts were lower in patients with LC and patients with LC plus HCC compared to CHB and HCC patients ($P < 0.001$). Platelet counts was also observed to be lowest among LC patients followed by LC + HCC, CHB and HCC patients ($P < 0.001$). The levels of ALT, AST, total and direct bilirubin were significantly higher in the AHB group compared to other patient groups (Table 1). In chronically affected patients, the liver enzyme levels such as ALT, AST and

Table 1 Characteristics of patients with HBV-related liver disease segregated according to clinical status

Characteristics	AHB (n = 29)	CHB (n = 73)	LC (n = 70)	HCC (n = 99)	LC + HCC (n = 25)	HC (n = 158)	P value
Age (median, range)	32 (17–70)	39.5 (20–76)	48 (17–74)	50 (15–79)	56 (37–81)	31 (19–38)	< 0.001
Gender (male/female)	23/6	55/18	54/16	84/15	25/0	112/46	< 0.001
Liver cirrhosis stage:							
Child-Pugh A (n,%)	NA	NA	22 (49%)[a]	NA	15 (60%)	NA	NA
Child-Pugh B (n,%)	NA	NA	12 (28%)[a]	NA	8 (32%)	NA	NA
Child-Pugh C (n,%)	NA	NA	10 (23%)[a]	NA	2 (8%)	NA	NA
RBC (×10^3/ml)	NA	6.7 (4.5–13.9)	6 (2.7–20.5)	5.8 (4–11)	5.7 (2.7–11)	NA	< 0.01
WBC (×10^6/ml)	NA	4.9 (4.1–5.3)	4.3 (2.3–6.7)	4.9 (4.2–6)	4.5 (3–6)	NA	< 0.001
PLT (×10^3/ml)	NA	168.5 (61–355)	87.5 (49–299)	196 (101–361)	122 (35–237)	NA	< 0.001
AST (IU/L)	1109 (115.5–4593)	143 (77–657)	71 (16.8–1059)	67 (14–371)	63 (25–655)	NA	< 0.001
ALT (IU/L)	861.5 (182–4425)	144 (89–1643)	57 (8–1426)	50.5 (3–471)	54 (22–551)	NA	< 0.001
Total-Bilirubin (mg/dl)	132 (21.8–558)	22.5 (12–412)	30.3 (6.5–722)	19 (5.1–282)	23 (9–185)	NA	< 0.001
Direct-Bilirubin (mg/dl)	117.3 (14.3–512)	12.4 (6.2–292.3)	14 (1.3–450)	8.8 (2–189.4)	8 (2–59)	NA	< 0.001
Albumin (g/L)	NA	42 (33–50)	32.5 (25–39)	39 (30–47)	38 (27–44)	NA	< 0.01
Prothrombin (%)	85 (50–120)	76 (26–122)	46 (15–100)	78 (37–100)	77 (19.6–117)	NA	< 0.01
HBV-DNA (log10 copies/ml)	3.96 (3.5–5.7)	4.2 (2.8–4.66)	4.1 (2.8–6.4)	3.98 (2.5–8.9)	6 (2.3–10.4)	NA	< 0.001
Alpha fetoprotein (IU/L)	NA	12.5 (2–151)	6.7 (1.2–1050)	96.7 (1.5–1050)	113 (2–300)	NA	< 0.001

Abbreviations: *AHB* acute hepatitis B, *CHB* chronic hepatitis B, *LC* liver cirrhosis, *HCC* hepatocellular carcinoma, *LC + HCC* patients with both LC and HCC, *HC* healthy control, *RBC* red blood cells, *WBC* white blood cells, *PLT* platelets, *AST and ALT* aspartate and alanine amino transferase, *AFP* alpha-fetoprotein, *IU* international unit, *NA* not applicable. Values given are medians and ranges. P values were calculated by Chi-squared test and Kruskal-Wallis test where appropriate. [a]Only patients with clear classification and Child-Pugh score available

albumin levels were higher compared to those with advanced liver diseases (LC, HCC) ($P < 0.001$). Also that total and direct bilirubin levels was higher, whereas albumin and prothrombin levels were lower in LC patients compared to the other groups ($P < 0.001$). As expected, the level of alpha-feto protein levels was observed to be elevated in patients with HCC than in patients without HCC ($P < 0.001$) (Table 1).

Soluble FGL2 levels in patients with HBV-related liver diseases
Soluble FGL2 levels were measured in different clinical subgroups of patients with HBV-related liver diseases and in healthy controls. We observed a mean of 91.1 ± 26.6 ng/ml in AHB, 77.2 ± 25.7 ng/ml in CHB, 85.2 ± 22.7 ng/ml in LC, 87.9 ± 24.8 ng/ml in HCC patients and 92.8 ± 14.1 ng/ml in LC + HCC patients. In healthy individuals, the mean was 62.4 ± 11.9 ng/ml. The results clearly show that sFGL2 levels were significantly elevated in patients with HBV-related liver diseases compared to controls ($P < 0.0001$) (Fig. 1). In the patient group, sFGL2 levels were increased in AHB compared to CHB patients ($P = 0.017$). The results indicate that sFGL2 levels are modulated according to the stage of HBV infection. Increased sFGL2 levels were observed in patients with advanced liver diseases such as LC, HCC patients and those with both LC and HCC compared to CHB patients ($P = 0.033$, 0.006, and 0.001, respectively).

There was no difference of sFGL2 levels in comparisons of LC with HCC patients ($P > 0.05$). Nevertheless, sFGL2 levels were higher in patients with both LC and HCC compared to those with LC or HCC alone, but the difference did not reach significance (Fig. 1).

In the patient group with chronic HBV-related liver diseases, we stratified the patients into subgroups with and without LC, and those with and without HCC. sFGL2 levels were significantly increased in the patients with LC compared to those without LC ($P < 0.0001$) (Fig. 2a). Patients with LC were further categorized as Child-Pugh-A, Child-Pugh-B and Child-Pugh-C based on Child-Pugh scores if available. Child-Pugh-C LC patients had higher sFGL2 levels, followed by Child-Pugh-B and Child-Pugh-A LC patients ($P = 0.024$) (Fig. 2b). Similarly, patients with HCC had significantly higher sFGL2 levels compared to the patients without HCC ($P = 0.009$) (Fig. 2c). Furthermore, we examined the expression of *FGL2* mRNA in tumor and adjacent non-tumor tissues. The relative expression of *FGL2* mRNA was significantly up-regulated in tumor tissues compared to adjacent non-tumor tissues ($P = 0.043$) (Fig. 2d). We then examined whether *FGL2* mRNA relative expression was associated with the development of HCC by analyzing *FGL2* mRNA relative expression according to the BCLC staging classification. However, *FGL2* mRNA relative expression did not differ between stage

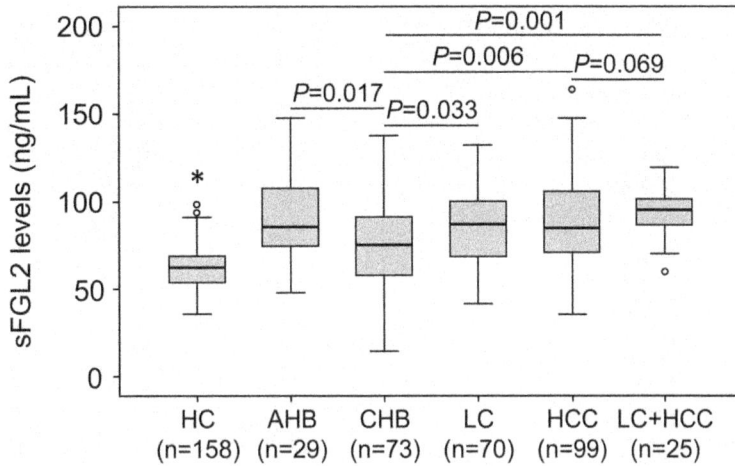

Fig. 1 sFGL2 levels in patients with HBV-related liver diseases and in healthy controls. sFGL2 levels were measured in study subjects and compared between subgroups. HC, healthy controls; AHB, acute hepatitis B; CHB, chronic hepatitis B; LC, patients with liver cirrhosis; HCC, patients with hepatocellular carcinoma; LC + HCC, patients with both liver cirrhosis and hepatocellular carcinoma. (*): $P < 0.0001$ for comparison with other groups. Box plots illustrate medians with inter-quartile range. P values were calculated by Mann-Whitney-Wilcoxon test

A and B HCC tissues as well as between the corresponding adjacent non-tumor tissues obtained from the same stage A and B HCC patients ($P > 0.05$) (Fig. 2e). These results indicate that sFGL2 levels are associated with advanced HBV-related liver diseases.

Correlation between sFGL2 levels and clinical parameters
We analyzed the correlations of sFGL2 levels with available clinical and laboratory parameters of HBV infection in HBV patients and observed a significant positive correlation of sFGL2 levels with HBV-DNA loads and with

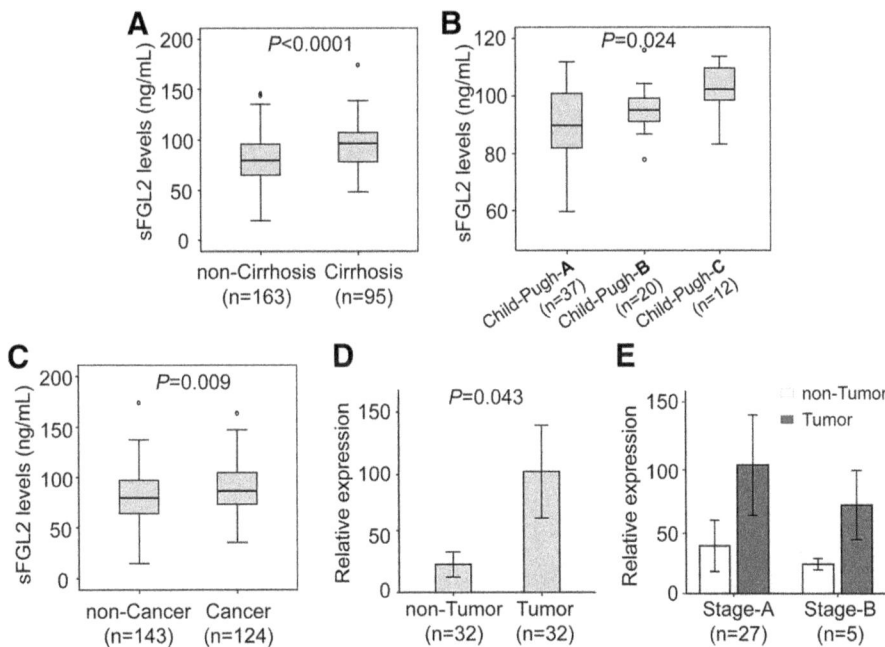

Fig. 2 sFGL2 levels in patients with HBV-related liver diseases and in healthy controls. sFGL2 levels were measured in study subjects and compared between subgroups. **a**: comparison between chronic patients with and without liver cirrhosis. **b**: comparison among different Child-Pugh groups of patients with liver cirrhosis. **c**: comparison between chronic patients with and without hepatocellular carcinoma. **d**: comparison of *FGL2* mRNA expression in tumour and adjacent non-tumour tissues. **e**: *FGL2* mRNA expression in stage-A and stage-B tumour and adjacent non-tumour tissues. Box plots illustrate medians with inter-quartile range. Comparisons of sFGL2 levels were performed using Mann-Whitney-Wilcoxon test or Kruskal-Wallis test, while comparisons of *FGL2* mRNA relative expression were performed using Paired-samples t test

AST levels (Spearman's rho = 0.21, P = 0.006, and Spearman's rho = 0.25, P = 0.023, respectively) (Fig. 3). sFGL2 levels were significantly and reversely correlated with platelet counts and albumin levels (Spearman's rho = − 0.27, P = 0.014, and Spearman's rho = − 0.24, P = 0.033, respectively) (Fig. 3). However, sFGL2 levels were either not or weakly only correlated with the levels of total and direct bilirubin, ALT and prothrombin.

Discussion

sFGL2 is a regulatory molecule of the immune system and involved in the pathogenesis of many diseases, including viral hepatitis [7, 14–16]. In this study, we have shown that sFGL2 levels are significantly altered in HBV-related liver diseases compared to healthy controls and are highest among patients with acute hepatitis B. sFGL2 levels are increased according to the clinical progression of chronic HBV-related liver diseases and are correlated with several clinical parameters such as AST, albumin, platelet counts and HBV-DNA loads. sFGL2 appears to play an important role in the clinical outcome of HBV infection and the progression of HBV-related liver diseases.

The findings that sFGL2 levels are increased according to the progression of chronic HBV-related liver diseases are in accordance with previous studies [14, 16, 19]. The observation that sFGL2 levels are strongly elevated in acute hepatitis B patients compared to those in CHB supports previous in vivo studies in mice showing that

infection with MHV3 induces FGL2 expression [11, 26]. Induction of FGL2 during viral infection has been established in animal models, showing that plasma FGL2 levels are considerably elevated 2 days after infection with lymphocytic choriomeningitis virus strain WE (LCMV-WE) [18]. In HCV infection, plasma FGL2 levels are extensively increased in patients with chronic hepatitis compared to healthy controls [19]. The increasing levels of sFGL2 in the acute phase of hepatitis in our study group supports the previous finding that FGL2 is involved in the pathogenesis and clinical outcome of fulminant hepatitis in animal models [27, 28].

Plasma FGL2 levels are higher in patients with HCV-related LC compared to those without cirrhosis and correlated with more severe cirrhosis [19]. Similarly, our results also indicate that sFGL2 levels are elevated in patients with HBV-related cirrhosis compared to those without cirrhosis, and sFGL2 levels are increased according to the stage of cirrhosis as assessed by Child-Pugh scores. However, sFGL2 levels are not different between patients with inactive alcoholic cirrhosis and healthy controls [19]. Furthermore, no association of sFGL2 levels with the stage of fibrosis and grade of steatosis were observed in patients with non-alcoholic fatty liver disease [16], indicating that increased sFGL2 levels are due to HBV and HCV infections rather than to the occurrence of cirrhosis [19]. FGL2 is over-expressed both at mRNA and protein levels in liver tissue from patients with more severe CHB [27]. A previous study

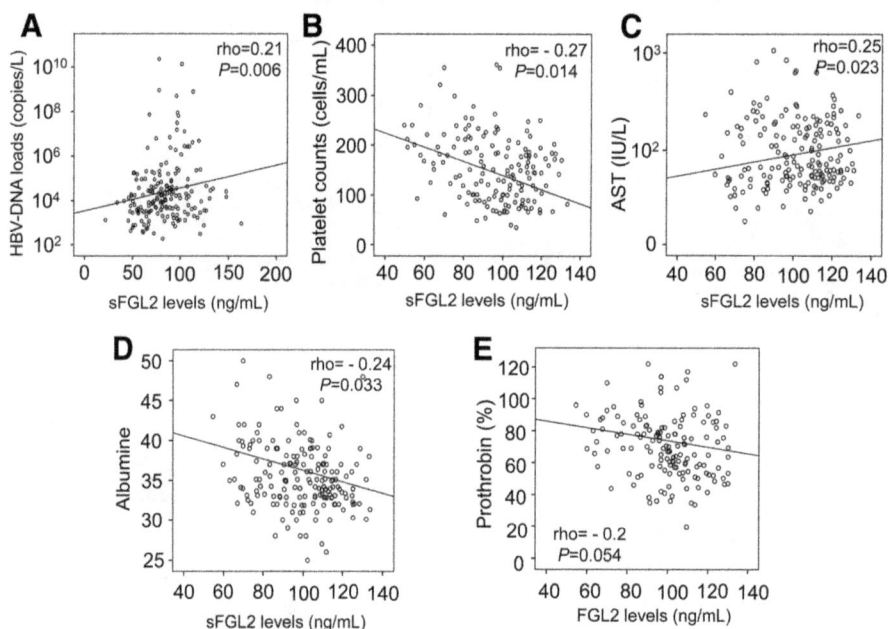

Fig. 3 Correlation of sFGL2 levels with clinical parameters of HBV infection. Correlations of FGL2 levels with different available clinical parameters were calculated by using Spearman's rank correlation coefficient test. The Spearman's rho and P value are also presented. **a**: between sFGL2 levels and HBV-DNA loads; **b**: between sFGL2 levels and platelet counts; **c**: between sFGL2 levels and aspartate amino transferase (AST) levels; **d**: between sFGL2 levels and albumin levels; and **e**: between sFGL2 levels and prothrombin

with a small sample size has shown that sFGL2 levels are higher in patients with HCC or LC compared to CHB patients, and that sFGL2 levels are increased in HCC patients with cirrhosis compared to those without cirrhosis [14]. Hepatic stellate cells express and secrete sFGL2, indicating that higher sFGL2 levels observed in LC patients are due to the production of sFGL2 by activated hepatic stellate cells in the cirrhotic liver [14]. Therefore, FGL2 plays a vital role during acute immune responses against HBV and HCV and is involved in the pathogenesis of the infections, particularly in the development of HBV-related cirrhosis.

Fibrin deposition and liver necrosis are decreased in FGL2-deficient mice infected with MHV-3 while the survival rate is increased, implying a crucial role of FGL2 in the pathogenesis of HBV infection [27]. FGL2 is involved in the immune responses against HBV infection as peritoneal macrophages from FGL2-deficient mice infected with MHV-3 lack a procoagulant response [27]. The $CD3^+CD4^-CD8^-$ double-negative T cells appear to contribute to the pathogenesis and clinical outcome of MHV-3-induced fulminant viral hepatitis via the immunoactivity of FGL2 in a mouse model [29]. The $CD4^+CD25^+$ regulatory T cells (Tregs) and their effector molecule FGL2 play a key role in susceptibility to HBV infection and in regulating the outcome of fulminant viral hepatitis in vivo [11]. Consistently, in a murine model of acute viral hepatitis caused by LCMV-WE, maturation of dendritic cells (DCs) and increased $CD8^+$ and $CD4^+$ T cells producing IFN-γ have been observed in FGL2 knock-out mice infected with LCMV-WE, demonstrating a crucial role of FGL2 in the immune response against hepatitis viruses [18].

FGL2 is also involved in the pathogenesis of chronic viral infection through regulation of the FcγRIIB/RIII immunosuppressive pathway, indicating that FGL2 might be a therapeutic target for chronic viral infection [30]. FGL2 together with C5aR and TNF-α contribute to coagulation and complement activation during MHV-3-induced fulminant hepatitis [31, 32]. FGL2 has been shown to induce fibrinogen deposition and procoagulant activity, which are commonly observed during liver injury [27, 31]. Clinically, sFGL2 levels are correlated with distinct clinical parameters of HBV infection (e.g. AST, albumin and, platelet counts and HBV-DNA loads) as observed in the present study and in HCV patients [19]. FGL2, as an effector of Treg cells, contributes to the inhibition of cellular immune responses (induced either by HBV or HCV) against virus replication. The above statement corroborate our findings that sFLG2 levels were thus positively correlated with viral loads and subsequently resulting in the unfavourable clinical outcome such as increased liver enzymes. Hence, sFGL2 may be an indicator of and/or

mediator for liver damage and progression of viral hepatitis and a potential target for intervention in fulminant and chronic hepatitis [11, 15, 18, 31].

FGL2 is not only highly expressed on the surface of macrophages, endothelial and dendritic cells, but also in solid tumors including HCC [25, 33, 34]. In line with previous studies [33, 34], up-regulation of FGL2 mRNA was observed in tumor tissues, compared to directly adjacent non-tumor tissues. Higher FGL2 expression was observed in programmed cell death protein 1 (PD-1)-deficient mice infected with MHV-3 compared to wildtype animals and FGL2 up-regulation is mediated by IL2, IFN-γ and TNF-α [34, 35]. This indicates that FGL2 is involved in controlling the immunopathological damage through PD-1 signaling, which is associated with various types of cancer [35]. Also, mFGL-2 appears to promote angiogenesis and tumorigenesis through the FGF-2/ERK (fibroblast growth factor-2/extracellular signal-regulated kinases) signaling pathway, but not by thrombin-mediated mechanism [36]. Importantly, FGL2 is over-expressed in colorectal carcinoma (CRC) and clear cell renal cell carcinoma (ccRCC) tumors compared to non-tumor tissues [25, 37], and the expression levels are associated with cell proliferation and invasion in vitro and with CRC progression and metastasis in vivo [37]. These findings are supported by our observation that plasma sFGL2 levels are increased in patients with HCC compared to those without HCC and healthy controls. Either FGL2 knockdown or intratumoral injection of an artificial microRNA targeting hFGL2 leads to a delayed proliferation of tumor cells and an inhibition of tumor growth and angiogenesis as well as improves survival in vivo [33, 38, 39]. In addition, increased FGL2 expression is significantly associated with poor prognosis in patients with ccRCC [25]. Therefore, sFGL2 and mFGL2 play an essential role in the tumorgenesis of HCC and may be considered a promising indicator for HCC prognosis and a potential target for HCC therapy. However, more studies are needed to evaluate the clinical potential of sFGL2 as well as the association of FGL2 mRNA expression with sFGL2 and mFGL2 in HCC.

Conclusions

sFGL2 levels are significantly induced by HBV infection and associated with the progression and clinical outcome of HBV-related liver diseases. sFGL2 levels may be an additional biomarker for monitoring progression and treatment of the diseases. The FGL2 gene and corresponding proteins (mFGL2 and sFGL2) may be a target for therapeutic intervention of HBV-related liver diseases.

Abbreviations
AHB: Acute hepatitis B; CHB: Chronic hepatitis B; HBV: Hepatitis B virus;
HC: Healthy control; HCC: Hepatocellular carcinoma; LC: Liver cirrhosis;
sFGL2: Fibrinogen-like protein 2

Acknowledgements
We thank all the patients and healthy individuals for their participation.

Funding
This study was funded by Vietnam National Foundation for Science and
Technology Development (NAFOSTED) under grant number 108.02–2017.15 to
Dr. Hoang Van Tong. Dr. Thirumalaisamy P. Velavan acknowledges the financial
support from Federal Ministry of Education and Research, Germany
(BMBF01DP17047) and from DAAD-PAGEL (57140033) for student fellow-
ship. The funder has no role in the study design, data collection and
analysis, decision to publish or preparation of the manuscript.

Authors' contributions
HVT and VTP designed and supervised the studies. HVT, NVB, NXH, MTB
and DTQ conducted the experiments. HAS, HVL, DQ, LHS and NLT evaluated
the clinical data and provided the clinical samples. HVT, CGM and VTP
analyzed the data and wrote the manuscript. All authors read and
approved the manuscript.

Competing interests
The authors declare that they have no competing interests.

Author details
[1]Institute of Biomedicine and Pharmacy, Vietnam Military Medical University,
222 Phung Hung, Ha Dong, Hanoi, Vietnam. [2]Department of
Pathophysiology, Vietnam Military Medical University, Hanoi, Vietnam.
[3]Institute of Tropical Medicine, University of Tübingen, Wilhelmstrasse 27,
72074 Tübingen, Germany. [4]108 Military Central Hospital, Hanoi, Vietnam.
[5]Vietnamese-German Center of Excellence in Medical Research, Hanoi,
Vietnam. [6]Medical Faculty, Duy Tan University, Da Nang, Vietnam.

References
1. WHO. Hepatitis B Fact sheet. 2017. Ref Type: Report.
2. Nguyen VT, Law MG, Dore GJ. An enormous hepatitis B virus-related liver
   disease burden projected in Vietnam by 2025. Liver Int. 2008;28:525–31.
3. Nguyen VT. Hepatitis B infection in Vietnam: current issues and future
   challenges. Asia Pac J Public Health. 2012;24:361–73.
4. El-Serag HB. Hepatocellular carcinoma. N Engl J Med. 2011;365:1118–27.
5. Rehermann B, Bertoletti A. Immunological aspects of antiviral therapy of
   chronic hepatitis B virus and hepatitis C virus infections. Hepatology. 2015;
   61:712–21.
6. Guerrieri F, Belloni L, Pediconi N, Levrero M. Molecular mechanisms of HBV-
   associated hepatocarcinogenesis. Semin Liver Dis. 2013;33:147–56.
7. Liu XG, Liu Y, Chen F. Soluble fibrinogen like protein 2 (sFGL2), the novel
   effector molecule for immunoregulation. Oncotarget. 2017;8(2):3711–23.
8. Yuwaraj S, Ding J, Liu M, Marsden PA, Levy GA. Genomic characterization,
   localization, and functional expression of FGL2, the human gene encoding
   fibroleukin: a novel human procoagulant. Genomics. 2001;71:330–8.
9. Levy GA, Liu M, Ding J, Yuwaraj S, Leibowitz J, Marsden PA, et al. Molecular
   and functional analysis of the human prothrombinase gene (HFGL2) and its
   role in viral hepatitis. Am J Pathol. 2000;156:1217–25.
10. Liu H, Yang PS, Zhu T, Manuel J, Zhang J, He W, et al. Characterization of
    fibrinogen-like protein 2 (FGL2): monomeric FGL2 has enhanced
    immunosuppressive activity in comparison to oligomeric FGL2. Int J
    Biochem Cell Biol. 2013;45:408–18.
11. Shalev I, Wong KM, Foerster K, Zhu Y, Chan C, Maknojia A, et al. The novel
    CD4+CD25+ regulatory T cell effector molecule fibrinogen-like protein 2
    contributes to the outcome of murine fulminant viral hepatitis. Hepatology.
    2009;49:387–97.
12. Wang L, Yang C, Xu M, Hu M, Wang X, Zhu T. The role of soluble
    fibrinogen-like protein 2 in transplantation: protection or damage.
    Transplantation. 2014;97:1201–6.
13. Zhao Z, Yang C, Tang Q, Zhao T, Jia Y, Ma Z, et al. Serum level of soluble
    fibrinogen-like protein 2 in renal allograft recipients with acute rejection: a
    preliminary study. Transplant Proc. 2012;44:2982–5.
14. Sun Y, Xi D, Ding W, Wang F, Zhou H, Ning Q. Soluble FGL2, a novel
    effector molecule of activated hepatic stellate cells, regulates T-cell
    function in cirrhotic patients with hepatocellular carcinoma. Hepatol Int.
    2014;8:567–75.
15. Shalev I, Selzner N, Helmy A, Foerster K, Adeyi OA, Grant DR, et al. The role
    of FGL2 in the pathogenesis and treatment of hepatitis C virus infection.
    Rambam Maimonides Med J. 2010;1:e0004.
16. Colak Y, Senates E, Ozturk O, Yilmaz Y, Coskunpinar E, Kahraman OT, et al.
    Plasma fibrinogen-like protein 2 levels in patients with non-alcoholic fatty
    liver disease. Hepatogastroenterology. 2011;58:2087–90.
17. Zhu C, Sun Y, Luo X, Yan W, Xi D, Ning Q. Novel mfgl2 antisense plasmid
    inhibits murine fgl2 expression and ameliorates murine hepatitis virus type
    3-induced fulminant hepatitis in BALB/cJ mice. Hum Gene Ther. 2006;17:
    589–600.
18. Khattar R, Luft O, Yavorska N, Shalev I, Phillips MJ, Adeyi O, et al. Targeted
    deletion of FGL2 leads to increased early viral replication and enhanced
    adaptive immunity in a murine model of acute viral hepatitis caused by
    LCMV WE. PLoS One. 2013;8:e72309.
19. Foerster K, Helmy A, Zhu Y, Khattar R, Adeyi OA, Wong KM, et al. The novel
    immunoregulatory molecule FGL2: a potential biomarker for severity of
    chronic hepatitis C virus infection. J Hepatol. 2010;53:608–15.
20. Van TH, Hoan NX, Binh MT, Quyen DT, Meyer CG, Song LH, et al. Interferon-
    stimulated gene 20 kDa protein serum levels and clinical outcome of
    hepatitis B virus-related liver diseases. Oncotarget. 2018;9:27858–71.
21. EASL clinical practice guidelines. Management of chronic hepatitis B virus
    infection. J Hepatol. 2012;57:167–85.
22. Bruix J, Sherman M. Management of hepatocellular carcinoma: an update.
    Hepatology. 2011;53:1020–2.
23. Cholongitas E, Papatheodoridis GV, Vangeli M, Terreni N, Patch D, Burroughs
    AK. Systematic review: the model for end-stage liver disease--should it
    replace child-Pugh's classification for assessing prognosis in cirrhosis?
    Aliment Pharmacol Ther. 2005;22:1079–89.
24. Hoan NX, Van TH, Giang DP, Cuong BK, Toan NL, Wedemeyer H, et al.
    SOCS3 genetic variants and promoter hypermethylation in patients with
    chronic hepatitis B. Oncotarget. 2017;8:17127–39.
25. Tang M, Cao X, Li P, Zhang K, Li Y, Zheng QY, et al. Increased expression of
    fibrinogen-like protein 2 is associated with poor prognosis in patients with
    clear cell renal cell carcinoma. Sci Rep. 2017;7:12676.
26. Zhu CL, Yan WM, Zhu F, Zhu YF, Xi D, Tian DY, et al. Fibrinogen-like protein
    2 fibroleukin expression and its correlation with disease progression in
    murine hepatitis virus type 3-induced fulminant hepatitis and in patients
    with severe viral hepatitis B. World J Gastroenterol. 2005;11:6936–40.
27. Marsden PA, Ning Q, Fung LS, Luo X, Chen Y, Mendicino M, et al. The Fgl2/
    fibroleukin prothrombinase contributes to immunologically mediated
    thrombosis in experimental and human viral hepatitis. J Clin Invest. 2003;
    112:58–66.
28. Yu H, Liu Y, Huang J, Wang H, Yan W, Xi D, et al. IL-33 protects murine viral
    fulminant hepatitis by targeting coagulation hallmark protein FGL2/
    fibroleukin expression. Mol Immunol. 2017;87:171–9.
29. Wu D, Wang H, Yan W, Chen T, Wang M, Han M, et al. A disparate subset of
    double-negative T cells contributes to the outcome of murine fulminant
    viral hepatitis via effector molecule fibrinogen-like protein 2. Immunol Res.
    2016;64:518–30.
30. Klingberg O, Khattar R, Farrokhi K, Ferri D, Yavorska N, Zhang J, et al.
    Inhibition of the FGL2:FcgammaRIIB/RIII immunosuppressive pathway
    enhances antiviral T cell and B cell responses leading to clearance of LCMV
    cl-13. Immunology. 2018;154(3):476–89.
31. Liu J, Tan Y, Zhang J, Zou L, Deng G, Xu X, et al. C5aR, TNF-alpha, and FGL2
    contribute to coagulation and complement activation in virus-induced
    fulminant hepatitis. J Hepatol. 2015;62:354–62.
32. Xu GL, Chen J, Yang F, Li GQ, Zheng LX, Wu YZ. C5a/C5aR pathway is
    essential for the pathogenesis of murine viral fulminant hepatitis by way of
    potentiating Fgl2/fibroleukin expression. Hepatology. 2014;60:114–24.
33. Liu Y, Xu L, Zeng Q, Wang J, Wang M, Xi D, et al. Downregulation of FGL2/
    prothrombinase delays HCCLM6 xenograft tumour growth and decreases
    tumour angiogenesis. Liver Int. 2012;32:1585 95.

34. Su K, Chen F, Yan WM, Zeng QL, Xu L, Xi D, et al. Fibrinogen-like protein 2/fibroleukin prothrombinase contributes to tumor hypercoagulability via IL-2 and IFN-gamma. World J Gastroenterol. 2008;14:5980–9.

35. Chen Y, Wu S, Guo G, Fei L, Guo S, Yang C, et al. Programmed death (PD)-1-deficient mice are extremely sensitive to murine hepatitis virus strain-3 (MHV-3) infection. PLoS Pathog. 2011;7:e1001347.

36. Rabizadeh E, Cherny I, Lederfein D, Sherman S, Binkovsky N, Rosenblat Y, et al. The cell-membrane prothrombinase, fibrinogen-like protein 2, promotes angiogenesis and tumor development. Thromb Res. 2015;136:118–24.

37. Qin WZ, Li QL, Chen WF, Xu MD, Zhang YQ, Zhong YS, et al. Overexpression of fibrinogen-like protein 2 induces epithelial-to-mesenchymal transition and promotes tumor progression in colorectal carcinoma. Med Oncol. 2014;31:181.

38. Wang M, Liu J, Xi D, Luo X, Ning Q. Adenovirus-mediated artificial microRNA against human fibrinogen like protein 2 inhibits hepatocellular carcinoma growth. J Gene Med. 2016;18:102–11.

39. Selzner N, Liu H, Boehnert MU, Adeyi OA, Shalev I, Bartczak AM, et al. FGL2/fibroleukin mediates hepatic reperfusion injury by induction of sinusoidal endothelial cell and hepatocyte apoptosis in mice. J Hepatol. 2012;56:153–9.

Permissions

All chapters in this book were first published in ID, by BioMed Central; hereby published with permission under the Creative Commons Attribution License or equivalent. Every chapter published in this book has been scrutinized by our experts. Their significance has been extensively debated. The topics covered herein carry significant findings which will fuel the growth of the discipline. They may even be implemented as practical applications or may be referred to as a beginning point for another development.

The contributors of this book come from diverse backgrounds, making this book a truly international effort. This book will bring forth new frontiers with its revolutionizing research information and detailed analysis of the nascent developments around the world.

We would like to thank all the contributing authors for lending their expertise to make the book truly unique. They have played a crucial role in the development of this book. Without their invaluable contributions this book wouldn't have been possible. They have made vital efforts to compile up to date information on the varied aspects of this subject to make this book a valuable addition to the collection of many professionals and students.

This book was conceptualized with the vision of imparting up-to-date information and advanced data in this field. To ensure the same, a matchless editorial board was set up. Every individual on the board went through rigorous rounds of assessment to prove their worth. After which they invested a large part of their time researching and compiling the most relevant data for our readers.

The editorial board has been involved in producing this book since its inception. They have spent rigorous hours researching and exploring the diverse topics which have resulted in the successful publishing of this book. They have passed on their knowledge of decades through this book. To expedite this challenging task, the publisher supported the team at every step. A small team of assistant editors was also appointed to further simplify the editing procedure and attain best results for the readers.

Apart from the editorial board, the designing team has also invested a significant amount of their time in understanding the subject and creating the most relevant covers. They scrutinized every image to scout for the most suitable representation of the subject and create an appropriate cover for the book.

The publishing team has been an ardent support to the editorial, designing and production team. Their endless efforts to recruit the best for this project, has resulted in the accomplishment of this book. They are a veteran in the field of academics and their pool of knowledge is as vast as their experience in printing. Their expertise and guidance has proved useful at every step. Their uncompromising quality standards have made this book an exceptional effort. Their encouragement from time to time has been an inspiration for everyone.

The publisher and the editorial board hope that this book will prove to be a valuable piece of knowledge for researchers, students, practitioners and scholars across the globe.

List of Contributors

Marta Iglis Oliveira
Programa de Pós-graduação em Ciências da Saúde, Universidade Federal de Pernambuco, Av. Prof. Moraes Rego 1235, Recife 50670-901, Brazil

Paulo Sérgio Ramos de Araújo
Programa de Pós-graduação em Ciências da Saúde, Universidade Federal de Pernambuco, Av. Prof. Moraes Rego 1235, Recife 50670-901, Brazil
Instituto Aggeu Magalhaes, FIOCRUZ, Av. Prof. Moraes Rego 1235, Recife 50670-901, Brazil

Claudia Fernanda de Lacerda Vidal
Instituto Aggeu Magalhaes, FIOCRUZ, Av. Prof. Moraes Rego 1235, Recife 50670-901, Brazil

Valter Romão de Souza Junior
Faculdade de Medicina do Recife, Universidade Federal de Pernambuco, Av. Prof. Moraes Rego, 1235, Recife, Pernambuco, Brazil

J. S. I. Schuffenecker
Laboratoire de Virologie, Institut des Agents Infectieux, Groupement Hospitalier Nord, Hospices Civils de Lyon, Lyon, France

M. Pichon, Casalegno, M. Valette, B. Lina, F. Morfin and L. Josset
Laboratoire de Virologie, Institut des Agents Infectieux, Groupement Hospitalier Nord, Hospices Civils de Lyon, Lyon, France
Univ Lyon, Université Lyon 1, Faculté de Médecine Lyon Est, CIRI, Inserm U1111 CNRS UMR5308, Virpath, Lyon, France
Centre National de Reference des virus respiratoires France Sud, Hospices Civils de Lyon, 103 Grande-Rue de la Croix Rousse, 69317 Lyon, France

A. Bal
Laboratoire de Virologie, Institut des Agents Infectieux, Groupement Hospitalier Nord, Hospices Civils de Lyon, Lyon, France
Univ Lyon, Université Lyon 1, Faculté de Médecine Lyon Est, CIRI, Inserm U1111 CNRS UMR5308, Virpath, Lyon, France
Centre National de Reference des virus respiratoires France Sud, Hospices Civils de Lyon, 103 Grande-Rue de la Croix Rousse, 69317 Lyon, France

Laboratoire Commun de Recherche HCL-bioMerieux, Centre Hospitalier Lyon Sud, Pierre-Bénite, France

G. Vilchez, V. Cheynet, G. Oriol, S. Trouillet-Assant and K. Brengel-Pesce
Laboratoire Commun de Recherche HCL-bioMerieux, Centre Hospitalier Lyon Sud, Pierre-Bénite, France

C. Picard
Unité de Biologie des Infections Virales Emergentes, Institut Pasteur, Lyon, France
CIRI Inserm U1111, CNRS 5308, ENS, UCBL, Faculté de Médecine Lyon Est, Université de Lyon, Lyon, France

L. Billard
INSERM UMR1078 "Génétique, Génomique Fonctionnelle et Biotechnologies", Axe Microbiota, Univ Brest, Brest, France

S. Vallet
INSERM UMR1078 "Génétique, Génomique Fonctionnelle et Biotechnologies", Axe Microbiota, Univ Brest, Brest, France
Département de Bactériologie-Virologie, Hygiène et Parasitologie-Mycologie, Pôle de Biologie-Pathologie, Centre Hospitalier Régional et Universitaire de Brest, Hôpital de la Cavale Blanche, Brest, France

Y. Gillet
Hospices Civils de Lyon, Urgences pédiatriques, Hôpital Femme Mère Enfant, Bron, France

Maria Mazzitelli, Carlo Torti, Chiara Costa, Vincenzo Pisani and Alessio Strazzulla
Unit of Infectious and Tropical Diseases, Department of Medical and Surgical Sciences, "Magna Graecia" University of Catanzaro, Viale Europa, 88100 Catanzaro, Italy

Jolanda Sabatino, Greta Luana D'Ascoli, Salvatore De Rosa and Ciro Indolfi
Cardiovascular Institute, Department of Medical and Surgical Sciences, "Magna Graecia" University of Catanzaro, Viale Europa, 88100 Catanzaro, Italy

Elena Raffetti
Unit of Hygiene, Epidemiology and Public Health, Department of Medical and Surgical Specialities, Radiological Sciences and Public Health, Viale Europa, 25123 Brescia, Italy

Alfredo Focà and Maria Carla Liberto
Institute of Microbiology, Department of Health Sciences, "Magna Graecia" University of Catanzaro, Viale Europa, 88100 Catanzaro, Italy

David T. Dunn, Leanne McCabe, Denise Ward and Sheena McCormack
MRC Clinical Trials Unit at UCL, London, UK

Mitzy Gafos
MRC Clinical Trials Unit at UCL, London, UK
Department of Global Health and Development, London School of Hygiene and Tropical Medicine, Faculty of Public Health and Policy, London, UK

Michelle M. Gabriel
MRC Clinical Trials Unit at UCL, London, UK
Trial Sponsor – University College London via MRC Clinical Trials Unit at UCL, Institute of Clinical Trials and Methodology, 90 High Holborn, 2nd Floor, London WC1V 6LJ, UK

Andrew Speakman, Fiona C. Lampe, Andrew Phillips and Alison J. Rodger
Centre for Clinical Research, Epidemiology, Modelling and Evaluation, Institute for Global Health, UCL, London, UK

T. Charles Witzel and Peter Weatherburn
Department of Social and Environmental Health Research, Sigma Research, Faculty of Public Health and Policy, London School of Hygiene and Tropical Medicine, London, UK

Justin Harbottle
Terrence Higgins Trust, London, UK

Simon Collins
HIV i-Base, London, UK

Fiona M. Burns
Royal Free London NHS Foundation Trust, London, UK

Déborah Ferreira Noronha de Castro Rocha, Luana Rocha da Cunha Rosa, Carla de Almeida Silva, Thaynara Lorrane Silva Martins, Regina Marcos André deMatos, Márcia Maria de Souza, Karlla Antonieta Amorim Caetano and Sheila Araujo Teles
Faculty of Nursing, Federal University of Goias/ Universidade Federal de Goiás, Goiânia, GO, Brazil

Brunna Rodrigues de Oliveira, Maria Bringel Martins and Megmar Aparecida dos Santos Carneiro
Institute of Tropical Pathology and Public Health, Federal University of Goias/Universidade Federal de Goiás, Goiânia, GO, Brazil

Juliana Pontes Soares and Ana Cristina de Oliveira e Silva
Faculty of Nursing, Federal University of Paraiba/ Universidade Federal da Paraíba, João Pessoa, PB, Brazil

Robert L. Cook
Department of Epidemiology, College of Public Health and Health Professions and College of Medicine, University of Florida, Gainesville, FL, USA

Reza Kamali Kakhki, Hosna Zare, Amin Hooshyar Chichaklu and Mahsa Sayyadi
Antimicrobial Resistance Research Center, Mashhad University of Medical Sciences, Mashhad, Iran

Alireza Neshani
Antimicrobial Resistance Research Center, Mashhad University of Medical Sciences, Mashhad, Iran
Student Research Committee, Mashhad University of Medical Sciences, Mashhad, Iran

Kiarash Ghazvini
Antimicrobial Resistance Research Center, Mashhad University of Medical Sciences, Mashhad, Iran
Department of Microbiology and Virology, School of Medicine, Mashhad University of Medical Sciences, Mashhad, Iran

Mojtaba Sankian
Immunology Research Center, School of Medicine, Mashhad University of Medical Sciences, Mashhad, Iran

Department of Microbiology and Virology, School of Medicine, Mashhad University of Medical Sciences, Mashhad, Iran

Eduard J. Sanders
Kenya Medical Research Institute, Centre for Geographic Medicine Research – Coast, Kenya Medical Research Institute, Kilifi, Kenya

Simon C. Masha
Kenya Medical Research Institute, Centre for Geographic Medicine Research – Coast, Kenya Medical Research Institute, Kilifi, Kenya
Laboratory Bacteriology Research, Faculty of Medicine and Health Sciences, Ghent University, De Pintelaan, 185 Ghent, Belgium
Faculty of Pure and Applied Sciences, Department of Biological Sciences, Pwani University, Kilifi, Kenya

Piet Cools and Mario Vaneechoutte
Laboratory Bacteriology Research, Faculty of Medicine and Health Sciences, Ghent University, De Pintelaan, 185 Ghent, Belgium

Patrick Descheemaeker and Marijke Reynders
Department of Laboratory Medicine, Medical Microbiology, AZ St-Jan Brugge-Oostende, Bruges, Belgium

Jing Miao, Weili Liu, Dong Yang, Zhiqiang Shen, Zhigang Qiu, Xiang Chen, Kunming Zhang, Hui Hu, Jing Yin, Zhongwei Yang, Junwen Li and Min Jin
Tianjin Institute of Environmental and Operational Medcine, Key Laboratory of Risk Assessment and Control for Environment and Food Safety, Tianjin 300050, China

Xuan Guo
Tianjin Institute of Environmental and Operational Medcine, Key Laboratory of Risk Assessment and Control for Environment and Food Safety, Tianjin 300050, China
Research Institution of Chemical Defense, Beijing 102205, China

Asfaw Ayalew, Zewdu Gashu, Tadesse Anteneh, Nebiyu Hiruy, Dereje Habte, Degu Jerene and Muluken Melese
Management Sciences for Health, Help Ethiopia Address the Low Performance of Tuberculosis (HEAL TB) Project, Bole Sub City, Kebele 02, House Number 708, Code 1250 Addis Ababa, Ethiopia

Genetu Alem
Amhara Regional Health Bureau, Bahir Dar, Ethiopia

Ilili Jemal
Oromia Regional Health Bureau, Addis Ababa, Ethiopia

Pedro G. Suarez
Management Sciences for Health, Health Programs Group, 4301 North Fairfax Drive, Suite 400, Arlington, VA 22203, USA

Danhuai Guo and Deqiang Wang
Computer Network Information Center, Chinese Academy of Sciences, 4th South Fourth Road Zhongguancun, Beijing 100190, China
University of Chinese Academy of Sciences, 19th Yuquan Road, Beijing 100049, China

Wenwu Yin and Hongjie Yu
Chinese Center for Disease Control and Prevention, 155 Changbai Road Changping District, Beijing 102206, China

Jean-Claude Thill
Department of Geography and Earth Sciences, The University of North Carolina at Charlotte, 9201 University City Blvd, Charlotte, NC 28223, USA

Weishi Yang
School of Geography and Planning, Sun Yat-sen University, Guangzhou 510275, China
Key Laboratory of Land Surface Pattern and Simulation, Institute of Geographic Sciences and Natural Resources Research, Chinese Academy of Sciences, Beijing 100101, China

Feng Chen
Department of East Asian Studies, The University of Arizona, 1512 E. First Street, Tucson, AZ 85719, USA

Megan E. Gray, Elizabeth T. Rogawski McQuade, W. Michael Scheld and Rebecca A. Dillingham
Division of Infectious Diseases and International Health, University of Virginia Health System, 801379, Charlottesville, Virginia 22908-1391, USA

David Sidebottom
Department of Public Health Sciences, Karolinska Institutet, Stockholm, Sweden

Susanne Strömdahl
Department of Public Health Sciences, Karolinska Institutet, Stockholm, Sweden
Department of Medical Sciences, Section of Infectious Diseases, Uppsala University, Uppsala, Sweden

Anna Mia Ekström
Department of Public Health Sciences, Karolinska Institutet, Stockholm, Sweden
Department of Infectious Diseases, Karolinska University Hospital, Stockholm, Sweden

Jin Li, Mingyu Tang, Bailu Du and Qing Cao
Department of Infectious Diseases, Shanghai Children's Medical Center, Shanghai Jiaotong University School of Medicine, Shanghai, China

Yue Tao and Xi Mo
The Laboratory of Pediatric Infectious Diseases, Pediatric Translational Medicine Institute, Shanghai Children's Medical Center, Shanghai Jiaotong University School of Medicine, Shanghai, China

Yijun Xia
Medical Affairs, Great China | bioMérieux (Shanghai) Company, Limited, Shanghai, China

Nicholas Petronella
Biostatistics and Modeling Division, Bureau of Food Surveillance and Science Integration, Food Directorate, Health Canada Ottawa, Ottawa, ON, Canada

Jennifer Ronholm
Department of Food Science and Agricultural Chemistry, Faculty of Agricultural and Environmental Sciences, Macdonald Campus, McGill University, Montreal, QC, Canada
Department of Animal Sciences, Faculty of Agricultural and Environmental Sciences, Macdonald Campus, McGill University, Montreal, QC, Canada

Menka Suresh, Jennifer Harlow, Oksana Mykytczuk, Nathalie Corneau, Sabah Bidawid and Neda Nasheri
National Food Virology Reference Centre, Bureau of Microbial Hazards, Food Directorate, Health Canada 251 Sir Frederick Banting Driveway, Ottawa, ON K1A 0K9, Canada

Komal Chacowry Pala, Stéphanie Baggio and Hans Wolff
Division of Prison Health, Geneva University Hospitals, University of Geneva, Chemin de Champ-Dollon 22, 1241 Puplinge, Geneva, Switzerland

Laurent Gétaz
Division of Prison Health, Geneva University Hospitals, University of Geneva, Chemin de Champ-Dollon 22, 1241 Puplinge, Geneva, Switzerland
Division of Tropical and Humanitarian Medicine, Geneva University Hospitals, University of Geneva, Geneva, Switzerland

Nguyen Toan Tran
Division of Prison Health, Geneva University Hospitals, University of Geneva, Chemin de Champ-Dollon 22, 1241 Puplinge, Geneva, Switzerland
Australian Centre for Public and Population Health Research, Faculty of Health, University of Technology, Sydney, Australia

François Girardin
Medical Direction and Division of Clinical Pharmacology, Toxicology Geneva University Hospitals, University of Geneva, Geneva, Switzerland

Vera Ehrenstein, Nickolaj Risbo Kristensen and Henrik Toft Sørensen
Department of Clinical Epidemiology, Aarhus University Hospital, Olof Palmes Allé 43-45, 8200 Aarhus N, Denmark

Brigitta Ursula Monz
F. Hoffmann-La Roche Ltd., Basel, Switzerland

Barry Clinch and Andy Kenwright
Roche Products Ltd., Welwyn Garden City, UK

Yvette Louise Schein
Perelman School of Medicine at the University of Pennsylvania, Philadelphia, PA, USA

Tesfaye Madebo
Department of Pulmonary Medicine, Stavanger University Hospital, Stavanger, Norway

Hilde Elise Andersen
Department of Pulmonary Medicine, TB unit, Stavanger University Hospital, Stavanger, Norway

Trude Margrete Arnesen
Department of Tuberculosis, Blood Borne and Sexually Transmitted Infections, Norwegian Institute of Public Health, Oslo, Norway

AnneMa Dyrhol-Riise
Department of Infectious Diseases, Oslo University Hospital, Oslo, Norway
Institute of Clinical Medicine, University of Oslo, Oslo, Norway
Dep. of Clinical Science, University of Bergen, Oslo, Norway

Hallgeir Tveiten
Department of Pulmonary Medicine, Oslo University Hospital, Oslo, Norway

Richard A. White
Department of Infectious Disease Epidemiology and Modelling, Norwegian Institute of Public Health, Oslo, Norway

Brita Askeland Winje
Department of Vaccine Preventable Diseases, Norwegian Institute of Public Health, Oslo, Norway

Ying Hu, Xiao-ni Zhong, Bin Peng and Yan Zhang
Department of Health Statistics and Information Management, School of Public Health and Management, Chongqing Medical University, Chongqing, China

Hao Liang
Department of Epidemiology and Medical Statistics, School of Public Health, Guangxi Medical University, Nanning, China

Jiang-hong Dai
Department of Epidemiology and Health Statistics, School of Public Health, Xinjiang Medical University, Xinjiang, China

Ju-ying Zhang
Department of Epidemiology and Medical Statistics, School of Public Health, Sichuan University, Sichuan, China

Ai-long Huang
Key Laboratory of Molecular Biology on Infectious Diseases, Ministry of Education, Chongqing Medical University, Chongqing, China

Bernhard Kerschberger, Qhubekani Mpala, Paola Andrea Díaz Uribe, Sydney Kalombola, Addis Bekele, Tiwonge Chawinga, Mukelo Mliba and Serge Mathurin Kabore
Medecins Sans Frontieres (OCG), Eveni, Lot No. 331, Sheffield Road, Industrial Area, Mbabane, Swaziland

Gugu Maphalala, Nomcebo Phugwayo and Sindisiwe Dlamini
Ministry of Health (National Reference Laboratory), Mbabane, Swaziland

Roberto de la Tour, Javier Goiri and Iza Ciglenecki
Medecins Sans Frontieres (OCG), Geneva, Switzerland

Nombuso Ntshalintshali
Clinton Health Access Initiative (CHAI), Mbabane, Swaziland

Emmanuel Fajardo
Medecins Sans Frontieres (Access Campaign), Geneva, Switzerland

Ming-Gui Wang, Miao-Miao Zhang, Yu Wang, Shou-Quan Wu, Meng Zhang and Jian-Qing He
Department of Respiratory and Critical Care Medicine, West China Hospital, Sichuan University, No. 37, Guo Xue Alley, Chengdu 610041, Sichuan Province, People's Republic of China

Jianhua Hu, Hong Zhao, Meifang Yang, Xuan Zhang, Hongyu Jia and Lanjuan Li
State Key Laboratory for Diagnosis and Treatment of Infectious Diseases, Collaborative Innovation Center for Diagnosis and Treatment of Infectious Diseases, The First Affiliated Hospital, College of Medicine, Zhejiang University, 79 QingChun Road, Hangzhou 310003, Zhejiang, China

Danfeng Lou and Hainv Gao
Shulan (Hangzhou) Hospital, 848 Dongxin Road, Hangzhou 310004, Zhejiang, China

Heng Sopheab and Chhorvann Chhea
School of Public Health at the National Institute of Public Health, Lot #80, Samdech Penn Nouth Blvd. Tuol Kork District, Phnom Penh, Cambodia

Sovannary Tuot
Center for Population and Health Research, KHANA, Phnom Penh, Cambodia

Jonathan A. Muir
Department of Epidemiology, University of Washington, Seattle, USA

Mauro José Costa Salles
Division of Infectious Diseases, Department of Internal Medicine Santa Casa de São Paulo School of Medical Sciences, Hospital da Irmandade da Santa Casa de Misericórdia de São Paulo, Rua Dr Cesáreo Mota Jr 112, , São Paulo, SP CEP: 01303-060, Brazil

Giselle Burlamaqui Klautau
Division of Infectious Diseases, Department of Internal Medicine Santa Casa de São Paulo School of Medical Sciences, Hospital da Irmandade da Santa Casa de Misericórdia de São Paulo, Rua Dr Cesáreo Mota Jr 112, , São Paulo, SP CEP: 01303-060, Brazil
Emílio Ribas Institute of Infectious Diseases, Av Dr Arnaldo 165, São Paulo, SP CEP: 01246-900, Brazil

Denise Silva Rodrigues
Clemente Ferreira Institute, Rua da Consolação 717, São Paulo, SP CEP: 01221-020, Brazil
Federal University of São Paulo (UNIFESP), Rua Sena Madureira 1500, São Paulo CEP: 04021-001, Brazil

Nadijane Valéria Ferreira da Mota and Marcelo Nascimento Burattini
Federal University of São Paulo (UNIFESP), Rua Sena Madureira 1500, São Paulo CEP: 04021-001, Brazil

Jinjian Fu, Yanling Ding, Shengfu Mo, Shaolin Xu and Peixu Qin
Department of Laboratory, Liuzhou Maternity and Child Healthcare Hospital, 50th Yingshan Road, Chengzhong District, Liuzhou 545001, China

Yongjiang Jiang
Department of Neonatology, Liuzhou Maternity and Child Health Care Hospital, Liuzhou 545001, China

Lyn Awad
Infectious Diseases and Antimicrobial Stewardship Clinical Pharmacist, Makassed General Hospital, Beirut, Lebanon

Hani Tamim
Department of Internal Medicine, American University of Beirut, Beirut, Lebanon

Dania Abdallah
Pharmacy Department, Makassed General Hospital, Beirut, Lebanon

Mohammad Salameh
Department of Internal Medicine, Makassed General Hospital, Beirut, Lebanon

Anas Mugharbil and Ahmad Ibrahim
Division of Hematology/Oncology, Department of Internal Medicine, Makassed General Hospital, Beirut, Lebanon

Tamima Jisr
Department of Laboratory Medicine, Makassed General Hospital, Beirut, Lebanon

Kamal Zahran
Middle East Institute of Health, Bsalim, Beirut, Lebanon

Nabila Droubi
Pharmacy Department, Makassed General Hospital, Beirut, Lebanon

Rima Moghnieh
Head of Antimicrobial Stewardship Program, Makassed General Hospital, Beirut, Lebanon

Jorge Rodrigues de Sousa
Instituto Evandro Chagas, Secretaria de Vigilância em Saúde, Ministério da Saúde, Ananindeua, PA, Brazil
Núcleo de Medicina Tropical, Universidade Federal do Pará, Belém, PA, Brazil

Juarez Antonio Simões Quaresma
Instituto Evandro Chagas, Secretaria de Vigilância em Saúde, Ministério da Saúde, Ananindeua, PA, Brazil
Núcleo de Medicina Tropical, Universidade Federal do Pará, Belém, PA, Brazil
Centro de Ciências Biológicas e da Saúde, Universidade do Estado do Pará, Belém, PA, Brazil
Instituto de Medicina Tropical de São Paulo, Universidade de São Paulo, São Paulo, SP, Brazil
Núcleo de Medicina Tropical, UFPA, Av. Generalíssimo Deodoro 92, Umarizal, Belém, Pará 66055-190, Brazil

Francisco Dias Lucena Neto
Centro de Ciências Biológicas e da Saúde, Universidade do Estado do Pará, Belém, PA, Brazil

Mirian Nacagami Sotto
Faculdade de Medicina, Universidade de São Paulo, São Paulo, SP, Brazil
Instituto de Medicina Tropical de São Paulo, Universidade de São Paulo, São Paulo, SP, Brazil

Mas Harithulfadhli Agus Ab Rahman, Suhaily Mohd Hairon, Mohd Nazri Shafei, Norazlin Idris, Surianti Sukeri, Wan Mohd Zahiruddin Wan Mohammad and Aziah Daud
Department of Community Medicine, School of Medical Sciences, Universiti Sains Malaysia, 16150 Kubang Kerian, Kelantan, Malaysia

Rukman Awang Hamat, Tengku Zetty Maztura Tengku Jamaluddin and Malina Osman
Department of Medical Microbiology and Parasitology, Faculty of Medicine and Health Sciences, Universiti Putra Malaysia, UPM, 43400 Serdang, Selangor, Malaysia

Zainudin A. Wahab
Health Department of Federal Territory Kuala Lumpur and Putrajaya, Jalan Cenderasari, 50590 Kuala Lumpur, Malaysia

Zawaha Idris
Health Promotion Unit, Penang State Health Department, Floor 7, Bangunan Persekutuan, Jalan Anson, 10400 Penang, Malaysia

Lei Zhang and Yong Wang
Department of Epidemiology, School of Public Health, Nanjing Medical University, Nanjing 211166, Jiangsu Province, China

Minghao Zhou
Department of Epidemiology, School of Public Health, Nanjing Medical University, Nanjing 211166, Jiangsu Province, China
Department of Expanded Programme on Immunization, Jiangsu Provincial Center for Disease Control and Prevention, Nanjing 210009, Jiangsu Province, China

Yuanbao Liu, Xiang Sun, Ying Hu, Xiuying Deng, Peishan Lu, Fenyang Tang and Zhiguo Wang
Department of Expanded Programme on Immunization, Jiangsu Provincial Center for Disease Control and Prevention, Nanjing 210009, Jiangsu Province, China

Wang Ma
First Affiliated Hospital of Nanjing Medical University, Nanjing 211166, Jiangsu Province, China

Sabrina Bakeera-Kitaka, Joseph Rujumba and Nicolette Nabukeera-Barungi
Department of Paediatrics and Child Health, School of Medicine, Makerere University College of Health Sciences, Kampala, Uganda

Mariama Mustapha
Department of Paediatrics and Child Health, School of Medicine, Makerere University College of Health Sciences, Kampala, Uganda
Ministry of Health and Sanitation, Freetown, Sierra Leone

Victor Musiime
Department of Paediatrics and Child Health, School of Medicine, Makerere University College of Health Sciences, Kampala, Uganda
Joint Clinical Research Centre, Kampala, Uganda

Nguyen Van Ba, Hoang Van Luong and Do Quyet
Institute of Biomedicine and Pharmacy, Vietnam Military Medical University, 222 Phung Hung, Ha Dong, Hanoi, Vietnam

Ho Anh Son
Institute of Biomedicine and Pharmacy, Vietnam Military Medical University, 222 Phung Hung, Ha Dong, Hanoi, Vietnam
Department of Pathophysiology, Vietnam Military Medical University, Hanoi, Vietnam

Hoang Van Tong
Institute of Biomedicine and Pharmacy, Vietnam Military Medical University, 222 Phung Hung, Ha Dong, Hanoi, Vietnam
Department of Pathophysiology, Vietnam Military Medical University, Hanoi, Vietnam
Institute of Tropical Medicine, University of Tübingen, Wilhelmstrasse 27, 72074 Tübingen, Germany

Nguyen Linh Toan
Department of Pathophysiology, Vietnam Military Medical University, Hanoi, Vietnam

Nghiem Xuan Hoan, Mai Thanh Binh and Dao Thanh Quyen
Institute of Tropical Medicine, University of Tübingen, Wilhelmstrasse 27, 72074 Tübingen, Germany

108 Military Central Hospital, Hanoi, Vietnam
Vietnamese-German Center of Excellence in Medical
Research, Hanoi, Vietnam

Christian G. Meyer and Thirumalaisamy P. Velavan
Institute of Tropical Medicine, University of Tübingen, Wilhelmstrasse 27, 72074 Tübingen, Germany

Vietnamese-German Center of Excellence in Medical
Research, Hanoi, Vietnam
Medical Faculty, Duy Tan University, Da Nang, Vietnam

Le Huu Song
108 Military Central Hospital, Hanoi, Vietnam
Vietnamese-German Center of Excellence in Medical
Research, Hanoi, Vietnam

Index

www.ingramcontent.com/pod-product-compliance
Lightning Source LLC
Chambersburg PA
CBHW061315190326
41458CB00011B/3809